MIGRAINE:
Manifestations, Pathogenesis, and Management

ROBERT A. DAVIDOFF, M.D.

Professor of Neurology, Physiology and
    Biophysics, and Molecular and
    Cellular Pharmacology
University of Miami School of Medicine

Chief, Neurology Service
Veterans Affairs Medical Center
Miami, Florida

 F.A. DAVIS COMPANY • Philadelphia

F. A. Davis Company
1915 Arch Street
Philadelphia, PA 19103

Printed in the United States of America

Last digit indicates print number: 10 9 8 7 6 5 4 3 2 1

Medical Editor: Robert W. Reinhardt
Developmental Editor: Bernice M. Wissler
Production Editor: Gail Shapiro
Cover Designer: Donald B. Freggens, Jr.

As new scientific information becomes available through basic and clinical research, recommended treatments and drug therapies undergo changes. The author(s) and publisher have done everything possible to make this book accurate, up to date, and in accord with accepted standards at the time of publication. The authors, editors, and publishers are not responsible for errors or omissions or for consequences from application of the book, and make no warranty, expressed or implied, in regard to the contents of the book. Any practice described in this book should be applied by the reader in accordance with professional standards of care used in regard to the unique circumstances that may apply in each situation. The reader is advised always to check product information (package inserts) for changes and new information regarding dose and contraindications before administering any drug. Caution is especially urged when using new or infrequently ordered drugs.

Library of Congress Cataloging-in-Publication Data

Davidoff, Robert A., 1934–
    Migraine : manifestations, pathogenesis, and management / Robert
A. Davidoff.
        p.   cm.
    Includes bibliographical references and index.
    ISBN 0-8036-2360-7
    1. Migraine.   I. Title.
    [DNLM: 1. Migraine.   WL 344 D249m   1994]
    RC392.D38   1995
    616.8'57—dc20
    DNLM/DLC
    for Library of Congress   94-16409
                                                         CIP

PREFACE

I have been intensely interested in the subject of headache for many years. This interest doubtless reflects personal experience. Not only have I been a life-long victim of migraine, but my wife and both children also suffer with the affliction. For many years I have skewed my clinical practice toward headache, so that the vast majority of my private patients are victims of migraine headaches. I am impressed not only with the intense pain and overall misery that can be caused by migraine, but also by the social, economic, and emotional morbidity that arise from a chronic disorder that can disable a patient at any time without warning. It also troubles me that in addition to those who actively seek treatment, migraine and associated headaches are a daily, weekly, or monthly fact of life to nameless millions who endure pain and discomfort in silence. Perhaps in response to the ubiquitous advertisements for over-the-counter preparations that promise to ease pounding headaches accompanied by upset stomachs, I have the suspicion that many migraineurs who could be helped instead believe that such headaches are a typical part of most people's lives.

Considering that headache pain may be the most common specific symptom for which patients in the United States seek medical care, the unsatisfactory and largely inadequate care received by the majority of patients with this disorder discourages me. In part, it is a consequence of the relative neglect of the subject until the last 10 or 15 years. In part, it is a function of the great amount of the physician's time and energy that the care of a patient with migraine requires. Migraine does not fit into the usual category of "high-tech" medicine practiced today. Most patients with migraine need few, if any, laboratory or imaging procedures. The average physician is ill-equipped either by schooling or residency training to cope with patients whose problems require dialogue, compassion, and understanding rather than laboratory examinations and procedures. Moreover, because migraine is a non-life-threatening condition, the physician can grow frustrated when patients return again and again, having failed to benefit from attempted treatment. As a result of all these factors, an unfortunate but widespread point of view prevails that migraine is merely a severe type of headache which consumes far more of an active doctor's time than its importance warrants.

On the other hand, I have been heartened by the determined efforts of a variety of clinical and bench scientists to understand migraine and its pathophysiology. Immense strides have been made in understanding the pathogenesis of pain and the pharmacology of various drugs which can benefit patients with migraine. Most physicians, however, have read very little about these new developments. For example, because the basic research findings on the subject are published in specialty journals or in journals largely inaccessible to most clinicians, the average neurologist is unaware of the strides made in understanding head pain and its treatment. As a result, far too many physicians fail to comprehend the complexities and variabilities of the condition.

The present volume focuses on migraine's myriad variations, its pathophysiology, and its treatment. The pages offer insights into the complex biological subject of migraine from the point of view of an author who suffers from migraine headaches, lives among a family of migraineurs, and is also both a concerned, practicing physician and a basic scientist. Underlying much of the book is the idea that the clinical significance of migraine and its treatment are intelligible only if the physician understands the anatomic, physiologic, pharmacologic, and psychological factors underlying both head pain and other manifestations of migraine.

ACKNOWLEDGMENTS

I wish to express my deepest gratitude to my wife Judith for her loving support, for her critical and logical approach to scholarship, for her ability to ask probing questions, for her editorial assistance, and for her patience with my shortcomings. I thank Drs. Cosimo Ajmone-Marsan, Terence Gerace, Bruce Nolan, Judith Post, and Norman J. Schatz for reviewing sections of the book.

ROBERT A. DAVIDOFF, M.D.

CONTENTS

Part I

CLINICAL ASPECTS

Chapter 1

EPIDEMIOLOGY OF MIGRAINE

DEFINITION OF MIGRAINE

It seems almost simpleminded to say that before migraine can be diagnosed, studied, or understood, it must be accurately described. Understanding migraine presupposes precise nomenclature and definitions. And yet, despite voluminous publications, we still lack a satisfactory *definition* of migraine. This is the case in large measure because our understanding of migraine depends primarily on clinical observations. In other words, migraine has been mainly delineated by neurologists and general practitioners of medicine who have treated substantial numbers of patients with complaints of headache and who have elicited a history of certain patterns of head pain and associated symptoms from these patients. A problem exists because attacks of migraine vary markedly among individuals and, even in a given person, particular symptoms may occur in one attack but not in another. But when clinicians describe migraine, they tend to cite *typical* attacks; accordingly, descriptions of migraine attacks and the attributes ascribed to the affliction are largely based on reports of representative bouts of headache in groups of patients self-selected by virtue of the fact that they have sought medical attention.

The many formal studies of migraine have largely been focused on patients chosen because they conform to preconceived ideas about various headache types. Research limited to patients chosen to correspond to headache types perpetuates existing biases in the definition and diagnosis of the disorder. The situation is made worse because a number of older definitions of migraine are too stringent, thus limiting our definition to what would usually be designated as *classic migraine*.

To counteract these limitations, some authorities have so expanded the concept of migraine that nearly any recurrent, severe headache would be included in the definition. Moreover, most of the definitions of migraine focus on severe attacks, omitting attacks in those patients with mild or moderate levels of head pain. Yet it does appear that a high percentage of patients with migraine have only mild headaches, and no one knows what percentage of the migraine population treat their migraine with over-the-counter (OTC) medication.[1279] It is quite conceivable that some of the "ordinary" headaches that almost every person suffers from time to time and at varying levels of intensity are migrainous. If that is the case, then migraine may be very common. And indeed, surveys in the general population have indicated that

3

headaches with at least some of the characteristics associated with migraine exist in a notable proportion of individuals.[1248]

In 1962 the Ad Hoc Committee on Classification of Headache, supported by the National Institute of Neurological Diseases and Blindness, made an attempt to inject order into the subject.[5] The classification published by the Ad Hoc Committee provided general guidelines for categorizing headaches based on clinical symptomatology. The committee defined *vascular headache of migraine type* as

recurrent attacks of headache, widely varied in intensity, frequency, and duration. The attacks are commonly unilateral in onset; are usually associated with anorexia and, sometimes, with nausea and vomiting; in some are preceded by, or associated with, conspicuous sensory, motor, and mood disturbances; and are often familial.

In 1970, the Research Group on Migraine and Headache of the World Federation of Neurology offered a definition whose similarity to that of the Ad Hoc Committee is inescapable:[2174]

[Migraine is] a familial disorder characterized by recurrent attacks of headache widely variable in intensity, frequency, and duration. Attacks are commonly unilateral and are usually associated with anorexia, nausea, and vomiting. In some cases they are preceded by, or associated with, neurological and mood disturbances.

These undertakings represented a considerable step forward in defining migraine and were used for years by many who study headache. However, the definitions are intrinsically unsatisfactory because they are actually descriptions of characteristic cases rather than precise definitions. Precise, unambiguous definitions would not include phrases such as "commonly unilateral," "usually associated with anorexia, nausea, and vomiting," and "in some are preceded by a warning." These definitions fail to incorporate symptoms suffered by migraineurs who have different patterns of head pain.

Presumably the principal limitations of these definitions arose from the fact that they were formulated by a group of headache experts who had investigated a small segment of the general population who had sought treatment for headache.

There is little difficulty using either of these definitions to diagnose a case of migraine that has all of the characteristic features. But because of the emphasis on three specific features generally attributed to migraine—warning signs of impending headache, unilateral head pain, and nausea and vomiting—which, as we shall see in subsequent chapters, are not invariably present in attacks of migraine, these definitions are often inadequate to determine whether a particular patient does or does not have migraine.

More recently the Headache Classification Committee of the International Headache Society (IHS) published an extensive document that offers a classification scheme with more precise definitions of various migraine syndromes.[917] The classification scheme specifies the attributes judged to be the optimum indicators that a headache is migrainous, and details whether or not they must be present if the headache is to be judged migrainous. The scheme stipulates that a certain *aggregate* of characteristic features must be present to establish a diagnosis of migraine. These features, which are discussed in more detail in chapter 3, include recurrence of attacks; a limited duration of each attack (from 4 to 72 hours); pain that has a unilateral location, a pulsating quality, an intensity sufficient to disrupt daily activities, and a sensitivity to routine physical activities; and an association with nausea, vomiting, photophobia, and phonophobia. The results of sophisticated laboratory tests are not included. The criteria do not contain equivocal terms such as "often," "usually," or "mostly." Moreover, this scheme has the distinct advantage that all definitions and diagnostic criteria are operational and use information accessible to the practicing physician. The diagnosis of primary headache disorders rests primarily on clinical analysis and assessment of symptoms, signs, and clinical course. The IHS classification scheme represented an important advance toward making headache diagnosis more objective. Nevertheless, the definition suffers from limitations because it specifies only typical, homogeneous headache syndromes, even though there are many transitional types of headaches that are difficult to diagnose as migrainous.[1372] The IHS classification scheme is too intricate for the ordinary physician to employ. Furthermore, the criteria are sufficiently inflexible that some patients with migraine do not meet them even though they respond to antimigrainous therapy.

Traditionally, migraine and *muscle contraction headaches (tension-type headaches, tension headaches)* have been considered distinct entities. Therefore, most classifications of headache have focused on symptoms supposedly specific to vasculature in migraine headaches and to musculature in tension headaches in order to differentiate these two types. Most clinicians are comfortable with this dichotomy and regard migraine and tension-type headaches as separate and independent clinical entities. Some epidemiologists and many clinicians, however, are skeptical about attempts to distinguish the two headache categories. Factor analysis of the responses of migraineurs to detailed questionnaires or analysis of patients in headache clinics have generated no one cluster of symptoms or set of variables frequently or strongly deemed characteristic of migraine headaches.* Most of the clinical variables, such as nausea and vomiting, unilateral head pain, visual symptoms before a headache, and response to ergots, are customarily believed to distinguish migraine from other types of recurrent headache, yet they do not

cluster together in a population of individuals with severe headaches. Moreover, excessive muscle contraction may not play a critical role in tension-type headache; several investigations have failed to demonstrate a consistent increase in muscle tension in patients with this complaint.[16,100,854,1591] Muscle contraction is at least as prominent in migraine as it is in tension-type headache.[634,1343,1583] Tenderness of pericranial muscles is a common finding in tension-type headache, but is also seen in patients during bouts of migraine.[315,1185,1273] Between attacks, migraine patients also have tender pericranial muscles. In addition, patients diagnosed as having tension-type headaches may have symptoms commonly ascribed to migraine; namely, a throbbing component of the head pain, nausea, phonophobia, and photophobia. Several groups of researchers question whether migraine and tension headaches are discrete headache entities that can be distinguished from each other.[517,518,2106,2201,2203]

Recently, a number of investigators have concentrated on the severity of headache rather than on a classification scheme that employs discrete categories with defined configurations of symptoms.[100,634,2102] According to this conception, migraine is considered to be one extreme in a spectrum of headache ranging from mild to severe and disabling. When headaches are distinguished by the level of severity of the attacks rather than by any unique constellation of symptoms, in general, the symptoms associated with more severe, more painful, and longer-duration headaches tend to be those traditionally used to characterize migraine.[336] A positive linear relationship exists between the severity of headache experienced by patients and the number of symptoms generally accepted as migrainous.[2107] Despite these observations, substantial overlap of symptoms customarily employed to classify headaches into the supposedly specific categories of migraine and muscle contraction headaches exists.[100,336,517,518,634] For

---

*References 517, 518, 546, 1552, 2201, 2203

example, patients unequivocally diagnosed as migraineurs experience symptoms considered diagnostic of muscle contraction more frequently than they suffer from migraine symptoms.[100,101] In addition, in the course of many headache attacks, the symptoms claimed to characterize muscle contraction headaches commonly coexist with symptoms ordinarily associated with migraine headaches.[336,1489] Muscle tenderness during the headache, for example, occurs both in attacks that would be diagnosed as migraine and in attacks that would be diagnosed as tension-type headaches. Thus, there may be a continuum of headache symptoms rather than discrete, identifiable, definable types of headaches. In other words, idiopathic headaches constitute an affliction with a multiplicity of symptoms of varying severity that can occur in different combinations. It is also possible that headache attacks characterized by symptoms of both migraine and tension headaches are *mixed headaches* with muscular contraction and vascular components coexisting in an attack. In fact, several authorities have stressed the notion that both migrainous and muscle contraction headaches frequently coexist during a particular headache attack.[1489,1606,2002]

Many of our present conceptions of migraine and its relationships to other neurologic and medical afflictions are based on epidemiologic data. Epidemiologic studies are used to help identify particular headache syndromes by ascertaining the distribution and correlates of headache-related phenomena in populations. Such studies can also suggest possible causes. The lack of an adequate definition for migraine has, however, undercut the validity of many epidemiologic studies, which are themselves the sources of the definition of the syndrome they seek to study. Given this circular process, it is no wonder that migraine has been so difficult to characterize.

The epidemiologic literature for migraine is extensive. The investigations, however, are difficult to summarize because they present inconsistent findings. For example, despite innumerable studies of the proportion *(prevalence)* of the population thought to suffer from migraine, it is nearly impossible to extract precise and reliable epidemiologic information about the prevalence of migraine headaches in a given group of individuals, in a community, or in a country.[2108] The major reason for such difficulties is that investigation of migraine has been impeded by methodologic obstacles, including:

1. *Lack of a universally accepted definition of migraine*
2. *No objective pathology*
3. *Lack of a diagnostic test.* Although a number of laboratory findings (abnormal platelet aggregation, changes in platelet enzyme content, and alterations in cerebral blood flow) have been described in patients with migraine, none are sufficiently precise to serve as a biological marker for the condition. In other words, no objective tests can be used to confirm the diagnosis of migraine.
4. *Differences in selection of case groups and in populations studied.* Many studies of migraine have included only individuals who sought treatment from physicians. In surveys of various communities, it has been estimated that fewer than one in four headache sufferers consults a physician.[1248] Data suggest that those individuals who do consult a physician are unlike those who do not seek medical attention.[1245,2108] For example, patients who pursue medical care appear to be members of a highly selected group who have more intense, protracted, or frequent headaches than the group of individuals who do not solicit medical attention. In addition, the two groups differ in other significant variables such as intelligence, income, psychological makeup, marital status, and sex.[1245,1256,2105] It is also probable that some groups of migraineurs are underrepresented in epidemiologic surveys consisting solely of patients who consult physicians for headache. These include individuals from lower socioeconomic groups.[1248] As a result, much information in clinical texts concerning

the epidemiology and clinical manifestations of migraine has been gathered from the impressions of clinicians who examined selected groups of migraineurs. Only a few studies have investigated a random sample of individuals from the general population.*

5. *Varying methods of data collection.* Both questionnaires and clinical interviews have been used to collect data.† Interviews have been performed by physicians or lay interviewers.[254,403,551,1307,1460] The validity of information collected by means of questionnaires and that obtained by clinical interviews performed by either experienced or inexperienced persons may differ substantially.[1643] Only easily understandable questions can be used in questionnaires, and the respondents must be capable of reading, writing, and comprehending instructions. Other possible problems with questionnaires include poor response rates and worry about the representativeness of responders to the population being studied. The prevalence of migraine may be overestimated when data are collected by means of self-administered questionnaires completed by self-selected respondents.[268] In contrast, although interviews are more flexible, preconceived notions may cause interviewers to bias data collection unintentionally.

DEMOGRAPHIC CHARACTERISTICS

The prevalence of headaches in the general population in the United States and Europe has been extensively investigated. In surveys of large populations, about 40% of men and about 50% of women have described severe, disabling headaches at some time in their lives *(lifetime prevalence).* [2197,2200] One study has indicated that only 4% of the total population has never had a head-

ache.[1644] It is difficult to obtain a figure for the prevalence of migraine, because some investigators studied lifetime prevalence, others reviewed different periods of time *(period prevalence),* and some did not specify the period of time.* It is therefore not surprising that the figures for the prevalence of migraine vary dramatically—from 1% to 31%.† Variation among studies may also, in part, reflect sociodemographic differences in the samples investigated.[1963] Most studies have concentrated on younger age-groups or only on women, and cannot be generalized to the general population.[488,1248,1307] There is a propensity to take a figure of 5% to 10% as an acceptable estimation of the proportion of individuals in the community who suffer from migraine at some time during their lives, even though these figures were largely derived from patients seen in clinics. The finding that only a minority of individuals afflicted with migraine have ever consulted a physician casts a doubt on these low estimates. It is probable that most cases of migraine are undiagnosed. A more reasonable estimate of the lifetime prevalence of migraine is probably about 15% to 20% of women and 10% to 15% of men. More recent data show that the prevalence of migraine is much higher than most earlier studies show—23% to 29% in women and 15% to 20% in men (Fig 1–1).[2107,2109] Another recent investigation has estimated that 17.6% of women and 5.7% of men have one or more migraine headaches per year.[1963] A prevalence study using the diagnostic criteria of the International Headache Society reported that 25% of women and 8% of men had a lifetime prevalence of migraine.[1644] It is also possible that much of the prevalence data in the literature underestimates the true proportion of migraineurs in the general population, because the data exclude individuals with modest degrees of head pain who may or may not have all of the

*References 254, 403, 433, 1461, 1644, 1963, 2102, 2107

†References 403, 1460, 1461, 1480, 1780, 2107, 2200

*References 442, 551, 967, 1237, 1460, 1582, 1644, 2102, 2107, 2200

†References 183, 268, 799, 1246, 1247, 1844, 2108

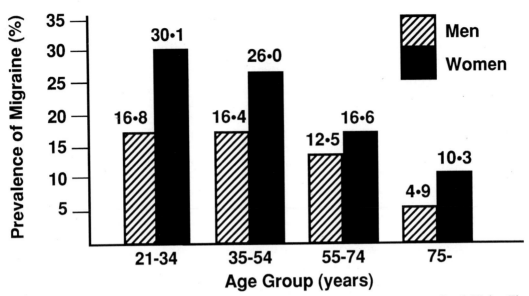

Figure 1–1. Prevalence of migraine in the year before a survey of men and women in South Wales. The data are based on clinical validation of questionnaires. (Adapted from Waters and O'Connor, p. 615, with permission.)

typical migrainous features during their attacks.

As far as we can tell, about 45% of cases of migraine emerge during childhood or during adolescence.[1450] In the remaining 55% of migraineurs, the first attack generally develops before age 40 years in at least 90% of patients.[1806] Migraine rarely begins after age 60 years. Migraine headaches are estimated to appear earlier in males than in females, and in both sexes cases of migraine with aura are more inclined to develop at an earlier age than cases of migraine without aura (Fig. 1–2).[1962]

Almost all clinical and epidemiologic investigations indicate that adult women are at greater risk for the development of migraine than adult men.* Although a precise assessment of frequency by sex is unavailable, it is estimated that the female-to-male ratio is approximately two or three to one.† The ratio varies with age (Fig. 1–3). Migraine headaches are believed to commonly begin in the same year as menarche, but this belief is largely based on the recall ability of adult women.[440] Studies carried out in young women of the association between onset of headache and menarche do not support the idea.[488] For women the frequency of headache is highest during their reproductive years (between age 25 and 45), whereas for men the frequency does not appreciably change between ages 20 and 65 years.[254] In addition, women consistently report more distress from their headaches than men do.[335,2107] Women indicate that their headaches are more severe and their attacks of longer duration than men.[335] Mild headaches are reportedly more common in men than in women.[2200] Female migraineurs are reported to have more frequent attacks than their male equivalents.[1963] Women are more likely to seek care for their headaches than men, but it is unclear whether this is caused by a greater intensity of symptoms in women or whether men have been socialized to restrain from consulting physicians.[335]

Clinicians and some epidemiologists traditionally accept the idea that migraine attacks become less frequent or disappear in middle age, but little quan-

*References 4, 362, 439, 1369, 1806, 2107
†References 254, 1172, 1460, 1644, 1806, 1963, 2102

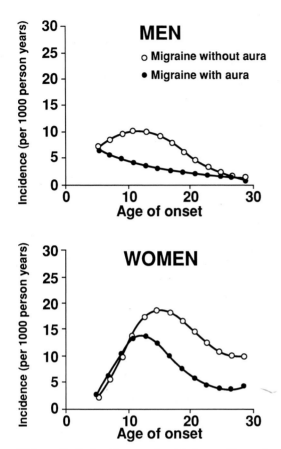

Figure 1–2. Incidence of migraine with and without aura in patients between 8 and 29 years of age. The upper curves in both graphs represent migraine without aura, and the lower curves, migraine with aura. (Adapted from Stewart WF, Linet MS, Celentano DD, Natta MV and Ziegler D: Age- and sex-specific incidence rates of migraine with and without visual aura. Am J Epidemiol 134:1111–1120, 1991, with permission.)

titative information exists with respect to this phenomenon.[799,1897,2107] In particular, it is unclear whether the frequency truly wanes in groups of older individuals or whether the characteristics of migraine undergo noticeable alterations.[254,362,440,2107] There is little doubt, however, that *some* migraineurs do cease having migraine attacks as they age. A number of factors presumably play a role in this phenomenon: in particular, a decrease of stress as a result of maturing, divorce, the end of childbearing, retirement, shift of occupation, and menopause. Other patients

note a change in the character of their attacks. Loss or reduction of vomiting and loss of the aura are the most common changes.[2146] Some older individuals, however, appear to experience a recurrence of classic migraine or are reported to develop migraine with concurrent neurologic symptoms *(late-life migrainous accompaniments).*[657] Nevertheless, the most common change is the metamorphosis from an episodic migrainous pattern of attacks in earlier life into a daily tension-type headache pattern in later life.[1335,1897]

Early anecdotal reports indicated that migraine was more common in intelligent or educated individuals.[28,2166] More recent accounts have shown that there is no major difference in intelligence between migraineurs and the rest of the population, but there is disagreement with regard to the prevalence of migraine among different socioeconomic classes.[183,1307,1461,2105] Patients from low socioeconomic groups are the most likely to go undiagnosed because of underutilization of medical care by these individuals. Recent data, however, suggest that migraine is much more common in both adults and children from lower income groups (Fig. 1–4).[1845,1963] Limited diet and stresses associated with restricted income may be factors involved in the increased frequency. The older clinical observations that migraine is more frequent in more intelligent individuals, in executives, in professionals, and in those better educated is probably attributable to overrepresentation in treatment samples. In other words, it is caused by the tendency of more intelligent individuals and those from higher socioeconomic classes to consult physicians more often for their migraine than less intelligent or less affluent people.[2102] It is now believed that marital situation, educational level, occupational category, and employment situation are not significantly correlated with migraine. Furthermore, the severity of migraine does not appear to depend on urban versus rural environment or region of the United States.[1963]

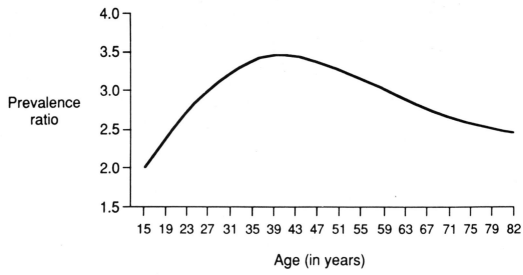

Figure 1–3. Prevalence ratio of female to male migraine sufferers by age. (From Stewart, WF and Lipton, RB: Migraine headache: epidemiology and health care utilization, Cephalalgia 13 (Suppl 12):41–46, 1993 by permission of Scandinavian University Press, Oslo, Norway. Copyright is held by Scandinavian University Press.)

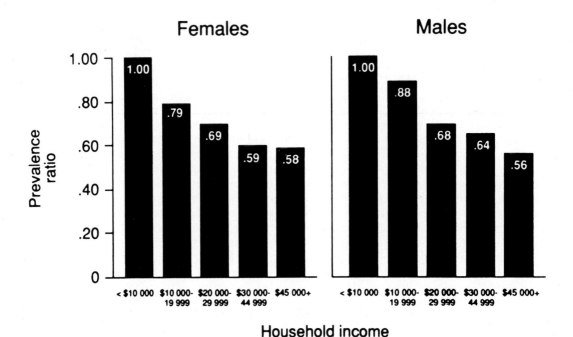

Figure 1–4. Prevalence ratio of migraine by income. (From Stewart, WF and Lipton, RB: Migraine headache: epidemiology and health care utilization, Cephalalgia 13 (Suppl 12):41–46, 1993 by permission of Scandinavian University Press, Oslo, Norway. Copyright is held by Scandinavian University Press.)

It is unclear whether or not the proportion of the population afflicted with migraine varies from society to society. The prevalence in China and in Japan appears to be far below that reported in most studies of Western populations, but whether this apparent difference is a result of biological or cultural differences between Eastern and Western societies is not known.[351,953] Migraine was thought to be rare among Africans, but recent studies have shown that figures for both adults and children from Africa are close to those for Europe and America.[1237,1485,1515] In addition, the epidemiologic characteristics of migraine in Africans are similar in most respects to those seen among Caucasians.[1515] In the United States there is no difference in prevalence between black and white women, but migraine appears to be less frequent in black men compared to white men.[1307,1963]

MIGRAINE IN CHILDREN

Observations that migraine frequently has different clinical patterns in children and adults complicates epidemiologic investigations in children. For example, headache is a less prominent feature of migraine attacks in children than in adults, and childhood migraine frequently has special features such as episodic vertigo, abdominal pain or vomiting, and autonomic symptoms. Although some estimates are higher, between 4% and 5% of children are thought to suffer from migraine.[488,1844,2054]

But children are less likely to have

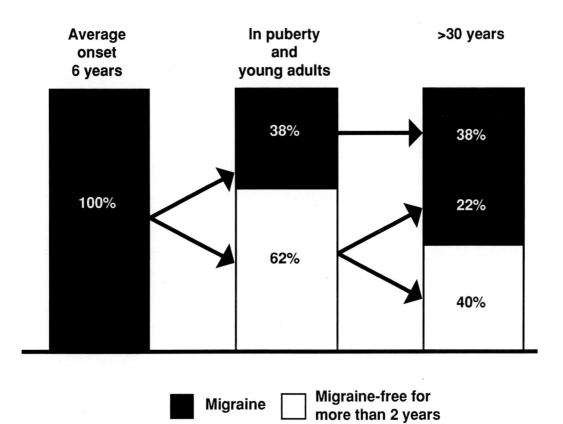

Figure 1–5. The course of migraine in 73 school children followed for 23 years. (Adapted from Bille, B: Migraine in childhood and its prognosis, Cephalalgia 1:71–75, 1981 by permission of Scandinavian University Press, Oslo, Norway. Copyright is held by Scandinavian University Press.)

their recurrent headaches diagnosed as migraine. This may reflect a lower prevalence of migraine in children, but it may also indicate that migraine in children can differ symptomatically from migraine in adults and go undiscovered by unsuspecting physicians. Furthermore, many children are brought for medical attention early in the course of their affliction before a recurring pattern typical of migraine has been established. In addition, the prevalence of common migraine invariably increases with age in childhood and peaks between ages 10 and 13 years.[183,440,1916,1962,2055] The first migraine headache in children is estimated to happen most often between ages 5 and 11 years, but published data vary and largely depend on the definition of migraine applied.[183,280,370,440] Children who subsequently develop typical attacks have been observed to have bouts characterized by nausea and signs of autonomic dysfunction in very early childhood.[117] Migraine has been reported in preschool children, toddlers, and even in infants.* Boys typically develop migraine at an earlier age than girls.[183,440] Most studies show that the prevalence of migraine in male children is the same, or slightly higher, than in female children,† but during adolescence migraine becomes considerably more prevalent in girls than in boys.[440]

The immediate prognosis for migraine in children appears to be good. More than 50% will improve in the 6-month period following the initial consultation regardless of the particular treatment or lack of treatment.[183,677,1615,1847] Many times this improvement is correlated with the end of the school year. The long-term prognosis is also believed to be good.[185] Long remissions are common (see Fig 1–5).[183,370,1844,1991] During puberty and young adult life, two thirds of childhood migraineurs have remissions for 2 years or longer, but in many, migraine

returns. More than half have migraine in middle age.

GENETIC AND FAMILIAL FACTORS

It is a clinical commonplace that migraine has a strong tendency to occur in certain families. The vast majority of migraine sufferers give a history of migraine—usually very similar to their own—in several family members. The average age of onset of migraine is younger in cases with a positive family history compared to cases without a reported family history.[1945] A family history can span several generations.[805] The idea of a family history of migraine has been accepted as so compelling that both the Ad Hoc Committee on Classification of Headache in 1962 and the Research Group on Migraine and Headache in 1970 included family history as a criterion for the diagnosis of migraine.[5,2174]

Considerable statistical evidence gathered in recent years supports earlier clinical observations that migraine headaches tend to run in families.[1246,1367] The high familial occurrence rate suggests that genetic factors play a part in the development of migraine. However, the patterns of migraine inheritance are complex; both the mode of inheritance of migraine and the role of genetic factors in the pathogenesis of the disorder are unclear. For example, several investigations of twins have demonstrated higher concordance ratios in monozygotic than in dizygotic twin pairs, but the concordance in most monozygotic twin studies is not very high.[909,1067,1279,2202] Also, although there is a higher prevalence of migraine in the maternal line of relatives than in the paternal line,[183] X-linked transmission has been excluded because male-to-male transmission does occur, if not quite as often. Several other genetic models have been proposed: autosomal dominant transmission with partial penetrance, autosomal recessive transmission, and polygenic transmis-

---

*References 183, 1615, 1843, 1846, 2055
†References 183, 1613, 1843, 1844, 1916, 1945

sion.[25,98,438,805,1651] It may even be that the mode of transmission does not fit any classic genetic model.[498,1611] The failure to identify a simple genetic mechanism does not rule out genetic determinants of migraine, but suggests either that not all migraine syndromes are genetically equivalent or that environmental factors also play a significant role. A reasonable hypothesis is that a number of genes render an individual more or less vulnerable to develop the affliction in response to a combination of environmental and internal trigger factors. In other words, what is probably inherited is a lowered biologic threshold to a variety of external and internal stimuli.

The approximate risk that offspring of migraineurs will develop migraine is based on family history. For example, it is reasonable to expect that when both parents are migraineurs, 70% of the children will develop migraine at some time in their lives. It is estimated that 45% of youngsters will eventually develop migraine when only one parent is affected. The risk seems to fall to less than 30% when close relatives suffer from migraine even though the parents are free from the malady.[1198] These estimates, however, presuppose accurate reporting. There is no way to know how many migraineurs have close relatives who treat mild headaches with OTC medications and are therefore unaware that their headaches are migraine headaches. In the many families where parents conceal illness from their children, even sophisticated adults may not know their parents were migraineurs. Adopted children and those from single-parent families may have no knowledge at all of family migraine.

MIGRAINE PERSONALITY

Clinicians have traditionally emphasized the association of migraine with a distinctive constellation of personality traits.[8,9,935] For over 50 years the migraineur has been viewed as a tense, compulsive, rigid, achievement-driven, perfectionist individual with an inflexible personality, full of resentment and aggression. This notion was fostered by the late H.G. Wolff and was accepted by many clinicians enthusiastic about the psychoanalytic theories prevalent at the time.[2166] Wolff and others contended that the migraineur maintained excessive self-control over a store of internalized anger and was unable to express aggressive feelings in a constructive manner.[248,711,717] Simply put, as a result of having a particular *migraine personality*, an individual was hypothesized to respond excessively to certain environmental stresses and to particular interpersonal relationships with a migraine attack. The attack itself was hypothesized to be a psychophysiologic expression of suppressed or repressed animosity and resentment that could not be expressed or resolved.[717]

Many migraineurs unquestionably do have intense, inflexible personalities, but so do many people without migraine headaches. Early studies that attempted to define a migraine personality were flawed. Most investigations concentrated on highly selected subjects with severe migraine who sought specialist medical help at a migraine clinic or who were referred by a community practitioner for psychiatric intervention. Depictions of personality were usually made on the basis of clinical interviews alone, and control groups were not used for comparison. Individuals with the so-called migraine personality are more likely to consult physicians and are presumably more committed to finding the cause of their discomfort *because* of their basic temperament. It is probable that these treatment-seeking groups have a higher proportion of individuals with traits of persistence, overconcern, and perfectionism. Investigations that have applied systematic measurement of these traits to large populations of migraine patients have not confirmed an association between a specific personality type and migraine.[403,701,1246] No one personality type can describe all migraine patients, and the personality manifestations in migraine patients are extremely variable.

PSYCHOLOGICAL FACTORS

Depression and Migraine

Although very few controlled investigations have systematically examined the association between migraine and depression, clinical authorities generally contend that depression is frequently associated with headaches, particularly in individuals who report a history of severe or disabling headache.* Children with migraine also appear to have a higher prevalence of depression.[50]

The relationship between depression and migraine is complex. Even though the exact mechanism by which depression might cause headaches has not been identified, it has been generally assumed that depression predisposes an individual to develop headaches. Nevertheless, it is unclear if depression causes headache or if the depression follows from the head pain. Many authorities believe that chronic pain is likely to be psychological in origin.[222,613] In many chronic pain sufferers, however, emotional disturbance has been shown to be a result of living with pain.[724] Convincing data indicate that any chronic pain is able to produce a wide range of psychosocial disturbances, including anxiety and depression.[2172] Patients become depressed as restrictions related to headache and the chronic incapacitation disrupt normal daily living and social functioning. Migraine patients and their relations often indicate that the depression is secondary to the severe and unremitting head pain.

Depression is often mentioned as an affective correlate of the headache itself. Thus, many patients develop alterations in mood and affect prior to an attack of migraine.[203] Migraineurs commonly note feelings of dejection, fatigue, and lethargy, or develop symptoms of frank depression with weeping spells that precede the actual attack of head pain by minutes, hours, or even days. In addition, patients who suffer from either headache or depression may complain of a number of similar somatic complaints, such as insomnia, appetite changes, irritability, and fatigue. Finally, as will be discussed in subsequent chapters, for some patients antidepressant medications decrease the frequency of, or even prevent, attacks of migraine. This suggests a neuropharmacologic connection between migraine and depression in some patients.

Anxiety and Migraine

A high proportion of persons with a history of migraine and major depression also have an anxiety disorder.[251] In many cases the anxiety disorder is manifest as panic attacks, but patients may also have phobias or generalized anxiety.[1370,1961] The anxiety disorder generally precedes the onset of migraine.[250] An increased frequency of suicide attempts among young adult patients with some forms of migraine has recently been reported.[249,251]

Recurrent Headaches and Behavior

A large proportion of chronic migraine sufferers alter their behavior and lifestyle.[1584,1585,1587] These changes may be pervasive, disruptive, and long-lasting. For example, migraineurs may change their jobs or may stop working entirely because the pain interferes with their ability to function. Some patients feel that headaches prevent them from having an adequate income. Many migraine sufferers discontinue specific leisure and recreational activities and curtail social activities with family and friends. They may avoid exercise, going to parties, having visitors, and shopping.[1587] The social isolation may be in-

---

*References 394, 499, 733, 935, 1368–1370

tense. Extraordinary efforts may be made to avoid bright lights, loud noise, and certain smells, such as perfumes. These changes may occur even when patients are free of pain. For example, chronic sufferers may develop stereotyped behavior that is more closely associated with anticipation or amplification of pain than with the pain ordeal itself. As a result, certain avoidance behaviors may develop that are unrelated to the average intensity, frequency, or duration of head pain. Many of these changes in behavior result less from severe and continued head pain than from an attempt to avoid headaches by curtailing exposure to environmental stresses. In contrast, many men and women with frequent, recurring migraine headaches learn to perform reasonably; many continue to work productively and seek medical services only sporadically.

SUMMARY

Although all clinicians realize that migraine is a common condition, most epidemiologic studies regarding the prevalence and demographics of migraine are imperfect because they have largely depended on inexact nomenclature and incomplete definitions. The new classification of headache disorders published by the International Headache Society represents a major step forward toward making headache diagnosis more objective. Much of our epidemiologic data may have to be reanalyzed using this classification scheme. Nonetheless, bearing in mind the problems of definition, certain generalities about migraine are agreed upon. Thus, migraine is a frequent cause of pain and dysfunction in all societies. All observers agree that adult women more frequently suffer from migraine than adult men. Migraine occurs in persons from all socioeconomic groups, but it may be more frequent in individuals from lower income groups. A family history positive for migraine is common, but the exact part that genetic transmission plays in the pathophysiology of migraine remains obscure. The proportion of the general population that suffers from migraine is still unclear. Clearly, epidemiologic data about migraine are important for clinical studies of pathophysiology and etiology.

Chapter 2

HEADACHE: INITIATORS, PRECIPITATORS, AND TRIGGERS

PSYCHOSOCIAL STRESS
DIETARY FACTORS
HUNGER AND HYPOGLYCEMIA
SLEEP
FATIGUE AND EXERTION
MEDICATIONS AND DRUGS
PHYSICAL AND ENVIRONMENTAL
   FACTORS
HORMONAL FLUCTUATIONS
ALLERGY
VIRAL/IMMUNOLOGIC DISORDERS
HEAD TRAUMA
DISORDERS OF THE NECK
ASSOCIATED MEDICAL CONDITIONS

An intrinsic biological substrate, presumably genetic, predisposes certain people to develop migraine headaches. Surprisingly, some individuals have episodes of migraine for years without ever knowing it. These, of course, are not patients with very severe pain or striking neurologic deficits. Rather, these may be youngsters who experience "Alice in Wonderland" symptoms, but dare not mention that the furniture in their rooms seems to shrink or grow larger for fear that people will think they are "weird." Most adults, on the other hand, have been exposed to so many television commercials about pounding headaches or headaches accompanied by upset stomachs that over the years they grow to assume such

headaches are part of everyone's life. Treating their headaches with over-the-counter (OTC) medications, they remain unaware that they suffer from migraine. Some of these migraineurs have mild, infrequent headaches and obtain adequate relief from the advertised medications. Others, with more frequent headaches, may unfortunately exacerbate their migraine headaches through overuse of analgesics.

Among those individuals who have been unaware that they suffer from migraine, and among those who have apparently never had an attack (but *do* have a genetic predisposition to develop migraine), an event may occur that triggers a headache perceived to be their first migraine. Blau has demonstrated that many individuals with migraine are convinced they can identify a specific occurrence that preceded their first attack.[205] Such initiating experiences are generally dramatic (although not necessarily bad). Examples include physical trauma such as a head injury, iatrogenic causes generally involving contraceptive pills or anti-anginal drugs that contain nitrates, or emotional pain such as a death in the family or a divorce. Even joyful life events such as a pregnancy or the birth of a baby can set off recurrent migraine headaches. Hormonal changes, of course, are factors in pregnancy and birth, but emotional stress is extremely important too. In fact, a large proportion of migraineurs experience their initial migraine headaches during an interval of emotional stress.[464] Once the first migraine attack has occurred, the individual has the capacity to develop further attacks.

In some migraineurs, biologic traits alone may be sufficient to *precipitate* recurrent attacks. The timing of their attacks follows an endogenous rhythm with no overt external initiators *(trigger factors, precipitating events).* Approximately 15% of migraineurs deny that trigger factors play a role in their headaches.[775] For most migrainous patients, however, both exogenous and endogenous factors trigger, or precipitate, migraine attacks (Table 2–1). Such factors include psychosocial conditions, dietary constituents, physical stimuli, changes in hormonal levels, or

Table 2–1 MAJOR PRECIPITANTS OF MIGRAINE ATTACKS

Precipitant	Examples
• Stress	
• Foodstuffs	Cheese, dairy products, chocolate, citrus fruits, pork, onions, seafood
• Food additives	MSG, nitrites, aspartame
• Alcohol	Red wines
• Hunger	
• Physical exertion	Excessive exercise, fatigue
• Visual stimuli	Bright lights, glare, stripes
• Auditory stimuli	Loud, blaring noise or music
• Olfactory stimuli	Perfumes, colognes, after-shave lotions, cigarette and cigar smoke, diesel and gasoline fumes, paint
• Weather changes	Alterations in barometric pressure
• Medications	Nitroglycerin, reserpine, oral contraceptives
• Hormonal changes	Menstruation, ovulation, pregnancy
• Sleep	Too much or too little
• Head trauma	

(Data from Selby and Lance,[1806] Van den Bergh, et al.,[205] Blau and Thavapalan,[219] and Linet and Stewart.[1247])

administration of medications. Trigger factors are not the cause of migraine in these patients, but are responsible for *inducing* attacks. It is tempting to speculate that migraineurs in general have a lowered threshold to commonplace stimuli—stimuli that do not provoke headaches in individuals without migraine. However, the catalog of factors reported to provoke migraine attacks is so extensive that we must infer either that subgroups of migraineurs exist who have different biologic abnormalities, or that a common, unique mechanism operates in migraineurs but gets triggered by a broad range of circumstances.

In therapeutic terms, it is crucial to identify trigger factors, because when specific influences are removed, many patients experience a significant decrease in the frequency of attacks.[219] Accordingly, many headaches may be prevented if a particular migraineur abstains from alcohol, eliminates chocolate, discontinues contraceptive pills, obtains adequate sleep, or eats three regular meals a day.

For some patients, sensitivity to a particular stimulus requires many years—or even decades—to evolve. For example, migraineurs may be able to drink some alcohol with impunity in their youth but cannot tolerate even a small quantity after 20 years of suffering from migraine. In contrast, what triggers an attack at one stage of life may no longer induce one at a later stage. In general, however, the number of trigger factors increases with age and with duration of disease.[2058] Identification of trigger factors in individual patients is hampered by the fact that exposure to a putative trigger does not always provoke an attack of migraine. Perhaps either a certain threshold dose, concentration, or exposure is necessary before an attack can occur; alternatively, initiation of attacks may be multifactorial, requiring simultaneous or serial exposure to several factors. The latter possibility is favored by the observation that during premenstrual and menstrual days, some women are sensitive to certain dietary factors that they can tolerate at other times of their cycle.[444]

About 85% of patients can identify specific trigger factors.[2058] The most prominent ones in adults include anxiety, frustration, or anger; fatigue or sleep disturbances; menstruation and ovulation; consumption of alcoholic beverages or certain foodstuffs; hunger; and a variety of sensory stimuli (see Table 2-1).[219,773,1540,1806,2058] In children, viral infections, changes in weather, watching television, and driving in an automobile appear to be important triggers. Precise figures as to the relative importance of specific trigger factors in the general population of migraineurs are difficult to obtain, however, because much of the data has been collected from patients attending special clinics. Moreover, in many studies the methods used to obtain the data are unspecified or incompletely described.

Many migraine precipitants also provoke headaches in non-migraineurs.[210] For example, hunger headaches, hangovers as a result of overindulgence in alcohol, premenstrual headaches, and so-called "stress headaches" are provoked by stimuli that also produce migraine headaches in migraineurs. Nitroglycerin prescribed for angina and nitrites present in preserved meats and fish produce a throbbing headache both in migraineurs and in some individuals without a history of migraine headaches. Nitroglycerin and nitrites, however, usually do not produce a complete migraine attack with all the associated features, such as nausea, vomiting, and photophobia.

How the majority of triggers precipitate migraine attacks is generally unclear, but there are theories to explain the effects of a few stimuli on susceptible people. Some chemical triggers such as alcohol, nitroglycerin, and nifedipine are hypothesized to produce vasodilatation. The traditional concept holds that the offending substance acts directly on the smooth muscle of arterial walls to cause vasodilatation, which is in turn responsible for the pain of the migraine attack. But the evidence linking the pain of migraine to dilated blood vessels is disputed. If vasodilatation is responsible for the pain, why do many potent cerebral vasodilators, such as CO_2 and papaverine, rarely cause headache? Moreover, many of the substances purported to produce headaches have only modest effects on blood vessels. The direct effects of alcohol on cerebral blood vessels, for example, are insignificant, producing only minor changes in cerebral blood flow.[1337] Yet alcohol clearly can trigger a bout of migraine. In sum, a vasodilatatory action is unlikely to be the *sole* mechanism responsible for the migraine headaches triggered by such agents as alcohol or nitroglycerin.

PSYCHOSOCIAL STRESS

There is little doubt that migraine has an organic basis, but psychological factors also play a crucial role in the development of migraine headache vis-à-vis the triggering of individual attacks, the ways chosen to deal with recurrent head pain, and the effects of chronic head pain on the personality. Psychological makeup interacts with biologic substrata in migraineurs to trigger, exacerbate, or maintain a headache state. Some authorities feel that migraine may be best regarded as a biopsychosocial illness. Accordingly, discrete, acute psychological events that evoke intense emotions may be a precipitant in almost three quarters of all severe attacks.[935,1115,1540,1806] Data also indicate that prolonged stress contributes to the frequency of migraine attacks.[935]

The relationship between stress and headaches is complex.[48,99,1236] A large number of individuals remember developing their first migraine attacks following a long period of emotional difficulty involving experiences of loss and bereavement, physical illness, or disruption of social support systems.[464] But although acutely stressful situations are believed responsible for many migraine attacks, there is no documentation that migraine sufferers are exposed to greater or more numerous stresses than individuals without headaches. Moreover, the precipitating stresses in many instances are part of everyday life—for example, anxieties about examinations or deadlines. Children frequently state that schoolwork (and in particular examinations) is a factor in the genesis of their headaches.[183] Adolescents complain that attending classes, doing homework, and preparing for exams are frequent causes of headache.[1923] Many attacks also occur in anticipation of some socially demanding duty, such as attending a large party or going on a family vacation; an attack of migraine frequently results in cancellation of the anxiety-provoking event. Some situations that are considered pleasurable or rewarding by most individuals may trigger headaches in susceptible patients. Winning a contest or receiving a raise in salary or a promotion fall into that category. An individual patient's reaction to each situation is idiosyncratic, determined by how the individual assesses that particular event.[598] It becomes stressful solely by virtue of the person's reaction. It is a reasonable hypothesis that migraineurs are predisposed by intrinsic biologic factors to experience more intense reactions to a given amount of stress than control subjects.[1586] There is also little doubt that acute stress can augment the intensity and duration of an ongoing migraine headache. Pain may also be identified by migraineurs as the most stressful aspect of their lives. Finally, sequelae of frequent migraine, such as marital difficulties, may be chronic stressors and exacerbate the headache problem.

Emotional triggers may precede migraine attacks by a considerable time period (2 or 3 days in some cases), but usually attacks occur on the day when stress levels are high, or 1 day later.[1130] In particular, clinical observations support the idea that patients with migraine have a penchant to develop headaches after the culmination of a stressful situation or event, during the *letdown* period of relaxation and repose. For example, many migraineurs develop headaches at the end of the school year, following the submission of a major report or paper, or when starting a holiday. Data conflict, however, as to whether or not headaches are more frequent during weekends than during weekdays.[1296,1418] Some workers have noted a weekly periodicity in the incidence of headache in populations of migraine patients, with an increased frequency of weekend headaches, but others have found no statistical association of headache with a particular day of the week.[414,817,1511] It is clear, however, that some individual patients have attacks predominantly during weekends. In these patients headaches may be related to relaxation after the workweek period of stress, increased consumption of alcohol, oversleeping, or caffeine withdrawal.[399]

DIETARY FACTORS

Perhaps as many as 45% of migraine patients believe that some or all attacks are induced by specific items of food.[773,1550,1806,2057] Understanding what role dietary factors play in the precipitation of migraine attacks is complicated both by a dearth of sound scientific study and by a plethora of misconceptions about diet in the popular press and on television. Determining which foods trigger headaches in the subgroup of migraine sufferers who *do* have dietary migraine is further complicated because particular foods may not provoke attacks on every occasion that they are ingested.

Investigations of the influence of diet on the frequency and severity of migraine attacks are challenging to perform. A diet trial cannot be carried out in a double-blind fashion. Not only is the placebo effect potent in such studies, but factors such as patient compliance and the inconveniences associated with a precisely altered diet are difficult to control. Most investigators have applied a time restriction of 24 hours as an outside limit when testing for reactions to foods, even though there are reports of delayed reactions.[444,754,879,1720,2205] Double-blind administration of the putative offending food in gelatin capsules has frequently resulted in negative results. However, food-induced attacks of migraine are typically dose-related, and gelatin capsules cannot deliver an adequate dose of the offending food. Moreover, dietary substances may interact with other susceptibility factors such as the degree of emotional or physical stress or (for women), the time in the menstrual cycle. In sum, definitive data about dietary migraine are challenging to procure.

In addition, the mechanisms of diet-provoked headache are obscure. Some of the foods commonly cited as triggering migraine attacks contain vasoactive amines. Many authorities feel that small amounts of these chemicals can precipitate an attack in susceptible individuals. Other foods that are reported to act as migraine precipitants do not contain amines. Some authorities hypothesize that food triggers migraine attacks via an allergic reaction, but, as reviewed below, a definite relationship between migraine and food allergy remains unproven.[597,824,1295,1407] It is also possible that the occurrence of a migraine attack after the consumption of a particular food may not be an idiosyncrasy, but may depend on a conditioned reflex to that food.

Vasoactive Amines

A variety of monoamines, such as p-tyramine, β-phenylethylamine, and octopamine are designated as *vasoactive amines* because they influence blood pressure. All have been thought to be migraine-triggering factors—in many cases, on the basis of insufficient evidence.

In normal individuals, oxidative deamination by monoamine oxidases (MAOs) and sulfate conjugation of the aromatic hydroxyl group by phenolsulfotransferases (PSTs) found in the bowel is believed to decrease the absorption of vasoactive amines found in foods. Once absorbed, however, vasoactive amines are enzymatically broken down in the body by two major mechanisms. The first is oxidative deamination of the side chain by MAOs found in the liver, and the second involves PSTs.

Migraineurs are postulated to have a deficiency of MAO activity. If this is so, the monoamine oxidizing deficiency would allow increased absorption of vasoactive substances and would also interfere with their breakdown. The only source of MAO-containing tissue that is readily available for clinical investigation is the platelet, and it only contains the B form of MAO. Compared to normal controls, some male migraine patients have lower MAO levels in the platelets during headache-free periods.[286,774,1750,1831] The idea that MAO deficiency is a causative factor in the production of dietary migraine is imperfect, however: the activity of the enzyme is not low in female migraine patients; the correlation between the levels of platelet MAO and the predisposition to dietary migraine is weak; and activity values overlap greatly between patients and control groups.[1430,1748] Finally, low platelet MAO activity is not confined solely to migraineurs; low levels of activity are found in patients with cluster headache, schizophrenia, and alcoholism.

PST enzymes are present in platelets in two forms, referred to as the monoamine (M)- and the phenol (P)-sulfating forms. The names refer to the preferred substrates for the two isoenzymes: M-PST specifically catalyzes the sulfation of monoamines, such as serotonin, dopamine, epinephrine, and norepinephrine; P-PST sulfates neutral amines, but no endogenous substrate has been found. Platelet levels of P-PST are relatively low in "dietary migraineurs" as compared to "non-dietary" migraineurs or controls.[772,1261,1892] M-PST is also diminished in the platelets of patients with dietary migraine, but less significantly so. If platelet PST activities reflect those elsewhere in the body, it is plausible that delayed detoxification of amines by PSTs may trigger dietary migraine, but the marked overlap of values between the levels of the enzyme in the platelets of those suffering from dietary migraine and in the platelets of controls substantially limits the appeal of this idea.

p-Tyramine

A large number of patients restrict their diets excessively to eliminate tyramine. Many patients are automatically placed on a tyramine-free diet by their physicians at the first visit despite the feeling that tyramine is probably not an effective migraine trigger in more than a small percentage of migraineurs.

p-Tyramine is a sympathomimetic amine. It has been postulated to trigger headaches in migraineurs indirectly by causing the release of norepinephrine and other catecholamines present in nerve endings and in the adrenal medulla. The release of catecholamines is responsible for the hypertensive reactions seen after p-tyramine is administered both to normal individuals and to patients taking MAO inhibitors. The transient increase in blood pressure seen after intravenous administration of p-tyramine occurs within 1 to 3 minutes; some migrainous individuals also experience migraine attacks 1 to 36 hours after such an infusion.[756] The difference in the latencies between the hypertensive and migrainogenic effects of p-tyramine suggests that the amine's role in the pathogenesis of migraine does not depend entirely on its ability to release catecholamines. This idea is supported by findings that pretreatment with the β-blocker propanolol reduces the headache but does not alter the pressor effect, whereas administration of an α-adrenergic antagonist before the intravenous administration of p-tyramine will reduce both the pressor effect and the headache.[754]

p-Tyramine is formed by decarboxylation of the amino acid tyrosine by the enzyme tyrosine decarboxylase. Tyrosine is a common amino acid, and small amounts of p-tyramine are found in many foods. In contrast, large quantities of p-tyramine are formed only in aged, fermented, or spoiled food products. For example, microorganisms containing tyrosine decarboxylase are necessary for the ripening of certain cheeses, for the curing of some sausages, and for the fermentation of sauerkraut.

Much of the literature indicating the presence of high concentrations of p-tyramine in specific foods is based on isolated and often unproven case reports of hypertensive crises that occurred after patients taking MAO inhibitors ate certain foods. It is true that hypertensive crises in patients on MAO inhibitors have been precipitated by ingestion of foods containing p-tyramine, but other hypertensive reactions were triggered by foods containing other vasoactive substances that have not been implicated as triggers of migraine. Largely on the basis of these case reports, a number of authorities have recommended that a variety of foods (such as aged cheese, yogurt, sour cream, chicken livers, sausages, bananas, avocados, canned figs, raisins, peanuts, soy sauce, pickled fish, fresh-baked breads, nuts, pork, vinegars, beans, and broad bean pods) be eliminated from the diet of all migraineurs because of their supposedly high p-tyramine content. Very rare but definite hypertensive reactions have occurred in patients on MAO inhibitors following ingestion of some of these foods, but in most cases, spoiled foods are thought to have been responsible. In other reports about MAO inhibitors, the hypertensive reactions were caused by constituents of the food other than p-tyramine. For example, broad bean pods, but not the seeds, contain L-dopa; banana pulp contains modest amounts of serotonin and dopamine and small amounts of L-dopa and norepinephrine.[639] It is not known whether or not these compounds trigger migraine attacks when administered orally, but they can certainly induce hypertensive reactions in patients taking MAO inhibitors. As a result, much conflicting and overcautious advice regarding p-tyramine endures and is frequently perpetuated in the migraine literature.

Some foods *do* contain high concentrations of the amine (Table 2–2). Matured and ripened cheeses such as Camembert, Brie, Cheddar, Emmenthaler, Parmesan, Roquefort, blue, brick, and Stilton contain large amounts of p-tyramine (up to 2000 μg/g).[1347] However, the tyramine content of different cheeses varies enormously, depending on such factors as the manufacturing process and the length of ripening. Long-matured cheeses (e.g., fully matured Cheddar) and blue-veined cheeses (e.g., Danish blue, blue Stilton) have the highest concentrations of tyramine.[617] Processed cheeses contain low concentrations of the amine, and cream cheese, cottage cheeses, yogurt, and sour cream have barely detectable levels unless these products have been allowed to ferment for extended periods. Dried salted herring (and possibly other dried fish) contain large amounts of p-tyramine, as do some sausages (some bolognas and salamis, pepper-

oni, summer sausage). Vacuum-packed pickled herring contains low levels of tyramine, but when opened and left unrefrigerated for even 2 hours, moderate levels of p-tyramine develop. Banana skins, but not the pulp, contain p-tyramine (65 μg/g); most people do not eat the skins. Fresh raspberries and very ripe avocados contain low to moderate amounts of the amine.[2050] Sauerkraut, yeast extracts (brewer's yeast), some brands of beers and ales, Chianti, and meat extracts contain variable amounts of p-tyramine.[1808] There are few data that p-tyramine is present in beans or bean pods, although soy sauce contains a trace. It is important to know, however, that foods normally containing a low concentration of p-tyramine may increase their content of the amine if spoilage occurs. For example, protein-containing foods that are not fresh or have been inadequately refrigerated or stored do contain high levels of p-tyramine. Badly stored chicken livers and beef livers are notorious offenders.

Controversy still surrounds the ability of p-tyramine to induce migraine attacks.[1129] Some studies have demonstrated that administration of p-tyramine can reliably produce migrainous symptoms in food-sensitive migraineurs, but other investigations have failed to show an infallible effect.[678,879,1399,1720,1879] Apparent conflicts in the findings of different studies appear to be caused at least in part by differences in procedures and patient selection. On balance, some clinical data support a role for p-tyramine sensitivity in a subgroup of migraine patients, but the data are not very conclusive. For example, cheeses containing p-tyramine have been implicated as headache-promoting foodstuffs in large numbers of food-sensitive patients.[215,1540,1550,1806]

Table 2–2 FOODS CONTAINING SUBSTANTIAL QUANTITIES OF p-TYRAMINE

- Matured and ripened cheeses (Camembert, Brie, Cheddar, Emmenthaler, Parmesan, Roquefort, blue, brick, and Stilton)
- Dried salted herring
- Sausages (bolognas and salamis, pepperoni, summer sausage)
- Sauerkraut
- Yeast extracts
- Badly stored protein-containing foods
- Some beers, ales, and Chiantis

(From Sens,[1808] Rice et al.,[1666] McCabe,[1347] and Evans et al.[617])

Chocolate

Chocolate is listed by many authors as a major precipitant of migraine attacks.* The headache may take as long as 24 hours to develop.[759] Chocolate is usually cited as being a more potent trigger in children than in adults.[183,1299] In fact, in children, chocolate is often identified as the only food or beverage recognized as a headache antecedent. It has been hypothesized, however, that some patients with putative chocolate-induced headaches may eat chocolate as a result of a craving experienced during a prodrome unrecognized as the actual beginning of an attack. When the headache develops, these individuals indicate that the bout was triggered by the chocolate, when in actuality, the eating of chocolate was not the cause, but a manifestation of an ongoing migraine attack.[210]

The biochemical explanation for the effects of chocolate is obscure. The agent in chocolate responsible for provoking headaches has been hypothesized to be the potent vasoactive amine β-phenylethylamine, which is also found in some cheeses and in red wine.[348,1798] The concentration of β-phenylethylamine and other amines in chocolate is low, however, suggesting that chocolate-induced migraine attacks are not related to β-phenylethylamine, or that chocolate-sensitive migraineurs are susceptible to exceedingly small amounts of β-phenylethylamine.[1007,1798] Reports concerning the ability of oral β-phenylethylamine to trigger headaches in patients who describe chocolate-provoked migraine attacks conflict.[1400,1750] Chocolate does contain a complex mixture of compounds that are potentially capable of affecting migraineurs, including a large number of phenolic compounds such as tyramine, octopamine, and serotonin.[1006] And although chocolate and other products derived from the cocoa tree also contain the methylxanthine derivative theobromine in uniquely high amounts, the ability of this substance to produce headaches has not been evaluated.

---

*References 215, 444, 879, 1400, 1540, 1550, 1806

Citrus Fruits

Citrus is one of the most frequently reported precipitants of migraine headache.[444,824,876,879] Citrus fruits contain at least two monoamines—octopamine (p-hydroxyphenylethanolamine) and synephrine.[1957,1958] Octopamine is a vasoactive amine capable of producing headaches in susceptible individuals.[754]

Alcohol

Between 20% and 50% of migraineurs believe that consumption of alcoholic beverages is a definite precipitant.[1540,1550,1806,2057] Moreover, alcoholic beverages are the dietary triggers most commonly reported by migraineurs. However, most migraine attacks provoked by alcoholic beverages are presumably not caused by the ethanol itself, but by the congeners present in the majority of alcoholic beverages. White wines, vodka, and light scotches and whiskeys have a low congener content, and these types of alcoholic beverages can be tolerated by some migraineurs when ingested in small amounts.[1260] In addition, most migraineurs believe that red wine is able to provoke migraine more easily than white wine does, even though their alcohol content is similar.[1259] The important agent in red wine has been postulated to be p-tyramine, but red wine and Chianti do not have a significantly higher p-tyramine content than white wine.[883] Complex phenol compounds (flavanoid phenols) have been suggested as alternative candidates because they are present in very much higher concentrations in red than in white wine, but there is no direct evidence for their involvement in migraine.[1260]

Monosodium Glutamate (MSG)

MSG is extensively employed as a flavor enhancer (Table 2–3). In addition to widespread use as a food additive by

Table 2–3 FOODSTUFFS THAT FREQUENTLY CONTAIN MONOSODIUM GLUTAMATE

- Fast-food hamburgers and fried chicken
- Frozen foods (especially dinner entrées)
- Canned, powdered, and dehydrated soups and bouillons
- Potato chips and prepared snacks
- Canned meats
- Diet foods and weight-loss products
- Cured and luncheon meats and sausages
- Poultry (frozen turkey) injected with "natural juices"
- Prepared sauces, salad dressings, mayonnaise, mustards, and gravies
- Gourmet salts and seasonings

(Adapted from Scopp[1799] with permission.)

Chinese chefs, it is incorporated in a large proportion of canned, frozen, diet, snack, and prepared foods. Soy sauce also contains substantial amounts of MSG. It is frequently difficult to identify the presence of MSG in prepared foods because a variety of terms are used by manufacturers to indicate that the product contains MSG. These terms include: "hydrolyzed vegetable protein" (8% to 20% MSG), "calcium caseinate" (4 to 20% MSG), "hydrolyzed plant protein," "protein hydrolysate," "natural flavor," "glutavene," "kombu extract," and "natural flavorings."[1799]

When ingested in sufficient quantities (3 to 5 grams), MSG induces adverse reactions in about one third of normal individuals (Chinese restaurant syndrome, Kwok's syndrome).[1659] Ninety percent of normal individuals will react to 10 grams of MSG. An average bowl of egg drop soup has 3 grams. A band-like headache and sudden feeling of tightness of the facial and jaw musculature are the most common symptoms. There are also reports of dizziness; diarrhea; nausea; abdominal cramps; paresthesias of the mucous membranes of the mouth and palate; flushing and sweating of the face; burning or pressure pain in the neck, shoulders, and chest; palpitations; and weakness. These symptoms develop within 20 minutes of ingestion.

A large number of migraineurs develop intense, throbbing, unilateral or bilateral headaches within 15 to 30 minutes after eating a food flavored with even *small* amounts of MSG. The amounts of MSG that produce headaches in susceptible migraineurs are generally insufficient to produce the complete Chinese restaurant syndrome. Many of these individuals cannot distinguish these attacks from their usual migraine attacks.

Nitrites

Sodium nitrite is employed as a food coloring and preservative in processed and cured meats and fish, such as frankfurters, bacon, ham, bologna, salami, pepperoni, sausages, corned beef, pastrami, and lox. A number of individuals develop headaches minutes to hours after ingesting products containing nitrites (hot dog headaches).[928] A nitrite-induced headache is typically bitemporal or bifrontal in location and is usually throbbing in nature. The headache is occasionally accompanied by facial flushing. Although the nitrite-provoked headaches share some features with migraine, it is unclear whether or not nitrite-provoked headaches represent migrainous events or are nonspecific vascular headaches.

Caffeine

Caffeine, a methylxanthine, is naturally present in coffee seeds (beans), tea leaves, and cocoa trees and is therefore present in foods and drinks made from derived products such as coffee, tea, cocoa, and chocolate. Cocoa products also contain theobromine, a methylxanthine related to caffeine. Tea contains theophylline.

One cup of coffee contains between 65 and 150 mg of caffeine, and one cup of tea contains between 35 and 75 mg of caffeine and 1 mg of theophylline. The exact amount depends on the alkaloid content of the coffee beans or tea leaves and the method of brewing. Drip-brewed coffee contains more caffeine than instant coffee. A cup of cocoa contains about 250 mg of theobromine and about 5 mg of caffeine per cup. Caffeine is added to cola drinks, numerous non-cola soft drinks, and many prescription and OTC analgesic medications. A 12-ounce bottle of a cola drink contains between 30 and 65 mg of caffeine. OTC drugs such as Anacin, Excedrin, and Empirin Compound include 32 to 66 mg of caffeine; Cafergot tablets have 100 mg, and 40 mg of caffeine are contained in prescription sedative/analgesic drugs such as Fiorinal and Esgic. In the United States the daily per capita caffeine consumption has been estimated to be about 240 mg, but it is much higher in England and Sweden (over 400 mg/day).[836]

Very few patients indicate that their migraine headaches are produced by the consumption of coffee or a caffeine-containing product. However, the continued ingestion of caffeine can produce physical dependence and physical symptoms of withdrawal on discontinuation of the usual intake. The most frequently reported symptom of caffeine withdrawal is headache, but drowsiness, fatigue, anxiety, irritability, restlessness, difficulty concentrating, clouded thinking, and nausea may also be present.[836] Throbbing headaches similar to migraine can be produced in migraineurs who consume moderate or even modest amounts of caffeine-containing products if the amount of caffeine is reduced suddenly. Characteristically it is promptly relieved by ingestion of more caffeine.

Caffeine withdrawal headaches usually occur 8 to 16 hours following cessation of caffeine intake. Such headaches usually peak at 24 to 48 hours, but may last for several days to a week. Individuals who ingest substantial quantities during the workweek may develop withdrawal headaches on weekends. For some migraineurs, caffeine deprivation may be responsible for the headaches they experience on awakening.

Artificial Sweeteners

Aspartame (NutraSweet, N-L-α-aspartyl-L-phenylalanine methyl ester) is used extensively as a synthetic sweetener in diet sodas, prepared foods, and desserts, and is used as a tabletop sugar substitute. Headache is the most frequent consumer complaint related to aspartame, and the compound has been cited by 8% of migraineurs as a precipitating factor.[1255] However, two clinical trials came to opposite conclusions concerning the significance of aspartame as a dietary trigger of headache.[1127,1771] The study that indicated that aspartame did not cause headache attacks was a rigidly controlled, double-blind inpatient study that presumably excluded a number of exogenous factors that may act synergistically with aspartame to trigger headaches.[1771] Until further data are reported, aspartame should be regarded as a potential headache trigger in selected patients.

HUNGER AND HYPOGLYCEMIA

Hunger that results from missing meals, eating inadequate meals, dieting, or fasting is recognized as a major precipitating factor.[212,444,1540] In a large survey of women with migraine, deprivation of food for 5 hours during the day or 13 hours during the night was reported to trigger migraine.[444] It has been posited that the major reason for the migraine headaches induced by fasting is hypoglycemia, even though low blood sugar is not a normal consequence of fasting,[212,372] and blood glucose levels do not fall before the onset of migraine headaches in patients with migraine related to fasting.[960] Thus, hypoglycemia per se does not appear to be the factor responsible for migraine induced by fasting.[1541,1629] Furthermore, administration of glucose to fasting migraineurs has been shown to have both beneficial and deleterious effects.[212,828,1310] Nonetheless, an evolving attack as a result of delay in eating may be ameliorated by eating a meal. The mechanism is unknown, but missing a meal may be only one incident in a time of excessive activity or stress that in itself would be likely to bring about a migraine attack. On the other hand, migraine attacks can be provoked in diabetics by insulin-induced hypoglycemia.

Many patients with migraine are said to have *reactive* (postprandial) hypoglycemic patterns discerned from the results of 5-hour glucose tolerance tests.[491] Reactive hypoglycemia represents an exaggeration of ordinary physiologic reactions. The blood glucose level ordinarily rises soon after the ingestion of food and then returns to normal. Hypoglycemia, with blood glucose levels of less than 50 mg/100 ml without accompanying symptoms, occurs in many normal individuals in response to the stimulus of a glucose load or a high-carbohydrate meal. In fact, low blood glucose values occur during the postprandial state in 25% of normal, asymptomatic individuals.[297] It may be that migraineurs are more sensitive to the effects of a high-carbohydrate meal than are non-migraineurs. Ingestion of large quantities of foods containing simple sugars has been said to cause attacks in some migraineurs. It is also possible that migraineurs are more sensitive to a modest reduction of blood sugar than other people are. Some patients have indicated that they experienced substantial improvement of migraine when they were placed on a frequent-feeding, high-protein diet.

SLEEP

Although for the great majority of migraineurs a brief period of sleep has therapeutic value in aborting attacks, too little sleep or excessive sleep can act as a stimulus for the precipitation of migrainous attacks.[204,1525] In particular, many migraine sufferers realize that they develop headaches on awakening on weekends and holidays, when they sleep later than they ordinarily do. For this reason, migraineurs should be strongly urged to awaken at a uniform time each day.

Some migraine patients are awakened from nocturnal sleep, or from a daytime nap, with a severe, throbbing headache. Awakening from nocturnal sleep with a headache is most common in the early-morning hours. A clear tendency for nocturnal migraine attacks to begin either during rapid eye movement (REM) sleep or immediately following REM sleep has been reported, even though this sleep phase only occupies about 15% to 20% of total sleep time.[493,494,990]

Sleep disorders are claimed to be more common in children with migraine than in children without it. For example, somnambulism, head banging, and night terrors may be more frequent in children with severe migraine.[112,183] The subject, however, has received little attention and requires further documentation.

FATIGUE AND EXERTION

Fatigue, whether it comes from exertion or from lack of adequate rest, can give rise to migraine headaches.[2058] In addition, any form of exercise may precipitate headaches in particular individuals *(benign exertional headache, effort migraine)*. Throbbing, bilateral headaches with typical migrainous features develop in some people only when their exercise is excessive or violent.[1319] The effort is generally protracted, uncharacteristically strenuous, physically stressful, and associated with exhaustion. Examples of reported activities include running, football, bowling, weight lifting, and dancing.[501,1319] Other factors include lack of a proper warm-up before exercise, dehydration, hypoglycemia, and exercising at high altitudes. In children the problem is more prevalent in boys, usually in relation to competitive sports and endurance contests.[183] But effort migraine can also occur during less intense, but more prolonged activity. This situation is commonly seen in poorly conditioned athletes.

These headaches may be triggered both in unconditioned persons and in athletes, particularly if activity is undertaken in hot, humid weather or at high altitudes. Attacks typically occur soon after the exercise. Such headaches may last from 5 minutes to 24 hours. Almost all of the patients either have migraine or have a family history of migraine. Patients with exercise-induced headaches usually have no demonstrable intracranial pathology, but should be assessed for the presence of lesions in the posterior fossa, arteriovenous malformations (AVMs), aneurysms, and pheochromocytomas.[1535]

Sexual Activity

A distressing type of headache that is usually considered a form of exertional headache is headache associated with sexual activity *(coital cephalgia, benign sex headache, benign orgasmic cephalgia).*[1593,1604] The problem affects men more commonly than women, and may pertain to the intensity of physical exertion in the sexual act. Because the same type of headache can come on when the individual is masturbating or playing a completely passive sexual role, however, perhaps the symptoms should be attributed to sexual excitement rather than to physical strain or exertion. Both exertional and sexual headaches have been documented in the same individuals.[1311,1534]

The most common type of head pain that arises during sexual activity typically occurs during, or slightly before, orgasm and is characterized by the abrupt onset of extremely severe, throbbing pain that may be accompanied by nausea, vomiting, and photophobia. The bout may last from minutes to several hours. The pain is usually bilateral and can be bioccipital, bifrontal, or holocephalic in location. Many patients have a personal or family history of migraine, and this type of coital headache is considered by some authorities to be a variant of migraine.[1311,1534,1604,1842]

MEDICATIONS AND DRUGS

Prescription Drugs

A number of prescribed drugs have the potential to induce either throbbing headaches or typical migraine attacks with all associated features in susceptible individuals, or a dull constant headache that may exacerbate preexisting migraine headaches. Frequently reported drugs are listed in Table 2–4. Information about the relative incidence of headache related to different drugs is sparse, however.[85]

Nitroglycerin can provoke intense, pulsating, bifrontal or bitemporal headaches in a reliable and dose-dependent fashion when used for the treatment of angina pectoris.[437,887] In normal individuals an immediate, short-lasting headache can be produced. Migraineurs are more sensitive to the headache-producing effects of nitroglycerin than are patients with tension headache or individuals without a history of headaches. The headaches may occur within minutes but may be delayed several hours after exposure to nitroglycerin. They may be transient but usually last for several hours. They can be associated with nausea and photophobia and often are indistinguishable from a spontaneous bout of migraine.

Parenteral administration of reserpine induces headache in most migraineurs, but only infrequently in normal control subjects.[63,419,667] Although the headache triggered by reserpine may duplicate the usual migraine of patients, reserpine does not reproduce the

Table 2–4 PRESCRIPTION MEDICATIONS REPORTED TO EXACERBATE OR INDUCE HEADACHE

VASODILATORS

Nitroglycerin, isosorbide dinitrate

ANTIHYPERTENSIVES

Reserpine, captopril, atenolol, metoprolol, prazosin

NONSTEROIDAL ANTI-INFLAMMATORY DRUGS

Indomethacin, diclofenac, piroxicam

H_2-RECEPTOR ANTAGONISTS

Cimetidine, ranitidine

CALCIUM CHANNEL BLOCKERS

Nifedipine, verapamil

HORMONAL PREPARATIONS

Contraceptives, danazol, estrogens, clomiphene

ANTIBIOTICS

Griseofulvin, trimethoprim-sulfamethoxazole

(Adapted from Solomon, 1991,[1895] with permission.)

aura in patients with classic migraine. The headache is often unilateral and throbbing in nature and is frequently associated with nausea and even vomiting.

After withdrawal of indomethacin, or within 24 hours after a single administration of the drug, a severe symmetrical, pulsating headache can result. The same is true for certain other nonsteroidal anti-inflammatory drugs (NSAIDs).

Illicit Drugs

Headaches are common in individuals who use cocaine, heroin, and marijuana, but little is known about headache and the use of other illicit drugs.[609] A wide variety of neurologic symptoms cause cocaine users to seek medical attention.[1278] Headaches are one of these symptoms.[1254] As many as 75% of cocaine users describe intense headaches, which they regard as related to the drug.[354,2101] The description of the headaches is variable from case to case, but new-onset migraine-like headache has been described as a consequence of cocaine use.[496,1764] In contrast, cocaine has also been reported to relieve migraine headaches in some chronic headache sufferers.[263,495] Self-medication of migraine with cocaine has even been demonstrated to be a factor in the development of cocaine addiction.[263] Heroin addicts have a significantly higher incidence of headache than do non-addicts.[477] Some heroin addicts complain of a severe throbbing headache associated with heroin intake, but others experience headaches more frequently during drug withdrawal. Some patients have been noted to develop bouts of migraine without aura after abruptly stopping marijuana after long-term use.[608]

PHYSICAL AND ENVIRONMENTAL FACTORS

A variety of physical or environmental factors may trigger migraine attacks. For many migraineurs, changes in weather, glare, noise, rhythmic movement, and strong smells are potent migrainogenic stimuli.[465]

Seasonal Factors and Changes in Weather

A number of patients report that their attacks have a seasonal periodicity. In other words, they have attacks mainly, if not exclusively, at certain times of the year.[252,803,1147] Different investigations have ascribed high attack rates to a variety of months and seasons, however, so it is difficult to attribute seasonal changes in migraine frequency to allergic factors such as changes in the levels of pollens or molds.

A large proportion of patients indicate that variations in weather patterns trigger bouts of migraine.[803] For example, many patients state that thunderstorms consistently precipitate attacks. For other migraineurs, cold weather; hot, dry winds (such as the mistral, the sirocco, the Chamsin, or the Santa Ana); the onset of humid, hot weather; or rapidly falling atmospheric pressure are significant factors. Bouts of migraine with aura are commonly noticed by migraineurs when they have been decompressed from a hyperbaric environment[44] or exposed to diminished barometric pressure during high-altitude flight or sojourns on mountains.[74,614] The reductions in barometric pressure during such activities are much larger than those that occur as a result of changes in weather. Furthermore, migraine frequency has also been reported to increase when the atmospheric pressure rises.[803] Some researchers find no change in the number of attacks at different levels of atmospheric pressure or during adverse weather conditions.[507,1147,1511,2155] It is safe to say that whatever part weather assumes in precipitating migraine attacks, its effects vary widely among individuals and among situations.

Visual and Auditory Stimuli

Prolonged exposure to the glare of intense light is a potent trigger for headaches in between 30% and 45% of migraine patients.[1806,2074] Exposure to sun is a particularly potent trigger, although reliable data regarding the length of exposure, the intensity of the sunlight, and the ambient temperature are not available. Many patients wear sunglasses much of the time, and many have learned to restrict exposure to strong light, especially that reflected from water or snow. As a result, they forgo summer beaches and ski vacations. Other patients report that exposure to flickering or flashing lights constitutes a specific provocative situation. They avoid flickering light in a cinema or from a television screen, lighting from fluorescent bulbs, repetitive flashes of photographic strobe lights, and night driving (because of oncoming automobile headlights). A proportion of migraineurs are bothered by viewing striped patterns.[1300] Although headaches are frequently reported by persons working for extended periods of time at computer display screens, the headaches are mainly generalized tension-type headaches resulting from postural abnormalities rather than migraine headaches.

Some migraineurs note that exposure to unpleasant, blaring noise will give them a migraine. They frequently emphasize the intensity, duration, and insistent beating quality of the noises that are produced by such varied stimuli as traffic, pneumatic drills, machines, and rock music bands.[723] Even sounds that are generally considered benign—for example, conversation in a large party or a crowded shopping mall—may induce headaches.

Motion and Motion Sickness

Motion is known to precipitate migraine, particularly in children. Between 9% and 15% of children with severe migraine report that traveling sets off their migraine headaches.[183,370] A number of authorities have indicated that both children and adults with migraine, and in particular classic migraine, have an increased vulnerability to develop motion sickness. The incidence is estimated to vary between 26% and 60%.[112,183,353,1087] There is dissent, however, because some experts do not find a significant excess of motion sickness in children with migraine.[488,1431] Nevertheless, it is widely believed that children with motion sickness often go on to develop migraine in later life.[353,1087,1153] Perhaps as many as 60% of adult migraineurs have a history of severe motion sickness in childhood.[1806]

Olfactory Stimuli

Many migraineurs are very sensitive to particular odors.[218] The smells may be those often considered to be unpleasant, such as cigarette and cigar smoke; paint, diesel, and gasoline fumes; tar and asphalt; newsprint; some detergents; furniture polishes; and ammonia, chlorine, and various industrial chemicals. Aromas most people find pleasant, such as perfumes, colognes, after-shave lotions, and fragrances added to hair sprays, shampoos, and other toiletries, may also be offenders.[1917] Many migraineurs are literally tortured by the inability of spouses and children to understand this type of problem. Bouts of migraine are uncontrollable when family members refuse to stop using certain fragrances and toiletries or to stop smoking in the bedroom and car. Other patients have difficulty in close-packed elevators or commuter trains, particularly in the early morning when perfumes, colognes, and after-shave lotions have recently been applied. Department stores, where perfume samples are liberally dispensed on passing customers, are offenders. Some migraineurs who are seriously affected by fragrances have found it necessary to avoid any gatherings where people are likely to be heavily scented.

Smoking

Data are inconsistent with regard to the frequency of smoking by migraineurs; in comparison to the general population, both a higher and lower incidence of smoking have been reported in different investigations.[350,633,1307,1537,2076] Study of a possible association between smoking and migraine is limited, but about one third of patients contend that smoking (as opposed to smelling the smoke of others) initiates or exacerbates their headache symptoms.[2076] In contrast, daily headaches are more common among patients who smoke than among those who do not.[106]

Ice Cream Headache

Ice cream headache (cold-stimulus headache) is transient head pain produced by eating ice cream or other frozen food, or drinking iced beverages.[1639] Application of a cold substance to either the palate or the posterior pharyngeal wall causes the pain, which develops within a minute of exposure, is usually bilateral, and is usually located in the frontal or anterior temporal regions. The orbit may be involved. It lasts for less than 5 minutes. About 30% to 40% of non-migraineurs experience ice cream headaches, but there is a division of opinion as to whether they are more frequent in patients with migraine.[186,538,1639] The incidence of ice cream headaches in migraineurs is said to vary from 27% to 93%.[538,1639] There is also dispute regarding correlation of the site of ice cream-induced pain and the usual site of headache pain.[186,548] In rare patients, an ice cream headache may trigger a bout of migraine.[186]

HORMONAL FLUCTUATIONS

Because migraine is an affliction so commonly found in women, it would not be unreasonable to expect to find it linked with cycles of hormonal change, such as menstruation, ovulation, pregnancy, and the early postpartum period. And indeed, these cycles have profound effects in determining the patterns and severity of migraine in a large proportion of female patients.[523,562] In addition, oral contraceptive medication and estrogen replacement therapy generally increase the frequency and severity of migraine.

Menstruation

As many as 60% of women migraineurs associate their headaches with menstruation or indicate that many of their attacks develop with a constant temporal relationship to menstruation.* Menstrual precipitation of migraine appears to be more firmly associated with common migraine than classic migraine.[1646] Fewer than 15% of woman will have their headaches exclusively at the time of menstruation.[616] This latter group of patients is more inclined to have had the onset of migraine at menarche, to have fluid retention and weight gain associated with menses, and to improve during pregnancy.[616,1450] The majority of migraine headaches related to menstruation occur just prior to, or during, menstruation. Rarely, migraine will occur immediately after the menstrual period. During menstruation, migraine is often associated with crampy menstrual pain (dysmenorrhea). Headaches associated with menses may occur alone or as part of the premenstrual syndrome (premenstrual tension syndrome, late luteal phase dysphoric disorder), which consists of some combination of depression, irritability, anxiety, mood swings, breast engorgement and tenderness, back ache, abdominal distension, and weight gain.

A number of women relate their migraine attacks to ovulation. These patients characteristically have bouts of migraine at mid-cycle. Migraine attacks that occur only during ovulation are rare.

The mechanism of menstrual precipitation of migraine is unclear, but most explanations have focused on the marked changes of estrogen and progesterone levels that characterize the menstrual cycle. Figure 2–1 illustrates the changes in plasma pituitary hormone, estradiol, and progesterone levels that occur during the normal menstrual cycle.[2018] Estrogens (estradiol) remain low during menses and for approximately a week after menstruation. Then they begin a gradual rise, which usually reaches its maximum in the periovulatory period, the day before the luteinizing hormone (LH) peak (LH surge). The LH peak is considered to be mid-cycle. After the LH surge, plasma estradiol levels fall rapidly for several days. There is a secondary increase in plasma estradiol levels that reaches its summit in the midpoint of the luteal phase of the cycle and then declines in the immediate premenstrual phase. Migraine generally occurs during or just after the simultaneous fall of progesterone or estradiol levels in women suffering from menstrual migraine, but the fall in estrogen levels appears to be the significant trigger. The natural decline in secretion of estrogens by the corpus luteum in the premenstrual phase, rather than the absolute level of the hormone, has been hypothesized as the causative migrainogenic factor.[1902] The basis for this rests largely on findings that the experimental injection of estrogen preparations to maintain a high plasma level of the hormone during the premenstrual and menstrual period does not postpone menstruation, but does delay the expected headaches until the estrogen level falls.[1904,1905] Clinical endeavors to prevent menstrual migraine by elevating estrogen

---

*References 1172, 1450, 1806, 2057, 2173

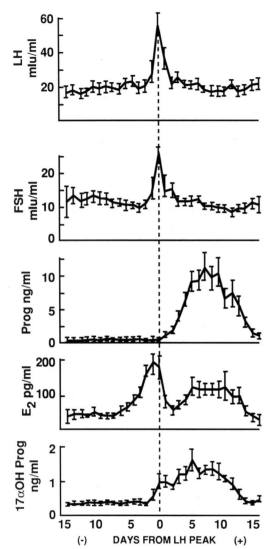

Figure 2–1. Daily changes in plasma concentrations of ovarian and pituitary hormones in women during normal menstrual cycles. Values are the mean and standard errors of the mean of results obtained in daily serum samples of nine normal women. Day O is the day of the mid-cycle LH peak. Ovulation occurs on day + 14 of the cycle. LH, luteinizing hormone; FSH, follicle stimulating hormone; Prog, progesterone; E₂, estradiol; 17αOH Prog, 17-hydroxyprogesterone. (Adapted from Thorneycroft IH et al.[2018] p 950, with permission.)

levels, however, have produced conflicting results.[475,1291,1904,1905] In addition, comparisons of estrogen levels among groups of women with menstrual migraine, with nonmenstrual migraine,

and without migraine have yielded results that are difficult to interpret and often contradictory.* In contrast, the drop in progesterone that precedes menstruation (see Figure 2–1) is not believed to be consequential in the timing of menstrual migraine. Experimental manipulation of progesterone levels during the menstrual cycle delays uterine bleeding but does not prevent the appearance of migraine at the expected time in the cycle.[1901] Some older studies did report that administration of progesterone preparations prevented menstrual migraine attacks.[443,826,1285,1858] Most studies have shown that testosterone, follicle-stimulating hormone (FSH), and LH levels are normal.[616]

Oral Contraceptives

Considerable attention has been paid to the effects of oral contraceptive agents on migraine ever since the early 1960s. When these medications were first used extensively, they were noted to initiate and to worsen migraine headaches in a number of patients. Oral contraceptives produce several different clinical effects in migraineurs.[1772,1840]

1. *New-onset migraine.* Between 10% and 30% of women with migraine develop headaches for the first time after starting oral contraceptives.[445,1144,1191] The headaches usually appear during the first few menstrual cycles, but sometimes they develop after prolonged oral contraceptive use. In general, migraine attacks occur on the pill-free days of a cycle, when the serum level of hormones drops.[445,800,1144,1191,2147] Discontinuation of the medication results in a marked improvement in a large number of patients, although the improvement is slow and may take months.[445,480,1144] A family history of migraine is much more common among individuals who suffer from headache while taking contraceptive medication than among individuals on the same medications without

---

headache.[1144,1191] Contraceptive medications apparently provoke headaches in women with a genetic predisposition to develop migraine.

2. *Exacerbation of preexisting migraine.* Both the severity and frequency of migraine headaches is reported to increase in up to half the women with previously established migraine.[445,480,1144,1285,2147] This worsening of their headaches is more likely to occur in patients who are multiparous, who are older than age 30, who have unusually long or short menstrual cycles, who had menstrual migraine before starting the pill, and who smoke.[445,825,1191] Most women who experience this intensification do so within the first several months of starting oral contraceptive medication.[1721] Discontinuance of the medication results in improvement over a period of months.[480,1144]

3. *Variation in the pattern of preexisting migraine.* Patients with common migraine may develop auras. Women whose pattern of attacks changes from common to classic migraine after starting contraceptive therapy appear to be at particularly high risk for the development of permanent neurologic deficits as a result of migrainous infarction.[165,176]

4. *Cerebral infarction.* Without regard to migraine, a twofold to tenfold greater frequency of thrombotic and hemorrhagic strokes has been reported in women taking oral contraceptives as compared to women of the same age not taking such medications.[1355,1603,1818] A *further* increased risk of stroke in migrainous patients taking oral contraceptives has been reported, but it is unclear by how much the risk of stroke is increased by the presence of migraine.[368,729,1315] The risk of migrainous infarction is even greater when women on contraceptive medication have other risk factors for stroke, such as hypertension or a lipid disorder. This is also the case for women who smoke, for multiparous women, and for women older than age 30.[445]

5. *Improvement of migraine.* Improvement of migraine is seen in a substantial minority of women. Cessation of migraine has been observed in almost 4% of female migraineurs taking oral contraceptives.[800,1191,1721]

It is difficult to determine which contraceptive drugs are more likely to cause headache and which are less likely, because the incidence of migraine varies so markedly among different studies. For the most part, current views of the undesirable side effects of oral contraceptives in migraineurs have generally been extrapolated from older data derived from studies of women taking preparations that contained higher concentrations of estrogens and progesterones than are currently in use. Almost all of the formulations now marketed contain less than 50 μg of estrogen and have a significantly lower incidence of serious side effects than the older products. Few data are available to show that a change in drug composition causes a decrease in the frequency of headaches. In the past 15 years, the incidence of stroke among all women who use oral contraceptives has fallen slightly.[1355,1602] However, whether this same decline in the rate of stroke occurs in women *with migraine* has not been examined separately. Furthermore, even if the use of preparations with lesser amounts of estrogen and progesterone has diminished the vascular risks of oral contraception, it has not eradicated them.

Pregnancy

Pregnancy can alter the pattern of established migraine. Although the response is highly variable, the traditional view is that for three quarters of patients, migraine tends to improve during pregnancy and may even cease, especially during the second and third trimesters.[303,616,1172,1285,1903] This remission rate is higher in women who are pregnant for the first time. Others have reported that migraine may worsen in pregnancy.[303,1903] Migraine is said to develop during the first trimester in 10%

to 15% of women without a history of prior migraine.*

During the week following delivery, 30% to 40% of all women develop headaches.[1595,1936,1937] The rapidly falling levels of estrogenic hormones following childbirth are thought responsible for postpartum headaches.[1936,1937] They usually last for more than a day, and not infrequently for 2 or 3 days.[1937] Although the majority of postpartum headaches are believed to be mild episodes of common migraine, there are instances of women who experience several bouts of classic migraine soon after delivery. Most of the women who suffer from postpartum headaches had migraine before their pregnancies or have a strong family history of migraine. Postpartum headaches can occur in women who have been free from migraine during the latter part of pregnancy, and unfortunately, when a pregnancy ends, preexisting migraine is often intensified.

The incidence of abortion, stillbirth, and congenital malformations among women with a history of migraine headaches is not higher than among non-migraineurs.[2089] It is unclear, however, whether or not there is an association between migraine and preeclamptic or eclamptic toxemia.[1700,2089]

Menopause

Even though there are widespread, anecdotal reports of impressive declines in the prevalence of migraine during or after menopause, almost half of female migraineurs appear not to notice any change in the frequency of their migraine headaches.[2146] In fact, for some women, vascular headaches commence or intensify during the postmenopausal period. Many women with clear-cut episodic migraine headaches in their earlier years develop daily headaches as they age; this may occur

in what might be called the "peri-menopausal" period, the group of years just before, during, and following menopause.

It is unclear whether the reduction of migraine headaches some postmenopausal women experience is a function of changes in hormonal status or merely a reflection of aging. Data gathered from migraineurs who undergo premature menopause induced by surgical oophorectomy are unenlightening in this regard. The procedure is reported to exacerbate migraine in about one third of cases, and either to have no effect or to improve migraine in about two thirds of women.[27] The effects of changing hormonal levels during menopause on the severity and frequency of migraine have not been clarified by studies on estrogen therapy in menopausal and premenopausal women. Both therapeutic improvement and increased incidence of headache have been reported in different series of women treated with estrogens.[93,309,347,452,1144] These disparate findings are presumably a function of the type and timing of the therapy. Cyclic estrogen therapy started at the time of menopause is reported to worsen headaches in many women, but daily replacement therapy may improve headaches.[1144]

ALLERGY

Numerous anecdotal reports and several case-control studies have shown that large numbers of migraine patients suffer from allergic disorders. These disorders include vasomotor rhinitis, asthma, hay fever, hives, and eczema.[1172,1407] Because both migraine and allergy are widespread conditions, however, significant numbers of migraineurs would be expected also to suffer from one or another allergic condition.[1172,1356] No increased prevalence of allergic symptoms is found in migraine patients when they are compared statistically to non-migraineurs; at least

---

*References 303, 341, 616, 1318, 1903, 2176

80% of migraineurs are free of any allergic disease.*

Allergy as a Cause of Migraine

Allergy—defined as hypersensitivity to an antigen accompanied by a specific immune response resulting in the production of IgE antibodies—is thought by many to cause migraine headaches. However, whether or not allergic migraine is a common phenomenon is still undetermined.[824,1407,1610] Much of the confusion has resulted from inadequate controls when investigating therapeutic measures, nor has the therapeutic potential of placebo been adequately considered. IgE-mediated reactions in patients who suffer from both migraine and allergic disease can produce migraine headaches, but only if the offending allergen causes a systemic reaction with some manifestations of anaphylaxis.[1074]

A large body of literature indicates that allergy to certain foods provokes migraine attacks. The list of foods asserted to cause migraine by allergic mechanisms is not only extensive, but also includes many common foods: wheat, oranges, eggs, milk and other dairy products, beef, pork, corn, yeast, soybeans, shellfish, onions, and peanuts.[824,993,1406] However, conclusions about the role of specific foods in individual patients have been based mainly on anecdotal evidence or on uncontrolled studies. Much weight has been placed on patient histories and on challenge tests that were performed without appropriate placebo controls. The problem is complicated by the fact that food has a complex composition in which the nutritional elements are amalgamated with a number of chemical constituents that occur naturally, are induced by the methods of handling foods (fermentation, canning, cooking), or are artificially added.

Elimination diets have been reported

to completely, or almost completely, relieve migraine headaches in a very high proportion of migraineurs.[597,824,1295,1407] This appears to be particularly so in children, reflecting the feeling that food allergy is a more frequent clinical problem in children. In some patients presumptive IgE-mediated headaches have been produced with double-blind placebo-controlled challenges of specific foods, but in many patients the effect of the putative offending food allergen is presumably dose-related, and insufficient allergen may be given in gelatin capsules.[597,1294] Yet even when the offending foods are identified by skin tests and by measurements of the serum levels of total IgE or of antigen-specific IgE by RAST (radioallergosorbent test), it is difficult to demonstrate an unequivocal immunologic component and to correlate it with the clinical picture.[597,1371,1610] The subject remains controversial. The polarization of allergists into "orthodox" (scientific) schools and "unorthodox" (clinical ecology) schools has further complicated and obscured the problem of allergy-triggered migraine.

Asthma

Although no significant association exists between headaches and typical asthma, the 4% to 20% of patients with aspirin-sensitive asthma appear to have a high incidence of migraine.[843] In these patients, ingestion of aspirin is followed within 1 to 2 hours with bronchoconstriction, rhinitis, or urticaria. They are also intolerant of other NSAIDs. Patients with this condition are also sensitive to tartrazine dye (yellow #5), which is used to color certain medications, and many have nasal polyps.

Hypersensitivity to Environmental Factors

Clinical ecologists are physicians who believe that some people may be-

---

*References 1172, 1356, 1371, 1955, 2203

come hypersensitive (or allergic) to environmental factors, such as polluted urban air, diesel exhaust, tobacco smoke, pesticides, plastics, newsprint, synthetic fabrics, perfumes, and food additives. They attribute a variety of physical and psychological symptoms to prolonged exposure to low levels of these common substances. Patients believed to be suffering from environmental illnesses are postulated to have a dysregulation of the immune system, and are treated with extreme dietary and environmental restrictions and provocation–neutralization techniques.

There is little doubt that exposure to many of the substances postulated to be factors in ecological illness can act as precipitants of migraine headaches in individual patients. There is also little doubt that environmental factors such as some chemicals and pollutants can influence general health. But there is a dearth of published investigations that allow a critical analysis of hypotheses regarding the relationship(s) between issues of clinical ecology and the development of allergy or the treatment with provocation–neutralization techniques.[302,620] More hard evidence is needed, and until it is available, the results of most clinical ecological treatment will continue to be viewed as the consequence either of placebo effects or of the removal of offending physical stimuli from the environment.

VIRAL/IMMUNOLOGIC DISORDERS

Acute viral infections are commonly accompanied by headache. Headaches lasting for the duration of an illness are typical accompaniments of systemic infectious disorders, such as influenza, infectious mononucleosis, measles, and mumps. The headache may resemble migraine but more often is persistent rather than episodic and aching rather than throbbing. Exceptions to this typical pattern occur in conditions such as cerebrospinal fluid (CSF) pleocytosis, chronic fatigue syndrome

(CFS), and acquired immunodeficiency syndrome (AIDS).

Cerebrospinal Fluid Pleocytosis

Several series of patients have been described who have developed a self-limited illness characterized by severe, throbbing headaches preceded and accompanied by sensory, motor, speech, and visual disturbances.[126,1697,1791] Both adults and children are affected. These patients do not necessarily have a history of migraine, although some do. CSF pleocytosis—generally lymphocytic and ranging from 12 to 350/mm^3—has been found. The CSF protein may also be high. The prognosis is good, and full and rapid recovery within a few days or weeks is the rule. The headaches and neurologic symptoms are thought to be evoked by a viral meningoencephalitis; both Epstein-Barr and cytomegaloviruses have been implicated in individual cases.[647,2056]

Chronic Fatigue Syndrome

Chronic fatigue syndrome (also known as the *chronic fatigue immunodysfunction syndrome,* [CFIDS]) is not a new problem. Over the past 50 years a number of reports have detailed sporadic or epidemic syndromes of fatigue associated with a flu-like illness. The reports have variously designated the problem as Iceland disease, benign myalgic encephalomyelitis, epidemic neuromyasthenia, and Royal Free Hospital disease. The disorder has attracted recent attention because of a major outbreak in the United States coupled with the strong realization that CFIDS is a widespread, largely underrecognized and underdiagnosed illness. The syndrome, which may be chronic or recurrent, is characterized by some combination of persistent and excessive fatigue, weakness, sore throat, myalgia, migratory arthralgia, hypersomnia or insomnia, and neuropsychological symptoms of memory loss, irritability, confusion, inability to concentrate, difficulty thinking, and depression.[969] Some patients are completely disabled by the fatigue, muscular weakness, and pain. More than 90% of patients with CFIDS complain of headache.[1965] The headache associated with CFIDS may manifest itself as a persistent daily headache or—in individuals with a previous history of migraine headaches—as much more frequent bouts of migraine.

The cause of CFIDS is unknown, but a number of studies have revealed humoral and cell-mediated immunologic abnormalities (e.g., reduced number of natural killer cells, partial hypogammaglobulinemias) that suggest that CFIDS is associated with disordered regulation of the immune system and persistent viral infection.[1264]

Acquired Immunodeficiency Syndrome

The human immunodeficiency virus (HIV) easily invades the central nervous system. A significant proportion of patients with AIDS complain of headache.[164,796,797,1345] Although many patients have benign headaches and some have the characteristics associated with migraine, headaches are more likely to herald a wide range of intracranial disorders. Most patients have a generalized or bilateral headache, most prominent in the frontal and occipital regions, and usually accompanied by some degree of nausea and vomiting. The headache is especially prominent in cases of HIV-related cryptococcal meningitis, in patients with systemic sepsis, and in those with intracranial mass lesions such as toxoplasmosis or abscess.

Systemic Lupus Erythematosus (SLE)

Headache is a common symptom in the acute phases of SLE and may even be the first manifestation of the disease.[245,1305] The majority of patients ex-

perience throbbing headaches that have many of the qualities of a typical migraine attack. Some patients report the presence of scintillating scotomas.[89,245,1013] The migraine-like symptoms are frequently related to exacerbations of SLE. Moreover, they appear to be caused by SLE rather than to represent the coincidental occurrence of the two conditions, for when adrenocorticosteroids are administered to manage other symptoms of SLE, they are very effective in controlling the headaches.[245]

ANTIPHOSPHOLIPID ANTIBODIES

Some workers have suggested that antiphospholipid antibodies found in large numbers of patients with SLE may produce changes in coagulation or cerebral circulation that are responsible for migraine in patients with SLE.[340,1233] Antiphospholipid antibodies are a heterogeneous groups of circulating polyclonal serum immunoglobulins of the IgG, IgM, or IgA subclasses. They are directed against a number of phospholipids. They consist of at least two types of antibodies: anticardiolipin antibodies and lupus anticoagulants. They are found not only in patients with SLE and related lupus-like autoimmune illnesses, but have also been recognized in patients without autoimmune disease.[1232,1274] It is widely held that an increased risk of thromboembolism is associated with these antibodies, most often affecting the cerebral circulation. Recent epidemiologic data indicate a lack of association between the presence of antiphospholipid antibodies in patients with SLE and the presence of migraine.[1305,1411]

Recently, the term "antiphospholipid syndrome" has been applied to a small group of patients with moderate to high levels of anticardiolipin antibodies who do not have SLE, but who have had recurrent episodes of thrombosis. Migraine headaches are frequent complaints of these patients.* Scintillating

---

*References 258, 963, 1012, 1233, 1674, 1825

scotomas, sensorimotor deficits, or confusion may be associated with the headaches. On occasion, the neurologic deficits may be prolonged. Some patients have chorea, livedo reticularis, and heart valve abnormalities. The syndrome has features of a systemic autoimmune disorder that overlaps with SLE.[84] The relationship between migraine and antiphospholipid antibodies has, however, been questioned.[937,1411] A large prospective study is necessary to define the putative role these antibodies play in migraine.

Nonspecific Immunity

Modest amounts of data indicate that immune mechanisms may be involved in the pathogenesis of migraine. However, documenting deficits in nonspecific immunity, elevated immunoglobulin levels, changes in lymphokine levels, or abnormalities of serum complement in migraine has caused controversy.† Both alterations in serum complement levels *and* normal levels have been reported. Accordingly, evidence is insufficient at present to support the idea that migraine has an immunopathologic basis. It is possible, however, that immunologic deficits develop as a consequence of migrainous episodes. This is a subject that needs further exploration.

HEAD TRAUMA

A bout of migraine may follow a sudden jar or blow to the head. Relatively trivial, blunt head trauma may rapidly induce symptoms of migraine, with attacks identical to those of classic or common migraine attacks[853] (see chapter 3). Headache is also the predominant symptom of the postconcussion syndrome. The headache usually emerges within 24 hours of the head injury and can take many forms. Even though for some patients post-trau-

matic headaches have features of migrainous headaches, post-traumatic migraine is reported as a rare condition.[150,1855,1986] This is probably not the case; in fact, recurrent bouts of migraine with and without aura are frequently initiated by blunt, closed head injury in susceptible individuals.[150,280,1379,2122] Post-traumatic migraine headaches have the same characteristics as bouts of migraine that do not follow head trauma, but may be accompanied by a postconcussion syndrome (see chapter 5).

DISORDERS OF THE NECK

Many patients suffer from headaches that are associated with pathologic problems in the cervical spine.[570] For example, cervical spondylosis can result in pain in the orbit and frontal regions. However, the cervical source of the pain is a matter of dispute. On the basis of generally vague evidence, a number of cervical structures—intervertebral and facet joints, ligaments, nerve roots, muscles—have been implicated as the origins of head pain.[108] Controversy notwithstanding, chronic pain in the cervical region can initiate migraine in individuals susceptible to the affliction or induce migraine attacks in patients with preexisting migraine. For these patients, appropriate treatment of the cervical abnormality can diminish the frequency of attacks.

Myofascial Trigger Points

When a myofascial trigger point involves the musculature of the head, neck, or shoulders, the pain is often referred to an area of the head or neck, where it can act as a stimulus for migraine attacks. In other words, the pain resulting from activation of particular myofascial trigger points may precipitate attacks of migraine. A great number of migraine episodes are initiated in such a manner, yet a surprising number of clinicians overlook this common

†References 147, 400, 1040, 1269–1271, 1415

phenomenon. Treating the myofascial problem may be the only way to offer the patient some relief from migraine.

A patient with a myofascial pain syndrome characteristically complains of a zone of persistent, dull, deep, aching pain localized in a specific muscle; in addition, a well-delineated, extremely sensitive trigger point—of which the patient may or may not be aware—can be demonstrated (Table 2–5).[1854,2032] The pain may have begun abruptly or gradually, ranging in intensity from a low-grade discomfort to extreme incapacitation. Pain may be present at rest or appear only after movements that stretch the muscle containing the trigger point.

Trigger points themselves are small, highly localized, extremely tender areas located in muscle or fascia. Each trigger point refers pain and tenderness in a predictable pattern. It is important to note, however, that the extended area of pain (the *referred pain zone*) generated by a trigger point may or may not include the muscle containing the trig-

Table 2–5 CLINICAL CHARACTERISTICS OF MYOFASCIAL PAIN

- Persistent, dull, deep, aching pain localized in a specific pattern in affected muscles
- Well-delineated, extremely sensitive trigger points
- Patient is startled or jumps on application of pressure to trigger point
- Referral of pain in a predictable pattern when a trigger point is pressed
- Reproduction of spontaneous pain complaint when a trigger point is pressed
- Tense cord or rope of muscle fibers palpable in affected muscle
- Alleviation of pain by stretching or injection of trigger point

ger point.[696] In fact, the pain is commonly located at a considerable distance from the trigger point.[696] As seen in Figure 2–2, each muscle has a distinct myofascial pain syndrome, with its own referred pain pattern specific for the trigger points in that muscle. Moreover, pain of this kind has a regional distribution that does not follow

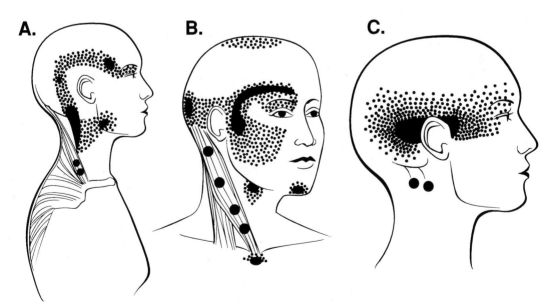

Figure 2–2. Representative myofascial pain syndromes of the head. Examples of locations of trigger points in selected muscles of the neck and shoulders, together with referred pain patterns. Trigger points are represented by large dots. The referred pain patterns are represented by smaller dots. (*A*) Upper trapezius muscle. (*B*) Sternocleidomastoid muscle. (*C*) Suboccipital muscles. (Adapted from Travell and Simons,[2032] pp 184, 203, 322, with permission.)

the pattern seen with radicular or peripheral nerve problems.[1093,1094,2031]

The major characteristic of a trigger point is that moderate, sustained pressure on the point reproduces or intensifies the spontaneous pain, causing a behavioral or verbal response from the patient. Characteristically the patient is startled or jumps when pressure is applied to the trigger point (jump-sign). Duplication of the patient's pain when pressure is exerted is the most compelling confirmation of an active trigger point. Trigger points are typically located in areas of muscle that are palpably firmer than the rest of the muscle. The trigger point itself may feel like a tense cord or rope of muscle fibers when the tip of the finger is rubbed perpendicular to the direction of the fibers. There is a restricted range of movement in the affected muscles—a restriction that prevents full lengthening of the muscles and that may induce alterations in posture and asymmetries of parts of the body. In addition, the affected muscles may atrophy.

The onset of a myofascial pain syndrome can sometimes be traced to an acute muscle overload, a twisting or straining movement, an overt injury or traumatic event such as an automobile accident, or a fall. Other times a sports activity in which a muscle or a group of muscles is used excessively or chronic mechanical overloading of a muscle, such as occurs in neck and shoulder muscles in patients with scoliosis, can account for the gradual development of this sort of pain. Frequently, however, there is no obvious precipitating event, and the patient is uncertain about the precise date of onset. The diagnosis of myofascial pain syndrome—especially when the onset is gradual—is challenging because there are few objective signs and no diagnostic laboratory tests. Routine laboratory tests demonstrate no abnormalities, nor is electromyographic examination of the involved muscles abnormal. Nevertheless, it is worthwhile to check for trigger points in patients whose history warrants it because such individuals can often be helped by physical therapy and other therapeutic modalities.

Occipital Neuralgia and Related Problems

In the pathogenesis of headache, the role of the greater occipital nerve (or its parent dorsal rami) is problematic. A number of syndromes implicating the occipital nerve have been reported, but occipital nerve involvement as a cause of headache is uncommon. Irritation of the greater occipital nerve has been postulated to cause a change in the character and frequency of migraine headaches.[60] When such irritation occurs, infrequent attacks of throbbing, hemicranial pain, most prominent in the frontotemporal region, are thought to convert to more frequent bouts of dull, steady, aching, severe pain that spreads throughout the occipital area on the affected side. The major migrainous feature that persists is the hemicranial nature of the pain. There is tenderness in the area of distribution of the greater occipital nerve.

Migraine with putative occipital nerve irritation should be distinguished from occipital neuralgia. The latter condition is thought to be caused by trauma, injury, inflammation, or compression of the occipital nerve somewhere along its course from the C-2 dorsal root to the periphery. Occipital neuralgia is characterized either by paroxysmal or continuous unilateral, burning or stabbing occipital pain that often radiates to the frontal region.[226,794,870,1004] Patients can have hypoalgesia, hyperalgesia, or dysesthesias in the distribution of the greater occipital nerve and circumscribed tenderness over the nerve as it crosses the superior nuchal line. Infiltration of the nerve with local anesthetic relieves the pain. Myofascial trigger points, however, can also cause occipital pain and may produce a clinical picture that closely mimics the symptoms of occipital neuralgia.[794,812]

Whiplash Injury

Whiplash and similar trauma to the cervical spine can exacerbate existing migraine or give rise to migraine-like headaches. Whiplash is a poorly understood phenomenon that commonly develops following extension–flexion injuries to the neck as a result of sudden acceleration–deceleration forces applied to the neck. Rear-end collision is considered the most typical mechanism. Transient occipital or cervical pain and stiffness lasting several hours to days is common and is generally ascribed to stretching of the cervical muscles and ligaments with or without contusion.[108,570] Limitation of neck movement, upper back pain, difficulties in carrying out everyday tasks, and headache are also frequent sequelae. Patients with traumatic disk protrusions and damage to the cord or nerve roots are usually excluded from the whiplash syndrome.[1545]

Controversy surrounds the chronic aspects of the syndrome. Many patients have intense and prolonged complaints following what appear to be minor injuries to the soft tissues of the neck.[1545] Headache is a common complaint following whiplash injury, but the mechanism causing it is poorly understood.[107] Some of the headaches following a whiplash represent the onset or exacerbation of migraine in individuals predisposed to develop the syndrome.[2122,2160] Other patients develop daily, dull, aching headaches; some of the latter groups have superimposed, periodic episodes of throbbing pain that seems typical of migraine. Severe cervical pain, muscular tenderness, and limitation of movement of the neck may also result from such injuries.[1777] Many develop myofascial trigger points in the cervical and shoulder musculature. Patients also complain of many symptoms characteristic of the *post-traumatic syndrome* or *postconcussion syndrome*, such as dizziness, tinnitus, depression, anxiety, and irritability, and cognitive alterations involving memory and attention span.[107,619] All of these latter symptoms also occur in patients recovering from head injury. Apparently the mechanical forces producing extension–flexion injuries can be transmitted to the skull to affect brain stem and cerebral structures.

The posterior cervical sympathetic syndrome of Barré[121] and the *migraine cervicale* of Bartschi-Rochaix[127] are two syndromes postulated to result from cervical injuries. Both syndromes have a clinical picture similar to that thought to result from whiplash and are believed to be produced by head trauma, particularly trauma that flexed the cervical spine. The symptoms of the posterior cervical sympathetic syndrome were postulated to be produced by irritation of the sympathetic nerve plexus surrounding the vertebral arteries; those of migraine cervicale to be caused by actual compression of the vertebral artery by osteophytes or trauma. Patients with both syndromes are said to have tenderness in the suboccipital region, spasm of the neck muscles, restriction of neck movements, and replication or escalation of the symptoms by neck movements. It is doubtful that these syndromes can be separated from the mass of patients with cervical trauma. The postulated pathology has never been demonstrated.

ASSOCIATED MEDICAL CONDITIONS

Migraine has been inconsistently linked with a heterogeneous group of medical problems such as mitral valve prolapse, multiple sclerosis, and hypertension. Some of these associations are based solely on case reports or small case series. Some are based on more sophisticated epidemiologic data. Neither migraine nor many of these conditions are uncommon; accordingly, their association in the same individuals may be explained by chance in some cases. In addition, the occurrence of migraine and another medical condition in the same individual does not necessarily indicate a common causal mechanism. A number of these investigations may have been biased because subjects with more than one disease are probably overrepresented in a hospital or clinical setting. But although it is difficult to interpret the importance of these postulated associations in view of the prevalence of migraine in the general population, some of the associations do appear significant.

Mitral Valve Prolapse

Mitral valve prolapse (MVP) is a common, but highly variable, clinical syndrome resulting from dysfunction of the mitral valve. It is thought to be a widespread cardiac abnormality; the results of both clinical and pathologic investigations have indicated that MVP has a prevalence of about 6% in the general population but is more common in women.[453,1281] Migraineurs are thought to have a substantially higher incidence of MVP: between one fifth and one quarter of patients with migraine are said to have the problem.[31,722,1257] Conversely, half of the patients with MVP are estimated to have migraine.[722] The basis for the association between migraine and MVP is unknown.

MVP results from excessive mitral valve tissue caused by myxomatous degeneration, usually confined to the posterior leaflet. In some patients regurgitation through the valve is increased by enlargement of the annulus and elongation of the chordae tendineae. The cause is unknown. The clinical picture varies among patients. Some have only a systolic click and murmur and mild prolapse of the posterior leaflet. Others develop a severe mitral regurgitation. Most patients are asymptomatic, but some patients suffer from arrhythmias and substernal chest pain.

Multiple Sclerosis

Early investigations of multiple sclerosis (MS) reached disparate conclusions about the frequency of headache in the condition.[564] More recent studies have shown that patients with demyelinating disease have a significantly higher prevalence of migraine compared with controls.[1680] Migraine attacks have even been reported to be a presenting symptom of the disease, and it is thought that an attack of MS may provoke migraine headaches in patients who are not established migraineurs.[688]

Hypertension

Data on the prevalence and significance of hypertension in patients with migraine are conflicting.[393,633,1307,2104,2123] The prevalence of migraine in the general hypertensive population has been found to be no higher than in the normotensive population, but there is contrary information that a very high incidence of hypertensive individuals have migraine.[1419,2092] If hypertension and migraine are present in an individual, a decrease of the blood pressure is said to alleviate both the frequency and severity of the headaches.[2028]

Dialysis

During a renal dialysis session, about 70% of patients develop headaches.[110,2079] The headache symptoms in patients with a past history of migraine resemble their previous attacks. The headaches begin between the second and third hours of dialysis and usually last a whole day.[110] The severity of the headache is directly related to length of the interval between periods of dialysis. The headaches are much more common than the group of neurologic signs and symptoms that have been designated the *dialysis disequilibrium syndrome.* This syndrome consists of nausea, muscle cramps, irritability, agitation, delirium, confusion, and seizures.[1690]

Platelet Disorders

Attacks of migraine have been reported in patients with blood dyscrasias involving platelets.[239] Patients with thrombocytopenic purpura have migraine attacks when there is a sudden decline in platelet count as a result of platelet destruction.[446] Moreover, a report has described a patient who began to have attacks of recurrent headache associated with transient neurologic symptoms that were indistinguishable from classic migraine when he developed essential thrombocythemia.[877]

SUMMARY

Many older physicians were educated at a time when migraine was believed to befall those with "migraine personalities." Chocolate, red wine, ripe cheese, and menstrual cycles could initiate or exacerbate headaches, but emotional makeup was the primary factor that separated migraineurs from the blissfully headache-free.

This chapter, I would hope, has provided a sense of how complicated the interaction between genetic substrate, external irritants, lifestyle practices, and medical conditions is. The genes that render some individuals susceptible to developing migraine have not even been identified, and altering them will not occur soon. But some external irritants can be avoided; exposure to others can be reduced; daily choices about meals, exercise, and sleep can be made; and certain physical problems can be addressed.

This is certainly not to say that all migraine headaches can be eliminated in all patients. But in most cases, the physician and the patient need to work together as detectives to ferret out the particular combinations of initiators, precipitators, and triggers that give rise to *that person's* migraine. Even the ideal dose of the ideal medication will be less than effective if the migraineur continues to live under the influence of factors that exacerbate his or her headaches.

Chapter 3

CLINICAL MANIFESTATIONS OF MIGRAINE

Migraine is characterized by the periodic emergence of attacks with a constellation of signs and symptoms of almost infinite variety. Most investigators have concentrated on headache as the defining variable, but head pain is only one component of a complex malady whose many features clearly comprise a generalized disorder. The systemic, neurologic, cognitive, affective, gastrointestinal, and autonomic symptoms that can accompany the headache indicate disturbed function of the cerebrum, brain stem, hypothalamus, eye, intracranial and extracranial vasculature, and autonomic nervous system. In any one migrainous individual, how-

ever, the nature of a particular attack can range from a few symptoms to a major siege in which all aspects of the disorder are manifest. As will become evident from the diverse clinical manifestations described in this chapter, migraine cannot be viewed simply as an intermittent annoyance. That may be the case for individuals who successfully treat themselves with over-the-counter (OTC) analgesics and who never seek a physician's care. But for a tremendous number of people, migraine must be thought of as a problem that can lead to profound, striking, and sometimes frightening alterations in the quality of life.

Although a number of neurologic problems are believed to be migrainous or to be associated with migraine, there is confusion as to whether or not these conditions are truly related to the routinely accepted migrainous syndromes of migraine with aura and migraine without aura. These conditions include ophthalmoplegic migraine, transient global amnesia, benign recurrent vertigo, benign paroxysmal torticollis in infancy, abdominal migraine, and cardiac migraine. At present, the status of these afflictions is ambiguous, but they are included in the present discussion for the sake of completeness.

Although emphasis is routinely placed on head pain, the typical attack of migraine consists of a sequence of events. Wolff divided typical migraine attacks into three phases: (1) pre-headache (2) headache, and (3) post-headache.[2167] Blau, however, has provided cogent evidence that attacks of migraine could be further subdivided into five stages: (1) prodrome, (2) aura, (3) headache, (4) resolution, and (5) postdrome.[207] In general, these stages blend into one another, and not every attack contains all five stages. Some bouts, in fact, exclude the head pain.

COMMON AND CLASSIC MIGRAINE (MIGRAINE WITHOUT AURA AND MIGRAINE WITH AURA)

The absence or presence of an aura—an episode of focal transient neurologic dysfunction—in the preheadache phase of a migraine attack has historically been used to separate migraine into two subtypes, which have been designated as *common migraine* and *classic migraine.* The term *common* merely implies that migraine without an aura is the most frequent variety. It has been estimated that approximately 80% of migraine sufferers have common migraine.[1806] About 70% of patients with classic migraine also have attacks without aura.[1628]

The terms *common migraine* and *classic migraine* have been replaced by the terms *migraine without aura* and *migraine with aura* in the scheme of the Headache Classification Committee of the International Headache Society (Table 3–1).[917] According to this scheme, the term *migraine with aura* also includes the following terms: *complicated migraine, migraine accompagneé, hemiplegic migraine, basilar migraine,* and *migraine aura without headache.* The diagnostic criteria for migraine without aura and migraine with aura are listed in Tables 3–2 and 3–3. By definition, well-defined episodes of focal neurologic dysfunction do not precede or accompany attacks of migraine without aura. In contrast, attacks of migraine with aura are associated with striking neurologic manifes-

Table 3–1 CLASSIFICATION OF MIGRAINE

1. Migraine
   1.1 Migraine without aura
   1.2 Migraine with aura
       1.2.1 Migraine with typical aura
       1.2.2 Migraine with prolonged aura
       1.2.3 Familial hemiplegic migraine
       1.2.4 Basilar migraine
       1.2.5 Migraine aura without headache
       1.2.6 Migraine with acute onset aura
   1.3 Ophthalmoplegic migraine
   1.4 Retinal migraine
   1.5 Childhood periodic syndromes that may be precursors to or associated with migraine
       1.5.1 Benign paroxysmal vertigo of childhood
       1.5.2 Alternating hemiplegia of childhood
   1.6 Complications of migraine
       1.6.1 Status migrainosus
       1.6.2 Migrainous infarction
   1.7 Migrainous disorder not fulfilling above criteria

From the Headache Classification Committee of the International Headache Society.[917]

tations, usually visual, but at times sensory, motor, vestibular, or cognitive. Although the absence or presence of the aura serves to separate migraine without aura from migraine with aura, the two types of migraine frequently coexist in the same patient, and both respond similarly to the same types of medication.[1628] One type may progress to another, or a person may have both types

Table 3–2 DIAGNOSTIC CRITERIA FOR MIGRAINE WITHOUT AURA (COMMON MIGRAINE)

- At least five attacks lasting 4–72 hours
- Headache has at least two of the following characteristics:
    Unilateral location
    Pulsating quality
    Moderate or severe intensity
    Aggravation by routine physical activity
- At least one of the following during headache:
    Nausea and/or vomiting
    Photophobia and phonophobia
- Normal neurologic exam and no evidence of organic disease that could cause headaches

Adapted from the Headache Classification Committee of the International Headache Society.[917]

**Table 3–3 DIAGNOSTIC CRITERIA FOR MIGRAINE WITH AURA
(CLASSIC MIGRAINE)**

- At least two attacks
- Aura must exhibit at least three of following characteristics:
  Fully reversible and indicative of focal cerebral cortical and/or brain stem dysfunction
  Gradual onset
  Duration less than 60 minutes
  Followed by headache with a free interval of less than 60 minutes, or headache may begin before
  or simultaneously with the aura
- Normal neurologic exam and no evidence of organic disease that could cause headaches

Adapted from the Headache Classification Committee of the International Headache Society.[917]

with the same frequency. The clinical impression is, however, that classic and common migraine may differ in some respects, but no agreement exists regarding the differences.[1296,1628,1646,1806] Patients with common migraine are thought to have more frequent and longer-lasting attacks.[1296,1628,1646] Common migraine attacks are believed to be more often associated with photophobia and vomiting, and to be accompanied by bilateral head pain.[1296,1806] It is unclear if attacks in patients with common migraine are more likely to be related to menses or to be precipitated by environmental situations, emotional states, and psychological stresses, and whether or not the duration, severity, and frequency of common and classic attacks differ in patients with headaches of both types.[1296]

PATTERN OF MIGRAINE ATTACKS

Attacks of migraine can show themselves in countless patterns.[1172,1489,1806] As discussed in chapter 2, many bouts are triggered when the migraineur is exposed to a stimulus noxious to that individual. An episode may begin at any time of the day or night. Some patients are awakened from sleep with an intense pounding headache. Not infrequently, patients awaken in the morning to discover that a headache is developing. In other patients migraine begins gradually early in the day and slowly increases in intensity. It does appear, however, that there may be a circadian variation in the onset of migraine attacks; most seem to develop early in the morning.[1894]

Similarly, the frequency of attacks varies greatly among individuals. More than half of the adult patients who visit neurologic clinics for their headaches have been estimated to endure between one and four attacks a month.[1806] Of clinic patients, 59% of females and 50% of males report one or more severe headaches per month.[1963] About 15% of clinic patients suffer more than 10 attacks a month. Similarly the frequency of headaches varies among migrainous children, from once monthly to two or three times a week.[183,370] In contrast, some individuals have had only two or three episodes in their entire lives. Moreover, the frequency of migraine may vary significantly throughout a patient's lifetime. For example, some patients may have periods of remission that last for months or even years. In other patients the attacks take on a cyclic pattern.[1358] For these individuals, headaches occur almost daily for a few weeks, after which there is an interval during which the patient is free, or relatively free, of headaches. The cycle may be repeated many times a year. Many of these individuals complain of depression during cycles.

Most texts state that migraine attacks do not develop daily, every other day, or even several times a week. Most patients with frequent headaches suffer from the chronic daily headache syndrome described later in this chapter. A subset of migraine patients do appear to have typical migraine headaches several times a week or even every day. It is felt that many patients experiencing more than one or two separate migraine attacks per week are overusing ergot-containing preparations or medications that incorporate sedatives and analgesics.[1759] In other cases, daily migraine appears to be related to intense emotional turmoil; depression; hormonal changes such as those resulting from the use of oral contraceptives, from menopause, or from hormonal treatment; the frequent consumption of a migraine-inducing food or alcohol; the use of a migraine-inducing medication such as nitroglycerin; or development of a systemic disease such as the chronic fatigue syndrome (CFS).

PREMONITORY SYMPTOMS (PRODROMES)

A number of migraineurs experience a variety of early systemic, mental, or psychological premonitory symptoms that precede the aura (if any) and the headache phase of a migraine attack. These symptoms are often very subtle and can anticipate the aura or head pain by several hours or even by days.[34,203,207,1646,2083] Such symptoms have been designated as *premonitory symptoms* or *prodromes,* but there has been confusion because the term *prodrome* has been used by some as a synonym for the term *aura.*[1167] However, prodromes and auras have different characteristics. Prodromal symptoms begin insidiously, may last several hours to days, and characteristically involve changes in mood, appetite, and energy levels. Auras develop abruptly, generally last minutes, and the symptoms indicate significant neurologic dysfunction with abnormalities of visual, somatosensory, motor, speech, or brain stem function. Prodromes may be more frequent than auras, but reports concerning the frequency of prodromes vary. They are reported in between as many as 30% to 80% of selected groups of migraineurs, but only in 12% to 16% of an unselected group.* However, prodromes are more common in patients with classic migraine than in patients with common migraine, and are more common in women than in men.[34] Some prodromes go unrecognized because they duplicate incidental discomforts that are part of ordinary life and are passed off with comments such as "It's one of those days" or "I got up on the wrong side of the bed." Many patients fail to associate prodromes with migraine attacks until the relationship between prodrome and headache is called to their notice. Furthermore, headaches do not consistently follow all prodromes in a given migraineur. In other words, migraineurs may have prodromal symptoms as the only manifestation of some of their migraine attacks.

Prodromal symptoms vary widely among patients. In addition, an individual may experience discrete sets of symptoms on different occasions. As seen in Table 3–4, prodromes may include changes in mood, behavior, or vigilance; symptoms suggestive of nervous system involvement; fatigue; gastrointestinal manifestations; and changes in fluid balance.[203,899,1751,1806,2083] A feeling of depression coupled to a sense of lassitude is the most consistent prodrome. Still other patients may develop symptoms often associated with the headache, such as photophobia and ill-defined blurring of vision. But some patients experience a feeling of well-being with increased energy and lucidity of thought; an increased appetite, particularly for sweets; and an unusual capability for work. One of my patients becomes unusually talkative the evening before some attacks. Except for yawning and irritability, a prodrome is unusual in children with migraine.

Some prodromal symptoms, such as feeling of increased energy or well-being, stop before the actual headache pain begins. These symptoms—designated as *nonevolutive symptoms*—are usually replaced by depression, lassitude, malaise, and difficulty with cognition. These *evolutive symptoms* usually continue through the headache and may even last into the postdrome.

---

*References 203, 1016, 1646, 1751, 2083

Table 3–4 MIGRAINE PRODROMES: PREMONITORY SYMPTOMS AND SIGNS

Changes in Mood or Behavior (mental state): irritability, difficulty thinking, overactivity, euphoria, excitement, depressive feelings, sluggishness, withdrawal, obsessional behavior, anxiety, apathy

Neurologic Symptoms: excessive yawning, trembling hands, phonophobia, photophobia, hyperosmia, blurred vision, accommodation disturbances, dysphasia, impaired concentration, dizziness, tinnitus

General Symptoms: excessive physical fatigue (or opposite: an unusual capacity for work), pallor, gooseflesh, shivering, aching muscles, increased urinary frequency, fluid retention

Symptoms Related to Head: cervical muscle stiffness or pain, heavy-headedness

Alimentary Symptoms: hunger, craving for food, bulimia, swollen or painful epigastrium, nausea, anorexia, constipation, increased frequency of bowel movement

Data from Amery et al.,[34] Blau,[207] and Waelkens.[2083]

MIGRAINOUS AURAS

Episodes of well-defined, transient, focal neurologic dysfunction—*auras*—accompany headaches at one time or another in about 20% of adult migraineurs. Auras are thought to be more common in adults than children with migraine.[118,183,370,956] Although visual auras have been reported in 40% to 50% of childhood migraineurs, others indicate that auras are uncommon in childhood.* Some patients have identical neurologic disturbances without an ensuing headache *(migraine aura without headache, acephalgic migraine).* In most patients the focal neurologic disturbance that constitutes the aura develops before the head pain commences, but on occasion an aura may appear or recur at the height of the headache. An aura is present before every migraine attack in some individuals, but in other patients, an aura accompanies only a small proportion of attacks.[2153] The intensity of auras varies among attacks; in some attacks the aura may be vivid and impressive, and in others, nearly indiscernible. By far the most frequently encountered auras consist of disturbances of vision, but an aura may consist of virtually any neurologic symptom (Table 3–5).[1034,1646] The symptoms of a migraine aura may remain constant from attack to attack in a particular patient, or they may vary in successive attacks in the same patient. For example, some patients have only visual auras preceding bouts; others may have a visual aura preceding one attack and a somatosensory aura preceding another. In addition, patients who suffer from migraine with aura not infrequently report progression from one type of aura to another.[1034] Thus, a patient may have a visual aura preceding the development of paresthesias in the hand and face. An aura generally lasts between 5 and 60 minutes.[109] In rare cases, the aura—particularly if it is visual—may reach its peak of intensity abruptly.[656]

Table 3–5 TYPES OF MIGRAINE AURAS

Sensory Disturbances
    Visual (scotomas, scintillating scotomas, photopsias)
    Somatosensory (cheiro-oral numbness/paresthesias)
    Olfactory
    Auditory
    Gustatory
Motor Abnormalities
    Hemiparesis
    Dysarthria
Aphasia
Vertigo
Behavioral and Perceptual Alterations
    Dreamy states
    Delirium
    Déjà vu/jamais vu
    Depersonalization
    Visual hallucinations
    Metamorphopsia
    Alice in Wonderland phenomena

*References 183, 280, 857, 955, 1615, 1843

Visual Symptoms

Disturbances of vision can be divided into two main types: positive visual phenomena with hallucinations and negative visual phenomena (scotomas), with partial obliteration or loss of vision in a portion or the whole of the visual field. Both positive and negative visual symptoms can arise from disturbances located either in the retina or in the occipital lobes. However, retinal disturbances with monocular symptoms are rare in comparison with visual disturbances caused by cerebral dysfunction. The latter characteristically produce bilateral abnormalities of visual function.

Photopsias are the simplest types of visual hallucinations (Fig. 3–1). Photopsias are white or colored geometrical figures in the visual fields.[1115] They consist of small spots or dots, stars, sparks, unformed flashes of light, streaks of light, wavy lines, or simple geometric forms and patterns. They frequently flicker, glisten, sparkle, or shimmer, and their margins are usually sharp. Many hundreds of dots or spots may be present at a time. Photopsias may be restricted to one part of the visual field, often arising in the central portion. In other cases they are noted temporally or are scattered throughout the entire visual field. They generally last from seconds to several minutes. Simple photopsias may also occur during the headache phase of the attack.

Migraine sufferers may develop almost any type of negative scotoma. They may have homonymous hemianopic or quadrantic field defects, central scotomas, tunnel vision, altitudinal visual defects, or even complete blindness.[1474,1860] Many migraineurs report patchy scotomas with irregular contours. Some patients report that only central vision is depressed or lost. Others indicate that the defect is limited to the periphery of the visual fields. A negative scotoma may completely escape observation even by a careful observer unless it blurs or obscures a target to which attention has been addressed. The loss of vision may materialize as the visual hallucinations subside, or visual loss may be present from the onset. In some cases a partial or complete loss of vision begins in the center and gradually increases in size, spreading outward to the periphery of the visual field. In other patients, vision is described as blurred, opaque, or foggy. These patients frequently state that their vision is distorted as if they were viewing shimmering or flickering objects through heated air or through a film of rippling water.

Scintillating scotomas are regarded as the most characteristic visual symp-

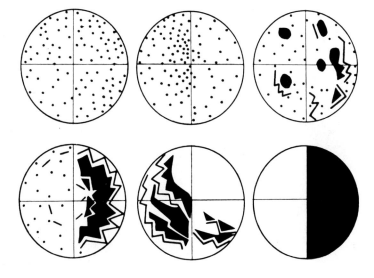

Figure 3–1. Characteristic types of visual auras. Upper row depicts different types of photopsias: *left*) diffuse, flickering spots or dots; *middle*) similar spots, but denser in the left hemifield of vision; *right*) so-called grouped dysopsias to the right. Lower row: *left*) fortification spectrum with scotoma in the right hemifield of vision and diffuse flickering spots in the left hemifield field of vision; *middle*) fortification spectrum with scotoma involving both fields of vision; *right*) complete right-sided homonymous hemianopia. (Adapted from Bücking, H and Baumgartner, G[274] p. 42, with permission.)

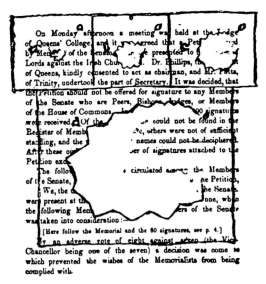

Figure 3–2. Drawing of a progressive central scotoma with a serrated edge. The scotoma progressively enlarges to occupy most of the central field of vision. Vision is intact outside the edge, but is lost within it. (From Gowers[809].)

toms that arise in patients with migraine (see Fig. 3–1). Such scotomas consist of an absent arc or band of vision (negative scotoma) with a shimmering or glittering zigzag border.[1667] Many migraineurs note that the visual abnormality begins in the center of the visual field with an ill-defined loss of vision or perception similar to that seen following the discharge of a photographic flashbulb.[29] During the next few minutes the area of disturbed vision slowly expands laterally and develops a

bright border (Fig. 3–2). The actual scotoma can take many different shapes, forms, and configurations (Fig. 3–3). It can assume diverse geometric designs but usually is perceived as a semicircular, crescent-shaped, or horseshoe-shaped visual defect bordered by moving, shiny streaks of light. The streaks of light may have a jagged or serrated outline. Because the hallucination frequently resembles the pattern formed by the bastions of a fort or by a medieval fortified town observed from above, it is called either a *fortification spectrum* (from the Latin *spectre* "to look or see") or a *teichopsia* (from the Greek *teikhos* "fortification" or "town wall" and *opsis* "vision"). It usually oscillates in brightness at a fast rate. The border may be white, gray, or colored. For most patients, the area of scintillation slowly enlarges as it expands laterally across the visual field. This gradual expansion over a period of 10 to 30 minutes has been termed *buildup*, and usually leaves an area of impaired or obscured vision behind it.[659] In a few instances there is no scotoma but only a scintillating border. Not all scintillating scotomas begin near the fixation point. A few patients invariably perceive teichopsias that start eccentrically or peripherally in their visual fields. All authorities accept the idea that hemianopic scintillating scotomas are the result of occipital cortical events. Of interest in this regard is the report of a patient with migrainous fortification

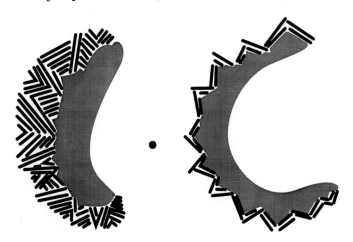

Figure 3–3. Diagrams of two types of fortification spectra. In each case the gray area represents a transient region of loss of vision. (From Richards, W: The fortification illusions of migraines. Sci Am 224:88–96, 1971. Copyright 1971 by Scientific American, Inc. all rights reserved.)

spectra that occurred after enucleation of both eyes.[29]

Patients frequently confuse homonymous photopsias and scintillations generated in the occipital cortex with monocular phenomena that originate in the retina or optic nerve. Monocular photopsias, usually of a fleeting nature, are described by patients with compressive, inflammatory, demyelinating, and vascular disease of the optic nerve and chiasm, and by patients with a variety of ocular problems such as posterior vitreous detachment, retinal detachment or tear, retinal emboli, and inflammation or infection of the retina or choroid.[1731] In contrast, photopsias that develop in a hemianopic pattern are almost always considered migrainous in etiology.[80]

Somatosensory and Motor Symptoms

A frequent aura in patients with classic migraine consists of sensory symptoms. These are second in frequency to visual symptoms and occur in over 40% of patients with classic migraine.[274,1034] This type of aura consists of a circumscribed feeling of numbness or of a sensation of tingling or pins and needles involving the hand, face, and tongue (*cheiro-oral* or *digitolingual paresthesias*) (Fig. 3–4).[1034] The radial or ulnar digits may be involved, and the paresthesias may ascend to include the entire hand and forearm. The paresthesias may *march* up an extremity, passing from one finger to another, and subsequently involve the whole hand. But most often the area of abnormal sensation begins in the fingers and then bypasses the arm and shoulder to involve the angle of the mouth, one half of the lips and tongue, the buccal mucosa, and the cheek. On occasion, the paresthesias are felt in the foot and the leg. In some cases, the numbness may be bilateral and extend to both hands, all four limbs, the circumoral region, and both sides of the tongue.[273,944] The somatosensory symptoms may be brief

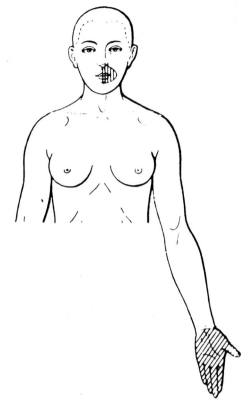

Figure 3–4. Cheiro-oral type of sensory loss involving the side of the mouth and the entire hand. (From Bruyn[267] p 157, with permission.)

and persist for only several seconds to minutes, but they typically take up to 30 minutes to develop fully. This leisurely expansion of sensory symptoms is analogous to the buildup of visual teichopsias. However, some patients report that the paresthesias appear at all sides simultaneously. The paresthesias in a forelimb may be accompanied by a subjective feeling of heaviness or clumsiness of the arm or hand. Mild, transient motor weakness is not uncommon, but severe paresis is an infrequent aura. Quite often paresis is associated with impaired coordination. Disorders of speech (*dysarthria*) may accompany paresthesias in some patients. Speech may be slow, slurred, faltering, or even stammering. The dysarthria is presumed to be secondary to sensory abnormalities of the tongue or mouth.

Migrainous limb pain has been described.[845,846] The clinical features suggest that it is of central origin. Some individuals have unilateral pain that sometimes alternates sides between attacks.

In the past, the cheiro-oral pattern of sensory disturbance has been attributed to dysfunction located in the postcentral gyrus of the parietal lobe, but lesions in this location do not cause this pattern of sensory symptoms.[404] There is evidence, however, that this remarkable pattern can be caused by lesions of the ventrobasal thalamus and brain stem or the operculum.[228,267,1944]

Vertigo

True rotational vertigo—the illusion of environmental movement (usually rotational)—alone or associated with nausea and vomiting, not infrequently constitutes a migraine aura.[1115,1806] Such vestibular symptoms usually last only a few minutes but can persist for an hour. In some individuals, the vestibular symptoms are accompanied by dysarthria, diplopia, and other symptoms of brain stem dysfunction, but in other patients the symptoms presumably originate in the labyrinth and are unaccompanied by evidence of brain stem involvement.

Nonvisual Hallucinations

Although visual hallucinations are extremely common, hallucinations of the other special senses are unusual in patients with migraine. Auditory hallucinations, however, can occur and generally consist of hissing, growling, or rumbling noises that, on occasion, are accompanied by dullness of sound or by diminished auditory acuity.[1729] More highly organized auditory hallucinations such as music are extremely rare. Migrainous olfactory hallucinations are also infrequent. The hallucinated smell is typically strong and usually, but not always, unpleasant. Hallucinations of burning rubber and decaying animal flesh have been described by patients. These olfactory phenomena can last anywhere from 5 minutes to 24 hours.[714]

Cognitive and Communicative Disturbances

On occasion, during more prolonged migrainous auras, patients become confused and disoriented as a result of major alterations of cerebral integrative functions.[1729] Dreamy states, delirium, intense feelings of *déjà vu* or *jamais vu* of extended duration, and transient states of depersonalization have been described, although most of the reports are not well documented. The mental symptoms may continue well into the headache phase.

Aphasia is well described as an aura of a migraine attack. Difficulties with word-finding (Broca's aphasia) appear to be the most common type. The aphasic symptoms tend to be mild and short-lasting. Alexia with and without agraphia can also occur.

Perceptual Alterations

In addition to photopsias and teichopsias, formed, complex visual hallucinations and disturbances of visual perception have been described by patients with migraine. The hallucinations may be exceedingly intricate, although geometric shapes far outnumber the formed visions. On occasion, the hallucinations consist of bizarre and elaborate apparitions of people and entire scenarios with distorted spatial relationships.[271] It is unclear how frequently these occur.[1116] In the Middle Ages, visions had otherworldly origins, so Hildegard of Bingen could freely describe them in her religious mystical writings. Hildegard was a twelfth-century nun who perceived countless visions that are now considered to be migrainous in nature (Fig. 3–5). Today, however, many patients may be reluctant to introduce the subject because of apprehension that the bizarre charac-

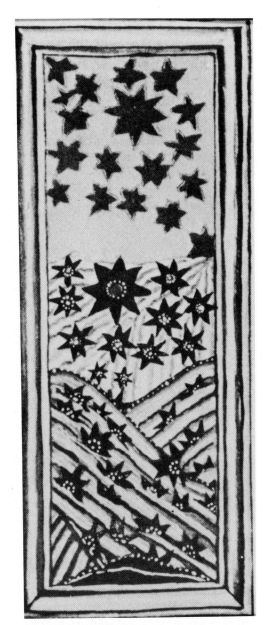

Figure 3–5. Illustration of a putative migrainous hallucination. Striking example of a visual hallucination (Vision of the Fall of the Angels) from a manuscript of Hildegard of Bingen's *Scivias* written at Bingen about 1180. The vision possesses an impressive similarity to the visual phenomena associated with an attack of classic migraine.

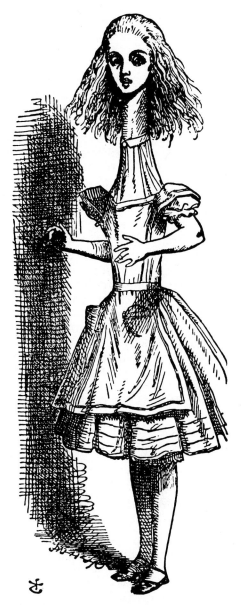

Figure 3–6. Drawing from the original edition of *Alice in Wonderland*. It illustrates the complex distortion in shape that can be associated with migraine.

teristics of their symptoms will cause attending physicians to regard them as irrational or possibly deranged.

Metamorphopsia is a well-described visual perceptual abnormality that oc-

curs as an aura in patients with classic migraine.[1115] Patients with metamorphopsia describe distortions and alterations of the shape and contours of an object. In addition, they may have accompanying illusions that structured objects have altered sizes, positions, or colors. The most common type of illusions are of changes in size—*microp-*

sia and *macropsia*—where part or all of the surroundings abruptly and momentarily appear either incongruously larger or smaller than their actual size.[29,857] Objects may also be perceived as being further away *(telopsia)*. Disturbances of visual perception are frequently experienced simultaneously with other neurologic symptoms such as photopsias or paresthesias.

Bizarre subjective perceptual alterations of the body shape or image also occur.[271] They are called *Alice in Wonderland phenomena* in the neurologic literature because during her travels in Wonderland, Alice occasionally becomes notably tall or short or distorted in shape (Fig. 3–6). *Macrosomatognosia* and *microsomatognosia*—perceptions that a part of the body is anomalously large or small—are acknowledged symptoms of migraine. Finally, some patients may have illusions of shrinking or elongation of the entire body, or the body may feel as if it is distorted in shape. Patients have described feeling as if a part of the body, such as the neck, the ear, or the hip, "balloons out," or the head feels as if it were enlarged and floating toward the ceiling.[1251]

Association of Different Aura Symptoms

Visual auras are the only types that regularly occur by themselves. Most other types—somatosensory, motor, speech, and communication symptoms—commonly follow visual auras.[109,274,944,1034] When two or more aura symptoms occur in a single attack, they regularly occur in succession and not concurrently.

MIGRAINOUS HEAD PAIN

Headache is generally considered the hallmark of the migraine attack. However, it must be stressed that headache is *never* the *only* symptom of a mi-

graine attack. Indeed, presence of headache pain is not even a characteristic of attacks in some individuals. The feature of migrainous head pain most often emphasized is its throbbing or pulsatile nature. Despite this emphasis, most attacks do not begin with throbbing pain. In their initial phases, the discomfort of many migraine attacks is characterized as a mild or dull, deep, steady ache or pressure sensation. The pain generally becomes more intense over a period of minutes to hours. It may then devleop the throbbing quality described by patients as "pounding," "hammering," "beating," or "banging." In those patients who do have such a throbbing component, the throbbing character of the pain is significantly correlated with its intensity. Frequently, pain of this kind reverts to a constant discomfort as the attack progresses. It is worth noting, however, that fewer than half of adult migraineurs have a pulsating component to their pain.[1489] Patients with steady head pain describe it as a "pressing," "squeezing," "splitting," or "vise-like" sensation and, less often, as a "sharp" or "sickening" pain. Whatever the quality, the duration of the head pain can vary from a few hours to several days. In general, the pain gradually subsides over a period of several hours and reportedly lasts for less than a day in two thirds of patients.[1806] Migrainous head pain usually has a shorter duration in children than in adults. It may last only 5 or 10 minutes or be sustained for several hours in children. The usual duration is 1 to 3 hours.[118]

It is typical for the intensity of the head pain to vary from attack to attack in the same patient. Sometimes the pain is so subtle that its existence is only perceived when the head is rapidly moved. During other attacks the pain may be of such intolerable intensity that the patient is totally incapacitated. In addition, the head pain usually fluctuates during a migraine attack. In some patients, the pain slowly waxes and wanes for the duration of the attack.

The word *migraine* is a French word derived from the Latin *hemicrania,* which in turn came from the Greek *hemikrania.* Put simply, etymology implies the presence of hemicranial or unilateral symptoms, and as a result undue emphasis has been placed on the necessity of a unilateral distribution of headache for diagnosis. Indeed, most definitions have stressed the unilateral nature of the head pain in migraine attacks,[5,917,2174] but migrainous head pain is strictly unilateral only in 56% to 68% of adult patients[1172,1489,1868] and 22% to 31% of childhood migraineurs.[118,183,370] If the pain is unilateral, the side involved in successive attacks may vary or the pain may recur consistently on the same side in each attack. About 20% of patients report that only one side of the head is involved throughout life.[1806] For some patients the pain involves one side for months, then switches to the opposite side, alternates sides, or becomes bilateral. In others, there is a relative proclivity for one side. Additionally, some patients state that headaches are consistently more painful and severe when a particular side of the head is involved; the episode is a mild one when the opposite side is involved. It is also possible for the pain to change from one side to the other during the course of an individual attack. Many patients say that the pain is bilateral and symmetrical, or that the pain involves the entire head. In other patients an initial hemicrania often develops into a holocranial headache.

One might expect that in migraine with aura the head pain would be invariably localized over the cerebral hemisphere from which the focal neurologic symptoms emanated, but one third to one half of patients with visual and sensory auras, when questioned after their attacks, indicate that they have *ipsilateral* headaches.* However, when patients are questioned during attacks, the vast majority indicate that the headaches are located on the side of

the cerebral hemisphere responsible for their aura symptoms.[1495]

In both adults and children, migrainous head pain most often involves the frontotemporal region of the head or is located in, around, or behind an eye. However, any region of the head or face may be affected—the parietal region, the base of the nose, the upper or lower jaw or teeth, the malar eminence, the upper anterior neck, and the postauricular region. The occiput and the vertex are less common loci of pain. The pain may persist in one sharply defined area, such as the medial wall of the orbit, or it may radiate to involve one half of the head. As a migraine attack continues, the process often involves the cervical paraspinal musculature and the trapezius muscles. Some patients, however, comment that their migraine attacks begin with a dull, aching pain in the neck and shoulders, which then radiates anteriorly to involve the temple or eye. The terms *mixed headache syndrome, combined headache,* or *vascular tension syndrome* have been used to designate the head pain suffered by the group of patients with features of both migraine and tension-type headache.[1753]

The scalp and the pericranial and cervical muscles often become tender during acute attacks.[540,1273,1489] These areas are more tender in patients with frequent headaches than they are in patients with few days of headache per month.[540] The sternocleidomastoid, cervical, and trapezius muscles are most frequently affected. The scalp tenderness is frequently present in the forehead, the temples, and the occiput, but is generally most severe at the locus of the headache.[540,1806] It may prevent the patient from lying on the affected side. Residual scalp and muscle tenderness may persist for a day or more after the acute attack has terminated.[540] The muscle and scalp tenderness has been traditionally ascribed to dilatation of extracranial arteries, but this idea is suspect because the temporal muscle blood flow does not significantly change during migraine attacks.[1033]

*References 109, 243, 1034, 1297, 1548, 1806

Another hypothesis suggests that muscle pain and tenderness are caused by reflex muscle spasm as a result of the migraine pain, but no data support this supposition. Recorded electromyogram (EMG) levels during attacks are not very great.[103,363] Patients with migraine may also have tender carotid and superficial temporal arteries on the same side as a hemicranial headache.[1640]

Migrainous pain is characteristically attenuated by lying still. An intense headache is, however, frequently made worse by a supine position, so that sitting upright or reclining with elevated head and shoulders provides some relief. The pain is increased in intensity by any physical activity or effort, by active or passive head movement, and by the transmitted impulse of coughing, sneezing, or vomiting. The pain may even be increased by the slightest movement of the bed or by the vibration caused by the steps of others in the room. In particular, many patients have observed that a dull, steady headache may develop an intense pulsatile quality when they bend forward, suddenly move their head, or perform Valsalva's maneuver. Physical exertion or lowering of the head may also result in the appearance of vertigo or photopsias.[1639]

In some patients manual compression of the superficial temporal artery produces transient abatement of pain.[214,545] A rare patient may even compress the ipsilateral carotid artery to procure some relief for a few minutes. Placing an ice pack on the scalp or neck decreases pain intensity in some migraineurs, although others favor the application of heat to the head. Still others have found that a hot shower or bath may reduce pain.

Lower-half Migraine and Carotidynia

Some patients find that their migrainous pain is *limited* to structures located below the level of the eyes; accordingly, this type of attack has been named *lower-half* or *facial migraine.* The pain of lower-half migraine is usually unilateral, involving the nostril, cheek, gums, and teeth. This syndrome has features usually associated with a migraine headache located in cranial structures, such as nausea, vomiting, and photophobia. Lower-half migraine is an unusual affliction and may be confounded with atypical facial pain, trigeminal neuralgia, or cluster headache. It is necessary to identify it and to distinguish it from these other entities, because lower-half migraine responds to the usual therapies for migraine.

Migrainous pain can also originate from the extracranial carotid artery in the neck.[1275,1640,1687] The term carotidynia is sometimes used to refer to this problem. The pain is throbbing and is either located in the neck, at the angle of the jaw, or in the jaw itself. The pain may radiate to the ipsilateral side of the face and ear and be associated with headache. The pain may occur in attacks lasting hours or days and recur several times a week or a month over a period of years. Conspicuous carotid pulsations and carotid tenderness or swelling of the neck are present on the side of the pain.

Ice Pick-like Pains

Superimposed on a migrainous headache may be severe, discrete, jabbing, sharp pains that have been compared to an ice pick, needle, knife, or nail. They have been designated by various terms: *ice pick-like pains, sharp short-lived head pains, idiopathic stabbing headaches, jabs and jolts, needle-in-the-eye syndrome,* and *ophthalmodynia periodica.*[917,1324,1641,1922] These pains characteristically occur around the orbit or the temple and less frequently in the occipital and parietal areas. Many patients experience these pains at the site of their customary headache. They are characteristically located on the side of the headache. Most patients experience only single jabs, although some may have volleys of jabs. Episodes occur up to 50 times a day and usually last from 5 to 10 seconds. This type of pain develops at times other than during a headache in more than 30% of migraineurs.[1641] Phenomena that appear identical to ice pick-like pains have also been reported by patients with cluster headaches and temporal arteritis.[602,865]

ASSOCIATED SYMPTOMS

Headache is typically the most dramatic occurrence in a migraine attack, but it is only one of a host of oppressive symptoms associated with the attack.

Photophobia, Phonophobia, and Osmophobia

Intolerance of light and noise are the most frequent symptoms associated with migrainous head pain. Between 80% and 90% of patients are believed to develop an amplified and usually unpleasant sensitivity to light during an attack.[539,1117,1806] The extreme intolerance to light usually consists of a combination of two quite different sensations: *photophobia* is pain induced or exacerbated by exposure of the eyes to light; *dazzle* is an uncomfortably or intolerably exaggerated sense of brightness. An excessive sensitivity to, and intolerance of, noise *(phonophobia)* is present in more than 80% of migraine patients.[1087] Sounds of moderate intensity, such as conversational speech, the noise of traffic, or the sound of a television, may seem unacceptably loud to a migraineur in the throes of an attack. In addition, patients frequently complain of a heightened sense of smell *(hyperosmia)* and an aversion to some odors *(osmophobia)*. During an attack patients may develop an exaggerated dislike for odors that are usually offensive, but frequently tolerable, such as cigarette smoke, and they also may experience an increased awareness of smells ordinarily perceived as pleasant, such as subtle perfumes.[218] Strong perfumes or colognes and heavily scented stationery or magazine advertisements may cause great distress. Food aromas may induce or accentuate nausea. Some patients feel that all smells acquire an intense and often foul quality.

Gastrointestinal Complaints

In the course of a migraine attack, the majority of patients complain of problems with their gastrointestinal tracts. Gastrointestinal disturbances are thought to be more common or more prominent in children, but this claim is difficult to confirm from published data.[956] Gastrointestinal symptoms usually begin after the inception of the pain, but may sometimes precede the headache. Whether the attacks are inconsequential or overwhelming, approximately 90% of patients report that they experience nausea.[1172] Nausea accompanied by vomiting affects more than half of adult migraineurs.[1172,1489,1806] Nausea and vomiting may affect over 90% of children with migraine.[370] Emesis may develop within an hour of the onset of the head pain, but it can also occur late in the course of an attack. In some migraine sufferers, the onset of vomiting ushers in a noticeable decline in the severity of the headache—even its conclusion. Certain patients intentionally induce vomiting to obtain respite from the head pain. In patients who suffer from prolonged, severe attacks, however, vomiting constitutes the most potentially harmful aspect of a migraine attack. It is the principal reason, in company with excessive sweating and diarrhea, for the intense fluid and electrolyte depletion, which can cause prostration.

Other gastrointestinal symptoms are also common. Diarrhea coexists with nausea and vomiting in between 10% and 20% of migraineurs.[1489] Some patients complain of constipation and abdominal distension. Others, particularly children, complain of abdominal pain accompanying the headache. Gastric emptying is delayed during migraine attacks, even in those patients who do not complain of vomiting.[241]

Autonomic Changes

Changes in the function of structures innervated by the autonomic nervous system are often seen during the course of an acute migraine attack. Most patients develop facial pallor.[214] Some individuals develop localized facial edema, which is most prominent in the temporal and periorbital regions. Dilatation of the superficial temporal artery is observed during the height of the pain in approximately one third of patients. On occasion, the forehead may become flushed and hot on the side of the hemicranial pain as a result of extracranial vasodilatation. Rarely, this process may be profound and may result in sufficient extravasation of blood to produce subconjunctival hemorrhages, epistaxis, or periorbital ecchymoses.[1919] Injection of the conjunctiva and lacrimation may be seen on the side of the headache. At least 20% of migraineurs complain of nasal congestion during migraine attacks.[209] The turbinates may be engorged and may lead both patient and physician to an erroneous diagnosis of sinus headache. Ptosis and miosis (Horner's syndrome) has been observed during the height of an attack in some individuals.[541,543] It can occur during attacks of migraine with or without aura. Horner's syndrome usually appears during the headache phase and is almost always on the side of the headache if the pain is hemicranial. It usually subsides when the headache is over, but may remain for hours or even days. In other patients, the pupil dilates on the side of the head pain.[1152]

Many patients complain of cold, clammy hands and feet and may feel cold all over or suffer from chills. In contrast, profuse sweating is a complaint in some patients, and fever occasionally occurs during attacks.[2165] Tachycardia is present in about 3% of patients during migraine attacks.[256] Hypertension, which is thought to be related to the pain, is frequently present. In other patients hypotension and bradycardia may occur.

Fluid Retention

Before an attack, approximately one half of migraine sufferers retain fluid and sodium. During a period lasting hours to days there may be a weight gain of 2–10 pounds, so that shoes, belts, and rings may feel tight.[1512,2167] Such fluid retention before an attack is more common in women than in men. Some patients may note oliguria as a prodromal symptom and experience polyuria either immediately after the inception of the head pain or during the recession of the headache. In the pre-headache phase the serum sodium level rises.[307] Decreased excretion of sodium and water is usually observed prior to and during the early phase of a migraine attack.[1790] As the attack subsides, sodium and water excretion increases. In addition, the serum osmolality is usually elevated just before a migraine attack and decreases during an attack.[1451] It is unlikely that retention of fluid and sodium is causally related to migraine attacks, because administration of diuretics does not typically prevent or modify the headache.

Dizziness

Patients who suffer from migraine frequently complain of what they call "dizziness" during attacks. Perhaps three quarters of migraineurs have vague, transitory periods of giddiness, light-headedness, heavy-headedness, or unsteadiness associated with some or all of their attacks.[1806] These symptoms are often initiated, or augmented, by changes in posture or head position such as rising from a horizontal or stooped position.[1087] They occur more frequently during the headache phase than during the prodrome or aura and may last from minutes to several hours. In some patients they persist as long as the headache. Other patients complain of true vertigo during an attack.[423,978]

Changes in Mental Status and Consciousness

Many migraineurs feel discouraged or even profoundly depressed during an attack. Others feel irascible, irritable, and hostile. A loss of control is common, and verbal stimuli that would, under normal circumstances, evoke little or no emotional response may trigger verbal outbursts. Many patients are well aware that they are behaving unreasonably, yet they are helpless to change their behavior. Most migraine sufferers sensibly and defensively crave isolation, seclusion, and darkness, and reject intimacy or even the presence of others. Yet even though most patients feel listless, apathetic, weak, and fatigued during an attack, some—notably stubborn and obsessional individuals—make no compromises with an attack and continue to work, with or without the help of analgesics. If an attack is severe enough, however, most migraineurs do retire to their beds, darken their rooms, decrease the ambient temperature, and lie still. Many are lethargic, drowsy, or even irresistibly sleepy.

Minor cognitive changes are frequent during migraine attacks. In particular, patients complain of reduced ability to concentrate, decreased capacity to comprehend the meaning and significance of a text or conversation, bradyphrenia, mild impairment of memory and attention, and an inability to think or express themselves clearly.[1117] Those migraineurs who persist in working often find that their work has to be carefully checked the next day because arithmetical and logical errors commonly characterize work performed during the course of a migraine attack.

Some patients develop a more severe organic mental syndrome during the headache phase of the attack. The problem is referred to as *dysphrenic migraine* by European clinicians.[272] Dysphrenic migraine is characterized by problems with abstract thought and orientation. Some patients have difficulty with word-finding, fashion paraphasias with the usage of incorrect words, make spelling errors, and suffer from dyscalculia. Migrainous alexia without agraphia has been documented during attacks.[181,664] Severe memory lapses may occur, with complete inability to remember a conversation or a discussion. Other patients suffer major alterations in consciousness that include twilight states, dreamy states, automatisms, delirium, and even stupor.[1215] Many of the latter problems have been associated with basilar migraine or hemiplegic migraine.

Varying patterns of mental confusion during migraine have been described in some patients for many years.[1172] A confusional state *(acute confusional migraine)* is reported to occur during migraine attacks, especially in children and in adolescents.[599,734] The confusion may be the dominant feature of the attack in children. It is not particularly common, and is more frequent in male than in female patients. Episodes are characterized by the acute onset of inattention, disorientation, distractability, bewilderment, and severe memory difficulties. These symptoms are often associated with agitation and purposeless irrational behavior. Some patients are violent and require physical restraint. Many patients are tremulous. These problems can be brief or can last up to 12 hours, but patients recover with no lasting sequelae.[610,734] The symptoms may wax and wane during the episode. Such a state may occur in the absence of head pain or in the presence of insignificant head pain, but usually occurs after the onset of a throbbing headache. The headache may be accompanied by the usual symptoms associated with attacks of migraine such as nausea and vomiting. In some patients a stuporous state may develop. Patients are frequently amnestic for the episode. Some cases occur after relatively trivial head truma. The diagnosis is typically made in retrospect, when other causes, such as acute toximetabolic encephalopathy and encephalitis, have been excluded.

Syncope is estimated to occur during bouts of headache in approximately 5% of adult patients with migraine.[1172] It is less frequent in children.[1615] The incidence is higher when one looks at individuals with basilar migraine (see below). Syncope appears most frequently when patients arise from bed. These losses of consciousness are transient and rarely last more than a minute. They are thought to be a consequence of postural hypotension caused by vasomotor instability combined with the fluid and electrolyte depletion that result from vomiting.[912] In support of this idea is the finding that many migraineurs have orthostatic symptoms between attacks.[1639]

TERMINATION OF MIGRAINE ATTACKS (POSTDROMIC STATE)

Many migraine attacks are terminated by sleep.[204,207] The pain may be eradicated by even a brief period of sleep in some patients, but in others a period of deep sleep lasting several hours is necessary. The period of sleep may occur during the day or night. As already noted, vomiting can terminate some patients' attacks. For most migraineurs, however, the pain gradually diminishes over a period of hours.[204]

The majority of migraineurs have a postdromal period after a headache, which can last several hours to several days.[204,211,1805] Many patients claim to feel "different." Most are extremely fatigued. Some feel weak, listless, or lethargic. This is particularly true if there has been much vomiting and diarrhea. Others are depressed. Many are incapable of performing imaginative or skilled activities because of impaired concentration, difficulty reading, weariness, and irritability during the postdromal period. Some patients limit their physical activities and cannot exert themselves. In contrast, many patients feel normal after attacks, and some even feel ebullient and enthusiastic.

COMPLICATED MIGRAINE

The designation *complicated migraine* has been used to refer to rare types of migraine with significant focal neurologic deficits and to migraine with neurologic deficits that persist well beyond the conclusion of the head pain and that may even endure permanently. Not only is the term *complicated migraine* an imprecise one, but definitions of it in the literature are often ambiguous. Many different names have been used for the same condition, and different terms have often described equivalent or analogous phenomena. For example, *migraine accompagneé* and *migraine associée* are terms used by French authors to refer to migraine with significant and long-lasting neurologic deficits.[273] The terms, however, are not without ambiguity, for they also refer to migraine with acute aura and to migraine attacks with the onset of neurologic signs after the debut of the headache. Most clinicians, however, accept *hemiplegic migraine, basilar migraine, retinal migraine,* and *ophthalmoplegic migraine* as types of migraine that may be complicated by prolonged neurologic deficits. In the new International Headache Society (IHS) classification, complicated migraine is now designated as *migraine with prolonged aura.* Migraine with prolonged aura is migraine in which the aura symptoms last more than 60 minutes, but less than a week. Results of neuroimaging studies are normal.[917] *Migrainous infarction* is migraine with aura symptoms not completely reversible within a week or associated with evidence of ischemic infarction on neuroimaging studies.[917] Attempts to diagnose the various types of *complicated migraine* in individual patients is confounded not only by inconsistent terminology, but also by the fact that non-migrainous conditions such as ischemic cerebral events can produce a syndrome of transient headache followed by persistent neurologic deficit—even in young individuals.[573]

Hemiplegic Migraine

The association of headache with prolonged unilateral sensory or motor deficits is a relatively uncommon syndrome that can be either sporadic or familial in origin.[243,2143] The presentation of the sporadic form of hemiplegic migraine superficially resembles migraine with aura. The problem typically starts in the teens or early twenties.[243] Most patients also experience attacks of common and classic migraine, which usually occur more frequently than the hemiplegic attacks.[944] When a hemiplegic migraine strikes, a hemisensory deficit or hemiparesis usually precedes the headache and persists throughout the headache phase of the attack. As the headache abates, the neurologic signs and symptoms may disappear, but, on occasion, the neurologic disturbances extend well beyond the headache itself, persisting for days or even for weeks. Complete recovery of motor and sensory function is the rule, although occasionally a degree of residual hemiparesis remains.[243,375] The question of cerebral infarction arises when neurologic signs persist for longer than 24 hours; it is difficult to decide when evaluating descriptions of cases in the older literature or in patients in whom appropriately timed computed tomographic (CT) scans have not been performed. It is common dogma that the same side of the body is affected in each attack in an individual, but, in fact, the hemiparesis and hemisensory deficits may alternate sides from one attack to another. Long-lasting unilateral sensory and motor symptoms may only occur in a single attack or may recur in subsequent attacks.

Although some authorities restrict the term *hemiplegic migraine* to specific attacks with severe, long-lasting hemiparesis, the spectrum of the affliction ranges from relatively brief unilateral paresthesias through modest numbness and weakness to profound hemiplegia. Sensory disturbances are the most frequent symptom in hemiplegic migraine and as a rule precede other symptoms.[243,944] Paresthesias that consist of tingling, numbness, or formication are common and invariably involve the hand. The arm may also feel heavy or clumsy, and it is also possible for the lower limb to be affected. A cheiro-oral or digitolingual distribution is frequently seen. Weakness of one side of the body is present in almost two thirds of patients.[243] It may come on rapidly, although seldom as suddenly as the hemiparesis caused by cerebral embolism. The hemiparesis may advance to become a fully developed hemiplegia and is usually much more severe than the amount of weakness observed in patients who are having a hemiparetic aura. Disturbances of speech and communication are frequent when the right side of the body is involved. Dysphasia or dysarthria accompany the hemiparesis in more than half of patients.[243,944] The dysphasia is typically of a mixed type, with difficulties of both expression and comprehension. Visual disturbances such as teichopsias or hemianopias in the appropriate homonymous fields are frequently noted. Indeed, visual symptoms in the ipsilateral field of vision may herald an attack.[944] An alteration in consciousness that varies from mild confusion to coma may be an attribute of an attack, especially when it occurs in a child.[2145] The headache component of an attack of hemiplegic migraine has all of the characteristics expected of migrainous head pain; it can consist of severe, throbbing pain, intensified by exertion and by bending over and, at times, accompanied by nausea and vomiting. It may last from a few hours to a few days. The headache involves the side of the head contralateral to the paresis in 47% of cases, but can be ipsilateral or even bilateral.[243] On rare occasions, the headache is inconspicuous or never develops at all. In a large proportion of young individuals with hemiplegic migraine, the frequency and severity of attacks decline with age and bouts of hemiplegia are often replaced by other forms of migraine.

It is difficult to make a diagnosis of hemiplegic migraine during the first attack because there is sometimes little to distinguish attacks of hemiplegic migraine from the syndromes produced by cerebral lesions caused by occlusive cerebral vascular disease, cardiac emboli, carotid dissection, cerebral hemorrhage, neoplasm, or vascular anomalies such as small intracerebral arteriovenous malformations. Only when there is a history of several attacks, particularly if the affected side of the body alternates, is the diagnosis apparent. Patients with the first attack require a full evaluation, particularly if the hemiplegia lasts 24 hours or longer.

Cerebral angiography has been performed during hemiparetic episodes and has usually revealed no abnormalities. Constriction of internal carotid and basilar arteries has been reported in a few cases.[1038] CT scanning and magnetic resonance imaging (MRI) ordinarily display no abnormalities. However, if permanent weakness occurs, neuroimaging studies may show a hypodense area of infarction. Regional cerebral blood flow studies have demonstrated a modest reduction in the blood flow of the hemisphere contralateral to the hemiparesis.[1038]

Hemiplegic migraine sometimes appears in several generations in a family.[2145] In these cases, the problem appears to be transmitted as an autosomal dominant trait.[770,1481] Of interest is the observation that not only is the same side of the body usually affected in an individual patient in all attacks, but that a familial history of attacks identical to those in affected individuals is also very common. Some authorities have indicated that the presentation of the familial form of hemiplegic migraine is more severe and prolonged, but this has been denied.[243,642,2145] Children with hemiplegic migraine may be intellectually impaired.[662]

Basilar Migraine

The term *basilar migraine (basilar artery migraine, Bickerstaff's migraine)* refers to a particular type of complicated migraine with aura symptoms that unquestionably arise from dysfunction of the brain stem or both occipital lobes (Table 3–6).[178] It was originally thought that basilar migraine predominantly affected adolescent girls.[173] Then, a number of reports stressed the frequency of its occurrence in children.[791,955] Current thought, however, recognizes that the affliction, although usually starting in the teenage years, occurs in all age-groups and in both sexes.[1969] Most cases have a family history of migraine, although not necessarily the basilar kind. Basilar attacks tend to become less common with time and, in the majority of patients, are eventually replaced by other, more common, varieties of migraine.

The sequence in which symptoms evolve during attacks of basilar migraine varies greatly among different patients, but most bouts are inaugurated by visual symptoms.[177] They are frequently bilateral, consisting of visual impairment or visual hallucinations in

Table 3–6 DIAGNOSTIC CRITERIA FOR BASILAR MIGRAINE

- Fulfills the criteria for migraine with aura
- Two or more of the following aura symptoms are present:
  Visual phenomena in temporal and nasal fields of both eyes
  Dysarthria
  Vertigo
  Tinnitus
  Decreased hearing
  Double vision
  Ataxia
  Bilateral paresthesias
  Bilateral pareses
  Decreased level of consciousness

Adapted from the Headache Classification Committee of the International Headache Society.[917]

the temporal and nasal fields of both eyes. Some patients may either lose vision completely or report its dimming or graying. Other patients describe dramatic visual hallucinations of unformed images or photopsias involving the whole of the visual fields. No matter what kind of visual symptoms occur, they are distinct from the usual case of migraine with aura, because even if the onset is hemianopic in basilar migraine, the symptoms eventually occur concurrently in both left and right visual fields.[955] Bilateral paresthesias or numbness of the extremities, the perioral region, and occasionally the tongue customarily follow the visual disturbances. Sensory abnormalities affect the hands and feet to just above the wrists and ankles. Varying combinations of vertigo, ataxia of gait, diplopia, dysarthria, difficulty with hearing, and tinnitus are usually present. These phenomena commonly last from 10 to 60 minutes, but can persist for hours or even days.[1969] They are followed by severe, bilateral, throbbing headache, predominantly in the occipital region. The pain, however, may extend down into the neck or radiate forward toward the vertex. During some attacks, it can spread to become holocephalic. The headache may last several hours or longer. Some patients in childhood or their early teens may endure the visual, sensory, and ataxic features of the syndrome without subsequently developing a headache. Nausea and vomiting is common and frequently prostrating.[177,955]

As might be expected from a condition in which the brain stem is affected, consciousness is altered—but only in a small proportion of patients with basilar migraine.[173,955,1188,1969] The disturbed consciousness ranges from mild drowsiness to extended coma, but prolonged amnesia, confusion, somnolence, stupor, and even syncope have been reported.[599,610,734,1215] The clinical picture may resemble sleep from which the patient can be aroused by vigorous stimulation. A curious, dreamlike, confusional state sometimes develops. In such cases, the symptoms generally occur just when the premonitory symptoms are subsiding and the headache is due to start. The abnormalities in sensorium are more common in younger patients. The symptoms are usually transient but have been known to last for days in some patients. Although not featured in the original reports of the syndrome, focal or generalized seizures are reported to develop during episodes of basilar migraine, especially when the episodes occur in children.[174] It is difficult to determine whether these cases represent a variety of basilar migraine or result from a coincidence of epilepsy and migraine. *Drop attacks* have also been reported in patients with basilar migraine. In these cases, even though the patients have intact sensoria, they suddenly lose postural tone, with resultant falling. Drop attacks usually occur at the point when the visual and brain stem symptoms are receding and the headache is slated to begin.

Permanent, albeit mild, complications can follow attacks of basilar migraine. It is uncommon, however, for major neurologic symptoms to outlast the headache, and it is exceptionally uncommon for a major neurologic deficit to be fixed (even though there have been a few case reports of lateral medullary and cerebellar infarctions following typical attacks).[375,1898,1969] Cochleovestibular abnormalities are frequent between attacks. Routine audiometry demonstrates a mild low-frequency hearing loss in many patients.[1501] A few patients have significant hearing loss. Positional nystagmus is seen on electronystagmographic (ENG) testing in a number of patients, and many have caloric abnormalities.[1501]

Basilar migraine must be distinguished from conditions that produce vertebrobasilar arterial insufficiency. The youth of most patients renders unlikely a diagnosis of occlusive cerebrovascular disease resulting from atherosclerosis and angiitis. Congenital malformations at the base of the brain such as Arnold-Chiari malformation, platybasia, and basilar impression could be responsible for episodic headache with alterations in brain stem and visual function. Patients with posterior fossa tumors, on the other hand, usually do not have an episodic course. An MRI or CT scan should rule out these possibilities. Patients who suffer from complex partial seizures may have recurrent attacks of visual and sensory disturbances accompanied by vertigo and followed by an alteration of consciousness and postictal headache. Such attacks, however, are of much briefer duration than are bouts of basilar migraine, and the headache is not a prominent feature of each attack. The diagnosis of basilar migraine in a particular patient is suggested by a family history of migraine coupled with an attack that is isolated or interspersed with more typical episodes of migraine, with or without aura.

Retinal Migraine

Retinal migraine is a form of complicated migraine characterized by repeated episodes of unilateral visual impairment (Table 3–7). A more precise designation of the condition would be *ocular migraine* or *anterior visual pathway migraine* because the ciliary or retinal circulations can be involved, and because the visual symptoms characteristic of attacks result from either

Table 3–7 DIAGNOSTIC CRITERIA FOR RETINAL MIGRAINE

- At least two attacks
- Monocular scotoma or blindness
  Completely reversible
  Lasts less than 60 minutes
  Confirmed by examination during attack or by patient's drawing of monocular field defect
- Headache preceding or following visual symptoms
- Normal ophthalmologic examination after an attack
- Embolism ruled out by appropriate studies

Adapted from the Headache Classification Committee of the International Headache Society.[917]

retinal or optic nerve dysfunction. The term *ophthalmic migraine* has also been used, but such a phrase can cause confusion, because some authorities use the term to characterize any migrainous visual disturbance, whether it results from ocular or from cerebral changes.

Retinal migraine is an unusual disorder, seen most often in young adults. Patients experience sudden monocular episodes of visual loss or photopsias. These recurrent episodes of sudden visual loss or impairment are frequently described as *blackouts, grayouts,* or *whiteouts.* But patients with this condition do not usually complain of a "curtain" dropping over the vision. The visual symptoms can accompany a migraine attack, or they may develop at other times in individuals with strong histories of migraine (see Table 3–6).[2037] When they accompany a typical migraine attack, the visual phenomena may occur before, during, or after the headache. They may be preceded by typical migrainous sensory symptoms. Patients also describe little sparkles of light in one eye, which may precede the disturbed vision. The duration of the visual abnormalities ranges from seconds to hours but, in most cases, lasts less than 30 minutes.[323] The headache may be a typical migrainous one, or may consist of a dull ache. The pain is characteristically retro-orbital and ipsilateral to the affected eye. Some patients have visual loss unaccompanied by headache.

Examination of the fundus during attacks has demonstrated constriction of retinal arterioles and venous narrowing. It may be that the venous narrowing is caused by active venous contraction or is secondary to diminished arteriolar inflow.[1119,2170]

Migrainous attacks of monocular visual loss may result in serious sequelae.[382,1992] Migrainous infarction of the anterior visual pathways can cause permanent visual field defects with central or centrocecal scotomas, altitudinal defects, constriction of the visual field, or even complete loss of vision in the affected eye. Ischemic optic neuropathy, central retinal artery or retinal artery branch occlusion, retinal vein occlusion, retinal pigmentary changes, and intraocular hemorrhage have been described as complications of this condition.[656,1005]

Patients with monocular visual alterations ascribed to migraine comprise a younger population than do patients with amaurosis fugax caused by atherosclerotic carotid artery disease. Even so, the clinical presentation of amaurosis fugax from embolic or atherosclerotic vascular disease is sufficiently inconstant to prevent a conclusive distinction from retinal migraine.[381,382,569] Points in favor of the diagnosis of retinal migraine include youth, a clear-cut personal and family history of migraine, no evidence of congenital or acquired valvular heart disease, lack of potential sources of emboli, and an absence of bruits or cardiac murmurs.

Ophthalmoplegic Migraine

Ophthalmoplegic migraine is a very rare condition, consisting of attacks of headache associated with partial or complete unilateral oculomotor palsy.[703,1539] The typical patient is a child or adolescent of either sex, although there is a strong male preponderance.[888] Most patients suffer their first attack before age 12, but there are reports of adults reaching their fourth or fifth decades before having an initial episode.[175,703,1539] Reports differ regarding a family history of migraine in patients with ophthalmoplegic migraine.[703,888]

The initial feature of an attack of ophthalmoplegic migraine is pain—pain that is always located on the same side as the subsequent ophthalmoplegia. The discomfort characteristically develops behind or above the eye, but, as the attack progresses, it may radiate to adjacent structures such as the cheek, temple, or forehead.[175] The pain is moderate to severe, continuous and non-throbbing, and is usually described as "boring" in nature. It increases in intensity over a 48-hour period and may persist for 1–4 days. In addition, in half the cases nausea and photophobia accompany the head pain.[888] As the headache reaches its peak, or as it begins to subside, the symptoms (diplopia) and signs (ptosis, extraocular muscle paresis, dilatation of the pupil) of ophthalmoplegia emerge on the affected side and progressively worsen. The first sign is usually ptosis. Paresis of the ocular muscles develops next. In many cases the condition progresses to total unilateral oculomotor nerve palsy. In most, but not all, patients, the reaction of the pupil to light is partially or totally lost and the pupil is dilated.[703,921,2073] The abducens and trochlear nerves are much less often affected than is the oculomotor nerve.[703] On rare occasions, the ophthalmic division of the trigeminal nerve may be involved.[703,1542]

The oculomotor paresis usually disappears over a period ranging from a week to a month or two. Some patients suffer multiple attacks without any residual deficit. But repeated ophthalmoplegic attacks may cause permanent damage to the oculomotor nerve, leaving a slight degree of ptosis, a sluggish pupil, or occasionally a residual, mild oculomotor paresis. Attacks can recur after the patient has been symptom-free for a period of several months to years, and when they do, the symptoms and signs may alternate sides. In children, ophthalmoplegic attacks become less frequent with time and are often replaced by the more common varieties of migraine.

The lesion responsible for the involvement of the oculomotor nerve is thought to be in or around the cavernous sinus. Edematous swelling of the wall of the intracavernous carotid artery has been hypothesized to compress the oculomotor and trigeminal nerves, but this supposition rests on meager arteriographic evidence.[175,2094] Subsequent reports of negative arteriograms during attacks do not support the intracavernous compression theory.[703] Alternatively, compression may occur in the posterior fossa, because the oculomotor nerve emerges from the brain stem between the posterior cerebral and the superior cerebellar arteries.[2067,2094] This notion does not, however, explain the occasional occurrence of abducens and trochlear nerve palsies. It has also been suggested that migrainous angiospasm of the small branch of the internal carotid artery, which supplies the oculomotor nerve, produces segmental ischemia of the nerve.[2073]

As indicated above, attacks of ophthalmoplegic migraine have a notably constant pattern both in the same patient and among different patients. If the pattern is not followed, other causes for the symptoms must be sought. In particular, one should suspect an aneurysm of the internal carotid artery on the main trunk or at the junction of the posterior communicating artery. The Tolosa-Hunt syndrome, a painful granulomatous inflammatory process that involves the cavernous sinus, the superior orbital fissure, or orbit and the enclosed cranial nerves, may also mimic ophthalmoplegic migraine. The clinical picture differs in that the headache and ophthalmoplegia occur simultaneously, and the duration of symptoms is more prolonged. Palsies of the oculomotor, trochlear, and abducens nerves, in any combination, are possible. The Tolosa-Hunt syndrome is most common in the fourth through the sixth decades of life.

The differential diagnosis also includes sphenoidal mucoceles or tumors, pituitary apoplexy, periarteritis with inflammation of the carotid siphon, and diabetic ophthalmoplegia. The diagnosis of ophthalmoplegic migraine should not offer problems if there is a history of previous attacks, especially if preceding occurrences involved the opposite side.

Migrainous Infarction

Long-lasting or permanent neurologic sequelae with evidence of ischemic infarction of the cerebrum or brain stem can occur during or following an attack of migraine.[231,375,529] When a patient with such a problem is young and has no evidence of artherosclerotic or embolic cerebrovascular disease and no hematologic problems, valvular heart disease, or vasculitis, the ischemic infarction is deemed migrainous. Cerebral infarction in childhood migraineurs is very uncommon, although migraine appears to represent a significant risk factor for stroke in children.[1696]

It is difficult to assess the risk of stroke in migraineurs because the proportion of migraineurs in a population of young stroke patients is generally reported to be comparable to the proportion of individuals with migraine in the general population.[369,904,950,1915] As a result, the conclusions of several retrospective surveys of strokes in young adults have been in conflict with regard to the importance of migraine as a risk factor.[369,904,950,1235,1915] For example, different investigations have acknowledged migraine as a potential cause of stroke in between 0% and 25% of young patients with cerebral infarction.* Because migraine is a common disease, it would be anticipated that 10% to 15% of patients with stroke would also suffer from migraine headaches.[125,931]

Although the number of well-described cases of cerebral infarction during or immediately following attacks of migraine is small, documentation supporting a causal linkage between migraine and stroke has been provided by the following:

1. *CT scan observations.* CT abnormalities similar to those seen in patients with non-migrainous stroke are noted in some patients with strokes associated with attacks of migraine.† However, similar lesions have been seen in the CT scans of migraineurs after attacks unaccompanied by neurologic deficits.[413,1002,1762] These lesions presumably represent subclinical

---

*References 229, 836, 950, 1308, 1730, 1885, 1915
†References 413, 529, 549, 1002, 1333, 1762

strokes. Evidence that the abnormalities are indeed infarcts is based on the general contour and topography of the affected regions. Low-density lesions are the most common abnormality, but cerebral edema has also been reported.[635,298,1322]

2. *Angiographic examinations.* Occlusion or narrowing of an appropriate intracranial artery in a few patients whose strokes occurred during a migraine attack has been verified by angiographic studies.[331,529,635] The most common occlusions have been of the posterior cerebral or middle cerebral arteries or one of their small branches.[259,529,1086,1633,1915] However, most migrainous infarcts are unaccompanied by angiographic evidence of arterial occlusion.[230,1544,1560,1699] Instances of arterial narrowing presumed to be caused by vasospasm have also been documented by arteriography, but are extremely rare.[554,1242,1321,1699]

3. *Pathological examinations.* Rare cases of putative migrainous cerebral infarction have been fatal and have been examined pathologically, showing either severe ischemia or infarction of brain tissue.[275,844,1230]

Strokes have been seen during attacks in patients with classic migraine[529] and in patients with common migraine, where neurologic deficits do not constitute part of a typical attack.[259,844] The risk is greatest in patients with classic migraine.[635,930] The bulk of the cases of infarction develop in women.[230,231,259] This female preponderance presumably is a reflection of the sex distribution of migraineurs, but it is in contrast to observations that the majority of cerebral infarctions in non-migraineurs younger than age 50 occur in men.[1885] Major factors that increase the probability that a migrainous patient will develop an infarction during an attack include the use of oral contraceptives, smoking, and discontinuation of migraine therapy.[635,904] It is unclear if the heavy use of ergotamine is a factor.[230,1699] The majority of strokes that take place during migraine attacks occur suddenly, but in some patients an incremental or gradual onset over 90 minutes to several days has been described.[635] In addition, stroke can develop in young migraine patients independent of an acute attack.[529] Epidemiologic data indicate an increased risk of developing an infarction unrelated to a migraine attack in patients who have classic migraine.[930]

A considerable proportion of migrainous infarcts involve areas of the brain supplied by the posterior cerebral artery.[259,375,929,1544,1730] In particular, the occipital lobes are affected more than other sites, which accounts for the findings that the most typical permanent neurologic deficits are visual in nature, such as homonymous field defects. Hemiplegia is also a common enduring deficit, however, and may be combined with an ipsilateral sensory deficit, dysphasia, or homonymous hemianopia.[635]

The diagnosis of migrainous stroke is difficult because headaches occur frequently in patients with ischemic thromboembolic cerebrovascular events.[573,1601] The incidence of headache in such patients is reported to vary from 25% to 44%.[568,1360] Many of these headaches have clinical features often associated with vascular headaches and can be confused with migraine.[569] In addition, there are reports of patients thought to have strokes related to acute attacks of migraine in whom later clinical events or autopsy established different mechanisms for the cerebral infarction.[1824] Migraineurs with cerebral infarction require a comprehensive assessment that includes hematologic, cardiologic, and arteriographic investigation. Cerebral infarction should not be attributed to migraine until all other diagnostic possibilities have been excluded.

Trauma-Triggered Migraine

As noted in chapter 2, minor or trivial head trauma can, on occasion, provoke an attack of migraine.[853] Similar episodes have been reported to occur after flexion–extension neck injuries.[2160] Soccer players who "head" the ball may experience blurring of vision within minutes followed by a headache (footballer's migraine).[1339] Most of the patients with trauma-triggered migraine have a personal or family history of migraine, and most are children or adolescents.[850] The attack usually begins within a few minutes of the trauma, but the symptoms can last from hours to days. The head pain has the characteristics of a vascular headache and is usually accompanied by nausea and vomiting. The headache may be preceded by, or associated with, visual disturbances, hemisensory disturbances, or hemiparesis. These latter attacks are said to be indistinguishable from attacks of classic or complicated migraine. An unusual syndrome of transient blindness with headache following head injury in children has been described.[225,834] In other patients, the headaches coexist with symptoms of confusion, agitation, incoherence, and somnolence that resemble attacks of acute confusional migraine.[850] Attacks of migraine without aura are less commonly seen following head trauma.

MIGRAINE EQUIVALENTS

The term migraine equivalents has often been used in an imprecise and ambiguous manner by different authorities. It has been used to specify two very different types of migrainous problems: first, a migraine aura without accompanying headache (acephalgic migraine), and second, a large number of poorly defined clinical syndromes, such as abdominal migraine and cardiac migraine, that are characterized by episodic, transient dysfunction of an organ system. The transient dysfunction is believed to be a substitute for a headache in some individuals with migraine or a familial predisposition to migraine. To make precise definitions more difficult, the same paroxysmal organ system dysfunctions are reported to occur simultaneously with, or alternating with, typical migraine headaches or may occur in individuals who have never had recurrent head pain.

Acephalgic Migraine

Individuals with acephalgic migraine (migraine sine hemicrania, abortive migraine, migraine dissociée) can have any of the neurologic symptoms—visual, sensory, motor, labyrinthine, or cognitive—that commonly occur as an aura, but they do not develop an accompanying or a subsequent headache.[2144] Acephalgic migraine is seen both in patients with a well-established history of migraine as well as in non-migrainous individuals with a strong family history of migraine. Attacks without headache may also alternate with episodes accompanied by headache. Some patients develop episodic neurologic dysfunction that resembles an aura, and that may be migrainous in origin, for the first time after age 45 (late-life migrainous accompaniments) (see below). It has been estimated that up to 20% of migraine attacks with aura may be unaccompanied by headache.[29,1034]

Although almost any neurologic symptom can recur in a migrainous pattern and yet be unaccompanied by headache, visual symptoms, such as scintillating scotomas, are the most common.[29,1150,1475,2144] Scotoma without headache occurs more frequently in men than in women.[29,2144] Some patients complain of repeated episodes of paresthesias of the face and hand, dysphasia, hemiparesis, or symptoms such as dysarthria and ataxia, which indicate involvement of the brain stem. Other patients have episodes of transient global amnesia (see below), which are presumed to be migrainous in some individuals. Still others suffer from repetitive vertiginous episodes (benign recurrent vertigo) (see below).

The diagnosis of acephalgic migraine must be considered when recurrent neurologic events occur in a young patient with either a history of migraine or a strong family history of migraine. However, the diagnosis of acephalgic migraine should be made in an older person only after organic disease of the brain and blood vessels has been excluded by appropriate investigations.

Late-life Migrainous Accompaniments

Fisher[657,659] described a large group of patients who developed episodes of neurologic dysfunction that included scintillating scotomas, paresthesias, dysarthria, aphasia, brain stem symptoms, and motor weakness for the first time after age 45. Although only one half of the patients had a history of recurring classic or common migraine and the episodes of neurologic dysfunction were often unaccompanied by headache, Fisher labeled these episodes *migrainous accompaniments* because they closely resembled the auras that accompany the migrainous episodes of young migraineurs. Suitable investigations eliminated embolic and occlusive cerebrovascular disease as a factor, and results of angiography were normal. Permanent neurologic sequelae were rarely observed in Fisher's patients, but a detailed follow-up was not provided.

Fisher's major objective in specifically designating these symptoms was to differentiate them from the symptoms seen during transient ischemic attacks (TIAs) caused by cerbrovascular disease. Fisher set forth a number of clinical criteria that could be used to support his diagnosis of migrainous accompaniments. These criteria included: (1) the presence of visual symptoms such as a scintillating scotoma; (2) gradual *buildup* or progressive expansion and enlargement of a scintillating visual scotoma over a period of 5–30 minutes; (3) a slow *march* of paresthesias from one area of the body to another; (4) the succession of consecutive accompaniments, as, for example, from visual to sensory; (5) the occurrence of two or more identical spells; (6) headache in association with the spell; (7) a generally benign course without permanent neurologic sequelae. These phenomena are unusual in cerebrovas-

cular disease, but not at all unique for migrainous attacks.

Fisher's approach to these problems has heuristic value. However, from a practical point of view the diagnosis of migrainous accompaniments can only be made after rigorous and exhaustive attempts have been made to exclude cerebral thrombosis, embolism, arterial dissection, subclavian steal, angiitis, thrombocythemia, polycythemia, hyperviscosity syndromes, the presence of anticardiolipins, and epilepsy. Few neurologists would consider the diagnosis unless angiography were performed and results were normal and unless the patient suffered from virtually identical occurrences over a period of several years without sequelae. In general, the diagnosis of late-life migrainous accompaniments should be made with extreme caution lest serious, but treatable, disease be missed.

Transient Global Amnesia (TGA)

Transient global amnesia is a clinical syndrome characterized by a sudden, but temporary, profound loss of short-term memory associated with severe retrograde amnesia for events during the attack.[311,1265] During an episode patients remain conscious but are bewildered, anxious, distressed, and, as a rule, cognizant of their memory difficulties. The registration and recall of current events are impaired. Other neurologic signs and symptoms are usually absent. Most attacks last less than 24 hours, and patients have no remaining abnormalities other than amnesia for events during the attack. Most patients suffer a single attack, although some do have repetitive episodes. The syndrome occurs most often in middle-aged people.

TGA is generally attributed to transient ischemia in the mesial temporal lobes and hippocampus caused by thromboembolic cerebrovascular disease; that is, a TIA within the vertebrobasilar system. There is evidence against the TIA theory: attacks are more extended than conventional TIAs, recurrent attacks are rare, and strokes within the appropriate vascular territory causing permanent memory loss are rare. In addition, TGA is not associated with the conventional risk factors for cerebrovascular disease.[961] Several authorities have advocated a migrainous cause for this syndrome.[312,408,468,961] Their rationale for viewing TGA as a "migrainous equivalent" includes the fact that a history of migraine is common (but not invariable) in patients with the syndrome.[408,961] The prevalence of migraine is significantly greater than in matched groups of normal controls and patients with conventional TIAs. Some episodes occur during typical migraine attacks, and headache and nausea are said to accompany or to immediately follow TGA in 20% to 40% of patients.[312,952,961] Migraine may play a causal role in a proportion of cases of TGA.

Benign Recurrent Vertigo

Complaints of dizziness and vertigo unassociated with headache are considerably more frequent in migraineurs than in non-migrainous individuals.[423,1153,1524,2110] A syndrome that consists of recurrent spontaneous episodes of vertigo in otherwise healthy children has been named *benign paroxysmal vertigo* by some who consider it a definite migraine equivalent.[596,641,1417,1876] This syndrome may be the first manifestation of migraine in younger children.[641] It may also occur as a autonomous event in children who have migraine headaches. The problem usually starts in early childhood, most often between ages 2 and 5 years. The attacks vary in frequency from once a month to several times a week. As a rule, the syndrome disappears after a few months or years or tends to evolve into a more common migraine syndrome in later life. It is characterized by very sudden and recurrent attacks of vertigo, accompanied by disequilibrium and ataxia, anxiety, and frequently nystagmus and vomiting. Pallor and sweating are common. The children wish to remain absolutely still. The attack may last from seconds to hours, but most frequently lasts from 1 to 5 minutes.

Adults, however, also suffer from recurrent, spontaneous episodes of vertigo that appear identical to the childhood condition. Here too, migraine may be the cause of the vertigo.[1417,1876] A family history of migraine is the rule, and a personal history of migraine—particularly classic migraine—is found in approximately one third of cases.[1087,1153] Women are most often affected. In some individuals, episodes may be an accompaniment of menstruation. Attacks can be precipitated by alcohol, lack of sleep, or emotional stress.[1876]

In general, the sensation of vertigo develops suddenly—typically on awakening in the morning. The vertigo may be sufficiently intense to force the patient back to bed. There may be nausea, vomiting, and hyperhidrosis, but cochlear symptoms such as tinnitus or focal neurologic symptoms do not occur. Positional or spontaneous nystagmus may be seen on ENG examination, and the caloric examination may be abnormal. An attack can last from a few minutes to more than 24 hours and usually subsides gradually. Patients who suffer in this way are usually asymptomatic between vertiginous events, but some patients have abnormalities in vestibular function during the headache-free interval.[1087] The frequency of attacks can vary from once daily to twice a year.

Benign Paroxysmal Torticollis in Infancy

Benign paroxysmal torticollis in infancy is a disorder characterized by recurrent episodes of head tilt.[871,1253,1886] The majority of infants with the problem appear pale, vomit, and are irritable or agitated during the episodes. The head tilt may be the only neurologic sign, but a bent trunk posture also may be present.[358] Older children can show signs of disequilibrium and unsteady gait and can complain of headache.[484] The nature of the neurologic dysfunction underlying paroxysmal torticollis is unknown, but the syndrome may be a variant of benign paroxysmal vertigo of childhood. Some children with paroxysmal torticollis later develop paroxysmal vertigo.[555] Some of the infants have symptoms of migraine or develop migraine later.[484]

Abdominal Migraine

Much controversy surrounds the concept of *abdominal migraine*.[957,1984] Some authorities doubt its existence; others consider the syndrome to be an epileptic phenomenon[94,343,1522,1559] or to be psychogenic.[398,1456] There is little controlled, prospectively collected information about these problems.

A high childhood incidence of pain or vomiting syndromes (cyclical vomiting in infancy, abdominal pain, bilious attacks) has been reported.[440] Perhaps 1 in 10 children of school age suffers from recurrent abdominal pain. Children with these problems suffer over a period of many years from prolonged, paroxysmal attacks of midline abdominal pain associated with lethargy, pallor, nausea, and sometimes vomiting, occasional diarrhea, and limb pains.[1983] The pain, which may be infrequent or recur several times a week, is intense enough to prevent the child from continuing with normal activities. The pain is usually described as a diffuse aching sensation, but at times it can become crampy or colicky. It may be difficult to localize but is usually said to be periumbilical in position. The pain may be mild or extremely severe and lasts from a few minutes to many hours. Most children choose to lie down in a dark room and endeavor to sleep. The diagnosis of *abdominal migraine* is made in some of these patients. Some reports indicate that many of the children have a positive family history for migraine, some suffer from concurrent

migraine or ultimately develop it, and some respond to specific antimigraine drugs.[869,1613,1614,1739] Other reports, however, show a low incidence of migraine in later life.[72,1663]

Some adult patients without identifiable intra-abdominal pathology suffer from recurrent attacks of abdominal pain with or without concurrent headache and have a personal or strong family history of typical migraine headaches.[333,1286,1752] Their episodes of pain usually start in childhood, but may begin in early adult life. For episodic abdominal pain in adults to be considered a migraine equivalent is, however, distinctly uncommon.

The central characteristic of the syndrome is upper abdominal, periumbilical, or epigastric pain of great severity accompanied by a variety of autonomic symptoms such as pallor or flushing (Table 3–8). The pain, which may have been preceded by a typical migrainous prodrome of listlessness, yawning, and drowsiness, may be crampy or steady and can last from 10 minutes to 2 days. In most cases the pain lasts 5 or 6 hours. The patients usually suffer from nausea and vomiting as well, and some also complain of bloating and diarrhea. Fever may be present, and the patient may be lethargic.

The physician should consider a diagnosis of abdominal migraine in an adult only if the patient has recurrent attacks of upper abdominal pain interspersed with more conventional symptoms of migraine, or if the abdominal discomfort is associated with a head-

Table 3–8 ABDOMINAL MIGRAINE (IN ADULTS)

- Frequent family history of migraine
- Frequent history of classic or common migraine in the patient
- Beginning of attacks of abdominal pain before age 40
- Recurrent, identical attacks of abdominal pain
- No abdominal symptoms between attacks
- Duration of attacks from 1 to several hours
- Pain usually localized in upper abdomen

Adapted from Lundberg,[1286] p 124, with permission.

ache. However, the diagnosis should not be made until appropriate investigations have eliminated the presence of all other possible pathologic abdominal processes. Various episodic abdominal conditions such as biliary disease, partial bowel obstruction, and the irritable bowel syndrome need to be excluded.

Cardiac Migraine

Some migraine attacks are said to be accompanied by angina. The condition has been called *cardiac migraine (thoracic migraine, precordial migraine).*[333,1229] The patients are said to experience typical anginal-type chest pain in association with migraine headaches. Their chest pain, however, is not related to exertion. Electrocardiograms usually show nonspecific T-wave abnormalities and occasionally ST-segment depression or elevation. The chest pain is relieved by sublingual nitroglycerin. Patients with this condition may also have symptoms suggestive of hypoglycemia, because they complain of palpitations, feelings of anxiety, tremulousness, diaphoresis, and dizziness; these symptoms are relieved by the administration of sugar.

Arterial spasm may play a part in these phenomena. For example, variant angina (Prinzmetal's angina) caused by coronary artery spasm may have a relationship with migraine in view of the high prevalence of migraine in patients with the condition.[1389,2113] Many patients with Prinzmetal's angina also have Raynaud's phenomenon, which is caused by digital arterial spasm. A frequent association between migraine with and without aura and Raynaud's phenomenon is also reported.[487,1484] A tendency for vasospasm may occur in different vascular beds at different times in the same patient with migraine.

Paroxysmal tachycardia has also been mentioned in the literature as a migraine equivalent. Patients with this condition complain of episodic palpitations.

CHRONIC DAILY HEADACHE SYNDROME

Approximately one half of patients with acute attacks of migraine also have frequent mild to moderate headaches in between major attacks of head pain. This is particularly true of the 15% of patients who suffer from more than 10 separate migraine attacks per month.[1806] These patients complain of a continuous, diffuse, dull discomfort—a constant aching, pressure, or tightness around the head and neck with periodic episodes of throbbing pain more typical of migraine. The pain may be bilateral or unilateral and frequently is frontal or frontotemporal in location.[1326] It frequently involves the neck. If it is unilateral, the daily pain tends to be on the side and at the same site as the migrainous attacks. The headache is already present in the morning when patients awake, and they typically are never headache-free during the day. Earlier in life, most of these patients only suffered from well-defined, intermittent migraine attacks separated by headache-free days. Most had episodic attacks of migraine without aura. The majority are women who developed migraine in childhood or adolescence. Most have a strong family history of migraine. Over a period of a decade or two, a continuous pain with the characteristics of a so-called *tension-type headache (muscle contraction headache)* evolves, with intermittent attacks of migraine with hemicrania, nausea, vomiting, and photophobia (Table 3–9). Some patients may develop the problem after only a few years or even months of

Table 3–9 CLINICAL FEATURES OF THE CHRONIC DAILY HEADACHE SYNDROME

- Daily or almost daily headaches
- Periodic episodes of throbbing migrainous pain
- Excessive, usually daily analgesic use
- Symptoms of depression and anxiety
- Disturbances of sleep
- Family history of headaches and depression

Adapted from Saper,[1753] p 285, with permission.

episodic headaches. Some patients apparently lose their episodic migraine attacks when the daily pain develops. In some patients the chronic daily headache syndrome developed in parallel with the appearance of migraine. This group of patients never suffered only from intermittent migraine attacks. This problem has received various designations: *chronic daily headache syndrome, transformational migraine, transformed migraine, evolutive migraine, migraine with interparoxysmal headache, mixed tension-vascular headache,* and *daily mixed headache.*[1334,1753,1757] The chronic daily headache is one of the most ubiquitous problems seen at headache clinics and in headache practices.

Although the continuous head pain in patients with the chronic daily headache syndrome is thought to be caused by excessive muscle contraction, it is unclear that this is the case. Muscles may indeed be a source of pain, and sustained voluntary or involuntary contraction of neck or head musculature is known to give rise to pain and stiffness. The characteristics of the pain—a deep, steady, dull ache or pressure rather than a throbbing pain—have been used as evidence that the pain is not vascular in origin. As a result, neurologists have usually presumed that these headaches are caused by excessive muscle contraction. However, EMG evidence indicates that the levels of pericranial muscle contraction are similar in patients with headaches having the clinical characteristics of either migraine and muscle contraction headache.[45,1312,1606] Furthermore, the correlation between the magnitude of frontalis muscle tension and the presence or severity of clinically diagnosed muscle contraction headache is inconsistent and variable.[615,1312,2002] Tension-type and migraine headaches may be difficult, if not impossible, to distinguish, and the development of a daily headache in patients with episodic migraine may not indicate that a new type of headache problem has developed.[100,2196,2201,2203]

The majority of patients who develop this problem use excessive amounts of OTC antipyretic and anti-inflammatory analgesics (aspirin, acetaminophen), prescribed analgesic–sedative (barbiturate) combination drugs, narcotic medications, or ergots.[106,823,1335,1753] Many of the medications contain caffeine. Any of these drugs taken in excessive amounts can cause and sustain headache.[514] The problem of drug-induced headache will be dealt with in more detail in chapter 8.

Frequently patients with drug-induced chronic daily headache complain of asthenia, anxiety, restlessness, fatigue, and depression. These symptoms accompany the development of the constant pain. Sleep disorders are common and include difficulty in initiating and maintaining sleep, and awakenings in early mornings with severe headache. Patients often complain of irritability and difficulties with memory and concentration.

Some patients develop daily headaches after the initiation of treatment with oral contraceptive or estrogen replacement therapy.[1335] Daily headaches are more common in patients who smoke. Many patients with daily headaches have an excessive caffeine intake. Chronicity may also coincide with menopause; with a traumatic event such as the death of a spouse or a parent, major surgery, or severe accident; or with an increased amount of stress produced by a change in employment or retirement, marital difficulties, or systemic illness.[106,1334] A number of these patients have evidence of cervical dysfunction (e.g., abnormal postures, trigger points) or temporomandibular joint dysfunction.

At least one fourth of patients with the chronic daily headache syndrome do not take an excessive amount of analgesic medication. Perhaps in some patients there is a natural progression of their clinical course with more frequent interictal headaches appearing between their migraine attacks. Eventually a chronic daily headache develops.

STATUS MIGRAINOSUS

Status migrainosus is the term applied to severe, unrelenting migraine attacks that last more than 72 hours. These attacks are refractory to the usual analgesics and are associated with nausa and protracted vomiting, prostration, and dehydration. Status migrainosus may necessitate repeated visits to the emergency room or physician's office for symptomatic alleviation of pain or may require hospitalization for correction of dehydration and pain relief.[390] Prolonged attacks of severe migraine of this type may be precipitated by severe emotional stresses; misuse of medications such as ergots, analgesics, and narcotics; dietary indiscretions; or alcohol abuse.[390]

MIGRAINE AND EPILEPSY

The relationship between migraine and epilepsy is still unclear. A number of investigators have reported a higher prevalence of all forms of epilepsy in a population comprised of patients with migraine.[132,959,1217,1225] Many early studies were flawed, however, by the use of poorly defined criteria for both epilepsy and migraine, and most were uncontrolled. A number of epidemiologic investigations have stressed the autonomous nature of most forms of epilepsy and migraine, and have indicated that the association of the two disorders in individual patients is largely fortuitous.[120,270,1172,1765] Nonetheless, epileptic seizures may occur during a migrainous aura or in association with a severe migraine attack in individuals who have both conditions.[38] This phenomenon is seen more often in childhood and adolescence, but can occur at any time of life. In rare instances patients with this problem develop recurrent seizures that are unconnected to their classic migraine attacks. Patients who have seizures that commence with a vascular headache or complex migraine symptoms have a high incidence of intracranial pathology such as an AVM or tumor.[1544] It has also been suggested that epilepsy may arise from a focal cerebral lesion caused by an episode of complicated migraine with infarction, but this sequence of events is exceptional.[38]

Occipital Lobe Epilepsy and Migraine

A syndrome characterized by severe, recurrent migraine headaches associated with transient visual disturbances, paroxysmal occipital spike and slow-wave abnormalities, and seizures has been noted in children and adolescents.[17,305,736,1520,1996] Headache and nausea are common after a seizure. Some of these patients have been thought to have basilar migraine because of the bilateral visual hallucinations and visual loss that accompany the recurrent throbbing headaches associated with nausea and vomiting. The interictal electroencephalograms (EEGs) of these patients, however, show prominent, repetitive epileptiform spike–wave activity confined to the posterior regions of one or both hemispheres. The epileptiform activity is present when the eyes are closed and is markedly attenuated when the eyes are opened.[1520] In contrast, the ictal EEG of some patients with basilar migraine demonstrates transient posterior slow-wave activity during attacks.[1523,1969,1977]

A similar clinical pattern has been seen in some forms of childhood occipital epilepsy with visual auras. In this latter group of patients, seizures are characterized by visual phenomena, often succeeded by sensory, motor, or psychomotor symptoms and postictal migraine headache and visceral symptoms. The EEGs in this group of patients are similar to those described above.

It is difficult to determine whether both groups of cases represent a special variety of basilar migraine, a coincidence of epilepsy and migraine, or an epileptic disorder.[483,1521] The latter supposition is probably correct in view of the excellent clinical response to anti-epileptic medication.

Rolandic (Centrotemporal) Epilepsy and Migraine

Benign rolandic epilepsy is generally a disease of childhood. Many children with this form of epilepsy either endure intense migrainous headaches during childhood or have an unusually high incidence of migraine in their families. The incidence of migraine in patients has been estimated to be between 63% and 80%.[191,1810]

Benign rolandic epilepsy is characterized by seizures that produce paresthesias affecting the tongue, lips, and cheeks, followed by tonic contractions or clonic jerks in the same areas as the paresthesias. The patients do not lose consciousness. The symptoms usually occur either during drowsiness or arousal. The diagnosis is confirmed by the EEG features. Slow, diphasic, high-voltage, pseudorhythmic, and unilateral spikes or sharp waves are seen in the rolandic or temporal area. They can be unilateral, but are often bilateral and independent. The syndrome is called benign because the natural history of the problem is one of regression.

Postictal Headaches

A headache that succeeds generalized tonic-clonic seizures is a well-described feature of major motor seizures.[1788] A similar headache can develop after minor motor seizures, although it is less frequently experienced. A postictal headache develops regularly in at least half of all epileptic individuals. It is generalized, moderately intense, and throbbing in nature. In some patients it has the characteristics of a migraine headache. Indeed, some migraineurs consider their postictal headaches to be identical to their independently occurring migrainous headaches.[132,1788,1998]

POSSIBLE MIGRAINE SYNDROMES

A few complicated, diverse conditions may present with recurring symptoms, which either are indistinguishable from migraine or are thought to be migrainous in nature. All of these conditions have a variety of other neurologic symptoms and signs.

Mitochondrial Encephalopathy Syndrome

Migraine-like attacks and seizures are found in patients with mitochondrial encephalopathies, a heterogeneous conglomerate of hereditary metabolic disorders. The *MELAS syndrome* (mitochondrial encephalopathy, lactic acidosis, and strokelike episodes)[1704] affects the central nervous system as well as muscle, and migrainous phenomena are prominent in many patients.[558] Progressive neurologic signs and symptoms such as hemiparesis, ataxia, seizures, ophthalmoplegia, dementia, visual and hearing loss, and pyramidal and extrapyramidal deficits are present in varying combinations. The migraine in these cases is usually classic in its features and severe in its presentation.[1410] The attacks of migraine may be followed by prolonged and often permanent neurologic deficits.[558]

Alternating Hemiplegia of Childhood

Alternating hemiplegia of childhood (paroxysmal hemiparesis of childhood) is a very rare condition. The affliction is characterized by repeated attacks of hemiplegia involving alternate or both sides of the body and lasting from a few minutes to a few days. The bouts of hemiplegia are associated with dystonic posturing (tonic fits), choreoathetoid movements, nystagmus and other ocular abnormalities, and autonomic disturbances such as tachycardia, mydriasis, and sweating.[527,1138] The tonic fits can occur independently of the hemiplegic episodes and can be unilateral or bilateral. They are accompanied by screaming, irritability, and sometimes brief episodes of loss of consciousness. After the onset of the affliction, which is usually before age 18 months, the child, who has been developing normally, shows evidence of mental retardation and neurologic deficits, which become increasingly noticeable with the passing of time.

Alternating hemiplegia has been proposed as a form of complicated migraine; the signs of the affliction suggest a paroxysmal vascular disturbance that affects structures supplied by the vertebrobasilar system.[791,986,2068] Evidence supporting this proposal is, however, modest, and the relation of alternating hemiplegia to migraine, if any, is uncertain.[483] Alternatively, alternating hemiplegia has been considered an epileptic problem, although paroxysmal EEG abnormalities have not been described.

Ornithine Transcarbamylase Deficiency

Deficiency of ornithine transcarbamylase, an enzyme in the urea cycle, is inherited with an X-linked recessive pattern.[1823] Males with the deficiency rarely survive the neonatal period, but a partial deficiency is seen in adult women. Migraine headaches are frequent after protein ingestion in these women.[764] Some patients have had an altered level of consciousness accompanying the headache.

SUMMARY

The material in this chapter reviews a variety of clinical phenomena that have been called "migrainous." The phenomena constitute a variegated lot, and many of them are far afield from the "ordinary" cases of migraine commonly seen in practitioners' offices. It is difficult to classify much of this material. The new classification of headache disorders published by the International Headache Society represents a considerable improvement for clinicians committed to the diagnosis and treatment of headaches. But even this classification scheme does not do justice to the extended array of migrainous manifestations. It is clear that even the entities of migraine with aura and migraine without aura—thought to be relatively well defined—consist of several stages or phases, some of which can occur as isolated entities. In the absence of headache the diagnosis becomes still more difficult. It is clear that the number of clinical phenomena that have been associated with migraine attacks is exceptionally broad. Going one step further, the clinical states designated as migraine equivalents and complicated migraine are controversial and challenging to define. In addition, it is dubious whether or not a number of other entities, such as ophthalmoplegic migraine, are caused by processes similar or identical to those responsible for migraine with aura and without aura. Moreover, it is unclear whether or not another group of clinical conditions that includes transient global amnesia, abdominal migraine, cardiac migraine, and alternating hemiplegia of childhood are migrainous in nature.

Chapter 4

EXAMINATION AND INVESTIGATION OF THE MIGRAINEUR

THE MIGRAINE HISTORY
CLINICAL EXAMINATION OF THE
  PATIENT WITH MIGRAINE
IMAGING PROCEDURES
ELECTROPHYSIOLOGIC STUDIES
OTHER DIAGNOSTIC TESTS

The *history* of a patient with migraine is considerably more important than the physical examination, because the diagnosis of migraine relies largely, if not entirely, on the patient's description of symptoms. Abnormal neurologic signs are unusual in cases of uncomplicated migraine. A comprehensive and detailed history does much to reassure the physician that the diagnosis of migraine is the correct one. But just as important, a comprehensive and detailed history does much to reassure the patient that the physician is interested and concerned. Because an effective physician–patient relationship is the key to successful management of migraineurs, the initial history-taking visit is the single most important chance to construct such rapport.[698] Many migraineurs have received unsatisfactory care from physicians in the past, and are therefore defensive about their problems. As a result, more than a few patients come to the initial consul-

tation with the negative expectation that the examining physician will be as unsympathetic and as unhelpful as previous physicians were. Extraordinary care may be necessary both to obtain a complete history and to establish an atmosphere of trust and optimism.

A number of factors have the potential to complicate the relationship between physicians and patients with migraine, especially if the physician does not suffer from headaches:

1. Physicians can easily lose patience with otherwise healthy individuals who have the misfortune to be afflicted with migraine. Most physicians have had no specific training in the treatment of headaches and have had little experience with the particular problems associated with migraine. Nonetheless, many physicians believe that patients with migraine can be approached in ways similar to those used for patients with other medical and neurologic complaints. This is generally not the case. Examination and subsequent management of the patient with migraine takes a great deal of time, perseverance, and compassion, which—as a result of the pressures of modern medicine—are commodities frequently in short supply.

Furthermore, patients may have already seen one or more ophthalmologists, allergists, neurologists, dentists, psychiatrists, radiologists, psychologists, physical therapists, chiropractors, and acupuncturists. Each of these practitioners has probably considered the headache to result from conditions he/she felt most knowledgeable about and therefore treated the patient accordingly. As a result, a single migraineur may have had extensive radiologic procedures, including computed tomography (CT) and magnetic resonance imaging (MRI) scans, or may have had glasses prescribed, as well as undergoing electroencephalograms (EEGs), biofeedback, allergy injections, manipulation of the neck, and sinus drainage—all without efficacy.

2. Migraine is not the type of easily remedied medical or surgical problem that most physicians prefer to treat. No laboratory results are sufficiently precise to serve as markers for this illness; as a result, migraine runs counter to the inclination of most physicians to search for a somatic illness that can be objectively confirmed. In other words, migraine is a "low-tech" condition. Unfortunately, however, much of the emphasis of modern medical training has been on "high-tech" diseases that generate reams of laboratory data. As a result, a poorly managed case of migraine will frustrate many modern physicians who have been trained to itemize an extensive list of differential diagnoses and then to exclude ("rule out") various possibilities by means of laboratory tests and special investigations. In contrast, the management of most patients with migraine requires only a comprehensive history and a careful examination; the vast majority of migraineurs can be evaluated appropriately and accurately without resorting to laboratory and radiographic procedures. And as society becomes increasingly concerned about escalating health care costs, this point needs stressing all the more—migraineurs need little in the way of technology, but much in regard to listening and asking the appropriate questions.

3. Unless the physician has taken sufficient time and expended adequate effort during the first visit to construct a degree of trust and empathy, patients will not be forthcoming with information, either about significant environmental and family problems or difficulties with excessive drug and medication use. Many patients disclose that their previous physicians indicated, either implicitly or explicitly, that they were "weaklings" for "giving in" to their problem, that they were exaggerating the severity of their symptoms, and that their "problem was all in the head"—an implication that patients were not suffering from *real* illnesses. "I wish I were in a wheelchair so that people would believe that I *really am ill*" is an often-heard complaint of migraineurs who suffer from frequent, recurrent headaches. In addition, many patients have had side effects from previously prescribed medication. If the prescribing physician has not taken the appropriate time or effort to prepare each patient for potential side effects, the patient may have grave misgivings about trying new medications. Unless you have the good fortune to be the very first professional a patient has consulted for headache, you may very well encounter an individual who is suspicious of all physicians. Patients appreciate physicians who are friendly and respectful, but many physicians have not learned to use empathy in their training or practice, and many feel that they do not have enough time to develop empathy.[236]

4. The expectations of physicians and patients are different (Table 4–1). Most physicians assume that headache patients primarily come for pain relief and medication.[1517] Although the majority of patients expect pain relief, most want an explanation of what is causing their pain, coupled with the presence of a thorough, knowledgeable physician who is willing to listen to their complaints patiently and with understanding.[364,1517] About two thirds of patients have fears about organic disease that can be dispelled during the initial consultation.[661]

Table 4–1 HEADACHE PATIENT NEEDS

• Explanation of genesis of pain	77%
• Relief of pain	69%
• Explanation about medication (side effects and how it works)	32%
• Complete neurologic examination	31%
• A physician willing to follow up the headache	26%
• Medication	20%
• Time to ask the physician questions	20%
• Treatment other than medication	18%
• A complete eye examination	11%
• Skull x-rays	8%
• Psychiatric examination	3%

Adapted from Packard,[1517] p 373, with permission.

THE MIGRAINE HISTORY

The correct antibiotic will cure an infection whether or not there is rapport between doctor and patient. So too, a bone will knit if properly set. Relief from severity and frequency of migraine attacks, however, can rarely be achieved unless a thorough history of the nature of that patient's suffering has been taken. The following information is necessary: a detailed medical, neurologic, and family history together with scrutiny of the occupational, social, domestic, emotional, dietetic, and environmental situation (Table 4–2). Much attention must be paid to the patient's past *medication history* and to the present intake of medications, including over-the-counter drugs. A complete roster should be made of all medications that have been tried in the past, the doses prescribed, the duration of use, and any therapeutic benefits or untoward side effects. Information about self-medication should be obtained. Female patients should be questioned about oral contraceptives and the effect, if any, of these agents on the frequency and severity of attacks. It is also imperative to investigate alcohol, tobacco, and so-called "recreational" drug use. Appropriate emphasis should be placed on the state of the patient's general health so as to determine whether the migraine should be considered an isolated affliction or part of a systemic disease. A complete review of systems is necessary, with particular stress on questions about the function of the eyes, ears, nose, throat, temporomandibular joints, and neck. Inquiry should also be made as to a family history of headaches.

A competent psychological assessment by the physician is critical for successful treatment of patients with migraine, but the scope and character of the psychological evaluation should vary with the needs of the patient.[8,9]

Table 4–2 SIGNIFICANT ELEMENTS OF HEADACHE HISTORY

- Number and types of headache present
- Age and circumstances of onset
- Frequency of headache
- Duration of attacks
- Usual time of onset
- Location and radiation of pain
- Quality and severity of pain
- Time and mode of onset of pain
- Premonitory or prodromal symptoms
- Aura
- Associated systemic and neurologic symptoms
- Precipitating factors
- Aggravating factors
- Relieving factors
- Postdromal symptoms
- Previous treatment and medications and therapeutic or idiosyncratic responses
- Present medication, including over-the-counter remedies
- Family history
- Previous workups, including neuroimaging procedures
- General health and past medical history
- Personal history, including social and marital relationships, occupation, habits, intake of alcohol, coffee, and "recreational" drugs, sleeping habits, and emotional factors

Data from Blau,[206] Lance,[1167] and Selby.[1805]

The stresses and events immediately preceding headaches must be noted. Psychological experiences or reactions that elicit powerful emotions are considered to be imoprtant precipitants in the majority of severe bouts of migraine. Prolonged stress also contributes to the frequency of migraine attacks; thus, data about social and marital relationships, family situation, educational qualifications, occupational responsibilities, and employment conditions belong in the history. In the case of children, information about parental and sibling relationships and school should be sought. It is also important to determine whether or not specific psychological problems are causative or result from the burden of contending with chronic, recurring headaches. If both appear to be the case, they may well be interconnected; chronic head pain and associated cognitive difficulties invariably make social and work situations more difficult to cope with.

The *migraine history* is naturally focused on the migraine attacks themselves, and especially on the pain of migraine attacks. However, all descriptions of pain are subjective, and many patients lack the verbal ability to describe exactly what they have felt. Most patients are sure that physicians have no idea of the magnitude of their suffering, and may select inappropriate or hyperbolic language that may confuse the physician and confound the diagnosis-making process. Accordingly, each physician must develop a questioning style that will aid patients in articulating the characteristics of their own attacks. For example, one might begin with an open-ended question such as "What are your headaches usually like?" If the answer is too vague to be useful, the physician must be prepared to step in with questions regarding location, type of pain, and consequences of pain, regarding changes in behavior or interference with activities that will guide the response.

The following points should be covered during the first meeting.[206,1167,1805] This must be done personally by the physician. A questionnaire filled out by the patient with or without the help of medical personnel is not sufficient, because history taking not only gives the physician insight into the patient's problems, but the act of taking a history through sensitive questioning also begins to build the bridge between patient and physician. (The 17 topics recommended here for taking a migraine history are treated only briefly because the characteristics of migraine attacks are treated in greater depth in chapter 3.)

1. *The frequency and type(s) of headache.* Migraine headaches can recur in regular or irregular patterns. The frequency ranges from a few times a year to several times a week. Some patients have several bouts of migraine followed by long periods of headache freedom. Other patients have headaches every week. Some women note an invariable relationship to their menses.

Migraine patients may suffer from more than one type of headache; some may interpret their varying symptoms as one type of headache of varying intensity. Conversely, some patients may believe that one type of headache that varies in severity represents several different types. About half of migraineurs have frequent or constant mild-to-moderate headaches in between major attacks of head pain. Many of these patients suffer from perpetual, dull discomfort punctuated by recurrent bouts of acute throbbing pain "typical" of migraine. The majority of patients who develop this problem use excessive amounts of pain medication and suffer from drug-induced headaches—one reason a thorough medication history is needed.

2. *The age of onset.* Migraine frequently commences in childhood or early adulthood. However, because migraine often has different symptoms at different ages, a patient may consider the first attack to be the first episode with severe pain or with a visual aura. That patient, under careful questioning about typical childhood symptoms, may disclose a history of migraine that began early in life. Headaches that have

their onset abruptly in later life are more likely to indicate a pathologic condition, whereas headaches lasting a period of many years or decades are usually benign.

3. *The circumstances of the first attack.* Not infrequently, the onset of migraine was preceded by such factors as a head injury, menarche, pregnancy, or the initial use of oral contraceptives.

4. *The temporal pattern of the headache.* Patients manifest great variation in the frequency of bouts (from 2 to 3 per year to 10 per month). It is important to determine the average frequency of attacks for each patient, because changes in the frequency of migraine attacks may indicate the development of an intracranial lesion in a previously migrainous patient. In addition, such information will be needed when judging if particular medications are efficacious or not.

5. *The usual time of onset of headaches.* Although episodes of migraine may develop at any time of the day or night, most develop early in the morning.

6. *Precipitating or trigger factors known to bring on bouts.* A variety of factors, separately or in combination, can set off migraine attacks in most patients. These include stressful psychosocial conditions, dietary constituents, missed meals, altered sleep schedules, physical stimuli, changes in hormonal levels, or administration of certain medications. The relationship of attacks to menstrual cycles must be explored. Every effort must be made to identify trigger factors, because a substantial reduction in the frequency of attacks may be produced when particular factors in the environment are altered or removed.

7. *The types of premonitory symptoms.* Many migraineurs notice a number of early systemic, mental, or psychological premonitory symptoms that antedate the headache stage of a migraine attack.

8. *The aura preceding the headache.* If auras form part of the pattern of attacks, the patient must be specifically questioned about symptoms referable to the visual, sensory, motor, vestibular, and communication systems.

9. *The location of the pain and its radiation.* Migrainous head pain is strictly unilateral in about two thirds of patients, but it may be bilateral or holocephalic in the other third. If the pain is unilateral, successive attacks of pain may alternate sides, or the pain may occur invariably on the same side. Any region of the head, face, or neck may be affected. The discomfort may affect unusual locations such as the vertex, the jaw, or the teeth. The presence of frontotemporal pain is not necessary for the diagnosis.

10. *The quality of the pain.* It is well to bear in mind that less than half of adult migraineurs experience a throbbing or pounding component to their pain. Often, attacks start with a dull headache, and later develop a throbbing quality. Many inexperienced physicians erroneously believe that a history of throbbing pain is necessary to make a diagnosis of migraine.

11. *The severity of the pain.* The severity of pain can best be determined by evaluating its consequences on the patient's daily activities. The intensity of the pain typically varies among attacks from an insignificant discomfort to an incapacitating problem of sufficient severity to require cessation of normal activities and confinement to bed.

12. *The duration of the pain.* The duration of acute migrainous pain can range from a few hours to several days, but in most patients the pain lasts for a day or less.

13. *The factors that exacerbate the pain.* Migrainous pain is characteristically augmented by physical activity or effort and by sudden head movement.

14. *The maneuvers that ease or relieve the pain.* Migrainous discomfort is typically reduced by lying or sitting still. Manual compression of the superficial temporal artery may result in brief alleviation of pain in a small number of patients. Some patients find that an ice pack reduces pain, but others favor the application of heat to the head.

15. *Neurologic symptoms associated with the attack.* Focal visual, sensory, motor, or speech disturbances may occur during attacks of complicated migraine. Changes in the mental status and consciousness ranging from minor cognitive changes to a severe organic mental syndrome with confusion can develop.

16. *Symptoms of gastrointestinal or autonomic dysfunction.* During an attack most patients suffer from photophobia and phonophobia and from nausea, vomiting, or other gastrointestinal symptoms, such as diarrhea. Autonomic symptoms, such as facial pallor, pupillary changes, and cold extremities, are common.

17. *The postdromal symptoms* Most migraineurs are notably fatigued or depressed for several hours to a day following an attack.

CLINICAL EXAMINATION OF THE PATIENT WITH MIGRAINE

Patients with recurrent head pain are examined under two distinctly different circumstances. Some examinations take place during an attack. In this case, even when migraine is strongly suspected, the emphasis should be placed on ruling out an acute intracranial problem such as meningitis, encephalitis, subarachnoid hemorrhage, or brain tumor, all of which may require immediate admission to the hospital for a diagnostic workup. Far more often, however, migraineurs are examined during an interictal period, when the clinician's task is to evaluate chronic or recurrent headaches. In both contexts, a full neurologic examination and a general physical examination are necessary to detect cases of organic disease that have presented with migraine-like headache.

Ictal Examination

Under these circumstances, it is often difficult to perform a complete neurologic examination with assessment of the mental status, cranial nerves, gait, coordination, power, reflexes, and sensation. Unfortunately, migrainous head pain is exacerbated by many of the procedures that comprise a routine neurologic examination. For example, inspection of the fundus produces extreme photophobic discomfort. Gait and muscle strength testing are difficult, because any maneuver that changes the position or causes jarring of the head aggravates the pain.

The examination must also include scrutiny, auscultation, and palpation of the skull; evaluation and visualization of ears, tympanic membranes, and mastoid areas; examination of the neck for range of motion and stiffness (meningeal signs must be tested for if the neck is stiff); examination of the nose; percussion and transillumination of the sinuses; evaluation of the eyes for evidence of increased intraocular pressure; and auscultation and palpation of the extracranial vessels.[1754]

The suffering of patients during a severe migraine attack is obvious (Fig. 4–1). They look ill, perhaps even moaning or quietly sobbing. These patients make every attempt to remain immobile, either lying flat or sitting propped up. Head movement is especially avoided. Their faces are usually pale or ashen; the skin is usually sweaty, whereas the extremities typically feel cold. Uncommonly, the forehead may be flushed and warm. In occasional patients, localized edema in the temporal and periorbital areas may be noted, and in some patients the superficial temporal vessels or the frontal and supraorbital vessels appear distended and prominent.[158] A slight fever and a small amount of neck stiffness may be present. The patient may be irritable or indifferent. A considerable degree of lethargy is not uncommon. Speech is frequently slow and hesitant, and may even be slurred and dysarthric. Evidence of cognitive impairment, or even a significant organic mental syndrome, may be present. Some patients have difficulties with word-finding.

As the pallor and sweating suggest,

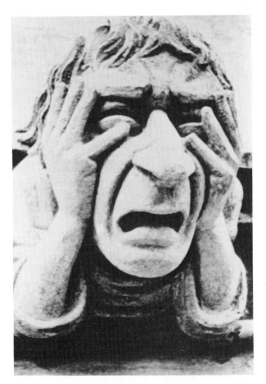

Figure 4–1. Gargoyle on Bell Tower, New College Oxford. A presumed 14th century rendition of a migraineur in the throes of an acute attack of migraine.

examination usually demonstrates evidence of autonomic nervous system involvement. The pupils are typically normal, but on occasion, one finds Horner's syndrome with ptosis or miosis. In some patients, the pupil is dilated on the side of the head pain.[1152] During some attacks, examination of the nose may show engorged turbines. The conjunctivae may be injected. Tachycardia and hypertension are often present, but hypotension and bradycardia are also possible.[256] Fever occurs rarely—usually in children.[2165] The pericranial and cervical muscles are often tender.[540,1273,1489] The sternocleidomastoid, trapezius, temporalis, and paracervical muscles are most commonly involved. Scalp tenderness is frequently present in the forehead, the temples, and the occiput.[540,1806] If the patient has complicated migraine, neurologic examination may reveal a hemiparesis, a hemisensory deficit, a homonymous hemianopia, decreased vision in one eye, or ophthalmoplegia.

Interictal Examination

Because the interictal diagnosis of migraine is almost always made on the basis of history, the neurologic examination itself is usually an anticlimax. Between attacks the results of neurologic examination of the migrainous patient should be essentially normal. Aniscoria may be seen more frequently in migraineurs than in the general population.[543,544] Examination of the head and neck may reveal residual tenderness of the scalp and the pericranial and cervical muscles for several days after an attack.[1273] A tender cervical carotid artery ipsilateral to the side of the hemicranial pain is present between attacks in a large proportion of patients with frequent migrainous attacks.[1640] The presence of well-defined, remarkably sensitive trigger points and tenderness in the distribution of the greater occipital nerve may be seen. Detection of other objective neurologic abnormalities between bouts casts suspicion on the diagnosis of migraine and indicates a need for additional studies.

IMAGING PROCEDURES

A confident diagnosis of migraine can usually be made on the basis of a comprehensive history, followed by a neurologic and general examination. For the vast majority of patients, laboratory tests are not necessary because only an exceedingly small number of patients with uncomplicated migraine have intracranial masses or other significant intracranial lesions.[321,413,1190,1762] Furthermore, the diagnostic assessment of migraineurs with normal findings on neurologic examination is expensive and unrewarding.[1190] Although CT scans and MRI scans show *nonspecific* abnormalities in a large number of migraine patients, these lesions are rarely significant, and accordingly their presence should alter neither the diagnosis nor the course of treatment. In sum, CT and MRI scans do not appear to be cost-effective procedures for the routine screening of patients with migraine headaches who are younger than age 45 and who have normal physical examinations (Table 4–3).* The same can be said for routine EEGs. Some patients, however, are convinced that they have serious intracranial lesions and feel that they require an elaborate workup. These patients need reassurance that their head pain does not result from an undetected tumor or other lesion. If the confidence of these patients has been gained, most can be convinced that they do not need unnecessary tests.

Far too many CT and MRI examinations are done simply because the tests are available, patients expect them, and physicians believe they are needed as protection against accusations of malpractice. Some situations do, however, warrant selected imaging procedures. These are listed on Table 4–4. When a migraineur has systemic symptoms such as fatigue, malaise, and muscle aching, appropriate examinations of blood must be ordered to rule out such conditions as systemic lupus erythematosus or chronic fatigue syndrome.

*References 321, 839, 1059, 1190, 1761, 1762, 2120

Table 4–4 INDICATIONS FOR LABORATORY EXAMINATIONS

- Recent worsening of the headache
- Increase in headache frequency
- Onset of headaches after age 50
- Abnormal neurologic examination
- History of complicated migraine
- Hemicrania consistently limited to one side
- Orbital or intracranial bruit
- Transient neurologic events without succeeding headaches
- First bout of basilar migraine, hemiplegic migraine, or ophthalmoplegic migraine
- Systemic symptoms such as fatigue and myalgia

Computed Tomographic Scans

CT studies of migraineurs both with and without focal neurologic deficits reveal abnormalities. The frequency of such abnormalities has ranged from 14% to 71% of the subjects, depending upon the study.* Most of the abnormalities are nonspecific, and consist of mild to modest ventricular enlargement sometimes associated with widening of the cerebral sulci.[549,1002,1148,1333] The changes in the brain are hypothesized to result from repeated attacks of migraine that lead to permanent changes in brain parenchyma.[1333] Scattered or

*References 102, 298, 299, 321, 1002, 1316, 1333, 1711

Table 4–3 COST-EFFECTIVENESS OF CT SCAN SCREENING

U.S. population = 246,043,000 in 1990.
According to Waters and O'Connor[2109]:
    80% of population report headaches.
    40% of population report severe headaches.
    20% of population report headaches compatible with migraine.
CT scans = $600 to $900
MRI scans = $1100 to $1500
CT Scans—Risks, Costs, Benefits:

Group	Deaths*	Cost	Benefit
Everyone	4920	$147 billion	??
All individuals with headaches	3936	$117 billion	??
All individuals with severe headaches	1968	$58 billion	??
All migraineurs	984	$29 billion	??

*1:50,000 die from dye reaction.
Adapted from Moore,[1413] p. 77 with permission.

focal areas of cerebral atrophy are sometimes found.[299,549,1761] The areas of localized atrophy are most frequently located in the temporal and parietal areas. The presence of CT abnormalities is not correlated with the duration, severity, or frequency of the migraine attacks, but CT abnormalities are more frequent in patients with classic migraine than in patients with common migraine.[413,549,1002,1762]

On occasion, CT scans demonstrate hypodense areas, which may or may not be enhanced following an injection of contrast material.[1002,1025] In general, these areas of low density have a limited "mass effect" relative to their size, are usually surrounded by meager amounts of edema, and are frequently transient in nature. Although they may involve any region of the brain, the occipital lobes are the most common sites. Hypodense areas are most often seen in individuals who have residual neurologic deficits after a migraine attack, but have also been noted in patients without apparent residual signs of neurologic dysfunction.[1002,1333] Because these lesions resemble those produced by ischemic processes, hypodense areas are thought to represent areas of cerebral ischemia.

Magnetic Resonance Imaging Scans

Parenchymal lesions have been demonstrated in the MRI scans of migraineurs. The prevalence of such abnormalities reportedly ranges from 5.5% to as many as 46% of patients, but they appear to be more frequent in patients with classic and basilar migraine.† These abnormalities consist mainly of multiple, bilateral, punctate white matter hyperintensities (white matter foci; unidentified bright objects) on both T2- and proton density-weighted images. Confluent lesions are more unusual.[630,645] The hyperintensities are es-

pecially prominent in the deep and periventricular white matter (Fig. 4–2). The presence of the lesions is not correlated with the frequency of attacks or the duration of the condition, but as the figure shows, the age of the individual is a major factor.[1009]

The presence of multiple, small, hyperintense foci is a nonspecific finding. Such abnormalities also show up in the scans of patients with multiple sclerosis, hypertensive small vessel disease, vasculitis, and multiple infarcts. In general, however, the lesions seen in scans of patients with migraine are smaller than the typical patches of demyelination seen in multiple sclerosis. An increased incidence of these foci is seen in scans in older individuals with and without migraine, but patchy foci of increased signal intensity in the white matter rarely occur in the brains of normal individuals under age 45.[246] The pathologic process responsible for the white matter hyperintensities is in some dispute. Hyperintensities are generally considered to reflect a pathologic increase in tissue water resulting in prolongation of T2 relaxation, but they have also been attributed to ischemic demyelination and to lacunar infarcts.[246,752,1654] Neuropathologic examinations of areas of the brains of nonmigrainous patients seen to contain hyperintensities on MRI images have shown a variegated picture that ranges from a lack of abnormalities to areas of incomplete white matter infarction or perivascular gliosis, demyelination, and atrophy without tissue necrosis. The significance of such lesions in the MRI scans of patients with migraine is simply not known.

On rare occasions, larger areas of signal abnormality are seen in scans of migraineurs. The findings consist of focal regions of increased signal intensity on T2-weighted studies. Such areas may also produce hypointense signals on T1-weighted images. These lesions are thought to represent areas of infarction.[1889,2198]

In sum, data collected so far from both CT and MRI scans of "ordinary" mig-

---

†References 506, 630, 1009, 1022, 1148, 1510, 1889

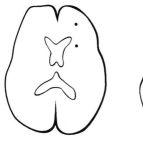
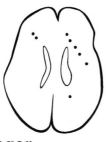
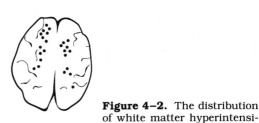

39 years or younger

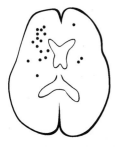
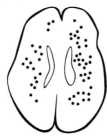
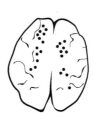

40 years or older

Figure 4–2. The distribution of white matter hyperintensities in MRI scans. In younger patients (≤39 years of age) the lesions are predominantly located in the centrum semiovale and the frontal white matter. With advancing age (≥40 years) the lesions extend to the deeper white matter at the level of the basal ganglia. (Adapted from magnetic resonance imaging in patients with migraine by Igarashi H, Sakai F, Kan S, Okada J and Tazaki Y, Cephalagia 11:69–74, 1991, by permission of Scandinavian University Press, Oslo, Norway, Copyright is held by Scandinavian University Press.)

raineurs are inconclusive. They do not shed light on the pathophysiologic processes involved in this condition or alter the physician's care of people afflicted with this common misery. Unless or until imaging procedures produce more useful information, they should be restricted to only those cases in which an abnormal lesion is suspected. All other patients should be reassured, on the basis of a careful history and physical examination, that they do not need expensive testing.

ELECTROPHYSIOLOGIC STUDIES

Electrophysiologic studies are certainly less expensive than imaging procedures, but their diagnostic value in patients with migraine is no more clear. Although many published reports indicate that EEGs and visual evoked potentials (VEPs) of migraineurs differ from non-migraineurs, few of the reported abnormalities are sufficiently specific to aid in the diagnosis of migraine. It would be fair to say that, at the present time, VEPs are to be considered experimental, and that the major clinical indication for performing an EEG in a particular migraineur is the need to determine whether a change of consciousness occurring in association with a migrainous headache is syncopal or epileptic in nature.

Electroencephalograms

Considering the modest value of the EEG in the diagnosis and management of most patients with migraine, it has been the focus of an extraordinary amount of attention.[1526,1745] Many researchers have reported an increased frequency of EEG abnormalities in migraineurs compared to the population of non-migraineurs. Although the prevalence of abnormal recordings in the interictal period has been reported to vary between 22% and 72%, most of these studies have been uncontrolled.* None of the abnormalities reported are exclusively found in patients with migraine. Furthermore, most workers have reported comparatively minor findings that have little specificity. In addition, the criteria for EEG abnormality vary from study to study. A number of older studies considered records pathological that contain findings now considered to be normal patterns or normal variants, such as posterior slowing and excessive hyperventilation responses.[1112,1745] Many studies display a paucity of age-, sex-, and medication-matched controls. Some older investigations presumably overestimated the proportion of migraineurs with EEG abnormalities, because their sample was biased by patients referred from headache clinics because of concomitant neurologic deficits or diseases, including epilepsy.

INTERICTAL EEG PATTERNS

The interictal EEG patterns most commonly reported are either disorganized traces dominated by abnormal fast and slow activity, or excessive slow activity that is usually diffuse but may be focal.[958,1526] Other reported patterns include focal spike or sharp waves, and abnormal responses during hyperventilation.[1877,2119] Paroxysmal abnormalities occur in the records of a few migrainous adults.[792,2119] and are noted with substantially higher frequency in the records of afflicted children.[2206] Focal EEG abnormalities occur with the highest frequency in patients who have focal cerebral hemispheric symptoms accompanying their attacks.[959] The degree and characteristics of the abnormalities seen in the EEGs of migraineurs may vary in serial tracings and, at times, even disappear. In contrast, at times the EEGs of patients with complicated migraine can show a persistent focus of slow wave changes that

*References 532, 710, 762, 959, 996, 1613, 1615, 1621, 1806, 1877, 1878, 1883, 2118, 2206

is related to the visual, motor, or sensory defects; this is an expression of a permanent cerebral lesion.[563,735,737] In addition, it is unclear whether or not the incidence of EEG abnormalities can be correlated with the severity or the frequency of migraine attacks or the duration of the affliction.[959,1057,1115,1883] An increased incidence of abnormalities is said to be present in patients with classic migraine, but this has not been confirmed.[959,1878]

Computer analysis of EEG data has shown some interictal abnormalities.[1046,1057,1851] Differences in power spectra between control individuals and patients with migraine have been described.[626,627,1782,1850] These power differences correspond to modest changes in background activity and, in general, indicate a degree of EEG slowing. Considerable overlap of findings exists between normal and patient groups. The value of EEG spectral analysis has significant limits in the diagnosis of migraine in individual patients.

ICTAL EEG PATTERNS

The EEG abnormalities occurring during bouts of common migraine have been poorly documented, but the data that are available show that ictal changes in the EEG are infrequent.[1203] In contrast, changes in the EEG are more frequent in patients during attacks of complicated migraine or of migraine with aura. Transient, slow-wave disturbances of high or low amplitude have been recorded from patients who have focal signs such as scotomas or hemiparesis, either occurring before or during attacks of migraine.[243,306,1691,2143] The slow waves may be diffuse, but are usually asymmetric, with a predominance of slow waves over the cerebral hemisphere contralateral to the neurologic deficit. The EEGs of some patients may show insubstantial changes such as asymmetric alpha activity.[1266] The abnormalities usually disappear concurrently with, or a few days to weeks after, clinical recovery.[243,306,1187,1691] The EEG of most patients with basilar migraine shows transient posterior slow-wave activity during attacks.[1523,1969,1977] There are a number of reports of children and adolescents with basilar artery migraine, paroxysmal occipital spike and slow-wave abnormalities, and seizures.[17,305,736,1520,1996] The epileptiform activity is present only when the eyes are closed. In contrast, the EEG of patients with acute confusional migraine demonstrates bilateral slow-wave activity.[1590,2093]

PHOTIC DRIVING

A number of reports indicate that the basic EEG rhythm of individuals with migraine is easily influenced by repetitive photic stimulation.[958,2060] *Photic driving* (also called *photic following*) is a rhythmic response present mainly in records from the posterior cerebral regions when an individual is subjected to intermittent photic stimulation. The rhythmic response occurs either at the same rate as the flash or at a subharmonic of the flash rate. Photic driving is a normal phenomenon when the rates of stimulation are in the alpha range. Migraineurs reportedly have augmented photic driving in response to high-frequency stimulation—a response that extends into the range above 20 flashes/sec (20 Hz). Its incidence in the migraine population is unclear, and its specificity for migraine is suspect.* However, power spectral analysis of the EEG during photic stimulation has demonstrated that the majority of patients with migraine display increased reactivity of the basic EEG rhythm to intermittent photic stimulation at rates ranging from 20 to 30 Hz.[1057,1470,1851] The precise import of the extended responses to repetitive photic stimulation in patients with migraine is also obscure.[1526] Nor is the phenomenon seen only in patients with migraine. Patients with anxiety, for example, show an equivalent enhancement of photic driving.[2051] And for many years, photic

driving up to 30 Hz has been demonstrated to occur in some non-migraineurs.[761]

Visual Evoked Potentials

Studies of *visual evoked potentials (visual evoked responses)* use a computer to separate background brain activity from stimulus-related potentials induced by a visual sensory input to the brain.[958,2058,2060] Two types of visual stimuli have been used in studies of migraineurs: flashes of bright light from a gas-filled strobe light,† and repetitive patterns, generally a checkerboard that alternates from black to white.[161,1098] VEPs are quantified by measuring the latencies and amplitudes of selected waveform peaks.

Despite the many useful clinical applications for pattern stimuli in neurologic testing, flash seems to be superior to pattern reversal for eliciting altered VEPs among patients with migraine. A number of studies show that VEPs evoked by repetitive flash stimulation are abnormal in migraineurs.* The reported abnormalities, however, have varied from study to study; accordingly, in patients with migraine, the amplitude of some component of the flash VEP was either somewhat greater or smaller, or the latency of a particular peak was somewhat delayed. A simple summary is impossible because differences among the series of subjects (e.g., age, sex, types of migraine), conditions of testing (e.g., wavelength, duration, luminance), and parameters of recording and averaging prevent comparison among flash stimulation studies. Although flash is a superior stimulus, repetitive patterns continue to yield data. Thus, the latencies and amplitudes of pattern reversal VEPs are also said to be increased in some patients who have migraine attacks, particularly if they

---

*References 801, 959, 1057, 1851, 1877, 2061

†References 801, 1218, 1219, 1288, 1470, 1670, 1883

*References 161, 742, 801, 1098, 1218, 1288, 1619, 1670

have migraine with visual auras. The frequency of abnormalities, however, again varies markedly among different series and, in addition, some workers have not found any significant differences between migraine patients and controls.[161,1098,1599,2060] In other words, because the frequency of abnormalities does not clearly correlate with the clinical picture, and because the reported abnormalities vary, VEPs are *not* useful diagnostic tools for the clinical assessment of patients with migraine headaches.

Unlike the visual evoked potential, the contingent negative variation (CNV) is an event-related, slow, negative cerebral potential recorded over the scalp during simple reaction-time tasks that are preceded by a warning stimulus. The amplitude of the CNV is reported to be increased in patients without aura between attacks, but more work is needed before the diagnostic value of the test can be evaluated.[1142,1289,1785]

If the data from either EEGs or VEPs consistently demonstrated a marked difference between migraineurs and non-migraineurs, we would have an extremely useful tool for determining *biological abnormality*. Unfortunately, despite the reams of data, and the actuality that many neurologists routinely order EEGs for new patients with migraine, electrophysiologic studies are of almost no use in the diagnosis and treatment of cases of ordinary migraine. Unless syncope or epilepsy occurs in connection with headache, such studies are unnecessary.

OTHER DIAGNOSTIC TESTS

Thermography

The facial thermogram of most normal, healthy individuals is symmetrical in pattern.[1174,1981] The warmest areas are near the inner canthi and the deep skin folds. The forehead is less warm, and the ears and nose are cooler than the rest of the facial structures.[705] In contrast, the forehead temperature of many migraineurs has a distinctive, interictal pattern. This pattern includes either a distinct *cold patch*—a discrete region of the forehead more than 0.5°C cooler than nearby areas—or a more widespread area of diminished temperature located on one side in the supraorbital region of the forehead. One or the other of these patterns is seen in 60% to 88% of patients with migraine.[1329,1979,1981] It also occurs, but is much less frequent, in patients with tension-type headaches and in control subjects.[1981] The distinctive thermographic findings have been reported to disappear in many patients following successful treatment,[2077,2078] but others have reported that the findings remain unchanged despite effective treatment.[1980]

Conflicting data also exist with regard to whether the face and scalp become cooler or warmer during migraine headaches. A lower facial temperature in the ipsilateral frontotemporal region was originally reported during unilateral bouts of migraine.[1174,1177,1329] More extensive observations during migraine attacks have indicated, however, that the ipsilateral frontotemporal region became approximately 1°C warmer compared to the contralateral side.[545,547,757] The increased temperature is significantly greater in that subgroup of migraine patients whose head pain is relieved by manual compression of the ipsilateral superficial temporal artery.

Most, if not all, severe attacks of migraine affect the autonomic nervous system in some way, producing pallor, cold extremities, and the like. But despite some provocative findings, especially with regard to the possibility of interictal asymmetric patterns, the merits of thermography in the diagnosis or management of patients with migraine remains to be demonstrated.

Angiography

At present, angiography is very rarely required for the evaluation of patients with migraine. Angiography infrequently, if ever, provides information about cases of migraine useful enough to justify the risk. When a migraineur has a normal neurologic exam and a normal CT or MRI scan, there is little or no justification to perform angiography. In the rare case when angiography is necessary, it is prudent to refrain from performing the test during an acute attack of migraine because of the difficulty in deciding—should a neurologic deficit ensue—whether it resulted from the procedure or was caused by the migraine attack itself. Because angiography is of so little clinical use, the following paragraphs simply summarize published data with regard to the angiograms of migraineurs.

Angiograms obtained to determine the cause of prolonged neurologic defects in migraineurs are generally normal, although in a few patients arterial branch occlusions or narrowings assumed to be caused by vasospasm have been demonstrated.* A negative study, however, does not exclude occlusion in small cerebral branch vessels not visualized by angiography. Different patients have lesions in different vessels, but lesions have been seen in all major cerebral arterial trunks in different patients.[331,529,635] Angiographic data obtained during an attack of migraine are limited, but are also usually reported as normal.† A few cases have shown filling of the posterior cerebral artery or upper part of the basilar artery.[1870,1871] With the exception of a few isolated case reports, vasospasm has not been demonstrated in migraine even when the angiography has been performed during a migraine aura documented to have low cerebral blood flow.‡

An increased risk from angiography in patients with migraine has been seen.[1097,1533] Deterioration of the neurologic status in patients with compli-

cated migraine has been reported in some patients.[662,976] Cortical blindness that resolved over several days has been seen following vertebral angiography, but is also reported to occur in non-migrainous individuals.[662,911] Many of the reported complications, however, are the result of direct carotid or vertebral arterial punctures and the use of older and more toxic radiographic contrast materials. Direct arterial punctures are not used now; accordingly, the risks of angiography in migraineurs are not believed to be higher than for patients in the general population.[1826] Less serious, but nevertheless unpleasant for the patient, is the development of bouts of migraine following arteriographic procedures. This has been well documented, particularly after direct puncture or catheterization of the carotid artery.[911,1028,1495] Acute attacks are also seen following injections delivered via a catheter from the femoral artery passed up to the internal carotid or vertebral artery. Headaches that mimic a patient's spontaneous attacks occur in about 50% of all migraineurs. The attack may develop preceding the injection of x-ray contrast material or after it. There may be a delay of about 30 to 60 minutes between carotid arterial puncture and the onset of aura symptoms.[1204,1205,1871]

Lumbar Puncture

The cerebrospinal fluid (CSF) pressure and the CSF itself are almost always normal during attacks of uncomplicated migraine.[2081] Even though transiently elevated protein levels (up to 150 mg/dL) and white blood cells in the CSF have been reported in patients with complicated migraine and migrainous infarction, lumbar puncture is rarely required for evaluation of patients with migraine headaches.[243,375,1141,1791] It should be reserved for those cases in which subarachnoid hemorrhage, meningitis, or encephalitis is suspected.

---

*References 230, 231, 375, 460, 1544, 1560, 1699
†References 231, 243, 375, 856, 1115, 1467, 1544, 1870, 1874, 1985
‡References 554, 695, 732, 1789, 1812, 1874

Neuropsychological Testing

Some migraineurs may show evidence of diminished higher cortical function in periods between attacks of migraine. Such abnormalities may consist of mild limitation of memory, difficulty with attention, slower reaction times, and decreased ability to abstract.[1117,1792,2149] As a result, patients with migraine may show impairment on batteries of standard neuropsychological tests compared to control individuals without headache.[979] It is unclear if such cognitive impairments have practical implications with regard to the individual's proficiency to maintain normal intellectual and occupational undertakings.

SUMMARY

The material in this chapter has been arranged in order of importance. It cannot be stressed too often or too emphatically that the migraine history is the cornerstone of the entire process of diagnosing and treating migraine patients. Migraine is not only diagnosed through talking, but the act of taking a detailed history, if done with sensitivity and patience, also begins to build an edifice of trust between patient and doctor. Treating migraine is an interactive process. Occasionally, the first medication prescribed will eliminate a patient's symptoms—but this is not the usual scenario. More typically, the patient will have to experiment with various lifestyle changes while the physician will have to try different drugs at a variety of doses. To avoid confounding variables, changes must be made step by step, not all at once. The migraineur must have confidence in the physician, or he or she will give up too soon, convinced that yet another physician has failed to help. The kind of physician–patient relationship needed to manage a difficult case of migraine cannot begin with a questionnaire followed by a perfunctory examination, the ordering of a great deal of expensive laboratory data, and a hurriedly written prescription. Examining a patient with migraine takes time, patience, and understanding.

Chapter 5

DIFFERENTIAL DIAGNOSIS

When a patient suffers from recurrent migraine attacks that consist of prodrome, aura, headache, and postdrome, the diagnosis is readily apparent. The diagnosis becomes still easier if the headache is unilateral and throbbing, exacerbated by activity, and accompanied by nausea, vomiting, and photophobia. Clinicians can feel even more confident about making a diagnosis of migraine if close relatives have similar headaches, and if the patient volunteers information that headaches can be precipitated by certain dietary indiscretions, hormonal changes, or exposure to specific environmental stimuli such as cigarette smoke, flash-

ing lights, or fragrances. But unfortunately, not all migraine attacks are textbook cases. Migraine often has diverse manifestations. Some patients describe an incomplete picture that can make diagnosis a challenge. Accordingly, for every headache that is not an unequivocal textbook case, the differential diagnosis must consider all conditions that might cause symptoms comparable to those of migraine. In this regard, quite a large number of headache-producing conditions are easy to rule out. But the clinician may find it considerably more difficult to distinguish tension-type headache and cluster headache from migraine, because these frequently occurring headaches often share characteristics with migraine headaches.

An extremely important factor in making a differential diagnosis of migraine is the duration of the symptoms. One group of clinical conditions must be kept in mind for patients who have had recurrent head pain for many years. In contrast, different clinical syndromes need consideration for any patient who is suffering from one of the following: an initial headache if the individual has no history of headaches; a headache that the patient describes as the worst of his or her life; a headache that has been present for only a few days, weeks, or months; or a significant change in the pattern of long-standing headaches. In any of these situations, it is obviously of prime importance to distinguish commonplace, "benign" headaches from head pain that signals imminent danger.

The circumstances of the examination are also germane to making a differential diagnosis. Accordingly, when a patient is initially seen during an acute attack, the diagnoses to consider are not the same as when a patient is first examined during an interictal period. The former situation requires rapid evaluation and response. A number of serious conditions, such as subarachnoid hemorrhage, meningitis, ischemic vascular events, and arterial dissections, must be differentiated from an acute bout of migraine. Other conditions, such as acute sinusitis, acute glaucoma, and optic neuritis, must also be considered. One must move quickly to rule out all serious causes for acute symptoms. If the patient is found to be experiencing a severe attack of migraine, action can then be taken to relieve suffering. In contrast, an interictal examination can be performed at a more leisurely pace, and appropriate emphasis can be placed on a meticulous history, which, if taken carefully and thoughtfully, usually reveals those patients who are migraineurs.

The differential diagnosis of migraine is made by considering every cause of repetitive head pain, together with a large number of conditions that can produce repeated focal neurologic symptoms or signs. One must include headaches that mimic migraine, but are actually the initial symptom of systemic or local intracranial and extracranial disorders. As can be seen by the roster of conditions considered in this chapter, the inventory can be considerable. For the differential diagnosis of relatively unusual types of migraine such as hemiplegic migraine, ophthalmoplegic migraine, basilar migraine, retinal migraine, and migrainous infarction, consult chapter 3. The focus here is on those types of headaches relevant to the differential diagnosis of the major subtypes of migraine—migraine with aura and migraine without aura.

TENSION-TYPE HEADACHES

Migraine and tension-type headaches (muscle contraction headaches, tension headaches, psychogenic headaches, stress headaches) have customarily been judged independent clinical entities. But, as indicated in chapter 1, many clinicians are dubious about endeavors to differentiate the two types of headaches completely. Several groups of researchers also feel that migraine and tension headaches may not be discrete headache entities. The International Headache Society has attempted to formalize the distinction between migraine and tension-type headaches.[917] Their distinction is, however, often difficult to make clinically, and for that reason, it may well come to pass that future "official" classification schemes will in some way link migraine and so-called tension-type headaches. A number of reasons account for the difficulty in distinguishing between migraine and tension-type headaches:

1. For many patients, tension-type headaches appear to precede or accompany their migraine attacks. Their bouts of head pain have features of both tension-type and migraine headaches (mixed headache syndrome).[1753]

2. Many patients complain of a continuous, diffuse, dull discomfort on which is superimposed periodic episodes of throbbing pain more typical of migraine (chronic daily headache syndrome).[1334,1757]

3. Large numbers of migraineurs experience two distinct types of headache at separate times—one that easily conforms to the criteria for migraine, and one that fulfills the criteria for tension-type headache.[1645]

4. Patients diagnosed as having tension-type headaches frequently have symptoms commonly ascribed to migraine—namely, a throbbing component of the head pain, anorexia, nausea, phonophobia, and photophobia.[100,1179] Frequently, however, the nausea results from the large quantity of analgesic medications so commonly

consumed by patients with this condition. Dizziness, lightheadedness, and fatigue are also common accompaniments of both types of head pain.[700]

5. The symptoms of a surprising number of patients give rise to ambiguous classifications.[1372]

6. Medications and other therapies that help migraineurs may similarly benefit patients diagnosed as having tension-type headaches.

These caveats to viewing tension-type headache as uniquely separate from migraine should cause diagnosticians to be skeptical when faced with written analyses of tension-type headaches and open-minded when examining patients presumed to suffer from them.

In contrast to claims of similarity between migraine and tension-type headaches, the International Headache Society promulgates what appear to be clear-cut criteria for tension-type headache[2203] (Table 5–1). And there are many patients who complain about a type of headache that meets these criteria. Individuals with such symptoms regularly describe their pain as a dull, aching sensation that feels as if a band were constricting their head. They commonly explain that their scalps are too tight, and that their heads seem to be squeezed in a vise or forced into a tight hat or headband.[700]

So-called tension-type headache pain is typically described as bilateral; more than half the patients claim it involves

the frontal, temporal, or frontotemporal regions.[704] But the pain may extend to the occipital region, and some patients provide accounts of occipital or occipitonuchal locations as the only site of pain. At times, however, the pain can—like many migraine attacks—be unilateral, and may even involve a localized area of the head. In other words, although a majority of patients have bilateral pain in the frontal or temporal area, location of the pain does not by itself identify this type of headache.

The pain is usually mild or moderate in intensity, characteristically waxing and waning throughout the entire day, and varying from day to day. It is not as intense as the pain associated with the usual case of migraine that brings a patient to a physician, and it is rarely severe enough to awaken a person from sleep. Patients generally describe tension-type headache pain as a steady ache or cramp, even though a throbbing component occurs in approximately one quarter of patients.[1179] But unlike the pain that characterizes migraine headaches, routine physical activity does not exacerbate the discomfort. And also in contrast to patients with migraine, most patients with tension-type headaches report few, if any, trigger factors other than emotional or psychological stress.

Some individuals with this type of headache complain of stiffness and tightness in the muscles of their necks. Neck discomfort often extends to the shoulders, involving the trapezius and even the upper back muscles. Scalp tenderness is frequently noted when combing or brushing hair. In addition, a sensation of tightness and aching in the face is a common complaint. Examination of the patient during a headache episode may not reveal any abnormalities. Tenderness of pericranial muscles, however, is a common finding, and appears similar to that seen in patients with migraine during an attack.[315,1185,1273] Passive and active movements of the neck may be limited as a result of marked cervical muscle contraction.

Table 5–1 DIAGNOSTIC CRITERIA FOR EPISODIC TENSION-TYPE HEADACHE

- Headache has at least two of the following characteristics:
  Pressing/tightening quality
  Mild to moderate intensity
  Bilateral location
  No aggravation by routine physical activity
- The following occur during headache:
  No nausea or vomiting
  Either photophobia or phonophobia
- Normal neurologic exam and no evidence of organic disease that could cause headaches

From the Headache Classification Committee of the International Headache Society.[917]

Tension-type headaches can be episodic (acute) or chronic. Episodic tension-type headaches are extremely common, consisting of recurrent bouts of headache that can last from minutes to days. These headaches are customarily mild, and are typically relieved by over-the-counter (OTC) analgesics. Most patients do not seek medical attention, nor do they lie down in quiet, dark rooms. As is the case with migraineurs, patients with episodic tension-type headaches ordinarily begin to suffer from them in adolescence or early adulthood.

In contrast to episodic bouts, chronic tension-type headache is unremitting. The pain has the distinction of being continuous for extended periods—for weeks, months, years, or even decades. It is noteworthy that many of the patients who develop chronic tension-type headaches begin as sufferers from intermittent attacks of migraine. After a period of years of intermittent but recurrent headache, they develop continuous pain with the characteristics of a tension-type headache. This phenomenon—the chronic daily headache syndrome—is considered in more detail in chapter 3. Again, as with migraine, women are afflicted with the problem more commonly than men.

The symptom that brings patients who presumably suffer from tension-type headaches to the doctor is probably the frequency or unremitting nature of the pain rather than its severity. In contrast, migraineurs with infrequent attacks often seek treatment if those infrequent attacks are very intense, whereas migraineurs with very frequent attacks may never see a physician if their attacks are less severe and respond reasonably well to OTC analgesics. The plethora of advertisements that focus on pounding headaches that upset one's stomach may lead many migraineurs to believe that such headaches are a normal part of life. Unless the bouts significantly interfere with functioning, this latter group may never mention them to a physician or may dismiss them during routine phys-

icals. In other words, physicians may be basing the distinctions between migraine and tension-type headaches on a skewed population: migraineurs who have severe attacks versus sufferers from tension-type headaches who have far less severe but very frequent attacks. If there were some way to factor in migraineurs who experience mild-to-moderate pain, we might find it far more difficult to distinguish these two afflictions.

In sum, the most striking difference between patients with chronic tension-type headache and most migraineurs is that the former have daily headaches—a pattern of suffering that distinguishes them from migraineurs, who endure clear-cut, severe, but discrete recurrent attacks of migraine. Some cases of *episodic* tension-type headache, however, can be exceedingly challenging to differentiate from common migraine—perhaps because they are different points on a single spectrum rather than different types of headache. After all, both groups of headaches may be recurrent, of long duration, nonthrobbing, bilateral, and of mild-to-moderate intensity. To complicate matters, either type can have throbbing pain. Both types can have associated nausea, photophobia, and phonophobia. Both can be associated with stiffness and tenderness of neck and shoulder musculature and with pericranial tenderness. At the extremes of the spectrum, migraine is easy to differentiate from tension-type headache. When the symptoms are more similar or overlap, the clinician may be presented with quite a challenge.

DISORDERS OF THE NECK, CRANIAL, AND EXTRACRANIAL STRUCTURES

Disorders of the Neck

In chapter 2, the issue was raised that pain in the cervical region could precipitate bouts of migraine in persons already vulnerable to the disorder. Migrainogenic pain of this sort is typically caused by cervical spine disease, myofascial syndromes involving the musculature of the neck and shoulders, or whiplash injury. In addition to triggering migraine attacks in susceptible individuals, degenerative or traumatic disease of the upper cervical spine, or myofascial syndromes, may cause a patient to develop associated, but non-migrainous head pain.[570]

Which of the various structures in the neck is the source of the pain remains a matter of dispute. Many individuals with extensive degenerative alterations in the cervical spine do not suffer from head pain; others afflicted with unrelenting, severe pain in the head have only minor changes observed on imaging studies. Accordingly, it is usually difficult to assert that a headache does, in fact, emanate from the cervical spine. Nonetheless, headaches associated with disorders of the neck have a number of properties that point to a source in the cervical spine or in surrounding soft tissues.[108,567,917] Among these symptoms are protracted neck and suboccipital or occipital pain; localized neck tenderness; a relationship between the headache and neck movement, specific cervical maneuvers, or sustained neck posture; resistance to, or restriction of, cervical movements; abnormal postures of the head and neck; intensification of the pain by deep, suboccipital pressure; and evidence from physical or radiologic examination of degeneration, or of injury to the cervical vertebrae or soft tissues.

Patients with cervical spondylosis or disk disease in the upper cervical spine often experience pain in their necks, shoulders, and heads. So do patients with anomalies or tumors of the craniovertebral junction, cervical canal stenosis, and cervical spine neoplasms. Those who suffer with pain from one of this group of disorders typically have abnormal findings on the neurologic examination.

But from whatever causes, pain associated with cervical disorders is characteristically constant and usually asymmetric. Most often, patients experience dull, aching discomfort, which may be confused with tension-type headaches. When intense, the pain can be referred to the forehead, orbits, or temples.[244] Some few patients have throbbing headaches, which may be construed as migraine. The presence of cervical features, however, should clarify the diagnosis.

MYOFASCIAL SYNDROMES

A myofascial trigger point in the musculature of the head, neck, or shoulders often produces pain that is referred to some area of the head. Such trigger points are most often located in the masseter, temporalis, pterygoid, splenius capitis, sternocleidomastoid, and trapezius muscles.[2030] In particular, trigger points in the trapezius muscle lead to temporal, frontal, or occipital headaches. These headaches are often misdiagnosed as "atypical" migraine.

Myofascial pain syndromes (as discussed in chapter 2) are characterized by circumscribed, exceedingly sensitive trigger points that produce localized or regional areas of dull, deep, aching pain.[1855,2032] The pain does not follow a radicular or peripheral nerve pattern, even though it may be perceived at a considerable distance from the trigger point.[696] The patterns of pain referral from trigger points have been well documented.[2032] Myofascial pain ranges from low-grade to incapacitating, and can be constant or intermittent in nature. For some patients, the pain exists at rest; for others, it emerges only when they move in particular ways. This syndrome should be easy to differentiate from migraine: myofascial pain characteristically occurs daily and is always associated with trigger points. Unlike migraine, it is rarely throbbing or associated with nausea or photophobia.

WHIPLASH INJURY

Whiplash or similar cervical injury may cause acute occipital and cervical aching together with limitation of cervical movement. Although these symptoms usually persist for days, chronic pain and stiffness lasting months or even years have been frequently reported. Some patients develop daily, dull, aching headaches accompanied by cervical pain, muscular tenderness, and limitation of movement of the neck. Unlike migraine, nausea, vomiting, and photophobia are not typical features. For further details about whiplash injury, see chapter 2.

CERVICOGENIC HEADACHE

A syndrome known as *cervicogenic headache* has become a fashionable diagnosis in Europe.[687,1863,1864] The syndrome is characterized by strictly unilateral, frontotemporal headaches. All episodes in an individual are confined to the same side of the head.[687,1864] The attacks are provoked by particular neck movements, coughing, sneezing, or pressure on tender spots in the neck. The latter are said to be located over the C-2 root, over the great occipital nerve, or over the transverse processes of C4-5. Signs and symptoms of cervical involvement, such as neck stiffness, pain, and restricted range of motion, are customary. Ipsilateral shoulder, arm, or hand pain can also be present. So-called cervicogenic headaches are infrequent, but when they do occur, they usually last for 1 to 3 days. The autonomic nervous system is often involved; accordingly, lacrimation, conjunctival injection, and rhinorrhea may occur on the side of the headache. During severe attacks, migrainous phenomena such as nausea, vomiting, phonophobia, and photophobia can develop.

The structures in the neck responsible for this kind of headache have not been specified. As indicated above, the symptoms of cervicogenic headache can be triggered by pressure on certain points in the neck or by cervical movement.[1580,1864] It is possible that pain referred from active myofascial trigger points located in cervical soft tissues is responsible for the clinical picture.[1024] Other possible causes of these headaches include C2-3 intervertebral disk injuries or dysfunction of the upper cervical synovial joints.[227] In this context, many patients with cervicogenic headaches have a history of trauma involving the neck, even though objective reports verifying changes in the cervical spine are sparse.

Cervicogenic attacks are considered headaches of cervical origin. However, the symptoms in many patients are very difficult, if not impossible, to differentiate from the symptoms of common migraine headaches.[1863] Moreover, many of the characteristics of cervicogenic headache, such as tenderness of neck muscles or limitation of neck movement, occur in patients with other headache syndromes. As a result, the diagnosis of cervicogenic headache should only be considered after all other causes of headache have been excluded. And because the diagnosis, although fashionable in Europe, is not popular in the United States, it is not often made. Instead, patients with this group of findings are more likely thought to be suffering from migraine, cervical spine disease, or myofascial syndromes.

Temporomandibular Joint Dysfunction

Disorders of the temporomandibular joint (TMJ) and the associated muscles of mastication are recognized as major sources of orofacial pain and headache.[811,849] TMJ pain and dysfunction result from two distinct entities: oromandibular dysfunction and temporomandibular joint disease. *Oromandibular dysfunction (myofascial pain–dysfunction syndrome, temporomandibular joint pain dysfunction syndrome, Costen's syndrome, craniomandibular dysfunction)* is primarily associated with pain of myofascial origin. One or more trigger points are thought to be present in the muscles of mastication. A number of etiologic components have been implicated in the syndrome. These include psychophysiologic factors such as stress and depression, malocclusion, misalignment of the jaws, habitual parafunction of the jaws (clenching and grinding of teeth, bruxism, fingernail biting, jaw posturing, frequent gum chewing, cheek biting), and abnormal head and neck posture.[766,926,1432,1740] The other TMJ disorder, *temporomandibular joint disease,* is caused by organic, intra-articular pathology. Intra-articular abnormalities include internal derangements of the articular disk, degenerative joint disease, traumatic or congenital lesions, inflammation, or other organic diseases that cause ankylosis and chronic dislocation. In addition, prolonged pathophysiologic disturbances of the muscles of mastication with persistent muscle spasm or continued jaw function with the condyle in an abnormal position may cause degenerative, structural changes in the TMJ.[2025]

The following signs and symptoms may be present in either form of TMJ dysfunction:

1. Recurrent pain, localized in the region of the TMJ; i.e., in the preauricular area, the mandible, or in the muscles of mastication. The latter muscles may feel tight after prolonged chewing. Patients commonly complain of deep ear pain or of pain spreading throughout the maxilla and mandible. Some individuals also experience neck pain and stiffness. The pain is frequently unilateral, but can be bilateral and involve both sides of the face or in both temples.[155,1661,2112] Wherever the pain is located, however, it is usually of moderate intensity, described as a persistent dull ache that often has a boring or gnawing quality. The pain seems to develop spontaneously, but is usually augmented by chewing, talking, or yawning. Its temporal pattern varies—some individuals endure their most intense pain in the morning, others in the afternoon, and still others have no fixed pattern.[1575]

2. Muscle tenderness when palpated. In particular, the masseter, temporalis, lateral pterygoid, sternocleidomastoid, and other neck muscles are involved.[1816]

3. TMJ tenderness.

4. Limited interincisal opening as a result of muscle spasm and fatigue, or as a result of a displaced joint meniscus. The inability to open the jaws can vary from a limitation of only a few millimeters to complete incapacity to separate the teeth. An opening of fewer than 40 mm is judged abnormal.

5. Lateral deviation of the jaw from the midline during opening. The shift of the mandible from the midline as the jaw opens can range from a barely detectable deviation to several millimeters.

6. Clicking of the joint during movement. Because 35% to 40% of normal adults have clicking sounds in the TMJ, this finding can only be used as a secondary diagnostic criterion.[719,2111] If no other symptoms are present, cases with joint sounds require no treatment.

7. Locking of the jaw.

Other symptoms include tinnitus or other vague ear symptoms and a sensation that one's bite is different. In addition, somatic and emotional changes are often associated with TMJ dysfunction.[718] Patients frequently complain of altered sleep patterns, fatigue, anxiety, and depression. In sum, the character and typical location of the pain, and the findings on examination of the jaw, together with the absence of nausea, vomiting, photophobia, and other usual symptoms, should be sufficient to differentiate TMJ dysfunction from migraine.

Trigeminal Neuralgia

Trigeminal neuralgia (tic douloureux) is characterized by brief episodes of severe, jabbing pains that radiate through the mandibular or maxillary divisions of the trigeminal nerve. Trigger zones are typically located around the nares and the mouth, prompting an attack when excited by even trivial stimuli. The characteristic temporal pattern of attacks make them easily distinguishable from migraine.

Ophthalmologic Headaches

The eyes are often indicted as sources for headache. Quite apart from actual pathology, many people are convinced that headaches are caused by reading in poor light, by reading in the wrong position, or even by reading too much. As far as medical facts are concerned, the frequency of headaches produced by primary disorders of the eye is certainly overestimated. But when a headache is actually attributable to an ocular or orbital cause, the patient's history and physical examination is almost always incompatible with migraine. It is true that bouts of classic migraine are often preceded by visual phenomena, and that migrainous pain is often located in or around the eye. Nevertheless, migraine headaches are quite different from ophthalmologic headaches or head pain. Unlike migraine, the pain caused by an ophthalmologic problem is correlated with use of the eyes or with apparent physical signs of ocular disease.

Eyestrain (asthenopia) arises from uncorrected refractive errors or from disturbances of ocular alignment (heterophoria). Many patients believe that either of these two conditions can be the basis for recurrent head pain. Eyestrain, however, is an infrequent cause of headache. It is possible for eyestrain to produce a feeling of heaviness or a mild, dull, aching pain around or behind the eyes that may radiate to the forehead and temples.[2026] But despite pain around the eyes or in the temples, eyestrain is not associated with symptoms characteristic of migraine—such as throbbing pain, photophobia, nausea, or vomiting.

Chronic glaucoma may cause severe, recurrent periorbital pain or a persistent, low-grade diffuse headache. Intermittent blurring of vision is common, but is dissimilar to the visual abnormalities that often precede attacks of migraine with aura. The impaired vision of chronic glaucoma lasts longer than the brief, blurred, or foggy vision that may be part of a migrainous aura. When the affected eye of a patient with chronic glaucoma is examined, there may be no overt findings. After several attacks, however, the optic nerve head may be pale and show cupping. A diagnosis of chronic glaucoma is established by tonometry.

In contrast to chronic glaucoma, acute narrow-angle glaucoma (angle-closure glaucoma) may be accompanied by acute pain and severe, generalized headache owing to a sudden rise in intraocular pressure. The condition occurs in middle-aged or elderly individuals who are anatomically predisposed to crowding of the anterior segment of the eye.[1277] Acute glaucoma can cause excruciating, prostrating eye and orbital pain, often accompanied by nausea, vomiting, and photophobia. The pain may involve the forehead and temple on the side of the affected eye. Vision can blur and fade, and a complaint of colored halos around lights is common. The nausea, vomiting, photophobia, and disturbances of vision may mimic a migraine attack, but careful physical examination should enable differentiation of the two conditions. Thus, in patients with acute narrow-angle glaucoma, the cornea may appear cloudy or gray because of edema, the pupil is often fixed to light and mid-dilated, and the conjunctiva appears red and inflamed. Minimal ocular compression demonstrates a hard rigid globe and intensifies the ocular and periocular pain.

Inflammatory disorders of the iris, ciliary body, and choroid—such as anterior uveitis–iritis and posterior uveitis–choroiditis—can cause head pain centered around the eye. The inflammation causes a dull, frequently severe, occasionally throbbing pain in and around the eye. The pain is usually persistent, although it typically fluctuates in intensity. Patients also experience sensitivity to light, blurring of vision, burning, and tearing.[149] Physical examination reveals findings quite unlike those seen in patients with migraine. The pupil is constricted because of spasm of the iris sphincter. The eye is red and tender to palpation.

Optic neuritis is another condition that may cause eye or orbital pain. Like the previous problems, its symptoms are also easily differentiated from migraine, both by history-taking and examination. Optic neuritis causes blurring or loss of vision in addition to pain. In some cases diagnosis is complicated because the pain precedes the visual symptoms by several days. The pain is usually located in, behind, or around the eye. Customarily the patient reports that the pain is increased by extreme movement of the globe. The eye and periorbital regions may be tender to mild pressure.

Sinusitis

An extraordinary number of patients complain of "sinus trouble," strongly convinced that their recurrent headaches are caused by chronic sinusitis.[188] Despite the strength of their convictions, most of these patients have inaccurate perceptions—partly the result of advertising media, which oversell so-called "sinus medications." Daily exposure to misleading advertising reinforces the belief many patients already have that all pains located in the frontal or periorbital regions are "sinus headaches." In reality, many are suffering from migraine associated with nasal congestion caused by turbinate swelling. But because many of these patients respond to "sinus medications" (which usually incorporate analgesics and decongestants), all too often they cannot be dissuaded from their convictions that they have sinus headaches.

Chronic sinusitis is an infrequent cause of headache or face pain. When it does cause headache, the pain is characterized by a dull ache or a feeling of pressure either over the affected sinus or over the midface. These symptoms are accompanied by intermittent nasal congestion and obstruction. Thick postnasal secretions are nearly always present. Because the pain is rarely throbbing, and because photophobia, nausea, and vomiting are unusual, differentiating chronic sinusitis from migraine should cause little difficulty.

Acute sinusitis can cause intense frontal or cheek pain. The pain is usually constant, dull, and aching, although occasionally it is throbbing or sharp. The pain is located over, or in the area of, the acutely inflamed sinus, but may radiate to other areas of the head, face, or neck—for example, around or behind the eyes, in the maxillary teeth, and in the vertex, temporal, or parietal areas of the cranium. Characteristically, the pain associated with acute sinusitis is augmented by bending forward, jarring the head, and straining. Fever, purulent nasal or postnasal discharge, productive cough, and pharyngitis are typical accompaniments. Percussion or digital pressure over the involved sinuses will produce discomfort or intensify the pain. Pathological findings on a computed tomographic (CT) scan or sinus x-rays confirm the diagnosis. This condition most often develops when the patient has an acute viral or bacterial upper respiratory infection. Acute sinusitis, however, has been documented in association with allergy, swimming, flying, dental repair, or trauma. Given its characteristics, there is little likelihood that acute sinusitis will be misdiagnosed as migraine.

CLUSTER HEADACHES

Cluster headache *(migrainous neuralgia, Horton's headache, histomic cephalgia, sphenopalatine neuralgia, vidian neuralgia, Sluder's neuralgia)* derives its name from the unique pattern of headaches: attacks occur frequently for weeks or months, but are separated by periods of remission that usually last months or even years. The clusters of headaches vary in duration. They usually last for a month or two, although some continue for 3 months or even longer.[1145,1173,1298] Most patients have one cluster of attacks per year. About 10% of patients suffer from chronic symptoms without any periods of remission—for them, "cluster headache" is a cruelly inaccurate designation.

During a cluster period, one or more attacks can occur daily.[1298] In the majority of cases the frequency ranges from fewer than one to as many as three per day, although a patient may be symptom-free for 2 or 3 days in a row. Some more unfortunate patients may have seven or eight bouts of head pain in a 24-hour period. Attacks can occur at any time of the day or night; nocturnal events are frequent.[1715] A typical attack lasts from 15 minutes to 3 hours. There is a predilection for the longer attacks to occur among women rather than among men.[1145] In contrast to migraine, only exceptionally does a bout of cluster headache last longer than 3 hours.[1173] However, documentation does reveal a range from between 5 minutes and 2 days.[819,1974]

The description of a cluster headache differs markedly from that of a migraine headache (Table 5–2). There is no prodrome or aura in cluster headaches.

Table 5–2 DIAGNOSTIC CRITERIA FOR CLUSTER HEADACHE

- At least five attacks
- Severe, unilateral orbital, supraorbital, or temple pain that lasts for 15–180 min
- Headache is associated with at least one of the following signs:
    Conjunctival injection
    Lacrimation
    Nasal congestion
    Rhinorrhea
    Forehead and facial sweating
    Miosis
    Ptosis
    Eyelid edema
- A frequency of attacks from one every other day to eight per day
- Normal neurologic exam and no evidence of another organic disease that could cause headaches

From the Headache Classification Committee of the International Headache Society.[917]

The pain is customarily of a nonpulsating type.[1173] It is typically specified as "deep," but patients use terms such as "boring" "squeezing," "pressing," "lancinating" "searing," "burning," "stabbing," "tearing," or "piercing," to describe the pain.[980,1173,1298] The intensity of pain is excruciating—usually said to be unbearable. It is considered much more severe than the pain of a typical migraine attack.

Cluster headache pain is unilateral in location. In a small number of patients, the side may change from one cluster period to another and, exceptionally, there are shifts from one side to the other during a single cluster period.[1145] Principally the pain affects the area in and around the orbit or the temple, but it may also begin in the face.[1298] The pain may spread to neighboring cranial and cervical regions such as the frontal area, cheek, mandibular angle, upper jaw, roof of the mouth, teeth, back of the neck, suboccipital area, and the front of the neck along the course of the carotid artery.[1145,1974] Occasional patients find that the pain affects the ear and the ipsilateral shoulder and arm. In addition, patients may note that some residual soreness in the area affected by the pain can persist for some time after an attack.

The pain is characteristically accompanied by supplemental symptoms and signs that indicate involvement of the autonomic nervous system on the side of the head pain.[542] These phenomena include conjunctival injection, lacrimation, nasal congestion, rhinorrhea, forehead and facial sweating, miosis, ptosis, and eyelid edema. Some few patients also develop symptoms commonly seen in migraineurs. Thus, photophobia can accompany attacks of cluster headache, although there is disagreement about its frequency, which is reported to vary between 5% and 72%.[1145,1974] Nausea can also occur, but again, there is no accord about the frequency (5.5% to 54%).[1145,1298] Vomiting is rare. The only focal neurologic manifestation of cluster headache is Horner's syndrome. This is generally transient, but after repeated attacks it may become permanent.[1457] The neurologic examination is otherwise normal.

The behavior of most patients during a cluster headache is very different from that of patients with migraine.[1145] Migraineurs typically wish to lie still in a quiet, dark room. The patient in the throes of a cluster headache is typically restless. Sufferers usually cannot bear to lie or sit still; instead they pace or walk about. Some patients are frankly agitated and may moan, cry, or even scream.[1298]

Cluster headaches may develop at any age, but the onset is generally in the second or third decades of life.[1145,1974] They are seen in children, and an onset after age 65 is not uncommon.[1135] In contrast to migraine, between 70% and 93% of patients are men.[1862]

Many men afflicted with cluster headaches have distinctive facial features.[818,820] Hazel eye color is common. The skin on their faces is characteristically thick, coarse, and markedly wrinkled, especially on the forehead. Often the facial skin has a pitted *peau d'orange* (orange peel) appearance or is telangiectatic. A plethoric appearance may be present. The men frequently have broad chins and skulls. These facial characteristics have been designated as "leonine."[820] In addition, the patients are often tall, well-built, and athletic in appearance.

In the vast majority of cases, cluster headache is easy to differentiate from migraine provided one takes an adequate history. Although, as in migraine, nausea and photophobia can accompany cluster headaches, most clinicians report these as infrequent occurrences. Other characteristics, however, provide clear contrast between migraine and cluster headache. The unique temporal pattern of attacks, the lack of a prodrome or aura, the severity of the pain, the behavior of patients during attacks, the obvious involvement of the autonomic nervous system—and often the patient's appearance—should readily allow one to make the diagnosis of cluster head-

ache. But all too often, appropriate questions regarding these phenomena are not asked and the patient goes misdiagnosed.

Paroxysmal Hemicrania

Paroxysmal hemicrania is an extremely rare disorder. Such attacks have pain characteristics, and associated autonomic symptoms and signs, similar to those of cluster headache.[1859,1861,1862] Paroxysmal hemicrania differs from cluster headache, however, in the shorter duration and greater frequency of the attacks. Bouts of paroxysmal hemicrania generally last between 5 and 30 minutes, and occur with a frequency greater than five a day. They may return as often as 30 times in a day.[70] And in contrast to cluster headaches, women are more frequently affected than men. Most cases are chronic (*chronic paroxysmal hemicrania*), although some patients have episodic hemicrania.[216] Indomethacin produces a dramatic response in all cases, and may therefore be used as therapeutic confirmation of the diagnosis.

UNRUPTURED ARTERIOVENOUS MALFORMATIONS AND MIGRAINOUS AURAS

The prevalence of migraine among patients with arteriovenous malformations (AVMs) is controversial. Although it is not often that one finds vascular headache accompanied by visual hallucinations (auras) of the migrainous type as the *sole* manifestations of an AVM, some consider migrainous auras to be frequent symptoms of occipital AVMs.* When such visual phenomena do occur in a patient with an AVM, they do not usually conform to the pattern,

---

*References 269, 852, 1401, 1807, 2039, 2097.

timing, appearance, and development expected of typical migrainous scintillations.[2039] The auras may follow the onset of headache, may be either fleeting or excessively prolonged, or may be restricted to a particular part of the visual field rather than spreading progressively across the visual field as they do before a migraine headache. In other words, although migraine and AVMs may sometimes coincide, more often it is relatively easy to distinguish them if a careful history is taken. On the other hand, convincing bouts of classic migraine have been reported to cease after excision of occipital AVMs.[1532,2038]

HEADACHES ASSOCIATED WITH HEAD TRAUMA

Between one third and one half of all patients who suffer head trauma develop headaches.[798] They typically emerge within 24 hours of the head injury, but can develop some days or weeks afterward.[463,1021] The headaches customarily become more intense for a period of days to weeks, and then progressively improve. Many patients, however, are left with head pain that lasts for years or even decades. Nor does the severity of the head injury determine the severity of the headache. Severe headache can follow even trivial head trauma. And because post-traumatic headache does not appear to be a single entity, it can take one of several forms:

1. *Tension-type headache.* The most frequently seen post-traumatic headache resembles tension-type headaches.[463] It is characterized by constant, non-throbbing, dull, diffuse, or bilateral discomfort.

2. *Migraine.* Although controversy exists with regard to its incidence, post-traumatic headaches in some patients have the features of migraine headaches.[150,280,1379,2122] In fact, a number of individuals who suffer from migraine are convinced they can identify an episode of head trauma that preceded their first attack.[205] Sometimes, particularly among children, a migraine attack emerges following a sudden cranial jolt or impact. This kind of attack can be accompanied by severe, but transient neurologic symptoms such as hemiparesis, somnolence, blindness, and brain stem signs.[853]

3. *Mixed headaches.* A number of patients may develop the combined symptoms of a daily tension-type headache with superimposed, distinct episodes of migraine.

4. *Cluster headaches.* About 10% of patients have a syndrome that seems to have all of the characteristics of cluster headache.[1660]

5. *Localized discomfort.* There are individuals who suffer from post-traumatic head pain characterized by localized discomfort that possesses a jabbing or neuralgic quality. At times, throbbing can occur. It is assumed that some of these problems result from entrapment of afferent nerve endings in scar tissue developing at the site of injury.

No matter what the type, post-traumatic headaches are often accompanied by a group of assorted symptoms that are relatively consistent, although they may vary considerably in severity among patients.[574] The collection of symptoms is either referred to as the *post-traumatic syndrome* or as the *postconcussion syndrome.*[619] Symptoms include true vertigo, non-specific dizziness, tinnitus, personality disturbances, depression, anxiety, irritability, apathy, cognitive symptoms such as impairment of memory and reduced attention span, insomnia, daytime sleepiness, easy fatigability, decreased libido, blurred vision, and intolerance to alcohol. Such symptoms usually develop within 24–48 hours after the trauma, but they may be delayed for many days. Unfortunately, the symptoms may persist for months or even years. Loss of consciousness, increased intracranial pressure, or electroencephalographic EEG changes during or following the original head trauma do not have to occur for the postconcussion syndrome to develop.

GIANT CELL ARTERITIS

Giant cell arteritis (temporal arteritis) is an inflammatory disease of the cranial arteries whose most common symptom is headache. In contrast to migraine, which most frequently develops before age 40, this condition almost always occurs in individuals older than age 50 years, affecting women more frequently than men.[806]

About three quarters of patients have scalp arteries (usually the superficial temporal artery) that are exquisitely tender to pressure, and that are swollen and cordlike to palpation. Impressive redness and swelling may overlay the branches of the superficial temporal artery on one or both sides. In addition, pulsation may be absent in distal branches, although it is usually possible to feel a pulse in the main trunk of the temporal artery.

The pain of giant cell arteritis is frequently felt in the scalp, especially over inflamed vessels. It usually involves one or both temporal regions, although it can occur in any region of the head.[1900] No specific quality characterizes the pain of this disease: it may be aching or boring, or even sharp in nature. Lancinating ice-pick pains have also been reported.[865] Throbbing may be present at first, but this symptom typically attenuates or even ceases after the early phase of the disease. Some patients describe a burning sensation—a feature most unlike other headaches that involve blood vessels. The headache of giant cell arteritis may be persistent or intermittent, but whatever form it takes, without treatment the headache tends to progress steadily over a prolonged course of months.

Visual changes can be an initial symptom of temporal arteritis. More often, however, they appear later in the course of the illness. When the visual symptoms do develop, it is with rapidity—over a period of minutes to hours. The usual cause of this problem is ischemic damage to the optic nerve and retina on one or both sides. Older studies reported that visual loss in untreated patients had a frequency up to 50%. In more recent investigations, the incidence is usually reported to be much lower—between 7% and 21%. The reduction in frequency is presumably a function both of earlier diagnosis and of effective treatment.

Polymyalgia rheumatica is frequently associated with giant cell arteritis.[918] Systemic signs and symptoms such as low-grade fever, malaise, anorexia, fatigue, night sweats, and weight loss may be part of the clinical picture.[300] Patients with polymyalgia rheumatica also complain of joint stiffness, and of muscular aching affecting the shoulders, neck, and hips. Their muscles may be tender and sometimes slightly weak. Atrophy, however, is unusual. These systemic symptoms may precede the headache of giant cell arteritis by several months.[900]

Another muscular problem that has been linked to temporal arteritis is jaw claudication. A history of jaw claudication is unusual among the general population, but is almost pathognomonic of giant cell arteritis.[982] This phenomenon consists of ischemic pain felt in the masticatory muscles when the patient chews; the pain is relieved by rest.

Frequently, the erythrocyte sedimentation rate (ESR) is strikingly elevated during the active phase of the disease. The mean elevation is 100 mm/hr. In 30% of cases, however, the ESR is below 40 mm/hr. And well-documented cases of giant cell arteritis with normal ESRs have also been seen.[2171]

In sum, giant cell arteritis can be clinically differentiated from migraine by several factors: advanced age at onset, the constant and usually progressive nature of the head pain, findings of inflammation of the temporal artery, frequent history of systemic symptoms, and elevated ESR. Confirmation is obtained by histopathologic examination of biopsy material from the temporal artery. When treated with steroids, the headache of giant cell arteritis usually recedes within 48 hours (Table 5–3).

Table 5–3 DIAGNOSTIC CRITERIA FOR GIANT CELL ARTERITIS

- One or more of the following:
  Swollen and tender scalp artery
  Elevated erythrocyte sedimentation rate
  Disappearance of headache within 48 h of steroid therapy
- Temporal artery biopsy showing giant cell arteritis

From the Headache Classification Committee of the International Headache Society.[917]

BENIGN INTRACRANIAL HYPERTENSION

Headaches that are occasionally difficult to differentiate from migraine can be caused by benign intracranial hypertension (pseudotumor cerebri, idiopathic intracranial hypertension, otitic hydrocephalus, serous meningitis, meningeal hydrops). This condition is characterized by increased intracranial pressure in the absence of focal lesions, hydrocephalus, intracranial infection, or hemorrhage.[1888]

As many as 94% of patients with benign intracranial hypertension complain of headache. Accordingly, headache is the most commonly reported symptom.[765,1051,1701,2121] Although the headache is usually generalized, some patients suffer from bitemporal, occipital, or even unilateral headaches. The character of the head pain also varies. In general, the pain is constant and relatively mild. Many patients, however, complain of throbbing head pain. But whichever kind of pain a patient suffers from, it is intensified by exertion, coughing, and straining, which raise intracranial pressure. In addition, the pain is frequently accompanied by nausea and vomiting. In view of this range of symptoms, an occasional patient who gives a history of throbbing headache with nausea and vomiting may appear to be a migraineur, when, in fact, benign intracranial hypertension is the cause of the symptoms. The question, then, is how does the clinician differentiate the former from the latter?

Most patients with benign intracranial hypertension have an additional symptom that distinguishes their condition from migraine; namely, gradually diminishing vision. This results from compression of optic structures, so that restricted peripheral visual fields, enlarged blind spots, visual blurring, and transient visual obscurations are produced. Papilledema is usually, but not always, present on funduscopic examination.[1918] In untreated cases one even sees hemorrhages and exudates. The results of neurologic examination are otherwise normal except for transient abducens palsy (Table 5–4).

The cerebrospinal fluid (CSF) does not have any chemical or cellular abnormalities, but the CSF pressure is elevated—usually in the range of 250–450 mm H_2O. Rare cases have normal resting CSF pressures, but continuous monitoring of such patients demonstrates transitory elevations of CSF pressure even when there is no activity or straining. For a diagnosis of benign intracranial hypertension to be made, neuroimaging studies should reveal no evidence of a mass lesion, ventricular enlargement, or venous sinus thrombosis.

Benign intracranial hypertension frequently occurs in overweight adoles-

Table 5–4 DIAGNOSTIC CRITERIA FOR BENIGN INTRACRANIAL HYPERTENSION

- Fulfills following criteria:
  Increased intracranial pressure (>200 mm H_2O)
  Normal neurologic exam except for papilledema and cranial nerve VI palsy
  No mass lesion or ventricular enlargement on neuroimaging
  Normal or low CSF protein concentration and normal cell count
  No evidence of venous sinus thrombosis
- Headache intensity related to variations of intracranial pressure

From the Headache Classification Committee of the International Headache Society.[917]

cent girls and in young women of child-bearing age.[1888] Although the condition may mimic migraine in some few patients, most patients have papilledema and should therefore cause no diagnostic difficulties. For those few patients without papilledema, the diagnosis may be more difficult. In these cases, the relative constancy of the headaches should alert the physician to look beyond migraine. So should a history lacking photophobia, phonophobia, and all of those symptoms that drive the typical migraineur to seek a quiet, dark room. Ultimately, however, diagnosis depends on CSF pressure examinations.

LOW CEREBROSPINAL FLUID PRESSURE

In contrast to the previous condition, headache can also be caused by low CSF pressure. The most common cause of low CSF pressure is leakage following a spinal puncture *(lumbar puncture headache)*. In that situation, the diagnosis is clear-cut. But an identical clinical picture can arise spontaneously *(primary intracranial hypotension, spontaneous intracranial hypotension)*.[1193] CSF can leak through the cribriform plate, the petrous bone, a basal skull defect, or a spontaneous tear in the spinal theca. When a leak develops through the cribriform plate or the petrous bone, the resultant CSF rhinorrhea or otorrhea may not be apparent to the patient. And when spinal thecal tear occurs, there may be no symptoms at all that the patient would be expected to notice. Accordingly, the etiology of the headache may be obscure, and from this point of view, diagnosis is made difficult. In terms of test findings, however, the CSF pressure is low—60 mm H_2O or less. The presence of a CSF leak may frequently be demonstrated by radionuclide cisternography.

Diagnosis of a low CSF pressure headache is first made clinically. In most cases the headache is dull, pulsating, and generalized, although it may be accentuated in the frontal or occipital regions. Neck stiffness, nausea, vomiting, tinnitus, and vertigo may be accompanying symptoms.[1627] The headache subsides after reclining or lying flat, but it is characteristically augmented by an erect position.[156,1994] This is the most telling symptom: headaches associated with low CSF pressure have such a characteristic relationship to position that the differentiation from migraine should cause few difficulties.

HYPERTENSION

Chronic, uncomplicated hypertension of a mild-to-moderate degree does not commonly result in headache.[97] In contrast, marked hypertension—when the diastolic blood pressure rises to more than 120 or 130 mm Hg—can cause headaches. Such levels of hypertension are usually seen in malignant (accelerated) hypertension associated with severe retinopathy. In these latter cases the resulting headache is temporally related to any rise in blood pressure and disappears within a few days after the blood pressure is lowered.

A hypertensive headache has no specific diagnostic features. Ordinarily it has a dull, throbbing quality, with generalized discomfort, although the occipital area may be a prominent site of head pain. This type of headache often develops or is most pronounced in the early morning, sometimes awakening the patient from sleep. Vomiting may also occur. The intensity lessens after 2 or 3 hours as the patient rises and starts to move about. Any undertaking, however, such as bending, stooping, coughing, or straining, which increases either the blood pressure or the intracranial pressure, may augment the headache. In sum, even though excessive hypertension has the capacity to cause headaches—some of which are accompanied by vomiting and worsen when the patient bends—there should be no problem in making a diagnosis. The height of the blood pressure and the lack of a typical migraineur's history clearly differentiate these two conditions.

Pheochromocytoma

Pheochromocytomas produce excessive amounts of pressor amines. The abnormally high levels of these amines cause abrupt rises in blood pressure, accompanied by headache and other dramatic symptoms. For many patients with these tumors, the precipitous and marked rise in blood pressure produces short-lasting, generalized, throbbing or pounding headaches that are alleviated as the hypertensive peak diminishes.[2015] During an attack, the patient may appear acutely ill—drenched in sweat, with cold extremities and dilated pupils. Especially severe episodes of headache may be attended by nausea, vomiting, tachycardia, palpitations, tremulousness, anxiety, and pallor.

The attacks of elevated blood pressure vary considerably in frequency, severity, and duration, depending on the patient. At least half of the headaches last less than 15 minutes, and the majority end within an hour.[2015] The headaches may occur without warning or may be precipitated by stimuli such as postural changes, physical exertion, or even emotional upsets. Headache associated with hypertension, palpitations, and diaphoresis strongly suggests the diagnosis of pheochromocytoma. This combination of symptoms should be sufficient to differentiate such headaches from migraine.

EXPANDING INTRACRANIAL LESIONS

Expanding intracranial lesions—tumors, abscesses, or hematomas—commonly produce headaches. Individuals with brain tumors report headaches as their primary symptom about 25% to 35% of the time. But despite these numbers, the majority of brain tumors call attention to themselves by other symptoms, whose prominence may mask the accompanying headache. Accordingly, headaches associated with intracranial masses typically increase in frequency and severity in parallel with the focal or generalized neurologic symptoms produced by the mass. If, for the purpose of this book, focus is placed on those patients whose intracranial lesions cause head pain, one usually finds it to be both modest and either episodic or transitory in nature. Some patients do experience pain that is persistent but easily relieved by OTC medications. Once the medication wears off, however, the head pain typically recurs. For other patients the discomfort is more severe, although rarely as intense as the head pain associated with a severe bout of migraine.[1712]

The headache associated with intracranial lesions usually has a deep, aching, steady, dull character. It may be intensified by coughing or straining, and is sometimes more severe when the patient is in an erect rather than in a recumbent position. For some patients the pain is worse in the early morning or even awakens them from sleep.[977] Most patients, however, experience their headaches at any time during the day or night.[977,1712]

The pain may be localized anywhere about the head. Supratentorial masses generally produce frontal or temporal head pain, whereas lesions in the posterior fossa characteristically cause occipitonuchal pain. When the headache is occipital or suboccipital, it is occasionally associated with stiff or aching neck muscles and tilting of the head toward the side of the tumor. Unless the pain is severe, nausea is usually slight. In children, however, vomiting is more frequent because many childhood tumors have a posterior location and so displace or compress the medulla.[977]

A mass that produces abrupt increases in intraventricular pressure can result in episodic headaches that can be confused with common migraine. Colloid cysts, intraventricular meningiomas, choroid plexus papillomas, and other intraventricular tumors can all generate this clinical picture.

These lesions can produce sudden, intense, bilateral headaches of great severity accompanied by nausea and vomiting, weakness of the legs, and possibly loss of consciousness. In a minority of cases, the pain is said to be both precipitated by, and relieved by, changes in posture.[1095,1258,1463] Vision may be blurred owing to the acute rise in intracranial pressure. Gait disturbances and papilledema sometimes occur. When this latter group of symptoms is present, there is no reason to consider migraine in the differential diagnosis.

Except for the masses mentioned in the previous paragraph, namely those that produce abrupt increases in intraventricular pressure, intracranial lesions do not usually cause episodic headaches that could be confused with classic migraine. Despite this general pattern, case reports have appeared indicating that brain tumors and other forms of intracranial pathology can mimic classic migraine.* Thus, migrainous auras have been described in patients with pituitary tumors, tumors of the lateral and third ventricle, and parasagittal tumors. Such cases are exceedingly rare, however, and their clinical descriptions of visual phenomena are so limited that it is difficult to determine whether or not the symptoms actually resemble migraine auras.[376,466,1776] Although some descriptions do appear to fulfill the International Headache Society criteria for migraine, the patients who experience them have headaches of recent onset.[1557] Differential diagnosis of this latter group, then, seems to depend on the migraineur's usually long-standing history of headache.

HEADACHES AS EMERGENCIES

Physicians commonly encounter patients suffering from acute headaches.

---

*References 1544, 1557, 1558, 1681, 1776.

Many of these patients are suffering from acute attacks of migraine, but in some cases there is reason to suspect an emergency. When this is so, appropriate diagnostic tests must be expeditiously performed and a diagnosis made as quickly as possible, because a delay may have disastrous consequences.

A thorough assessment is imperative under several circumstances (Table 5–5): when the patient complains that the headache: (1) is the first one of its kind, (2) is the most severe headache that he or she has ever had, or (3) represents a distinct change in the pattern of his or her usual recurrent headaches. Notice must be taken if a migraineur complains of new neurologic symptoms or is found to have focal neurologic signs. Particular attention is also necessary when any patient has signs of meningeal irritation, alterations either in mental status or in alertness, changes in the eye grounds, unexplained vomiting, or fever. A history of previous head trauma, a systemic malignancy, or bleeding disorder should suggest the possibility of serious intracranial pathology. These latter patients need an extensive neurologic evaluation, including CT scan or magnetic resonance imaging and lumbar puncture.

Table 5–5 SIGNS AND SYMPTOMS OF HIGH-RISK ACUTE HEADACHES

- Severe, crippling headache in a patient without a history of significant headaches
- Uncommon presentation of headache in a patient with a history of chronic headaches (e.g., unusual severity, precipitous onset, changed sensorium)
- Appearance of a new neurologic symptom
- Presence of a neurologic deficit
- Change in mental status
- Nuchal rigidity or other signs of meningeal irritation
- Alterations in the eye grounds, such as papilledema or hemorrhages
- Fever
- Unexplained vomiting
- History of head trauma, malignancy, or coagulopathy
- Precipitation of headache by exertion or coitus
- Excessive elevation of blood pressure

Headaches Associated with Aneurysms and AVMs

As a rule, unruptured intracranial aneurysms and AVMs are nonpainful and accordingly are not connected to long histories of frequent headaches. Evidence that unruptured AVMs and aneurysms cause chronic, recurrent headaches is for the most part anecdotal and retrospective. In contrast, there are trustworthy reports that aneurysms and AVMs in the head can produce pain. Frequently, such pain is associated with neurologic symptoms that develop if and when one of these lesions expands.

Acute or subacute headaches, however, are another matter. Among patients whose aneurysms rupture, between 30% and 60% experience the sudden onset of excruciating, generalized or hemicranial headaches (sentinel headaches) 1 or 2 days prior to aneurysmal rupture. Such headaches can even antedate the rupture of an aneurysm and the subsequent subarachnoid hemorrhage by several days—or even by weeks.* Whatever the time frame, these headaches persist until the actual rupture occurs. Subacute headache pain associated with an unruptured aneurysm has been ascribed to expansion of an aneurysm, to leaks that warn of impending hemorrhage, or to bleeding confined to the arterial wall. These headaches may be accompanied by nausea and vomiting, particularly if the lesion is located in the posterior fossa.[2084] Both acute and subacute pain, in the absence of rupture, may be challenging to differentiate from migraine, but the constancy of the headache is a major cue.

Rupture of either an AVM or an aneurysm produces an extremely intense headache, which is most likely to develop abruptly, although it may occasionally evolve incrementally over a period of several hours. The pain is reported to be extreme or cataclysmic. It is usually diffuse, but may become lateralized. A decreased level of consciousness, vomiting, seizures, and focal neurologic signs are common—their development depending on the locus of the rupture and on whether or not the rupture is accompanied by intracerebral hemorrhage. Examination of the patient may additionally show nuchal rigidity, and retinal or preretinal hemorrhages.

The seriousness of an acute rupture is obvious. Nor is the condition difficult to recognize. Lesser, noncatastrophic, subarachnoid hemorrhage from aneurysms or AVMs can present a greater diagnostic challenge. The symptoms may mimic migraine, producing a localized headache accompanied by nausea and vomiting. The absence of a history of migraine should cause the physician to look further. A CT scan that shows subarachnoid blood, and lumbar puncture that yields bloody spinal fluid will lead to the proper diagnosis. If, however, a long-time migraineur develops a noncatastrophic, subarachnoid hemorrhage with migraine-like symptoms, diagnosis is more problematic. In this case, the extraordinary severity of the head pain should provide the necessary clue for the physician to initiate the relevant diagnostic measures.

Thunderclap Headaches

Thunderclap headache is the term used to designate the sudden onset of a severe and unusual headache whose symptoms make it appear to be caused by a subarachnoid hemorrhage, even though the patient's CSF is clear and the CT scan shows no subarachnoid blood.[461,1306] Angiography in most patients with this type of headache does not show an aneurysm.[1306,2150] Seventeen percent experience recurrent thunderclap headaches.[2150] The characteristics of a thunderclap headache necessitate an emergency workup even though the data ultimately reveal that

---

*References 552, 1113, 1213, 1483, 2084.

there was no emergency. The cause of these headaches is obscure, but they are so unlike migraine that they should present no problem with regard to differential diagnosis.

Headaches Secondary to Meningeal Infection

Infection of the meninges is a source of acute, intense headache. Nuchal rigidity together with severe headache and fever are characteristic of meningitis. Most of the time the headache is generalized, but it sometimes predominates in frontal or occipital areas. The pain may extend into the neck and frequently also extends down the back. A change in the level of consciousness, photophobia, nausea, and vomiting are also typical of this condition. Viruses, bacteria, fungi, and the tubercle bacillus may be causative agents. Firm diagnosis rests on clinical evaluation and lumbar puncture.

Headaches Associated with Ischemic Vascular Disease

Headache is a common accompaniment of acute, ischemic cerebrovascular disease: ischemic stroke, cerebral embolism, intracerebral hemorrhage, and transient ischemic attacks (TIAs).[568,569,807,1601] Headache in patients with cerebrovascular disease typically signifies involvement of large vessels rather than small-vessel disease or lacunar infarction.[655,807] Episodic headaches may precede an ischemic ictus by days, weeks, or even months. In these cases diagnosis of headache is subject to uncertainty, especially when the patient has no previous history of an ischemic cerebral event.[569,807]

The headache pain in ischemic cerebrovascular disease is ipsilateral to the side of the involved blood vessels. The headaches are equally inclined to be rapid or gradual in onset. They frequently last minutes to hours, although on occasion they can last for days. The quality of the pain differs widely among patients. They are variously described as throbbing or steady, and range in severity from trivial to severe.[807,1601] In a manner similar to migraine, the headaches' intensity is increased by bending, straining, or jarring the head.[568] Vomiting is infrequent.

As far as differential diagnosis is concerned, many headaches associated with ischemic cerebrovascular disease are enough unlike migraine that they present no confusion. However, some older patients, either with no prior history of migraine or with a newly changed pattern of headaches, may describe episodic, throbbing headaches. These headaches may suggest migraine. The physician, therefore, must be cautious when evaluating older patients with new or recently altered headaches. Although migraine may emerge at any age, the first diagnosis that comes to mind in an elderly individual without antecedent attacks should not be migraine. Ischemic cerebrovascular disease should be ruled out.

Carotid and Vertebral Artery Dissection

Head pain together with focal ischemic neurologic deficits can result from carotid artery dissection.[658,2136] Dissection can occur either spontaneously or as a result of trauma to the head or neck. In addition to head pain, an ipsilateral Horner's syndrome and neck pain are frequently seen. The head pain typically precedes the neurologic deficit by as much as a week or two. It is hemicranial, located in orbital, periorbital, or frontal regions. This type of headache is usually slowly progressive and can be quite severe.[658] The pain can be either steady or throbbing. At times, patients may have several attacks of short-lasting, incapacitating head pain.[2136] Dissection of the vertebral arteries can cause pain in the upper neck or occiput. The pain is associated with signs of brain stem or cerebellar infarction. Because the pain caused by arterial dissection can mimic that of migraine, angiographic evidence that shows narrowing of the artery and findings consistent with dissection within the arterial wall are needed to establish a diagnosis.

Toxic Vascular Headaches

The phrase *toxic vascular headache* is applied to a headache caused by intense cerebral vasodilatation resulting from a high fever of any cause. Most such headaches appear as part of a systemic viral or bacterial infection, such as influenza or typhoid. The pain of toxic vascular headache is not distinctive. Patients describe it as dull, deep, and aching in quality. At times it may have a throbbing component. The pain is almost always bilateral, possibly localized to the frontotemporal regions of the head, the back of the head, or the occipitocervical region. Ocular or retroorbital pain worsened by eye movement is a characteristic accompaniment. Patients with toxic vascular headaches do not have classical signs of meningeal irritation, but they may have cervical myalgia or neck stiffness (meningismus) that limits neck movement. If the symptoms are severe enough to suspect bacterial meningitis, such patients must receive immediate investigation and urgent treatment.

SUMMARY

As the material reviewed in this chapter indicates, a number of clinical conditions produce symptoms that can be confused with those considered to be diagnostic of migraine. Some of these conditions, especially tension-type headaches, are intimately related to migraine. Others are the result of particular systemic or localized disease processes. Although the clinician making a diagnosis of migraine must be wary of a number of these conditions, a diagnosis of migraine can generally be made based almost entirely on a comprehensive and detailed history.

Part II

PATHO-PHYSIOLOGY OF MIGRAINE

Chapter 6

VASCULAR CHANGES AND THE AURA

CEREBRAL BLOOD FLOW
INTERICTAL CEREBRAL BLOOD
    FLOW
CHANGES IN CEREBRAL BLOOD
    FLOW DURING THE AURA
SPREADING OLIGEMIA DURING
    ATTACKS OF MIGRAINE WITH
    AURA
SPREADING DEPRESSION
ISCHEMIA AND VASOSPASM
CONTROL OF CEREBRAL
    CIRCULATION

The first comprehensive set of assumptions about the cause of migrainous symptoms resulted from the pioneering experimental efforts of Harold G. Wolff and his associates. Their speculations are well summarized in Wolff's 1963 monograph.[2167] Wolff hypothesized that vasoconstriction of intracranial vessels reduces blood flow, resulting in cerebral hypoxia. This cerebral hypoxia was thought responsible for the neurologic deficits that characterize migrainous auras. Wolff also assumed that vasodilatation of the cranial circulation follows the vasoconstriction, so that nerve endings in vascular walls are stretched, giving rise to the head pain of a migraine attack.[822,2045] The vasodilatation was conceived of as a reactive hyperemia generated by the preceding cerebral hypoxia. In sum, Wolff considered migraine to be a primary vascular problem.

Wolff's arguments in support of the vascular origin of migraine symptoms were based on indirect evidence because appropriate research techniques to study cerebral blood flow (CBF) directly were not available at the time. His observations included the following:

1. The visual auras of classic migraine transiently regressed when cerebral vasodilatation was induced by administration of amyl nitrate or by inhalation of a gas mixture containing 10% CO_2 and 90% O_2.[1301]

2. During the headache, the amplitude of the pulse of the superficial temporal artery increased, and concomitantly the throbbing or pounding quality of the pain in most attacks of migraine correlated with these increases in pulse amplitude.

3. Ergotamine, which reduced the pulsations of the superficial temporal artery, relieved the pain.[822]

Not all of these observations stand up under scrutiny. For example, in some of Wolff's recordings, the superficial temporal arterial pulsations are of equivalent amplitude both before and during a severe headache.[202] Nor have other investigators been able to verify a significant correlation between the magnitude of the temporal artery pulse and the intensity of head pain.[247] Moreover, the vascular theory of migraine fails to explain the genesis of prodromal events, many of which are likely to stem from central nervous system events. And, in addition, some of the drugs used successfully to treat migraine attacks have little or no effect on blood vessels.

Despite these caveats, Wolff's ideas dominated scientific analysis of the cause of migraine symptoms for many decades. And debate still rages over the validity of his beliefs; the status of his *primary vascular hypothesis* as the cause of migraine symptoms is uncertain. An alternative view—the so-called *primary neuronal hypothesis*—has been in competition with Wolff's for many years. This hypothesis posits that migraine is primarily a process originating in the brain parenchyma, and that any involvement of cephalic blood vessels is a secondary phenomenon. In the last decade or so, the primary neuronal hypothesis has risen in prominence, until it has come to dominate much present-day thinking about causation of migraine symptoms.

The primary neuronal hypothesis owes its present popularity to modern technology. New opportunities to investigate the role of vascular factors in migraine arose with the development of techniques to measure regional cerebral blood flow (rCBF)—CBF in discrete regions of the brain. Such methods are based on determining either regional cerebral uptake or estimating the clearance of radioisotopes. Measurements of rCBF furnish a potential method to delineate vascular abnormalities that occur during migraine. And, indeed, experimentation seeking to link migraine auras to changes in CBF has yielded some extremely interesting data. But just as Wolff's arguments require caveats, we must also examine the newer data critically.

First of all, it must be realized that there is no ideal method for measuring rCBF during acute, spontaneous migraine attacks, and it is often difficult to obtain repeated measurements during the course of any one experimentally induced attack.[691] Each of the methods of measuring CBF has disadvantages; the following sections will enumerate the more obvious ones. To our inability to obtain perfect measurements of CBF during spontaneous attacks of classic migraine, we must add disagreements over methods of analyzing the data. The same data analyzed two different ways can point in opposite directions. Fi-

nally, we must remain aware, as we think about the primary vascular hypothesis versus the primary neuronal hypothesis, that these two propositions are not necessarily competitors. Neither fully explains the aura, but they are not mutually exclusive. Indeed, there are indications that both vascular and neurogenic phenomena must be invoked to explain the large body of clinical and experimental observations about migraine attacks.

CEREBRAL BLOOD FLOW

CBF is usually expressed as a quotient whose numerator is cerebral perfusion pressure and whose denominator is cerebrovascular resistance. Cerebral perfusion pressure is taken as the difference between the systemic arterial pressure and the cerebral venous pressure. The cerebral venous pressure is normally very low when compared to the systemic arterial pressure, and for practical purposes the cerebral perfusion pressure can be considered as a function of the mean systemic arterial pressure. Determining cerebrovascular resistance is somewhat more complicated.

Measurements of rCBF provide data about the performance of only part of the cerebrovascular system—that part of the brain perfusion supplied by the cerebral precapillary resistance vessels, which provide the major resistance to blood flow. In most circulations the arterioles provide most of the resistance. But because large cerebral arterial branches are long, whereas cerebral arterioles are comparatively much shorter, large arteries may in fact account for a substantial portion of the vascular resistance in the brain. In the resting state, the large extracranial and surface vessels of the brain are estimated to constitute between 39% and 51% of the total cerebrovascular resistance. Under normal conditions, small vessels less than 400 μm in diameter account for the remaining resistance to flow. Debate exists, however, about the relative contributions of small and large arteries to resistance changes under various physiologic and pathologic conditions.[922,1815,1966] In addition, the cerebral circulation appears to lack the precapillary sphincters that are responsible for substantial resistance to blood flow in other circulations. Finally, although the meningeal circulation appears to have an abundance of arteriovenous shunts, the importance of such shunts for regulating CBF in the human carotid circulation is uncertain.[1050,1100,1703]

Radioactive Xenon (^{133}Xe) Methods

The tracer most widely used to measure CBF is the γ emitter ^{133}Xe. This inert gas can be inhaled or administered by either intravenous or intracarotid injection of a bolus of saline solution containing the radioisotope. When the ^{133}Xe arrives at the brain, it diffuses freely across capillary walls and rapidly dissolves in the brain tissue. Recirculation is assumed to be negligible. Subsequently, unlabeled arterial blood washes out (*clears*) the radioisotope from the tissue. The rate of clearance depends on the rate of cerebral perfusion. External measurements are made over the brain using one or more stationary scintillation detectors. An individual detector views a distinct region of the brain through a lead collimator. Only the superficial layers of the brain can be seen because ^{133}Xe photons have low energy. Those photons released in deeper layers are absorbed by overlying brain tissue to a considerable degree and do not reach the scintillation detectors.

The methods that use inhalation or intravenous injection of ^{133}Xe are noninvasive, but suffer from a number of technical shortcomings. These shortcomings derive from extracerebral con-

tamination caused by the presence of radioisotope in the cranial air passages (when inhalation is used) or by the labeling of soft tissues outside the cranial cavity, and to intracerebral contamination produced by scattered counts of radioactivity from the contralateral cerebral hemisphere.[233,692] All of these factors limit the accuracy of the measurements.

The injection of ^{133}Xe via the internal carotid artery reduces the problem of extracerebral contamination but the technique necessitates preparation. Moreover, the method is invasive, requiring the insertion of an indwelling catheter into the internal carotid artery. Puncture of the carotid artery appears to provoke migraine attacks in many migraine patients, particularly those who are prone to bouts of migraine with aura. Use of this method has, however, made it feasible to investigate CBF just before the onset of induced attacks, during the aura, and during the headache phase of an attack in an individual patient. These serial data are limited to one hemisphere labeled during a study.

Tomographic Evaluation

In humans, rCBF has been assessed tomographically via both single-photon emission computerized tomography (SPECT) and positron emission tomography (PET). As a result of its tomographic features, the SPECT technique permits visualization of rCBF in gray and white matter at several transverse levels. Early studies determined brain activity after inhalation or intravenous injection of ^{133}Xe. More recently, other SPECT tracers have been used, one of the most popular being ^{99m}Tc-HMPAO (^{99m}technetium-D,L-hexamethyl-propylene-amine-oxime). The latter has reasonable radiation characteristics for SPECT imaging, but it is firmly retained in the brain for several hours, so that serial studies are hard to perform. Complications resulting from radioactivity that emanates from extracerebral structures and from superimposition of different tissue layers are eliminated by SPECT techniques, but the spatial resolution is limited.

PET is a powerful technique for measuring changes in rCBF and in oxygen and glucose metabolism. But because of the cumbersome technology, it is exceedingly difficult to apply to the study of unpredictable, spontaneous bouts of migraine. It has been used in only a few patients, and unfortunately the findings have not appreciably added to our comprehension of the pathophysiology of migraine.

INTERICTAL CEREBRAL BLOOD FLOW

Although migraineurs have usually been considered to have normal cerebral perfusion between attacks, a number of conflicting reports have shown both increased blood flow (hyperperfusion) and decreased blood flow (hypoperfusion) in various brain regions.* By and large, the alterations in CBF are minor and are typcially less prominent in patients with common migraine than in those with classic migraine. One estimate is that one quarter of all patients show persistent changes in the posterior parts of the hemisphere usually involved during attacks of classic migraine.[693] It is unclear if the rCBF changes observed during interictal periods are the result of permanent neurologic dysfunction caused by repeated, transient episodes of reduced CBF, or if they reflect abnormal vascular regulation between attacks. As expected, a high proportion of patients with complicated migraine have reduced CBF in damaged regions of the brain thought responsible for the neurologic symptoms.[1773-1775]

CHANGES IN CEREBRAL BLOOD FLOW DURING THE AURA

Auras accompany headaches at one time or another in about 20% of adult migraineurs, even though most migraineurs with aura do *not* experience aura symptoms before every bout of migraine. It is conceivable, however, that the pathophysiologic occurrences responsible for the aura are present during all migraine attacks, but are not sufficiently intense to generate neurologic deficits in the majority of individuals. Should this prove true, the distinction between classic and common migraine would have to be replaced with a continuum based on the frequency, severity, and variety of aura symptoms.

If changes in rCBF are the basis for the neurologic deficits that characterize the aura of classic migraine, then such changes should correlate with the symptoms of the migraine attack. The earliest investigations of cerebral perfusion during spontaneous migraine attacks did indeed demonstrate significant decreases in rCBF during the aura and preheadache phases of the attack.[1471,1472,1871] Later studies also supported the view that rCBF is reduced during the aura in attacks of classic or complicated migraine.† Because of differences in methodology and inherent technical difficulties in studying acute migraine attacks, however, reports have varied with regard to both the frequency and the regularity of the changes in rCBF. Widespread reductions, bilateral reductions, and focal reductions of CBF have all been reported. Thus, when compiled, the results from a number of investigations imply that the association between focal symptoms and changes in CBF is *not* as clear-cut as had been thought. Even so, the results of rCBF studies have been

---

*References 1124, 1126, 1160, 1234, 1331, 1678, 1736, 1773–1775, 2135

†References 856, 1068, 1331, 1467, 1736, 1849, 1870

used to buttress the hypothesis that arterial vasospasm is the initial event in the genesis of the migrainous aura.

SPREADING OLIGEMIA DURING ATTACKS OF MIGRAINE WITH AURA

Although each method has limitations, techniques for measuring rCBF have progressed dramatically in the last two decades, especially with regard to the use of multiple scintillation detectors. These computerized, multi-detector systems now make it feasible to acquire very detailed accounts of the sequence and spatial qualities of vascular events in the brain during bouts of migraine. The most credible studies of CBF during attacks of migraine are those of Olesen and his colleagues in Copenhagen. Their investigations involve catheterization of a carotid artery—a technique that enables ^{133}Xe to be injected at the same time that rCBF is measured in 254 areas of one cerebral hemisphere. Almost all the attacks that Olesen's group studied were triggered by the procedure, and as a result they have been able to perform serial measurements and thereby to determine the progression of changes during migraine attacks.

Recorded changes in CBF have been documented at least 5–15 min before patients noted the first symptoms of the migrainous aura (Fig. 6–1).* These changes have consisted of unilateral rCBF reductions (hypoperfusion), which Olesen's group designated by the term *oligemia.* Oligemic changes appear to be restricted to the neocortex.[1203] The oligemic changes start posteriorly, but because the intracarotid injection method studies are confined to the vascular territory of the internal carotid artery, whether or not the CBF reductions are initiated in the occipital lobes has not been determined. When the area of hypoperfusion expanded during a study, aura symptoms usually ensued, but no consistent relationship could be demonstrated between reduction in CBF and the appearance of aura symptoms. Moreover, aura symptoms regularly disappeared by the time the reductions in CBF attained a maximum. In addition, the hypoperfused state often prevailed even though the patient had no residual neurologic deficits.[1204,1874] In fact, not only did the oligemia outlive the aura, but CBF reductions typically persisted for the first 4–6 hours of the attack.

When migraine attacks were induced and studied with the methods just described, data revealed that decrements in CBF encompassed the parietal, temporal, central, and posterior frontal regions of the cortex. In contrast, the

---

*References 1204, 1205, 1495, 1496, 1874

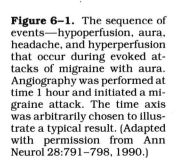

Figure 6–1. The sequence of events—hypoperfusion, aura, headache, and hyperperfusion that occur during evoked attacks of migraine with aura. Angiography was performed at time 1 hour and initiated a migraine attack. The time axis was arbitrarily chosen to illustrate a typical result. (Adapted with permission from Ann Neurol 28:791–798, 1990.)

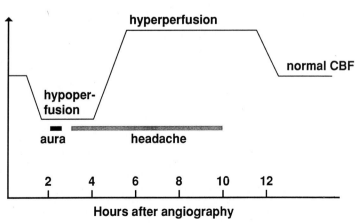

territory of the anterior cerebral artery was not typically involved. The decrease in rCBF began posteriorly, and appeared to spread anteriorly; the term *spreading oligemia (spreading hypoperfusion)* has been used to describe this phenomenon (Fig. 6–2). The reduced CBF has been estimated to move with a velocity of 2–3 mm/min and appears to transgress the vascular boundaries of the major cerebral arteries. This suggests that the reduced flow results from constriction of arterioles rather than from a process involving the large arterial vessels. The data also appear to show that major cytoarchitectonic boundaries or major foldings of the brain (such as the lateral and central sulci) constrained progression of the hypoperfusion. On occasion, a short-lasting, focal hyperperfusion (hyperemia) was seen in the initial stages of the attack before the oligemia was noted.[695,1496] The hyperemia appears to arise posteriorly, presumably in the occipital area, and to spread forward. Its significance is unclear because it has not been seen in all patients.

Olesen and his colleagues have stressed the point that the CBF reduction is modest—on average to a level of 40 mL/100 g/min—and well above the threshold for ischemia. They considered the magnitude of the reduction insufficient to explain the development of focal neurologic symptoms.

Vascular reactivity to various stimuli during migraine attacks has been studied by a number of investigators, including the Copenhagen group. The cerebral vasodilator response to changes in P_{CO_2} is impaired during the aura.[1737,1849] Such an impairment may be limited to hypoperfused areas of the brain.[1205] Some investigators found a reduced response of cerebral vessels to

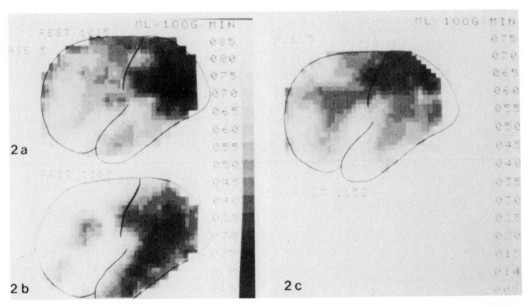

Figure 6–2. Changes in rCBF during an attack of classical migraine measured by intracarotid injection of ^{133}Xe and a 254-channel scintillation camera. The figure show computer-generated, gray-scaled images. A scale on the right indicates the relationship between the shades of gray and the rCBF (mL/100 g/min). The patient's nose is to the left. The attack was triggered by the carotid puncture. (A) The patient had no symptoms, but rCBF was reduced in the posterior parietal region. (B) Thirty minutes later, the patient was experiencing paresthesias and mild paresis of the right arm. The area of hypoperfusion had spread anteriorly to involve the temporal lobe. A small area of hypoperfusion is also evident in the frontal lobe. (C) One hr later, the patient was suffering from a throbbing, left-sided headache, but the neurologic signs and symptoms had disappeared. The anterior area of hypoperfusion spread to occupy much of the frontal lobe. (Adapted from Lauritzen,[1200] with permission.)

changes of systemic blood pressure (*cerebral autoregulation*), whereas in other studies, rCBF remained constant in response to an elevation of blood pressure.[566,1205,1736,1737] Physiologic activation by stimuli such as moving a hand or speaking did not increase CBF in cerebral regions affected by the migrainous process when the flow in these regions was diminished.[1205]

The observations made by Olesen and his co-workers using intracarotid ^{133}Xe provide considerable food for thought. Their data, however, might be open to criticism on the grounds that the attacks they studied were all triggered by the procedure. Carotid puncture has uncertain effects on CBF and may even have affected the results. Accordingly, one could question whether or not the changes in rCBF recorded with the ^{133}Xe technique develop during

spontaneous bouts of migraine. But SPECT studies of patients with spontaneous attacks have been performed by the same group of investigators. These studies have shown essentially the same findings—namely, unilateral regions of hypoperfusion of the cerebral cortex contralateral to the side of the focal neurologic symptoms (Fig. 6–3).[1203] The SPECT studies complement the ^{133}Xe studies very well.

In sum, the important and seminal investigations of Olesen and his co-workers appear to show that:

1. The decrease in CBF during attacks of migraine with aura is modest—estimated to be 25% to 30% with the intracarotid ^{133}Xe technique and 20% with SPECT studies. The reduction is not considered sufficient to produce ischemic changes in the brain during migraine attacks. Accordingly,

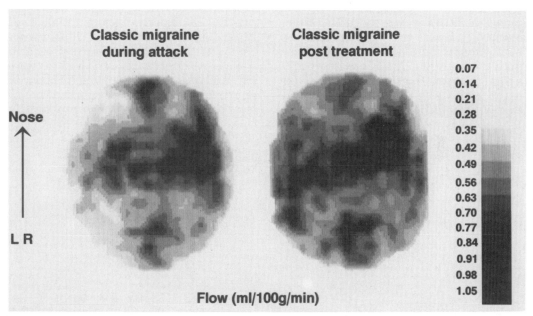

Figure 6–3. Changes in rCBF during a spontaneous attack of classic migraine measured by SPECT following ^{133}Xe inhalation. The figure shows computer-generated, gray-scaled images. The figures are transverse images and the patient's nose is facing up. Tomograms were taken 5 cm above the orbitomeatal line. A scale on the right indicates the relationship between the shades of gray and the rCBF (ml/100 g/min). (*Left*) Examination performed one hour after onset of attack of migraine with aura consisting of right-sided visual scintillations, right hemiparesis and hypesthesia, and speech difficulties. Reduced blood flow is present in the left temporal, parietal, and frontal cortex. The blood flow remained reduced for the next hour, and then normalized after treatment. (*Right*) Examination between attacks. Blood flow is normal except for the left insula, which showed some residual hypoperfusion. (Adapted from Lauritzen,[1200].)

ischemia is not thought to be the cause of the neurologic symptoms that comprise the aura.

2. The area of oligemia appears to expand in size and to spread anteriorly as the attack progresses.

3. The anterior spread of the reduced CBF is independent of the boundaries of the major cerebral artery territories. This finding has been interpreted to mean that vasospasm of a major cerebral artery supplying a discrete area of the cerebral cortex is unlikely to be the cause of the blood flow reduction.

4. A poor correlation has been found between the prolonged time course of the reduced rCBF and the considerably shorter duration of focal neurologic symptoms.

The aggregate of these findings persuaded Olesen and his colleagues that a vascular cause of migraine with aura is unlikely. They believe that the oligemia is not caused by a primary vascular process, but is *neurogenically* determined. In other words, both the oligemia and the aura are considered to be *responses* to some type of primary neuronal dysfunction. A neuronal process is thought to be the fundamental event in the genesis of migraine attacks (at least of attacks of migraine with aura),

and the reduced rCBF is considered an epiphenomenon—a process correlated with the depression of neuronal activity but not responsible for the production of symptoms. A phenomenon called *cortical spreading depression* is posited as the process causing the aura symptoms, the spreading oligemia, and, after a delay, the headache.[1200,1201,1492] The same conclusion had been reached earlier, but on the basis of different evidence.[730,1194,1210,1393] For example, the psychophysiologist Lashley, on the basis of his knowledge of the retinotopic organization of the visual system, estimated that the process responsible for his own scintillating scotomas traveled in a wave across the occipital cortex at a rate of 2–3 mm/min (Fig. 6–4).[1194] Lashley's calculations have been confirmed, and the patterns have been related to the functional organization of the striate cortex.[1667] A few years after Lashley made his observations, Leão described a neurologic process in experimental animals that he designated *spreading depression*. He found that various stimuli produced a wave of depressed neuronal activity extending across the exposed cortex at approximately the same rate that Lashley had estimated.[1208] Leão proposed a

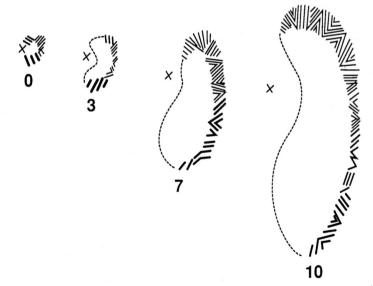

Figure 6–4. Successive observations of an expanding scintillating scotoma. The progressive involvement of the visual field was plotted at intervals indicated in minutes. The fixation point is marked by an X. The short, straight lines oscillate. The area within the dotted lines is the scotoma (from Lashley[1194]).

possible relationship between spreading depression and spread of the migrainous aura.[1210] Thus, a number of pieces of data have been used to circumstantially relate spreading depression and spreading oligemia.

SPREADING DEPRESSION

The spreading depression Leão found in the exposed cerebral cortices of experimental animals such as rats and rabbits is doubtless a pathologic response to various kinds of stimuli, including local electrical or mechanical stimulation, local application of either L-glutamate or other excitatory amino acids, or high concentrations of potassium chloride.[278,1309,1473] Any of these stimuli set up a transient wave front that suppresses both evoked and spontaneous neuronal activity. This depression spreads in all directions from its site of origin. It slowly propagates at a rate of 2–3 mm/min across the surface of the cortex. Neurons are markedly depolarized during the process. Simultaneously, a large, predominantly negative, DC potential develops in the extracellular space.[1209] The DC potential shift and the neuronal depression are accompanied by large ion fluxes in and out of cells (Fig. 6–5). In particular, the extracellular K^+ concentration increases from a resting level of 3 mM to as high as 50 mM.[885,1139] In contrast, the concentration of extracellular Ca^{++} decreases from 1.3 mM to 0.07 mM and Na^+ declines from 154 to 59 mM. These ionic changes suggest that the function of cortical neuronal membranes is abolished during spreading depression. The process is transient but fully reversible.

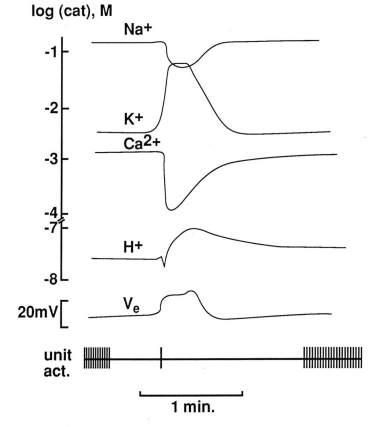

Figure 6–5. Changes in extracellular ionic concentrations, DC potential, and neuronal firing during spreading depression elicited in rat cortex. The process was initiated by a needle stab in the frontal cortex. The concentration of extracellular K^+ markedly increases; the levels of Na^+, Ca^{2+}, and H^+ diminish. Recording of the discharges of a single cortical neuron (unit activity) indicates that cessation of firing precedes a striking burst of high-frequency spike activity which accompanies the onset of the spreading depression. The neuron is totally silent for more than one minute. V_e is the DC potential, which is predominantly negative in the extracellular space. Slow recovery occurs over a period of more than a minute. (Adapted from Lauritzen, M: Cortical spreading depression as a putative migraine mechanism. Trends Neurosci 10:8–12, 1987, with permission.)

Return of the extracellular ionic concentrations to normal levels requires active ionic transport across the cell membranes.

Spreading depression in the cortex of experimental animals is accompanied by marked blood flow changes. At the beginning of the process, cortical blood flow increases for 1–2 minutes as a consequence of pial vasodilatation.[886] Following this increase, cortical blood flow is reduced by about 20%–30%, presumably because small blood vessels constrict.[1199,1206] The reduction persists for about 90 minutes. Blood pressure autoregulation remains normal, but cortical vessels do not respond in an ordinary manner to changes in p_{CO_2}. These blood flow changes are similar to those Olesen and his coworkers found in patients with migraine.

Mechanism of Spreading Depression

The mechanism of spreading depression is imperfectly understood, but appears to involve K^+ ions and the neurotransmitter L-glutamic acid. Enhanced neuronal excitation, coupled with firing in a localized region of the cortex, is known to result in the local buildup of K^+ in the extracellular space.[1907] The increased extracellular K^+ is thought to depolarize adjacent inactive neurons, causing the process to spread. In other words, spreading depression is hypothesized to result from release of K^+ and its subsequent diffusion through the extracellular space.[813] But in addition to K^+, the excitatory neurotransmitter L-glutamic acid is released during spreading depression.[2063] Activation of neuronal receptors by the release of endogenous L-glutamic acid can also initiate movements of Na^+, K^+, and Ca^{++} ions. Some or all of this ionic movement may play an important role in the genesis and expansion of spreading depression. At this point, no one knows whether the phenomenon is caused by the actions of K^+ or L-glutamate alone, or by their interactions.

The Spreading Depression Hypothesis and Migraine

The migration of the visual aura described by Lashley must have a physiologic foundation, but whether or not such migration parallels spreading depression is an open question (Fig. 6–6).[1194] The notion that spreading depression is responsible for initiating attacks of migraine with aura is supported by superficial similarities between spreading oligemia in humans and certain phenomena associated with spreading depression in animal models. For example, the areas of hypoperfusion in migraine are reported to expand progressively in size just as spreading depression does in rats. Moreover, the modest CBF reductions in migraine reported by the Copenhagen group are approximately the same as the level found in rats during spreading depression.[1206] And finally, the hypoperfusion associated with spreading depression continues for 1–2 hours in rats, and the oligemia in migraine patients persists for 1 to several hours in man.

Whether or not spreading depression in animal experiments is similar to the phenomena observed in humans during the aura is, however, questionable. Although spreading depression can be easily provoked by cortical stimuli in lower animals with a smooth cerebral cortex, such as rats and rabbits, it is more difficult to elicit in animals with convoluted cortical surfaces, such as cats and monkeys. Spontaneous, unprovoked spreading depression is not observed in experimental animals. Furthermore, spreading depression has never been convincingly demonstrated in the human neocortex.[771] A single example of the phenomenon appearing intraoperatively in the human hippocampus and caudate nucleus has been reported, but it has not been confirmed.[1927] Finally, because spreading depression is a completely reversible phenomenon, it explains neither the frequent persistence of neurologic deficits after attacks of classic migraine nor

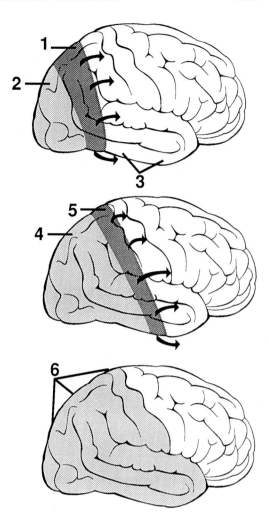

Figure 6–6. Diagram illustrating the hypothesis of progression of classic migraine proposed by the Copenhagen group. Lateral views show the human brain at approximately 30-minute intervals following the onset of an attack. The diagrams presuppose that spreading depression occurs in humans and that it is responsible for both the changes in blood flow and the focal neurologic symptoms and signs seen during the aura. The lighter dotted area represents the region of hypoperfusion, the darker dotted area is the region of disturbed neuronal function accompanying the hypothesized spreading depression, and the arrows indicate the direction of progression of the hypothesized spreading depression. The postulated spreading depression (1) is thought to be evoked at the occipital pole of the brain during the onset of the attack and to progress anteriorly. At the region of the spreading depression, temporary changes in ionic concentrations and neuronal firing are postulated to occur and to be responsible for the development of focal symptoms. In the region previously affected by the hypothesized spreading depression (2), CBF is depressed for 2 to 6 hours. The CBF in regions uninvaded by the hypothesized spreading depression (3) continues to be normal. The area of oligemia (4) progressively extends as the hypothesized spreading depression (5) shifts more anteriorly. The spreading depression is hypothesized to stop at the central sulcus. Still later, the hypothesized spreading depression has stopped, but a persistent reduction of CBF remains (6). At this point, the patient no longer has focal neurologic symptoms, but suffers from headache. (Adapted from Lauritzen[1200] with permission.)

the long-lasting focal abnormalities demonstrated by the use of electroencephalography (EEG) and computed tomography (CT) scans.

Magnetoencephalography (MEG)

The electrical currents in the brain can generate external magnetic fields in some geometric situations. MEG is a technique that has been used to locate the magnetic sources in the brain responsible for the magnetic field. Because it produces such dramatic changes in the electrical activity of the brain, spreading depression causes a strong magnetic field. If spreading depression occurs in humans, it should produce changes in cranial MEG recordings.[731,1482] And indeed, slow, long-duration (10–30 minutes), large-amplitude magnetic field changes have been recorded both between and during attacks in migraine patients with and without aura. These changes have not been noted in patients suffering from other forms of headache or in normal controls.[116] Although these shifts are very similar to shifts observed in MEG studies in experimental animals with spreading depression, the specificity of the signals is unknown. It is still too early to state that the occurrence of spreading depression has been demonstrated by MEG during the aura of attacks of classic migraine.

ISCHEMIA AND VASOSPASM

For over a decade, the Copenhagen group has provided us with some very interesting data. But because they used soft radiation sources such as ^{133}Xe, their conclusions about rCBF are open to alternative interpretations. The phenomenon known as scattered radiation (*Compton scatter*) raises questions about what their data may mean.[1873,1874] Compton scatter occurs because not all photons are emitted in a linear direction between the nuclide and the particular gamma-ray detector that is measuring radioactivity over a localized region of brain. Instead, some of the photons emitted by the nuclide may interact with orbital electrons, thereby losing energy, and changing direction in unpredictable ways. As a result, the photons may be recorded by a detector that is focused on another part of the cerebrum (Fig. 6–7). Radiation scattered from other areas especially complicates analysis from regions of the brain where blood flow is locally reduced when compared with the surrounding tissue. If adjacent areas of brain have equivalent blood flow, Compton scatter from one area would balance scatter from another. But areas of hypoperfusion give off far less scattered radiation than do areas with normal blood flow. Probes located over the area of low CBF will register two types of radiation—one from the area of low flow and representing the precise flow in the area, and a second scattered from the nonaffected parts of the cerebrum. Accordingly, scatter from a nearby area with greater blood flow can result in an overestimation of actual blood flow in hypoperfused regions of the brain. Most published studies of rCBF in migraine have paid insufficient attention to the consequences of this phenomenon.

Possible errors caused by Compton

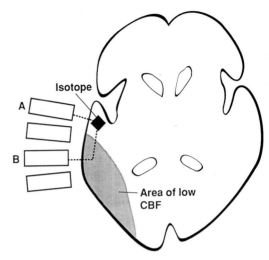

Figure 6–7. The effects of Compton scatter on measurements of rCBF. The isotope from an area of brain that has a normal blood flow is registered by detector A and represents undistorted blood flow in the area. Other photons from the same area are deflected and are recorded by detector B, which overlies an area of reduced CBF (hatched area). This latter radiation (Compton scatter) is recorded as if it originated from the area of low CBF. Compton scatter produces an overestimation of rCBF in the low-flow area. (Adapted from Skyhøj: Olsen, T and Olesen, J: Regional cerebral blood flow in migraine and cluster headache. In Olesen, J and Edvinsson, L (eds): Basic Mechanisms of Headache. Elsevier, Amsterdam, 1988, pp 377–391 with permission.)

scatter may give rise to data that appear to show spreading oligemia, when it could be just as reasonable to construe the data as indicative of a localized area of brain tissue involved in an *ischemic* process that gradually increases with time. Such a fixed area of brain might, in actuality, be the territory of a single cerebral artery affected by vasospasm that causes progressive ischemia.[1873,1874] If this is so, the aura symptoms may result when the CBF in the low-flow area decreases below the ischemic threshold. The idea of spreading oligemia has been widely embraced, perhaps because it is easy to explain. Understanding the implications of Compton scatter requires facility with complicated mathematics. Complexity, however, is no reason to dismiss material with potentially important implications. It may well be that spreading oligemia is an artifact caused by scattered radiation.

When Compton scatter was *not* taken into account, only modest reductions of CBF—approximately 25% (40 mL/100 g/min)—were estimated to occur during the aura.[41,1203,1204,1496] These levels correspond to the oligemic flow levels seen when spreading depression is induced in experimental animals. It is crucial, however, to recognize that these levels are well above both the threshold for ischemia and the threshold affecting normal neuronal function.[1202,1605,2036] In other words, if Compton scatter is not going to be factored into the analysis of CBF data, calculations of rCBF during the aura are going to show that the blood supply should be sufficient to meet the energy demands of the tissue. By using their data in this way, researchers are *inevitably* led to some explanation other than cerebral ischemia to account for the neurologic deficits. That other explanation is spreading depression. Data analysis that ignores Compton scatter thus supports the primary neuronal hypothesis about the aura.

In contrast, when Compton scatter was taken into consideration, estimations of the amount of focal reduction in CBF averaged 50% or more—reductions that correspond to a blood flow of 20–25 mL/100 g/min.[1873–1875] This is only slightly above a level of CBF that would be *insufficient* to maintain normal cortical electrical activity.[1817,2036] In this context, ischemia, and not spreading depression, is likely to be the primary cause of the neurologic deficits that comprise the aura.[1874] The CBF data, when Compton scatter is taken into account, suggest a primary vascular origin for migraine.

These alternative hypotheses are based on differing interpretations of the same data. And there is a further complication—namely, that the validity of the correction factors for Compton scatter is controversial.[435] At the present time, then, we are not clear as to whether the decreased CBF recorded during migrainous auras is caused by a neurogenic process such as spreading depression or by a vascular process such as vasoconstriction. While this research continues, should we seek elsewhere for additional data that negate or support an ischemic process?

From a clinical point of view, the characteristic picture of the aura with gradual expansion of a scintillating scotoma or the spread of paresthesias in the arm and face is rarely seen in cerebrovascular diseases that produce ischemia.[656] But even without correction for radiation scatter, small areas of ischemia in perfused oligemic regions of the brain have been noted both in some patients with classic migraine and in patients with hemiplegic migraine.[695,1204] These observations lead to questions about migrainous changes and other cerebral pathology that involves ischemia.

Clinical Studies and Cerebral Ischemia

The studies just described aim at demonstrating the merit of the primary neuronal hypothesis. Other bits and pieces of data from a variety of sources point toward and away from an ischemic process as the cause of the migraine aura. Among the data that must be considered are CT scans and angiograms of patients suffering from complicated migraine. Angiography performed during the aura phase of an attack is also worth study. Laboratory examination of cerebrospinal fluid and clinical examination of ocular and conjunctival vessels also yield useful data. Finally, PET and magnetic resonance spectroscopy (MRS) add some data. The question, of course, is whether data from all these sources point in a consistent direction. If not, do they suggest directions for further study?

Most clinicians would ascribe various migrainous phenomena to an ischemic process. Among the phenomena are neurologic deficits that occasionally persist well beyond the end of a migraine headache and may even persist permanently. Also on the list are protracted, focal EEG abnormalities or hypodense areas on CT scans. Of particular importance in ascribing these phenomena to an ischemic process is the observation that alterations in the CT scan seen after such episodes are identical in general contour and topography to those seen in patients with non-migrainous stroke.

Traditionally, the cerebral ischemia putatively responsible for migrainous infarction is thought to be caused by vasospasm. This proposition—based more on intuition than experimental evidence—remains controversial.[243,656,1992] Most angiographic investigations performed after an attack characterized by long-lasting or permanent neurologic changes have not demonstrated arterial occlusion.[230,375,1544,1560,1699] A small number of angiograms performed in patients with presumed migrainous infarction have shown occlusion or narrowing of an appropriate intracranial artery.[331,529,635] Absent the ability either to predict which headache will result in permanent deficits or to perform angiography during that attack, ascribing the migrainous infarction to ischemia (caused by spasm of an intracranial artery) is difficult to prove. But in the context of comparing the primary neuronal and primary vascular hypotheses, one would not expect spreading depression to produce persisting neurologic deficits, as it is a totally reversible process that does not injure neurons. In general, the electrophysiologic changes that characterize spreading depression are completed within 15 minutes following the initiation of the process.

Cerebral angiography has also been performed in conjunction with rCBF measurements during the aura.[695,1496,1874] Significant changes in arterial diameter could not be related to the occurrence of aura symptoms. In some cases, however, reflux into the vertebrobasilar system has been described. Reflux may be caused either by increased vascular resistance in the carotid system or by decreased vascular resistance in the vertebrobasilar territory, or by a combination of both. Other arteriographic studies of cases of classic and complicated migraine have not shown changes in arterial diameter.[656] Only rare examples of arterial narrowing ascribed to vasospasm have been seen during attacks of migraine accompanied by neurologic deficits.* The finding of normal arteriograms during bouts of classic migraine implies that if ischemia is the process causing the neurologic deficits, it is not occurring in the arteries. Arteriolar vasconstriction, in contrast to arterial vasoconstriction, may be the responsible process.

Cerebrospinal fluid (CSF) taken from classic migraine patients during attacks has shown both marked increases of lactate and significant decreases of bicarbonate levels.[1870] The presence of cerebral lactic acidosis suggests anaerobic glucose metabolism, such as would occur during ischemic hypoxia. Other investigations have shown increased concentration of the amino acid gamma-aminobutyric acid (GABA) and of cAMP (cyclic AMP; 3',5'-adenosine monophosphate).[2126,2127] These changes in GABA and cAMP are similar to those seen after brain hypoxia, and accordingly support the hypothesis that ischemia does occur during migraine attacks.

The vessels of the optic fundus are branches of the ophthalmic artery, which in turn is derived from the internal carotid artery. In contrast, the conjunctival circulation consists of an anastomosis of branches from both the internal and external carotid circulations. If changes in carotid blood flow occur during attacks of migraine, the vessels of the fundus or of the conjunctiva might be expected to show alterations in diameter. Unfortunately, vari-

---

*References 554, 732, 1242, 1699, 1789, 1812

ous studies have not produced a coherent picture of vascular changes during migraine. The vessels of the optic fundus either show no significant changes or only minor variations during migraine attacks.[2167] And although the conjunctival vessels are reported to show changes in their caliber during bouts of migraine, there is no agreement as to the significance of the changes. Most observers have noted dilatation of conjunctival blood vessels accompanied by reduced blood flow and aggregation of red cells.[213,456,1513,2043,2168] These investigations of conjunctival blood flow are compatible with a reduction in capillary flow in the carotid system during migraine attacks.

Positron Emission Tomography (PET)

PET studies, which can measure rCBF and the metabolism of oxygen and glucose, should provide definitive answers regarding the presence or absence of ischemia during the aura.

A PET study performed on one subject late in a spontaneous attack of migraine with aura showed a focal reduction in CBF. The reduced rCBF, however, was compensated for by an increase in oxygen extraction. The cerebral oxygen consumption was normal.[940] These findings, although inconclusive, suggest that neither metabolic depression nor ischemia was present in this patient. In a second patient with the same condition, both the oxygen extraction and oxygen metabolism were normal. PET studies performed during the early stages of reserpine-induced attacks of both classic and common migraine have shown a global decrease in the cerebral metabolism of glucose.[1728] In patients with aura, the changes were not confined to the hemisphere presumed to be site of the process responsible for the aura. These findings, thus, neither support nor negate the presence of ischemia.

Magnetic Resonance Spectroscopy (MRS)

Although still an experimental tool, MRS allows noninvasive, in vivo measurements of the spectra of high-energy phosphate compounds in human brains. These measurements can provide important information about the energy status of the human brain. The results of studies using in vivo ^{31}P-MRS in migraineurs show evidence of disordered brain energy metabolism during attacks of classic, but not common, migraine. The disordered brain energy status has also been documented during interictal periods in patients who had experienced previous episodes of migraine accompanied by prolonged aura,[113,114,2130] leading to the conclusion that high-energy phosphate production is impaired in patients with classic migraine. Similar changes in phosphate metabolism can be found during ischemia caused by non-migrainous conditions. In contrast to data suggesting an ischemic process, the in vivo spectroscopic studies showed no evidence of acidotic intracellular pH shifts during migraine attacks. Intracellular acidosis would be expected in cerebral ischemia.

The results of these spectroscopic investigations may, however, also indicate that under stressful conditions, the brains of patients with migraine have a decreased capability to contend with metabolic demands. Similar metabolic defects are present in platelets and in muscle biopsies of some patients with classic and complicated migraine.[113,1398,1409] Whether or not this defect in energy metabolism is causative in migraine attacks remains to be established, but the results support the possibility that cerebral ischemia is easily provoked during attacks of migraine.

CONTROL OF CEREBRAL CIRCULATION

The regulation of cerebral blood vessel diameter, resistance, and flow is a complex mechanism that includes metabolic, neural, and endothelial components. Several major factors play roles in the process:

1. *The level of local metabolites and chemical regulators (metabolic coupling).* Blood flow in the brain has been linked to local neuronal activity and to metabolism. Cerebral blood vessels are very responsive to the levels of different metabolites and to chemical stimuli such as changes in CO_2 tension and the concentration of perivascular H^+. A tight correlation between local O_2 consumption and blood flow has been shown both in humans and in experimental animals. In general, the blood flow is adjusted locally in response to the moment-to-moment needs of the tissue. A number of chemicals such as arachidonic acid metabolites, bradykinin, adenosine, and histamine are released by neurons, endothelium, platelets, and mast cells. These substances have also been proposed as local regulators of CBF.

2. *CBF autoregulation.* Autoregulation pertains to the ability of the brain to preserve a constant CBF despite fluctuations in systemic arterial pressure. Although the mechanism of autoregulation is unclear, liberation of vasoactive metabolites or chemicals—possibly induced by nascent local tissue hypoxia—is a reasonable hypothesis.[1131] Alternatively, maintenance of constant CBF in the face of changes in blood pressure could reflect a myogenic mechanism initiated by changes in the stretch of vascular smooth muscle. This view implies that the control of brain blood flow occurs at the level of small arteries and arterioles.

3. *Neural influences exerted by the release of various types of transmitters for perivascular nerves.* Cerebral arteries and arterioles are innervated by a dense network of perivascular nerve fibers that come from a number of sources both extrinsic and intrinsic to the brain. These sources include extensive sympathetic innervation from the superior cervical ganglia, modest parasympathetic nerve supply from the sphenopalatine and otic ganglia, supply from the trigeminovascular system, innervation from brain stem nuclei, including the locus coeruleus and the raphe nuclei, and fibers originating in the basal forebrain. These nerve fibers contain a number of neurotransmitters such as norepinephrine, acetylcholine, neuropeptide Y, vasoactive intestinal peptide, serotonin (5-hydroxytryptamine; 5-HT), substance P, neurokinin A, calcitonin gene-related peptide, and others.

4. *Endothelial control of cerebrovascular tone.* Findings that endothelial cells synthesize and release substances that produce vasodilatation and vasoconstriction have led researchers to realize that the endothelium plays a major and hitherto unrecognized part in the regulation of vascular tone. The endothelium was shown to secrete substances that can mediate both relaxant and vasoconstrictive responses. With regard to relaxant properties, after specific receptors were activated by a variety of neurohumoral agents (such as acetylcholine, substance P, bradykinin, serotonin, histamine), endothelium-dependent vasodilatation occurred both in isolated arteries and in arteries in vivo.[1287] The substance released by endothelial cells and believed responsible for the relaxation has been termed *endothelium-derived relaxing factor* (EDRF) (Fig. 6–8). EDRF is now thought to be nitric oxide (NO).[1010] L-Arginine, by means of the enzyme NO synthase, synthesizes NO. NO then activates guanylate cyclase—the enzyme that catalyzes the synthesis of cyclic GMP (cGMP)—in vascular smooth muscle cells. cGMP, acting as a second messenger, is thought to underlie the smooth-muscle–relaxing properties of NO.

The functional role of NO in the neural regulation of the cerebral circulation is as yet unclear. Studying the problem is complicated for several reasons. First, endothelium-dependent relaxations vary among different blood vessels.[716] In addition, we do not know whether or not neurotransmitter sub-

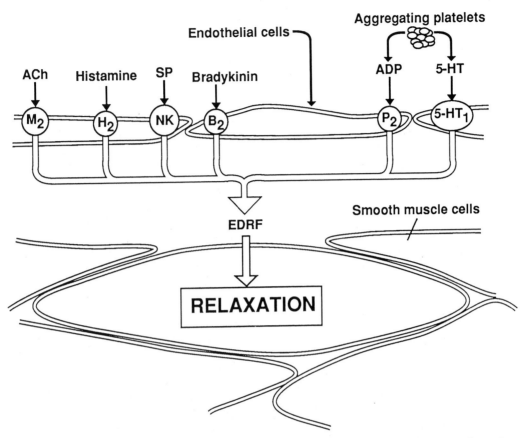

Figure 6–8. Neurohumoral mediators and transmitters cause the release of endothelium-derived relaxing factor (EDRF). These substances activate specific receptors located on endothelial cells. ACh, acetylcholine; M_2, muscarinic receptor; H_2, histaminergic receptor; SP, substance P; NK, substance P receptor; B_2, bradykinin receptor; ADP, adenosine diphosphate; P_2, purinergic receptor; 5-HT, serotonin; 5-HT$_1$, serotonergic receptor. (Modified with permission from Lüscher, TF and Vanhoutte, PM: The Endothelium: Modulator of Cardiovascular Function, 1990. Copyright CRC Press, Inc., Boca Raton, FL.)

stances released from autonomic or other nerve terminals located in the adventitia and media of large, thick-walled cerebral vessels reach the endothelium, thereby causing the release of NO. Researchers consider it probable, however, that neurally released neurotransmitters reach the endothelium in microvessels, and it can be verified that exogenous neurotransmitters and drugs reach receptors located on the endothelium. Besides gaps in our knowledge of how neurotransmitters affect the endothelium, there are other difficulties in studying the relationship between endothelium and neural regulation of cerebral circulation. As indicated above, NO mediates the actions of several endogenously released, non-neurotransmitter neurohumoral agents, such as bradykinin and histamine. These agents have complex actions, which will be discussed later in this chapter. Finally, endothelium-dependent responses vary among species. This variation obviously can confound extrapolation of data from one group of experiments to another.

Endothelial cells also synthesize and release one or more potent vasoconstrictor peptides now designated *endothelins*. Three endothelin isoforms with vasoactive properties have been characterized, although only one form—endothelin-1—is expressed in endothelial tissue.[1011,2186] All three types of endothelin cause potent and sustained vasoconstriction of cerebral arteries in vitro and in vivo.[1732] These responses occur when specific receptors located on the smooth muscle cells of cerebral vessels are activated. Endothelin is produced by endothelial cells at a slow rate, and circulating levels of the substance are extremely low.[611] In addition, plasma endothelin is rapidly degraded by endopeptidases. Various organs, particularly the lungs, remove endothelin from plasma by rapid uptake. But despite a very short half-life, the biological effects of endothelins are long-lasting, presumably reflecting their effectiveness in occupying receptors.

Major efforts have been expended to determine whether or not dysfunction of the structures that innervate intracranial vessels is responsible for some or all of the symptoms of migraine. Most authorities have concentrated on neuronal innervation in the pathogenesis of migraine, and have not stressed the roles of local metabolites, autoregulation, or endothelial activity in the pathophysiology of migraine. Although these three topics need much more consideration, the following discussion will, of necessity, present data that are currently available: namely, information about neural influences on cerebrovascular structures.

Autonomic Innervation of the Cranial Vasculature

The intracranial circulation is innervated by both sympathetic and parasympathetic fibers, following a distinctly different pattern of innervation for each. Pial and parenchymal vessels receive sympathetic adrenergic nerve fibers; the supply by parasympathetic cholinergic nerves is apparently confined to extraparenchymal arteries. As the two following sections will indicate, a great deal is known about the pharmacologic and physiologic features of

the autonomic innervation of the cerebral circulation. Much less is known about its functional importance in the regulation of CBF.

SYMPATHETIC INNERVATION

Norepinephrine has been considered the primary transmitter for most of the perivascular sympathetic nerves. An abundant supply of noradrenergic sympathetic fibers surrounds intracranial arteries, including large pial and small parenchymal arterioles.[589] In contrast, veins have a less dense sympathetic innervation. Moreover, arterioles are not all innervated to the same degree. The density of noradrenergic sympathetic innervation varies among different regions of the brain. Accordingly, much denser innervation of arterioles can be found in the parietal cortex than in the occipital cortex.[593] Denervation experiments have shown that the majority of sympathetic fibers originate in the superior cervical ganglia (Fig. 6–9).[892,1516] A comparatively sparse contribution—mainly to the more caudal arteries of the circle of Willis—is derived from the stellate ganglion. Noradrenergic fibers from the locus coeruleus also contribute to the innervation of the cranial vasculature (see below).

In general, stimulation of the superior cervical trunk results in constriction of pial arteries, larger arterioles, and veins, but produces little or no change in the diameter of smaller arteries.[2116] In contrast, perivascular application of norepinephrine evokes some degree of constriction in all cranial arteries, arterioles, and veins.[592,1155] But although they all constrict, cerebral arteries are much less sensitive to exogenous norepinephrine and to sympathetic stimulation than are peripheral arteries. Binding studies of radioactive adrenergic ligands indicate that both α_1- and α_2-adrenoceptors are present in cerebral arteries.[2053] The α_1-adrenoceptor antagonists, however, are the compounds that block norepinephrine-induced contractions.[2021] Cerebral arteries in vitro can also undergo β-adrenoceptor–

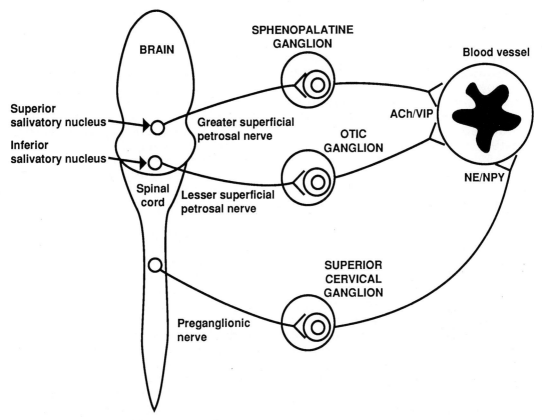

Figure 6–9. The autonomic innervation of the cerebral vasculature. The source of the sympathetic innervation is the spinal cord (*lower left*). The cervical sympathetic preganglionic nerve innervates the superior cervical ganglion, which then supplies the major blood vessels. Both norepinephrine (NE) and neuropeptide Y (NPY) are co-localized in the postganglionic adrenergic nerves. The preganglionic parasympathetic nerves originate in the superior and inferior salivatory nuclei (*upper left*) and project as the greater and lesser superficial petrosal nerves to the sphenopalatine and otic ganglia. Both acetylcholine (ACh) and vasoactive intestinal polypeptide (VIP) are co-localized in the parasympathetic postganglionic cholinergic nerves (Modified from Hara, et al[889] with permission.)

mediated vasodilatation in response to application of exogenous norepinephrine. A combination of β_1- and β_2-adrenoceptors have been demonstrated on human pial arteries.[576] But despite these findings, activation of β-adrenoceptors by norepinephrine released from nerve fibers in vivo has not yet been definitely shown.

Recent evidence shows that norepinephrine is not the only transmitter substance released from sympathetic nerve terminals. Most sympathetic postganglionic perivascular nerves also contain *neuropeptide Y* (NPY).[26,578,582,583,1563] Not only is NPY a potent constrictor of cerebral and pial ar-

teries, but it also has complex interactions with norepinephrine.[575,583] NPY has direct postjunctional actions that enhance blood vessel contractions whether neurally evoked or produced by exogenous norepinephrine. But NPY also has prejunctional effects that limit the release of norepinephrine from nerve terminals.[575,583] Obviously there is a complex connection between NPY and norepinephrine. In most situations, however, the postjunctional potentiating actions prevail over the prejunctional inhibition of norepinephrine release.

A dual role has been postulated for adenosine 5′-triphosphate (ATP). It is believed to function both as a co-transmitter with norepinephrine in sympathetic nerves that supply cerebral blood vessels, and as a neurotransmitter in some nonadrenergic, noncholinergic autonomic nerves.[19,281] ATP, released as a co-transmitter with norepinephrine from perivascular sympathetic nerves, is a potent vasoconstrictor. Elucidating the precise roles ATP and related purine compounds play in regulating cerebral circulation is complicated in part by questions about their origins. Some experiments indicate that in addition to release from perivascular nerves themselves, ATP and other purines may also be released from endothelial cells and platelets.[673,893,1438,1439] ATP, entering the blood from some endothelial cells and acting on the same and other endothelial cells, is believed to lead to the release of EDRF, which in turn dilates arteries.[282] The same mechanism presumably causes endothelium-dependent vasodilatation when adenine nucleotides are secreted by activated platelets.[989] In contrast, ATP originating in nerve terminals can influence vascular tone by acting at several different sites and on at least two different blood vessel receptors. When acting on prejunctional P_1 purinergic receptors, ATP may inhibit its own release as well as that of norepinephrine.[1970] ATP may also activate two kinds of postsynaptic purinergic receptors. ATP activation of P_1-receptors located on smooth muscle cells and of P_2-receptors located on endothelium cells causes vasodilatation. In contrast, activation of P_2-receptors located on smooth muscle may cause vascular contraction.[1099] This compound, then, is released from multiple sources, functions alone and as a co-transmitter, affects its own release, and causes both vasoconstriction and vasodilatation. Full clarification of how ATP works will doubtless add much to current knowledge about cerebral circulation.

When we turn from pharmacologic and physiologic data about sympathetic control of the cerebral circulation to the topic of regulation of CBF, the circumstances are quite different. Despite decades of study, the role of the extrinsic sympathetic system in regulating CBF is unclear.[923] Section of the cerebrovascular sympathetic supply has little effect on CBF. Under some experimental conditions, electrical stimulation of the cervical sympathetic nerves caused moderate constriction of cerebral arteries and veins and moderate decrease in CBF. Under most conditions, however, CBF was only slightly reduced or not reduced at all.[284,897,924,1026] This is somewhat surprising, since, as described above, sympathetic fibers secrete a number of neurotransmitters with powerful actions on blood vessels. One would have expected that cutting or stimulating these fibers would have had more pronounced effects on CBF. Since it did not, another hypothesis is needed—one more compatible with available data. Despite the density of the innervation, it would seem that under normal conditions cerebral blood vessels have little resting sympathetic tone and that the sympathetic nervous system has only minimal influence on CBF. It may be that the sympathetic innervation functions as a vasoconstrictor system to modulate increases in flow evoked by hypertension or intense metabolic stimuli.[182,1436] How migraine might fit into the workings of this system is unknown.

PARASYMPATHETIC INNERVATION

As just discussed, our present knowledge about the sympathetic innervation of the cerebral circulation is limited—especially with regard to its functional role in regulating CBF. The case for the parasympathetic nerve supply is still less clear, even though some evidence points to a connection between migraine and parasympathetic innervation that is more direct than any connection postulated between the sympathetic innervation and such headaches. What follows is an account of what is presently believed about the parasympathetic system.

A cholinergic parasympathetic innervation of the cerebral blood vessels has been described for many years. Even so, the physiologic role of this innervation in regulating CBF remains a subject of controversy.[172] Immunohistochemical mapping studies have elucidated to some degree the origins and pathways of cranial parasympathetic nerves. Preganglionic parasympathetic neurons are present in the superior and inferior salivatory nuclei situated rostral to the dorsal motor vagus nucleus (see Fig. 6–9). Postganglionic cholinergic parasympathetic fibers that innervate supratentorial vessels arise in large part from the sphenopalatine ganglion and are distributed by means of the greater superficial petrosal branch of the facial nerve. Other parts of the postganglionic parasympathetic innervation arise from several sources. Fibers from the otic ganglion involve the lesser superficial petrosal nerve.[891,892,2096] Some parasympathetic nerves originate in local microgang lia. Postganglionic parasympathetic innervation of the basilar artery comes mainly from cell bodies in the vagal ganglia, with some contribution from the sphenopalatine ganglia.[79]

Exogenous acetylcholine produces modest vasodilatation both in the cephalic circulation and in cerebral microvessels.[586,925] In microvessels, the dilatation is dependent on the release of EDRF, whereas in large conduit vessels, where the diffusion distances between perivascular nerve terminals and endothelial cells are longer, neurogenically released acetylcholine is thought not to reach the endothelium.[1694] In these latter structures, evidence suggests that the cholinergic system dilates vessels indirectly by activating prejunctional nicotinic receptors that inhibit the release of norepinephrine from adjacent sympathetic nerve endings.[91,586]

As in the case of norepinephrine's contribution to sympathetic function, the role played by acetylcholine in parasympathetic function is still unclear. Cholinergic mechanisms have indeed been implicated in the control of the cerebral arterial system. In the 1930s, cerebral vasodilatation was observed in vivo following electrical stimulation of the facial or greater superficial petrosal nerves; the phenomenon was confirmed in later studies.[355,432,1026,1592] More recent research, however, has failed to support these findings.[283,1802] The reported discrepancies may in part relate to species differences and methodologic considerations, but whatever their source, the discrepancies limit our ability to draw firm conclusions. It does appear, however, that acetylcholine is involved in resting cerebral vascular tone. This conclusion is reasonable because data from experimental animals have shown that the cholinesterase inhibitor physostigmine increases cortical blood flow.[1802]

Vasoactive intestinal polypeptide (VIP) is co-localized with acetylcholine in the terminals of some populations of parasympathetic nerves. Many VIP fibers emanate from the sphenopalatine ganglion, with contributions from the otic ganglion.[890,1284,1976,2096] These fibers are believed to innervate mostly extracerebral vessels. Other VIP fibers, however, especially those derived from perikarya in local ganglia (microganglia) around the internal carotid artery in the cavernous sinus, appear to innervate cerebral vessels. Nerve fibers containing VIP form a prominent plexus in the walls of both cerebral and extracerebral blood vessels.[580,760] VIP-containing fibers are also found on all the vessels of the circle of Willis, but are most prominent on the anterior vessels.[1192]

With regard to function, VIP causes relaxation of isolated cerebral arteries, arterioles, and veins by activating specific VIP receptors.[580,2020] This vasodilatation does not depend on an intact endothelium and is most prominent in small arteries. As expected, intracarotid infusion of VIP causes modest increases of CBF in primates.[585]

Parasympathetic neurons in the greater superficial petrosal nerve–sphenopalatine ganglion pathway may become activated by impulses from trigeminal nociceptive fibers. The pathway is believed to involve a reflex arc whose afferent limb consists of trigeminal primary afferent fibers that synapse in the brain stem and connect the spinal trigeminal nucleus with the superior and inferior salivatory nuclei.[784] Should this be the case, activation of pain fibers during a headache would result in dilatation of vessels innervated by the parasympathetic system.

Trigeminovascular Fibers and Cerebral Blood Flow Regulation

Neural influences from the trigeminovascular system are also exerted on the cerebral circulation. Trigeminovascular fibers constitute an afferent sensory system; in addition to its sensory role, the trigeminovascular system has cerebral vasomotor functions. Afferent nociceptive trigeminal fibers that innervate dural and pial vessels both store and secrete neuropeptides. These neuropeptides—particularly substance P, neurokinin A, and calcitonin gene-related peptide—function as neurotransmitters.* We have known that trigeminovascular fibers release neurotransmitter peptides on secondary neurons in the brain stem and spinal cord. But (as will be discussed in detail in the next chapter) it has now become apparent that such fibers also release neuropeptides peripherally from their free endings on blood vessels. All of these peptides have potent vasomotor effects on cerebral blood vessels. In particular, direct evidence that these peptides have cerebral vasodilatory properties has been provided by stimulation experiments. Thus, when the trigeminal ganglion is stimulated, blood flow increases both in the frontal and parietal areas of the cerebrum, as well as in the external carotid territory.[2027] In addition, substance P, neurokinin A, and calcitonin gene-related peptide induce relaxation of

human cerebrovascular smooth muscle.[594,1349]

Despite the actions just described, trigeminal axons appear to play only a modest role in the moment-to-moment control of the cerebral circulation.[1350,1429,1738] Perhaps the trigeminovascular system functions to reestablish normal vascular diameter and sufficient cerebral perfusion when there is intense cerebral vasoconstriction—such as that which may occur during the migraine aura.[590] Here again, we must await further data.

Brain Stem Effects on the Cranial Circulation

Evidence has accumulated in recent years that activation of a number of sites within the brain stem alters CBF.[784,1814] The locus coeruleus is the origin of noradrenergic neurons, and the raphe nuclei are the origin of serotonergic neurons, both of which innervate the intracranial vasculature. We will consider current knowledge about these two areas relative to their effects on cranial blood flow and whether activity in these areas is reasonably implicated in the pathogenesis of migraine symptoms.

LOCUS COERULEUS

Central—as opposed to sympathetic—noradrenergic innervation of the brain arises from several discrete collections of cells that are distributed from the rostral pons to the caudal medulla.[1414] The most prominent body of central noradrenergic neurons is located within the *nucleus locus coeruleus*, a prominent, pigmented nucleus located in the caudal pons. Although the locus coeruleus is a small nucleus, highly collateralized branches innervate the entire neuraxis, including forebrain, brain stem, cerebellum, and spinal cord.[1414] In addition to synaptic contacts on neurons, noradrenergic fibers from the locus coeruleus occasionally lie in close apposition to small

---

*References 882, 1263, 1350, 2049, 2184

intraparenchymal microvessels, capillaries, and venules, especially those in the brain stem.[469,905,906,1978] This intraparenchymal innervation is predominantly ipsilateral. Doubt exists, however, as to whether or not fibers from the locus coeruleus innervate large cerebrovascular vessels.[588]

The locus coeruleus is considered by some to be the central counterpart of the sympathetic ganglia, innervating the cerebrovascular system in much the same way that sympathetic nerves supply peripheral vascular beds. But investigations of the influence of the locus coeruleus on CBF in experimental animals have not always been in agreement. A number of studies have shown, however, that electrical stimulation of the locus coeruleus produces both a rapid, but modest, decrease in ipsilateral CBF as a result of vasoconstriction and increased vascular resistance in the internal carotid circulation.* CBF in cats is reduced, especially in the ipsilateral occipital cortex, by approximately 35%.[776] The vasoconstriction that gives rise to this reduction is reported to be mediated by α_2-adrenoceptors.[783] Such results imply that the innervation from the locus coeruleus has a contrictor action on cerebral blood vessels mediated by α-adrenoceptors in a manner analogous to the sympathetic innervation of peripheral blood vessels. These findings, however, are not clear-cut; other investigations have suggested that β-adrenergic receptors, but not α-adrenergic receptors, are present on microvessels.[896,1449]

Unlike the work just discussed, some research does not reveal any alterations of CBF when the locus coeruleus is stimulated.[429,1664] These studies found that stimulation of the parabrachial nucleus—a structure adjacent to, and intermingled with, the neurons of the locus coeruleus—produces cerebral cortical vasoconstriction in a manner similar to that reported by previous investigators to follow locus coeruleus stimulation.[1664] These results imply that the changes in CBF that reportedly accompany electrical stimulation in the region of the locus coeruleus may well be confounded by—or even actually be caused by—unintended stimulation of the parabrachial nucleus.[1664]

RAPHE NUCLEI

Serotonin-containing central nervous system neurons are mostly confined to the *raphe nuclei,* collections of cells in the median and paramedian zones of the brain stem.[1940] Some serotonin-containing cell bodies are also found in the reticular formation. From these sites, highly branched ascending and descending axons project to virtually the entire central nervous system. Serotonin acts as a central neurotransmitter *and* has potent vasoactive properties, but whether or not serotonin-containing nerve fibers of central origin are present on either large or small pial vessels is controversial. Both histochemical and biochemical evidence supports the idea that cerebrovascular nerves containing serotonin originate in the raphe nuclei. Thus, both biochemical studies and fluorescence histochemical investigations have revealed a system of perivascular nerves that contain serotonin.[579,1768] Cerebral blood vessels at all levels of the cerebrovascular tree—large pial and cerebral arteries, arterioles, and microvessels—have been shown by immunocytochemical and neurochemical techniques to be innervated by serotonin-containing fibers believed to originate from mesencephalic raphe nuclei.[512,513,1662,1768,1939] But other investigations have shown that serotonin-containing cerebrovascular nerves are not visualized unless the blood vessels have been previously incubated with exogenous serotonin. Observations showing the presence of such nerves may have to be reinterpreted because vessels may have been contaminated by serotonin released into the CSF or extracellular space during dissections.

---

*References 470, 776, 780, 1084, 1180, 1623, 1624

In addition, a number of recent studies have shown that fibers appearing to contain serotonin are localized in the sympathetic nerve plexus of major pial arteries.[342,1017] The presence of serotonin in sympathetic nerves may result from its uptake into such nerves that use norepinephrine as a neurotransmitter. Alternatively, it is possible that serotonin is synthesized by sympathetic fibers, or that a small number of serotonergic sympathetic neurons are present in the superior cervical ganglion.

Experiments on both human and animal blood vessels show that exogenous serotonin can produce both vasoconstriction and vasodilatation.[966,2065] The complex actions presumably reflect, in part, a diversity of serotonin receptors on the extracranial and intracranial vasculature. In addition to multiple types of serotonin receptors, the response to applied perivascular serotonin also seems to depend on the region of the cerebrovascular tree studied and its preexisting vascular tone. To complicate matters even more, different anatomic segments of the same artery may have varying responses to serotonin.[2022] But with regard to isolated, large pre– and post–circle-of-Willis arteries (even though it is still unclear which receptor is involved), low concentrations of perivascular serotonin produce a predominantly contractile response.[1527] Depending on the species, different serotonin binding sites have been implicated in the cerebral vasoconstrictive actions of serotonin.[1529] In general, systemically administered serotonin is a potent constrictor of extracranial arteries in monkeys and humans, but it has minimal effects on the intracranial circulation. Moreover, intravascular serotonin does not significantly change blood flow in humans or other primates provided the blood–brain barrier is intact.*

The role of the raphe nuclei in the functional control of CBF remains a matter of controversy. Stimulation of the dorsal raphe nucleus in the midbrain does affect the caliber of intracerebral vessels, but the changes produced in CBF depend on the type and level of anesthesia used in the experiments.[235,412] Most studies have shown that the major effect of raphe stimulation is vasodilatation of both the extracerebral and the intracerebral circulations, with an increase in CBF.[411,783,786] Some studies, however, have reported decreases in CBF after raphe stimulation and increases in CBF after administration of a neurotoxin that destroys serotonergic neurons.[235,1346]

Stimulation of both the locus coeruleus and the raphe nuclei at certain frequencies augments extracranial blood flow in ways comparable to the increases reported in migrainous patients during the headache.* The pathway involved is indirect, comprised of connections with the parasympathetic outflow through the facial nerve. The pathway exits in the facial nerve from the brain stem. It involves a route from the greater superficial petrosal branch of the facial nerve to the sphenopalatine and otic ganglia, from which vasodilator fibers are distributed to blood vessels.[781,782] The vasodilator fibers ending on intracerebral vessels may secrete VIP as their transmitter.[786]

Alterations in Brain Stem Activity as a Cause of Migraine

Alterations in the activity of the brain stem monoamine systems have been causally implicated in the vascular processes that not only occur during migraine attacks, but also are relevant to the genesis of migrainous events (Fig. 6–10).[784,1171,2125] As indicated above, stimulation of the locus coeruleus or the dorsal raphe can change both cerebral and extracranial blood flow. In particular, the locus coeruleus is hypothesized to cause constriction of the ipsi-

---

*References 898, 1175, 1496, 1925, 1926

*References 780, 781, 783, 785, 786, 1163, 1180

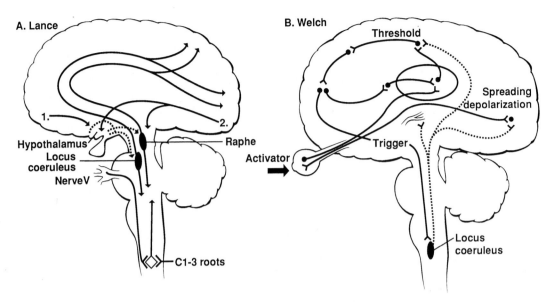

Figure 6–10. Theoretical models proposed to explain the initiation of migraine attacks. (*A*) The Lance Hypothesis. The bout of migraine may be triggered by emotion or stress (*1*), by an intense afferent stimulus such as flickering light (*2*), or by an "internal clock" located in the area of the hypothalamus. Projections to the raphe nuclei and locus coeruleus may cause alterations in rCBF (related to the aura), or may depress the endogenous pain control system (related to the head pain). (Adapted from Lance[1169] with permission.) (*B*) The Welch Hypothesis. An "activator" of the migraine attack (such as a visual stimulus) elicits a cerebral process that determines whether or not the (proposed) orbitofrontal-brain stem pathway is activated. If the threshold is reached, activity in this pathway is postulated to initiate activity in the locus coeruleus. The projection of the locus coeruleus to the occipital cortex causes changes in neuronal function (and possibly spreading depression or depolarization). The locus coeruleus may also affect the threshold for activation of the frontal lobes. (Adapted from Welch[2129] with permission.)

lateral cranial blood vessels when norepinephrine released by axons from the nucleus binds to α-adrenoceptors. Decreased blood flow in the occipital cortex induced by neural activity in the locus coeruleus is presumed to result in the aura of classic migraine. In addition, various migraine triggers or precipitating factors are hypothesized to excite appropriate cerebral areas. For example, strong flashing visual stimuli activate the primary visual cortex; emotional stress activates the limbic system. Impulses from these cerebral areas are then postulated to be relayed via the hypothalamus or the orbitofrontal cortex to influence the locus coeruleus and the raphe nuclei.

All of these events, taken together, form the brain stem neural hypothesis of migraine. This hypothesis is attractive because it accounts for the vascular changes associated with migraine. Un-

fortunately, many details are lacking. For example, no direct connections have been found between the hypothalamus or orbitofrontal cortex and the locus coeruleus (although the raphe nuclei receive input from the hypothalamic region). In fact, the locus coeruleus has a remarkably restricted set of afferents. Its major inputs, located in the rostral medulla, consist of the nucleus paragigantocellularis and the nucleus prepositus hypoglossi.[87,88] Moreover, the structures projecting to these latter nuclei are not known with precision, although the nucleus paragigantocellularis has been shown to function as an intersection for neural circuitry pertaining to environmental stimuli (particularly noxious ones) and central autonomic function.

Whatever its connections may be, specific behavioral and sensory events are reported to evoke concerted activity among neurons in the locus coeruleus. In particular, a rapid burst of action potentials occurs in locus coeruleus neurons in response to sudden shifts in attention to external sensory stimuli.[86,669] Accordingly, it has been hypothesized that if the excitability of the locus coeruleus is increased sufficiently, discharges along its diffuse projections to the ipsilateral cerebral cortex will result in inhibition of cortical neuronal activity and in vasoconstriction, which is most marked in the posterior cerebrum. The latter effects set off a chain of events producing the aura.[1084] Whether the locus coeruleus or the adjacent nucleus parabrachialis is responsible for the putative effects of locus coeruleus stimulation challenges the brain-stem neural hypothesis of migraine. Direct experimentation cannot stave off this challenge because it is difficult to examine the function of the locus coeruleus in humans. But the contingent negative variation—a slow, negative cerebral potential dependent on a noradrenergic input, which could well originate from the locus coeruleus—has been shown to be altered in migraineurs.[1289] If future studies convincingly link this potential change to the locus coeruleus, the brain-stem neural hypothesis will be strengthened.

In contrast to adrenergic neurons in the locus coeruleus, the activity of serotonergic neurons in the raphe nuclei displays a notably regular discharge pattern, even when there are extensive changes in the behavioral state of the animal.[1019] Exposure of an awake animal to differing stressors results in very little variation in the firing rate of raphe neurons. And the firing rate remains steady even while marked changes take place in a number of physiologic systems. It is difficult to see how neurons that respond in this manner would modulate the responses to internal and environmental migrainogenic stimuli. The question remains, then, whether or not these brain stem structures are involved in the pathogenesis of migraine. The raphe nuclei and the locus coeru-leus, however, do have the ability to cause dilatation of the extracranial vasculature.[785] And because dilatation of branches of the superficial temporal artery is seen in approximately one third of patients during attacks of migraine, this may be a factor in the production of the migrainous syndrome in some individuals.[545]

Basal Nucleus

Although the anatomic connections between the cholinergic fibers derived from the basal forebrain (basal nucleus of Meynert, substantia innominata) and the cerebral vessels are still unsatisfactorily defined, stimulation of the basal nucleus substantially increases cortical blood flow in the ipsilateral cerebral hemisphere.[179,1157] That the effects are a result of activating both muscarinic and nicotinic receptors is verified by the attenuation of the increase in CBF after administration of either the muscarinic cholinergic receptor antagonist atropine or the nicotinic antagonist mecamylamine.[179,450] The role of the basal nucleus in the pathophysiology of migraine is unknown.

Other Factors Regulating Cerebral Blood Flow

A number of chemical substances such as arachidonic acid metabolites, bradykinin, histamine, and adenosine have potent effects on the cerebral circulation. Accordingly, discussion of their *vascular actions* belongs in this chapter. Some of these chemicals, however, are thought to be involved not only in the regulation of CBF, but also in the genesis of head pain by virtue of their effects on trigeminal nociceptive terminals. Chapter 7, because it focuses on the pathophysiology of migrainous head pain, will take up the topic of how some of these compounds interact with the trigeminal nociceptive system.

ARACHIDONIC ACID
METABOLITES

Arachidonic acid is present in virtually all cells esterified in the sn-2 position of membrane glycerophospholipids. It can be liberated by a number of phospholipases (especially phospholipase A_2). Various stimuli, particularly injury and inflammation, can activate these phospholipases, as can some chemicals such as bradykinin and histamine.[1064,1065] Arachidonic acid liberated from cell membranes by the action of phospholipases is rapidly metabolized by three principal pathways—the cyclooxygenase pathway, the lipoxygenase pathway, and the cytochrome P-450 epoxygenase pathway (Fig. 6–11).[1882] These pathways in the arachidonic acid cascade produce a group of unsaturated fatty acids called eicosanoids.[867,1741,1743] The eicosanoids are synthesized not only by brain tissue, but also in the walls of cerebral blood vessels and in platelets.

Little if anything is known about products of the cytochrome P-450 epoxygenase pathway of the arachidonic acid cascade with regard to migraine. We know a bit more about whether migraine is affected by leukotrienes formed by the lipoxygenase pathway of arachidonic acid metabolism.[1742] Leukotrienes have pronounced vasomotor effects and, in general, produce a substantial constriction of pial vessels.[1693] Leukotriene concentrations are increased after cerebral ischemia, and transient elevations of specific leukotrienes (LTB$_4$ and LTC$_4$) have been measured during attacks of classic migraine.[744]

What these findings mean for migraine is unclear. Far more is known about the cyclooxygenase limb of the arachidonic acid cascade. This limb produces *prostanoids*—particularly *prostaglandins, prostacyclin* (PGI$_2$), and *thromboxane A$_2$* (TXA$_2$).[1452] Different cell types have widely varying capacities to synthesize prostanoids. For

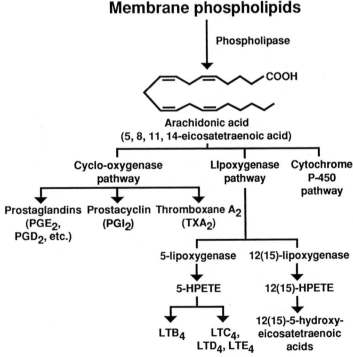

Figure 6–11. Current concepts of arachidonic acid metabolism. Shown are three multienzyme pathways required for synthesis of eicosanoids. 5-HPETE, 5-S-eicosatrienic acid; 12(15)-HPETE, 12(15)-S-hydroxyeicosatetraenoic acid; LTB$_4$, Leukotriene B$_4$; LTC$_4$, Leukotriene C$_4$; LTD$_4$, leukotriene D$_4$; LTE$_4$, leukotriene E$_4$.

example, arachidonic acid is mainly converted to PGI_2 by endothelial cells in blood vessel walls and to TXA_2 in platelets. Some of the actions of prostanoids do indeed seem relevant to the study of migraine.

The effects of prostanoids on the cranial blood vessels are complex: different prostanoids have differing effects on different vascular beds.[2052,2142] For example, the prostaglandin PGE_2 reduces cerebral blood flow, but increases extracranial blood flow.[1588] The prostaglandin PGE_1 is considered a potent vasodilator of most vascular beds, although whether it dilates or constricts the internal carotid vasculature in experimental animals is a matter of dispute.[482,985,1554,2131] Human data in this regard show that intracarotid infusion of PGE_1 causes both a slight increase in CBF and a marked dilatation of extracranial blood vessels.[1488] In physiologically relevant concentrations, PGI_2 has been demonstrated to be a potent cerebral vasodilator, whereas TXA_2 is a potent vasoconstrictor of cerebral arteries.[1588,1589] In addition, endothelial-cell–synthesized PGI_2 prevents platelet adhesion to the endothelium, whereas platelet-derived TXA_2 augments platelet aggregation and adhesion to the capillary wall. Because of this wide variety of contradictory actions, it is difficult to predict the net result on a particular blood vessel when the arachidonic acid cascade is activated.

Prostaglandins and prostacyclin have been implicated in the development of migraine headaches ever since it was reported that prolonged infusions cause headaches. When individuals who do not ordinarily suffer from migraine receive infusion of some prostaglandins (such as PGE_1), they develop severe and frequently throbbing headaches. These bouts are usually bifrontal, and like many attacks of migraine, are accompanied by nausea, vomiting, and autonomic symptoms such as flushing and sweating.[167,314,1479,1549,1987] Abdominal cramps also accompany the headaches. In some cases, the headaches are prefaced by visual phenom-

ena such as flashing lights, which are suggestive of migrainous auras. In contrast, when prostacyclin is infused, it causes less dramatic phenomena— namely nonspecific, dull, throbbing headaches.

The overproduction of prostanoids by the endothelium of cranial arteries has been proposed as an intrinsic abnormality in migraineurs.[1377] Some investigators have reported prostaglandin-like biologic activity in the CSF of migraine patients during severe attacks. Others, however, have been unable to detect such substances.[1,58,124,1747] Data also conflict with regard to changes in prostanoid levels in the blood of migraineurs during attacks.[58,741,1089] Although experimental data are not clear-cut, prophylactic use of drugs that inhibit prostaglandin synthesis—such as aspirin and nonsteroidal anti-inflammatory drugs— can suppress the symptoms of migraine.[625,1386,2124]

Although attempts have been made to formulate a prostaglandin hypothesis of migraine, the full range of symptoms from which migraineurs suffer cannot be explained by variations in prostaglandin levels alone.[314] However, some migrainous phenomena—particularly sensitization of intracranial nociceptive pain endings—may be explained by local changes in arachidonic acid metabolism. This topic will be discussed in the next chapter.

BRADYKININ

The peptide bradykinin is derived when the enzyme kallikrein acts on inactive precursors, the α_2-globulins called kininogens.[1080] Because all the components of the kallikrein system are present in both the blood and the brain, the peptide can be formed in either tissue.[2087] Bradykinin has been detected in axons and neuronal somas in both the hypothalamus and cerebral cortex.[384] Although this peptide is known to be released in the brain during ischemia or injury and from the plasma by inflammatory processes, no data that measure blood bradykinin levels during bouts of migraine are available. Raised CSF bradykinin levels have been reported in a small minority of patients during migraine attacks.[345]

Bradykinin relaxes cerebral arteries and arterioles through a EDRF-mediated process. In particular, bradykinin is a reportedly potent dilator of pial arteries when it is applied to the perivascular side. Relaxing effects of this peptide have also been recorded in isolated extraparenchymal and intraparenchymal cerebral arteries.[425,2085,2138,2139] In addition to its direct action on endothelium, bradykinin also stimulates cyclooxygenase, leading endothelial cells to produce PGI_2. Correspondingly, inhibitors of cyclooxygenase blunt the response of a number of arteries to bradykinin. This suggests that the release of vasodilator prostanoids such as PGI_2 contributes to bradykinin's endothelium-dependent relaxations.[352]

Bradykinin exerts its effects via two types of kininergic receptors, B_1 and B_2. Most actions of bradykinin are mediated through the B_2 receptor, described in a wide variety of arteries and veins; its activation produces relaxation of cerebral vessels. In addition, the receptor linked to the release of EDRF belongs to the B_2 subtype.[1653,2087] The B_1 receptor is not expressed to any significant extent in normal tissues. It is found in only a few vessels. Activation of the B_1 receptor produces mainly contraction.[1655] Thus, the physiologic role for this receptor is unclear. B_1 receptors may be synthesized in larger numbers after tissue injury or inflammation.[1654] The relationship of bradykinin to the development of aura symptoms is speculative.

HISTAMINE

The role of histamine in migraine headache is still a subject of debate. Experimental headaches can be produced by intravenous administration of histamine.* Such headaches are bifrontal

---

*References 359, 612, 670, 702, 1468, 1797

and bioccipital in location and throbbing in nature. Moreover, migraine patients are more sensitive to the effects of histamine than are control subjects, and migraineurs react to smaller concentrations of the amine.[1137] In addition, histamine infusions frequently cause migraineurs to develop pain first on the side of the head that is customarily affected during their migraine attacks.[1828] In some of these regards, histamine headaches correspond to migraine attacks. If these observations were the only ones available, researchers would want unequivocally to focus on histamine's role in the pathogenesis of migraine. Other findings, however, undercut them. For example, the experimental headaches are not associated with nausea or other symptoms characteristic of migraine. They are accompanied by facial flushing. Moreover, histamine-induced headaches are pharmacologically different from migraine. They can be terminated by the administration of H_1 receptor antagonists, whereas migraine headaches are unaffected by such drugs.[1137] In contrast, histamine headaches are immune to doses of ergotamine, which can abort migraine attacks. Clearly, histamine-induced headaches are not identical to migraine.

Interestingly, the effects of histamine seem to depend on which arterial circulation is used for infusion of the amine. Injection into the common or external carotid artery causes throbbing head pain, whereas injection into the internal carotid artery does not produce any headache, nor does it alter rCBF.[1137,1827] These data suggest that the origin of histamine head pain is in the extracranial circulation.

Histamine is found both in histaminergic nerves and in the granules of mast cells. Because of their perivascular locations around arterioles in the meninges and in the brain, the mast cells are regarded as the main source of the histamine that acts on blood vessels.[526] Perivascular application of the amine in situ dilates pial and intraparenchymal arteries.[424,472,838,2086] It also causes dilatation of arterioles and particularly of capillaries.[838,2086] The blood–brain barrier is impermeable to histamine. Intravascular histamine, however, can act on endothelial receptors, which then release EDRF.[1486] The resultant histamine-caused, endothelium-dependent vasodilatation has been demonstrated in a variety of isolated arteries, including human preparations. Which histamine receptors—H_1 or H_2—are involved in these processes is debated. Analysis of the problem is complicated by observations that different histamine receptors—or different ratios of H_1 and H_2 receptors—may be present in different-sized vessels.

Studies of histamine metabolism in connection with migraine have been largely inconclusive. Blood histamine levels have been reported as both normal and high during spontaneous migraine attacks. Both normal and increased urinary secretion of histamine and histamine metabolites have been seen during attacks.[61,1268,1865] Of interest, skin biopsies taken from the involved side of the head of patients with migraine have degranulated mast cells; increased numbers of basophils and degranulated basophils are found in the blood taken from the temple on the side affected by the headache.[1827,2017] Between attacks, histamine levels are reportedly higher in migraineurs than in control subjects.[66,861,920] But despite these associations between histamine and migraine phenomena, combined H_1- and H_2-receptor blockade provides poor prophylaxis for migraine headaches.[69] All in all, although the amine may represent one element in the pathogenetic process, little support exists for the idea that histamine is responsible for the pathophysiologic events known to occur during the migraine aura.

ADENOSINE

Adenosine is another dilator of cerebral vessels. It has strong vasodilator effects when applied to pial arteries and arterioles in vitro or topically by superfusion in vivo.[168,587] The effect is mediated by A_2 receptor subtypes. Intact endothelium is not required for adenosine-induced relaxation of cerebral arteries. Levels of adenosine and other related purine compounds (AMP and cAMP) are rapidly raised during ischemia, such as that which may occur during the migrainous aura.[168] If local CBF falls below 25 mL/100 g/min, adenosine concentrations are transiently elevated. Such decreased levels of CBF may be present during the aura.[858,2195] Under such conditions, it is believed that purines are released mainly by endothelial cells, although aggregating platelets and perivascular nerves may contribute. Whether these phenomena are pertinent to the migrainous process is yet to be discovered.

SUMMARY

Studies from a number of laboratories have documented CBF changes in the brains of patients who suffer from classic migraine. Although reductions of CBF during the aura have been repeatedly noted, data vary with regard to the nature and degree of the reduction. And despite enormous amounts of effort, we can still only theorize as to whether these changes in CBF are primary or secondary events in migraine. The next two chapters will explore what is known and what is speculated about other aspects of the pathophysiology of migraine headaches.

Chapter 7

HEAD PAIN AND ASSOCIATED SYMPTOMS

Because the extracranial circulation was accessible to study, Harold G. Wolff and his colleagues focused on the role of vasodilatation of the superficial temporal artery and other branches of the external carotid artery in the genesis of head pain.[822,2043,2045] Most neurologists have accepted Wolff's ideas—including the concept that migraine pain is a condition caused primarily by distension of branches of the external, and possibly the internal, carotid artery. Wolff himself hypothesized that other factors were necessary for the production of pain, in particular, the accumulation of certain neuropeptides within and in the vicinity of the vessel walls. Nevertheless, most neurologists have continued to assume that vasodilatation is sufficient to excite pain-sensitive nerve endings (*nociceptive nerve endings, nociceptors*) in the arterial walls.[344,2169] As this chapter will demonstrate, experimental proof is available for alternative explanations.

LOCUS OF MIGRAINE PAIN

A number of clinical observations undermine the claim that vasodilatation accompanied by increased pulsations of arteries, especially extracranial arteries, is the primary cause of migraine pain in most patients.[214] First, pulsating or throbbing pain is not pathognomonic of a primary vascular origin of pain. Pulsating pain is felt after injury or inflammation in a number of structures and represents a vascular response to inflammation in either vessels or in their surrounding structures. Second, pulsating pain is present in only about half of migraine patients.[1489] Studies performed subsequent to Wolff's have shown one of two conditions: (1) *no* consistent difference between the pulsations on the headache and the headache-free sides of the head, or (2) the pulse amplitude of the frontal branch of the superficial temporal artery is larger on the side of a unilateral headache in only a minority of migraineurs who experience pulsating pain.[247,545,943] Third, if extracranial vasodilatation is the cause of pain, patients might be expected to be flushed during bouts of migraine, but migraineurs are most often pale or even ashen; flushing during attacks is unusual.[214] In line with this, we lack convincing evidence that changes occur in extracranial blood flow to skin and muscle during bouts of migraine.[607,1032,1033,1736] And finally, if vasodilatation of the superficial temporal artery is the major factor in pain production, one would expect that manual compression of the superficial temporal artery would eliminate pain in all migraine sufferers. In fact, compression of the artery temporarily reduces the pain in only a minority of patients.[214,545] Similarly, occlusion of extracranial vessels by means of a blood pressure cuff placed around the head and elevated above the systemic blood pressure does not alleviate the headache in most patients.[214]

Some of these findings can be explained by the observation that those patients whose throbbing headache can be attenuated by application of pressure over the superficial arteries appear to form a separate subgroup with larger pulsations of the frontal branch of the superficial temporal artery and thermographic evidence of increased facial blood flow on the side of the headache.[545,546] All these data lead to the conclusion that dilatation of the superficial temporal artery and its branches is not a major cause of the pain of migraine headache in the majority of patients.[545,546] Clinical evidence that the pain has an intracranial component is derived from the observations that almost all patients suffer more intensely from head movement, particularly when the head is rapidly rotated or jolted.[214]

Intracranial Sources of Migraine Pain

Headache-like pain can be evoked in neurosurgical patients by electrical stimulation or distension of the main trunks of the dural arteries, of dural sinuses and their tributary veins, and of the proximal segments of the large pial arteries comprising the circle of Willis.* In contrast, the pial arteries and veins located over the convexity of the cerebral hemispheres are much less sensitive. The dura—in particular, the supratentorial dura covering the cerebral

convexities—is relatively insensitive to pain, except along the margins of the dural sinuses, the sites where cerebral veins enter these sinuses, and along the course of the meningeal arteries.[1556,1647,2163] Pain is not produced by stimulating the skull, the choroid plexus, the ventricular ependyma, the brain parenchyma, or the cerebral veins.

Pain resulting from stimulation of intracranial arteries is referred to specific loci, such as the ipsilateral temple; forehead; retro-orbital, periorbital, and frontal regions; and is reported to be throbbing, aching, or boring in nature. Moreover, specific patterns of pain referral have been reported. Thus, stimulation of the circle of Willis, the proximal anterior cerebral artery, and the middle cerebral artery produces pain in, behind, or around the ipsilateral eye. Disturbance of the posterior cerebral artery elicits pain located in retro-orbital or parietal regions. Stimulation of the intracranial part of the internal carotid artery leads to pain within, behind, or above the eye. Parietotemporal, orbital, or auricular pain is produced by stimulation of the middle meningeal artery, and orbital pain by stimulation of the anterior meningeal artery. All these data indicate that nociceptive transmission from supratentorial structures is carried by perivascular pial and dural afferents and referred to the somatic receptive fields of the trigeminal nerve. In contrast, stimulation of the vertebral and basilar arteries induces pain in the back of the head and in the neck. These latter results show that, at least in part, nociceptive impulses from certain posterior structures involve referral of pain to areas innervated by cervical roots.

Clinical observations suggest that dural venous sinuses located close to the midline (or possibly tributary veins) are the loci of the process causing migraine headache in some patients. Thus, in many migraineurs the pain is bilateral. In some migraineurs, it is steady and aching in quality rather than pulsating. In many, it is augmented by performance of maneuvers

*References 629, 637, 1455, 1468, 1555, 1556, 1647

such as bending over, coughing, sneezing, breath holding, or straining—all of which increase intracranial venous pressure. All of these characteristics are expected of a process affecting dural venous sinuses. It is not unexpected, then, that stimuli applied to large veins at the base of the brain and to the sagittal and transverse sinuses or their tributary veins produce orbital and frontal pain.

In sum, the dural and pial vasculature appears to be the most plausible location for the pain-generating process that leads to misery for the majority of migraineurs. Central pain pathways, however, have also been implicated as candidates for pain production. For example, some patients develop headaches immediately after electrodes are implanted in the periaqueductal gray matter or in the somatosensory portion of the thalamus.[1638] These post-implantation headaches can occur in patients not previously troubled by headaches; for some individuals, they persist for months to years. The headaches resemble migraine headaches. Some patients are reported to develop both a pattern of intermittent, recurrent, pounding headaches and a syndrome that includes visual disturbances, nausea, and vomiting. The pain was exaggerated by administration of serotonin precursors in one patient and alleviated by reserpine and ergotamine in other patients. Thus, perturbation of selected areas of the central nervous system (CNS) may produce head pain that has some of the characteristics of migraine. The implications of these findings for cases of "ordinary" migraine need investigation.

AFFERENT TRIGEMINAL AND CERVICAL SYSTEMS

The data reviewed in the previous section indicate that the pain of most, if not all, migraine attacks is produced in intracranial vascular structures. The following sections take a closer look at these structures. After outlining their innervation in general, and with particular regard for the central terminations of afferent fibers, the discussion will show that pain from intracranial structures in man is mediated by perivascular pial and dural nociceptive terminals, that nociceptive information is conveyed by trigeminal and dorsal root afferent fibers that use peptides as neurotransmitters, and that pain arising from intracranial vessels is referred to specific somatic receptive fields of the trigeminal nerve.

The periadventitial tissue and the superficial adventitia of pial and dural blood vessels contains abundant plexuses of small-diameter myelinated and unmyelinated nerve fibers, as well as some larger myelinated fibers.[426,1556] Many of the fibers are sensory in origin, in that they are axons of ipsilateral, small- and medium-sized, primary afferent neurons located in the trigeminal ganglia and upper cervical dorsal root ganglia.* The dura itself also has a trigeminal sensory innervation, which is most dense along the border of the superior sagittal sinus.[52] Much of this innervation consists of unmyelinated C fibers.

Nociceptive afferent fibers from arteries and venous sinuses above the tentorium arrive in the brain stem chiefly via the trigeminal (fifth) cranial nerve, whereas the fibers from vessels below the tentorium are carried primarily through the upper cervical nerves. Although all three divisions of the trigeminal nerve are involved in transmitting nociceptive information from intracranial blood vessels, branches of the ophthalmic (V_1) division are the major source of pain-sensitive afferents.[1353,1556,1934] Results from surgical procedures verify the importance of the ophthalmic division in generating migrainous pain. For instance, surgical treatment of migraine headache has shown that the head pain can be attenuated by trigeminal rhizotomy, gasserian alcohol injection, or bulbar tractotomy. The most effective therapeutic

*References 1092, 1341, 1342, 1466, 1476

outcomes, however, are realized when the skin supplied by the first trigeminal division is rendered anesthetic.*

The *Gasserian ganglion (trigeminal ganglion, semilunar ganglion)*—the location of the pseudounipolar primary afferent cell bodies of the trigeminal nerve—is located on the petrous bone near its apex in the middle cerebral fossa. As expected, the ophthalmic division of the Gasserian ganglion is the source of most of the cell bodies of afferent axons that innervate dural and pial vessels. Dural, and probably pial, arteries, however, are also innervated in part by the maxillary (V_2) and mandibular (V_3) divisions of the ganglion.†

The exact pathway connecting the trigeminal ganglia and the cerebral vessels is a matter of some dispute. Innervation of the cerebral vessels may involve at least six different nerves or groups of nerve fibers:‡

1. The *nervus tentorii (tentorial nerve of Arnold)* innervates the superior surface of the tentorium cerebelli;

the posterior portion of the falx cerebri; the walls of the sagittal, transverse, and straight sinuses; and the torcular Herophili (Fig. 7–1). Older descriptions of the nerve indicated that it arose from the ophthalmic branch of the trigeminal nerve proximal to the superior orbital fissure.[637,1353,1556] And indeed, in the schematic drawing of Fig. 7–1, the dotted line of the *nervus tentorii* does appear to branch off the first division of trigeminal nerve. The tentorial nerve may, however, be a branch of the cavernous plexus of nerves rather than a direct branch of the ophthalmic nerve.[1713] The cavernous plexus consists of an intermingling of trigeminal and autonomic fibers lying in the connective tissue surrounding the ophthalmic and abducens nerves in the lateral wall of the cavernous sinus. Afferents from the plexus are dispensed directly to the internal carotid artery and are distributed along its intracranial branches to reach dural and venous structures.

2. The *anterior meningeal nerves (anterior and posterior ethmoidal nerves)* are branches of the intraorbital portion of the ophthalmic branch of the

---

*References 422, 629, 1498, 1555, 1702, 2140
†References 52, 79, 1342, 1476, 1856, 1933
‡References 1110, 1111, 1353, 1556, 2029

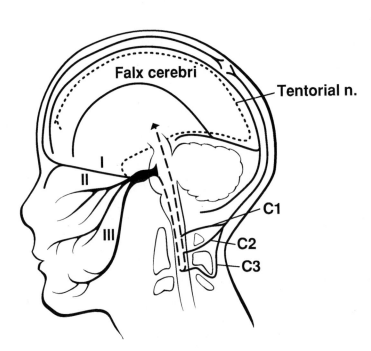

Figure 7–1. Schematic diagram of the three divisions of the trigeminal nerve, the Gasserian ganglion, and the upper cervical nerve roots. The three interrupted lines indicate the route taken by the descending spinal tract of the trigeminal nerve, the path taken by crossed second-order nerves ascending to rostral structures such as the thalamus, and the position taken by the tentorial nerve. The first cervical nerve root is inconstant. (Adapted from Lance, JW: Mechanism and Management of Headache. ed. 4. Butterworth, London, 1982, with permission.)

trigeminal nerve. They enter the cranium as nasociliary nerves through the cribiform plate. This small group of fibers carries painful impulses from the anterior cranial fossa and the anterior aspect of the falx cerebri to the Gasserian ganglion.

3. The *nervus spinosus of Luschka* is a recurrent branch of the extracranial part of the mandibular nerve. The *nervus spinosus* enters the cranial cavity via the foramen spinosum.[1353,1556] It joins the middle meningeal artery, and supplies both the dura of the anterior and middle cranial fossae and the dura overlying the lateral convexity of the cerebrum.

4. The *middle meningeal nerves* (*nervus meningeus medius*) emerge from the intracranial portion of the maxillary nerve to accompany the frontal branch of the middle meningeal artery. These nerves innervate the dura of the anterior middle fossa and the sphenoid ridge.

5. The major innervation of the rostral pial vessels in primates comes from the *ophthalmic division of the trigeminal nerve.*[1342,1714,1856] Two or three short, fine branches of the intracavernous part of the ophthalmic nerve appear to join the cavernous plexus. The maxillary nerve also appears to contribute fibers to pial vessels via an orbitociliary branch. These latter fibers are thought to pass caudally through the infraorbital fissure to join the fibers from the ophthalmic division in the cavernous plexus and to innervate the internal carotid artery and its branches.[892]

6. Several satellite miniganglia are located on the internal carotid artery at sites in the carotid canal and in the cavernous sinus. These structures may also be a source of intracranial vessel innervation. Composed of neurons that resemble those of the trigeminal ganglion, the miniganglia are believed to contain cell bodies of some trigeminal afferent fibers.[329,1714,1976] The miniganglia are of various sizes: some contain less than 20 neurons; others contain several hundred neurons.

Not only is there dispute about how cerebral vessels are innervated, but there is also some confusion about where certain other afferent nerve fibers originate. Under question are the nociceptors responsible for supplying painful sensation to the dura mater lining the posterior cranial fossa, the dural blood vessels of the posterior fossa, and the basilar and vertebral arteries. At various times, researchers have believed that alone, or in various combinations, the facial, glossopharyngeal, vagal, spinal accessory, sympathetic, or the upper three cervical nerves supplied these structures.[1090,1092,1101] Now, however, a consensus has been reached with regard to the posterior fossa—namely, that it receives afferent innervation from fibers arising chiefly from cell bodies in the upper three cervical dorsal root ganglia, but with variable contributions from the trigeminal nerve.* The branches of the cervical nerves, however, frequently travel to the posterior fossa with the tenth and twelfth cranial nerves. The tenth cranial nerve may also supply a small number of afferents to the basilar artery.[1090]

Some midline vascular structures are innervated by bilaterally projecting sensory fibers. The superior sagittal sinus, for example, receives bilateral trigeminal ganglion innervation.[1342] The anterior cerebral arteries and the rostral basilar artery also receive projections from both trigeminal ganglia.[1735]

Central Terminations of Afferent Fibers—Anatomic Considerations

The primary afferent trigeminal nociceptive axons exit from the gasserian ganglion in the trigeminal sensory root (*portio major*). The root passes through the posterior cranial fossa to enter the anterolateral portion of the pons. Anatomic data indicate that the nociceptive

*References 78, 79, 1090, 1092, 1110, 1111, 1735

axons, or branches of these axons, descend caudally to join the bundle of fibers designated as the *spinal tract of the trigeminal nerve.* At the caudal end of the medulla oblongata, the spinal tract merges into the tract of Lissauer in the spinal cord. Terminal and collateral branches of the spinal tract are given to the *nucleus of the descending tract of the trigeminal nerve.* But recent investigations have shown that the upper spinal segments are also involved in the central termination of afferent fibers from pain-sensitive intracranial structures. Thus, a moderate number of trigeminal fibers extend as far down as the second or third cervical segment, and histologic data appear to show that these fibers terminate in the cervical dorsal horn.[78,1023,1821] That considerable overlap exists between the trigeminal and cervical distributions is shown by findings that these same areas of the gray matter of the cervical dorsal horn that receive trigeminal afferents also receive ramifications from the first three cervical dorsal roots.

From the dorsal horn of the spinal cord the nucleus of the descending trigeminal tract extends rostrally to the principal trigeminal sensory nucleus in the pons.[1503] This descending nucleus is divided in a rostral to caudal direction into three subnuclei—the nucleus oralis, the nucleus interpolaris, and the nucleus caudalis (Fig. 7–2). The last of these, the *nucleus caudalis*, has traditionally been perceived as the fundamental locus from which pain information was relayed to more rostral levels of the central nervous system. The perception that the nucleus caudalis is involved in transmitting painful sensations is based in large part on data collected from patients after lesions were made in their spinal trigeminal tracts for the purpose of treating trigeminal neuralgia. These patients lost their ability to perceive pain in areas of the face innervated by the trigeminal nerve. And indeed, this perception makes sense because not only is the nucleus caudalis a rostral continuation of

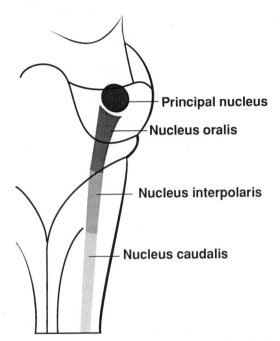

Figure 7–2. The subdivisions of the trigeminal sensory nucleus. The upper portion is the main (principal) sensory nucleus. Caudal to the main nucleus are the three subdivisions of the nucleus of the descending trigeminal tract: the nucleus oralis, the nucleus interpolaris, and the nucleus caudalis. The latter nucleus is continuous with the dorsal horn. (Modified from Olszewski, J: On the anatomical and functional organization of the spinal trigeminal nucleus. J Comp Neurol 92:401–413, 1950; copyright John Wiley & Sons, 1950; reprinted by permission of Wiley-Liss, a division of John Wiley & Sons, Inc.)

the dorsal horn, but it also has morphologic similarities to the dorsal horn. In addition, neurons in the nucleus caudalis usually function in ways comparable to those of nociceptive neurons in the dorsal horn. Moreover, most unmyelinated trigeminal afferent fibers—those fibers putatively involved in nociceptive mechanisms—terminate in the nucleus caudalis. All of these factors support the traditional view that connected pain pathways to the nucleus caudalis. Recent data suggest that the anatomy of these pain pathways differs somewhat from the traditional view. There are indications that large numbers of unmyelinated projections from pial arteries are present in the nucleus interpolaris, and that the nucleus interpolaris, and possibly the nucleus oralis, also function in the processing of nociceptive information from intracranial structures.[78]

Central Terminations of Afferent Fibers—Physiologic Data

Physiologic investigations of the firing patterns of individual brain stem and spinal neurons have demonstrated that the accepted perceptions of the synaptic terminations of trigeminal fibers must be modified. Activation of pain-sensitive intracranial structures such as the superior sagittal sinus and the middle meningeal artery causes neuronal discharges in two *main* locations:

1. the traditional brain stem areas, including the nucleus caudalis and, to a lesser extent, the nucleus interpolaris,[457,458,530,1964] and

2. a newly described spinal area *lateral* to the dorsal horn in the second cervical segment.[78,1162,1165,2193] This spinal area is located in the region of the lateral cervical nucleus. Activation of neurons in this region of the spinal cord following stimulation of intracranial pain-sensitive structures has been confirmed by autoradiographic metabolic studies.[787]

The input to both areas involves the trigeminal system, but the spinal area also receives contributions from cervical dorsal roots.[789] Both areas project to the thalamus.[54]

In sum, pain in intracranial structures is subserved by cranial and upper cervical nerves. Nociceptive fibers from intracranial structures such as the dural and pial arteries and the dural sinuses synapse on neurons located in several subdivisions of the nucleus of the descending trigeminal tract and in the dorsal horn and lateral cervical nucleus of the cervical spinal cord. Both trigeminal and cervical afferents are involved.

Thalamic and Cortical Projections

The axons from cells in the nucleus caudalis and in the cervical spinal cord project via the *trigeminothalamic tract* (*quintothalmic tract*) to the contralateral thalamus (Fig. 7–3). Electrophysiologic and anatomic studies have shown that the major site for axons from these nuclei to terminate is the classic sensory-receiving nucleus of the thalamus—the *ventroposteromedial nucleus* (VPM)—and its ventral periphery.[458,713,789,1964,2193] All units in VPM excited by vascular stimulation also have facial receptive fields, particularly in areas of the face supplied by the ophthalmic division of the trigeminal nerve.[2193] Moreover, electrophysiologic studies have revealed that in other areas of the thalamus neurons respond to intracranial vascular stimulation. These thalamic areas include the medial part of the posterior complex (an ill-defined group of cells in the caudal thalamus at the mesodiencephalic junction) and the intralaminar nuclei (consisting of several small cell groups in the internal medullary lamina).[458,789,1964,2193]

Neurons in VPM and in the posterior complex excited by trigeminothalamic afferents project to the ipsilateral primary somatosensory cortex in the postcentral gyrus. All of the intralaminar nuclei have diffuse cortical projections, particularly to the frontal lobe and the limbic system.[1052]

Various characteristics of noxious events may be "processed" differently in different areas of the brain. The pathways that discriminate sensory aspects of noxious events and are responsible for determining the location, type, and intensity of the nociceptive input to the CNS are hypothesized to involve VPM and the primary somatosensory cortex.[1363] In contrast, the unpleasant feelings associated with pain—the so-called affective–motivational aspects of pain—are thought to involve the intralaminar nuclei and their projections to the frontal lobe and limbic system.[1363]

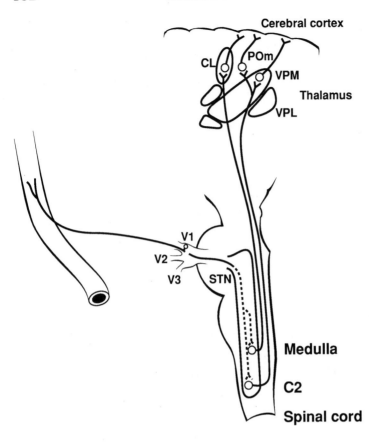

Figure 7–3. The pathways taken by nociceptive information from intracranial vessels. The primary afferent neuron is a bipolar cell located in the Gasserian ganglion that makes synaptic connections on neurons in the subnucleus caudalis (medulla) and the second cervical segment (C2). Axons of the medullary and spinal neurons cross and then ascend in the trigeminothalamic tract to the thalamus to synapse on cells in the ventroposteromedial nucleus (VPM), the medial nucleus of the posterior complex (POm), and the centrolateral nucleus (CL). Axons of thalamic neurons project to the sensory cortex. (Adapted from Goadsby,[789] p 370, with permission.)

Afferent Transmitters

As noted in the previous chapter, many of the nociceptive trigeminal and upper cervical sensory primary afferent fibers innervating the cranial vasculature contain and secrete neuropeptides. These neuropeptides include substance P, neurokinin A, and calcitonin gene-related peptide.* Much recent data indicate that in the trigeminal system—and in other afferent systems— these peptides act as nociceptive neurotransmitters in a large number of unmyelinated C fibers, and possibly in some thinly myelinated Aδ fibers. Immunohistochemical techniques have demonstrated that in pial arteries and veins and in the dura there is a delicate, but moderately dense, network of substance P-containing, neurokinin A-

containing, and calcitonin gene-related peptide-containing fibers and varicose terminals.[594,2049] The density of peptide-containing nerve fibers and terminals is higher in the proximal parts of the circle of Willis and in the vertebrobasilar system than in more distal arterial structures.[1976] The trigeminal afferent nerve fibers that innervate the cerebrovascular bed admost always contain more than one peptide. For example, all trigeminal afferents that contain substance P or neurokinin A also contain calcitonin gene-related peptide. Cholecystokinin has also been identified within trigeminal fibers projecting to intracranial vessels. Its role, however, has not been determined.

Cell bodies containing substance P and calcitonin gene-related peptide are located in several locations. Among them are the trigeminal ganglion, the C-2 dorsal root ganglion, and the internal carotid microganglia.[79,378,473,1976,2049]

---

*References 577, 581, 582, 881, 1262, 1263, 1338, 1350, 1424, 2041, 2049, 2098

As in the afferent fibers, these two peptides coexist in many of the same nerve cells, but a subset of trigeminal ganglion cells and nerve fibers contain calcitonin gene-related peptide but not substance P.* Unilateral trigeminal ganglionectomy substantially reduces the levels of all peptides in the rostral intracranial vessels, an indication that the trigeminal ganglion is the major source of the afferent peptide-containing fibers.[1263,1350,2185] Cerebrovascular substance P-containing nerve fibers appear to originate mainly in the ophthalmic division of the trigeminal ganglion.[1263,1341,1342,1733] It has been estimated that substance P is a putative transmitter in 15% to 20% of the neurons in the trigeminal ganglion.[1262,2185]

Referred Pain

Mechanical and electrical stimulation of pial and dural arteries and of venous sinuses produces pain in temporal, retro-orbital and periorbital, frontal, occipital, and cervical regions. The locations of such pain support a concept that pain arising from intracra-

___

*References 847, 882, 1216, 1477, 1976, 1997, 2049

nial vascular structures is *referred to somatic receptive fields* of the trigeminal nerve.† In other words the source of the pain is not the place where the pain is actually perceived. Two major mechanisms have been proposed to explain the referral of such pain:

1. *The branched primary afferent hypothesis of Sinclair.*[1857] Sinclair postulated that some primary afferent fibers bifurcated, furnishing branches to both somatic and visceral structures (Fig. 7–4A). As a result of this bifurcation, Sinclair suggested, sensory messages from a somatic structure (such as the skin of the temple) and a visceral structure (such as an intracranial blood vessel) were carried by the same afferent, so that the message from the visceral branch could be misinterpreted by the brain and localized as pain in the temple. Branching of primary afferents does indeed occur. Some trigeminal ganglion cells send axon collaterals to innervate more than one intracranial vessel.[1427,1476] For example, trigeminal ganglion neurons innervating the middle meningeal artery may also send projections to innervate the middle cerebral artery. However, axonal branches of single afferent trigeminal neurons do

___

†References 629, 637, 1468, 1555, 1556, 1647

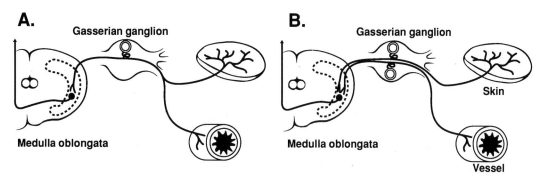

Figure 7–4. Theories of Referred Pain. (*A*) Branched primary afferent theory. A single primary trigeminal afferent branches to supply both an intracranial artery and the skin. The artery is the source of pain, but the pain is perceived in the skin. The existence of such branched fibers in the trigeminal system has not been documented. (*B*) Convergence-projection hypothesis. Primary afferents from skin and from intracranial vessels converge on the same medullary pain-projection neurons in the trigeminal nucleus caudalis. The brain mistakenly "projects" to the skin the sensation arising in the afferent from the intracranial artery. Such convergence of afferents from peripheral and intracranial structures has been demonstrated in the trigeminal system. (Modified from Fields, HL: Pain, McGraw-Hill, New York, 1987, with permission of McGraw-Hill.)

not innervate both intracranial and extracranial structures. Accordingly, the lack of appropriate neural connections negates the theory.[238,1352,1476]

2. *The convergence–projection hypothesis of Ruch.*[1708] Ruch presumed that referred sensation was caused by the synaptic connections of both visceral and somatic afferents onto the same relay neurons. If the trigeminal vascular afferents project onto nociceptive relay neurons that also receive somatic inputs from skin and muscle, impulses from either input could be capable of initiating activity in the same trigeminal relay cells (Fig. 7–4B). The relay cells could, in turn, project to rostral sensory areas in the brain. The convergence–projection theory is generally thought to supply the best explanation of referred headache pain because electrophysiologic studies have demonstrated that both vascular and somatic afferents do synapse on single neurons within the nucleus caudalis.[1964] Thus activation of intracranial afferents could excite sensory pathways also excited by somatic afferents. This process is thought to elicit a sensory experience at the somatic input rather than at the vascular origin of the noxious stimulus.

TWO THEORIES OF THE SOURCE OF MIGRAINOUS HEAD PAIN

Vasodilatation that stretches nociceptors located within the walls of blood vessels has been accepted for many years as the process responsible for activating vascular nociceptors and producing the head pain of a migraine attack. But more recently the trigeminovascular system has been implicated in a process of neurogenic inflammation responsible for sensitizing nociceptive nerve fibers, thereby causing migrainous head pain. The following sections consider these two possibilities in light of recent research.

Cerebral Blood Flow During Migrainous Head Pain

If, as earlier theories postulated, a change in the caliber of intracerebral vessels plays an important role in producing migrainous pain, variations in blood flow might be expected to correlate with the severity of the head pain. And indeed, a number of authorities have described both focal and global hyperemia during the headache phase of common and classic migraine attacks.* Other investigators, however, have found hyperemia to occur only in some patients.[856,1944] Focal cortical oligemia with a patch of hyperemia was demonstrated in two cases of spontaneous common migraine.[748] Moreover, it is important to note that although a number of studies demonstrated changes in blood flow during headaches, oftentimes the changes were bilateral and symmetrical even when the patients experienced unilateral headaches.[1124–1126,1376]

The concept of hyperemia during the headache phase of migraine has been challenged by the Copenhagen group of investigators. These workers have documented that the onset of hyperemic changes in cerebral blood flow (CBF) bears a poor temporal relationship to the development of head pain in patients with classic migraine.[1204,1496,1870,1874] In contrast to assertions attributing pain to arterial dilatation, the Copenhagen group found that the head pain usually develops at a time when regional cerebral blood flow (rCBF) is reduced. Moreover, in cases of migraine with aura, although pain typically emerges when the aura recedes, hyperemia characteristically takes many hours to develop and may persist for many hours or even days—long after migrainous head pain has disappeared.[41,848,1376] As for attacks of common migraine, these researchers have shown that such headaches, although

---

*References 566, 748, 1068, 1124–1126, 1331, 1378, 1467, 1471, 1472, 1736, 1870, 1871

clearly painful, are commonly unaccompanied by significant changes in CBF.[1204,1206,1496,1874] The sum total of these results indicates that it is extremely unlikely for intracranial vasodilatation that causes changes in CBF to be solely responsible for the head pain of a migraine attack. More information is needed to account for the discrepancies between results from investigators who have concluded that hyperemia is associated with headache and those who have not. In particular, we need to learn the extent to which these differences may be a consequence of studying CBF at different times after the onset of an attack.

There are also a few studies of blood vessel diameter changes during the headache phase of migraine. For example, dilatation of secondary and tertiary branches of the internal carotid artery on one side was demonstrated by serial angiography of one case during a possible migraine attack.[1321]

Inferences about possible changes in the diameter of intracranial vessels have been made using transcranial Doppler ultrasonography (TCD). TCD is a comparatively recent, noninvasive, ultrasonic technique that permits measurement of blood velocity in the large intracranial vessels.[490,2190] These arteries can be insonated through the skull. Commercially available TCD devices employ a probe that emits an ultrasound signal, which is reflected from the red blood cells traveling through the arteries at the base of the brain. The reflected signal is received by the same probe and transmitted to a computer that uses the Doppler shift principle to calculate blood velocity, thus providing information about peak flow velocity, pulsatility, and the waveform of the arterial blood flow. One drawback to TCD technology is that it cannot detect changed blood velocity in the meningeal and dural arteries—vessels strongly implicated in the genesis of migrainous head pain. But because TCD is noninvasive, one would hope that the data it can generate about blood flow

will provide important insights. Unfortunately, blood velocity and the diameter of blood vessels are inconstantly related. An increased blood flow velocity may be caused by vasodilatation accompanied by increased CBF, but it could also occur in a situation in which CBF has been lowered as the result of reduction in the diameter of the arterial lumen, caused, for example, by arterial spasm or by arterial stenosis.

During bouts of migraine, increases in velocity have been reported by some authors.[672,1536,1686,2013] There is, however, a marked heterogeneity of responses, and many patients show either decreased Doppler velocities or no change in velocity during attacks.[694,1536,2207] Moreover, neither vasodilatation nor vasoconstriction correlates with the locus of the aura or of the headache. And in addition, little data are available regarding possible sequential changes in velocity during the evolution of an attack. To some extent, the controversy appears to reflect a lack of standardized examination procedures. It is possible that velocity changes may, in part, be secondary phenomena caused by a stress reaction or a reaction to pain. TCD has not yet added much to our understanding of the pathophysiologic changes in blood flow that occur during migraine, particularly with regard to the changes that may occur during the aura. In contrast, consistent changes reflecting dilatation have been observed in patients during cluster headache and following administration of glycerol trinitrate.[427]

Recent investigations undertaken during spontaneous, unilateral migraine attacks have simultaneously measured rCBF in middle cerebral arteries by means of single-photon emission computerized tomography with ^{133}Xe inhalation and blood velocity by means of TCD. These studies showed that the middle cerebral artery velocity was significantly slower on the headache side than on the unaffected side at a time when the rCBF was unchanged.[694] The lower velocity in the feeding artery in the face of normal rCBF in the territory of brain supplied by that artery can best be explained by dilatation of the middle cerebral artery during the headache. As indicated above, however, other studies have shown enhanced Doppler flow velocities in some patients during migraine attacks.[672,1536,1686] Moreover, measurement of blood flow by the ^{133}Xe inhalation technique has been shown to significantly alter middle cerebral artery blood flow velocities.[1716] If experimental results are inconsistent, and if the experimental technique is capable of interfering with the process being measured, there can be no consistent objective data that unequivocally supports an hypothesis that intracranial vasodilatation is responsible for migraine headache pain.

In sum, substantial and convincing evidence linking intracranial vasodilatation in either cerebral conductance arteries or arterioles and the pain of migraine headache is lacking. By itself, distension of large pial and dural arteries appears unlikely to be sufficient to induce headache pain. Additional explanations will have to be sought.

Neurogenic Inflammation and Vascular Pain

The elegant investigations of Moskowitz and his colleagues have shed a different light on the mechanisms that cause head pain during migraine attacks. Their work appears to have brought us closer to an understanding of the processes involved in the generation of headache.[1420-1422] Moskowitz has proposed that *neurogenic inflammation* plays a preeminent role in the production of the pain associated with migraine headaches.[1420,1426] This process consists of vascular dilatation, enhanced leakage or extravasation of plasma proteins across the endothelium with subsequent edema formation in vessel walls, and a complex chain of chemical and physiologic events that excites, sensitizes, and lowers the threshold of the trigeminal nociceptive

terminals. Because neurogenic inflammation is produced by activation of trigeminal nociceptive fibers in vessels of the dura, it would appear that the process involves the trigeminovascular system.[525,894] Neurogenic inflammation presumably occurs also in the walls of large vessels equipped with vasa vasorum—structures in which inflammation may develop at the microvascular level, producing protein extravasation with subsequent edema formation and sensitization of nociceptive terminals in the large vessels.

The basis for the inflammatory hypothesis rests on findings that under experimental conditions, mechanical or chemical stimulation of craniovascular nociceptive nerve endings, or antidromic electrical stimulation of the trigeminovascular system, produces neurogenic inflammation involving the vessels of the dura (Fig. 7–5).[1303,1425] Plasma extravasation with enhanced transcytosis and subsequent perivascular edema formation, platelet aggregation, and mast cell activation all follow activation of the trigeminovascular system.

When nociceptive afferents are excited and fire, neuropeptides are released centrally onto second-order neurons in the nucleus caudalis of the brain stem and in the dorsal horn of the spinal cord. The neuropeptides cause these second-order neurons to transmit nociceptive signals to the central nervous system. Discharging nociceptive afferents, however, also have the unique ability to release neuropeptides from their *peripheral* perivascular terminals—the so-called *efferent function* of afferent terminals.[975] In other words, impulses proceed both antidromically and orthodromically on activation of these nerves. Furthermore, the process spreads from one nerve terminal to another by means of *axon reflexes*.[1428] When nerve impulses traveling orthodromically in an afferent nerve fiber reach a branch point, they are thought to fire antidromically in collateral branches. In turn, when the action potential reaches the peripheral

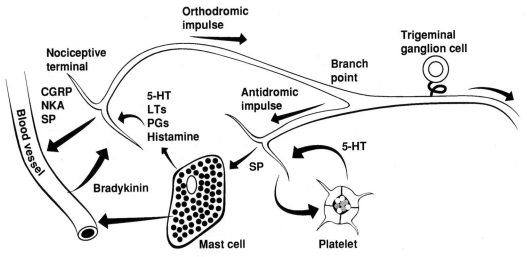

Figure 7–5. Some of the putative events involved in the activation and sensitization of intracranial nociceptor terminals. Following activation of a nociceptive terminal, impulses are generated in the terminal and propagate orthodromically. Axon reflexes are produced when the impulse reaches a branch point and is propagated antidromically into another terminal branch. This results in the release of neuropeptides including substance P (SP), neurokinin A (NKA), and calcitonin gene-related peptide (CGRP). SP and other peptides act on the blood vessels to induce vasodilatation and plasma extravasation. The interstitial levels of bradykinin, synthesized from plasma proteins, rise. SP also causes the release of histamine and other substances from mast cells, and serotonin (5-HT) from platelets.

terminals of the collateral branch, it causes the release of neuropeptides. The process may also spread from one intracranial vessel to another because, as mentioned above, trigeminal fibers send branches to innervate more than one intracranial vessel.

The claim that neurogenic inflammation involves the antidromic release of neuropeptides from intracranial trigeminovascular nociceptive nerve terminals and the subsequent development of neurogenic inflammation is supported by a number of findings:

1. Electrical stimulation of the trigeminal ganglion in experimental animals causes the antidromic release of substance P and calcitonin gene-related peptide, and also results in elevated levels of these peptides in blood draining from the sagittal sinus.[1425]

2. Activation of nociceptive craniovascular afferents by electrical stimulation of the superior sagittal sinus results in elevated levels of calcitonin gene-related peptide in external jugular-vein blood.[2192]

3. Neurogenic inflammation manifested by leakage of plasma proteins from dural blood vessels is observed following trigeminal ganglion stimulation, and during infusions of substance P or neurokinin A.

4. Capsaicin (8-methyl N-vanillyl-6-noneamide), the active ingredient of hot peppers, which is known to depolarize unmyelinated nociceptive afferent nerves and to cause the release of neuropeptides from nerve endings, produces neurogenic inflammation in the dura.[679,726,991]

5. Intracranial neurogenic inflammation is not observed in experimental animals lacking unmyelinated C fibers.[1303]

The connection between release of neuropeptides and migraine attacks in humans is provided by findings that calcitonin gene-related peptide is elevated in the cranial circulation during acute attacks of migraine with or without aura.[778] In addition, during surgery for trigeminal neuralgia, stimulation of the trigeminal ganglion by thermocoagulation causes the release of substance P and calcitonin gene-related peptide into external jugular vein blood.[777]

As mentioned in the previous chapter, substance P, neurokinin A, and calcitonin gene-related peptide are vasoactive substances and potent dilators of cerebral and pial blood vessels as well as potent initiators of neurogenic inflammation.[581,582,591,595] These peptides, however, differ in their actions. Calcitonin gene-related peptide provokes a more powerful dilatation of pial arterioles in vivo than does substance P; in contrast, substance P dilates pial veins, whereas calcitonin gene-related peptide does not.[595,1350] Moreover, the dilatation induced by substance P depends on an intact vascular endothelium; the action of calcitonin gene-related peptide is independent of the vascular endothelium and is exerted directly on smooth muscle.[881]

Substance P and neurokinin A cause protein leakage through vascular walls, presumably by acting directly on receptors located on postcapillary venule endothelium. Following trigeminal stimulation, both vacuolation and an increased number of cytoplasmic vesicles thought to be responsible for transporting plasma proteins across the vessel wall are seen in the endothelium of postcapillary venules.[524] Some venules also show subintimal edema. Arterioles do not often show such alterations. Calcitonin gene-related peptide does not cause such plasma extravasation by itself, but it potentiates the extravasation produced by both substance P and neurokinin A.

The topic under consideration here is the possible relationship between neurogenic inflammation and migrainous head pain. Factors that alter nociceptors in other parts of the body, however, may shed light on the processes occurring in painful intracranial vascular structures. In skin, muscle, joints, and viscera, neurogenic inflammation affects the properties of nociceptive terminals. An attractive proposal is that nociceptor terminals are chemosensitive. Accordingly, they are activated by neuropeptides and by a number of pain-producing chemicals (*algesic* or *algogenic chemicals;* i.e., *inflammatory mediators*) released as a result of the inflammatory process. Perivascular nerve endings, mast cells, plasma, platelets, blood vessels, and tissue cells secrete the various inflammatory mediators: among them are histamine, arachidonic acid metabolites, bradykinin, and serotonin. All of these are known to affect the properties of chemosensitive nociceptive nerve terminals either directly or indirectly and to contribute to the inflammatory response in peripheral tissues. These substances either initiate neuronal discharge or alter the threshold and responsiveness of the terminals to subsequent physical or chemical stimuli (*sensitization*). The pain these substances produce is capable of outlasting the stimulus. Moskowitz has proposed that the same processes that occur in peripheral tissues such as skin, muscle, joints, and viscera also take place in the trigeminovascular system, giving rise to prolonged activation and sensitization of cranial vascular nociceptors and to the perception of pain.

PLATELET ACTIVATION

Aggregation and degranulation of platelets have been reported to occur following activation of unmyelinated trigeminal nerve fibers.[291] These changes may be relevant to the platelet abnormalities (increased spontaneous aggregation, serotonin release) seen during attacks of migraine.

MAST CELLS AND HISTAMINE

Histamine released by mast cells produces dilatation of arterioles and capillaries, a process that involves both H_1 and H_2 receptors.[838,2086] Histamine also causes plasma extravasation by an action on postcapillary venules. H_1 receptors are clearly important in this latter response, whereas the role of H_2 receptors is uncertain. Although it is clearly involved in neurogenic inflammation, the compound is unable to excite peripheral nociceptive sensory endings directly.[1088,1166,1497] To complicate the picture, the major sources of histamine—the mast cells—synthesize and secrete numerous other powerful inflammatory mediators such as prostaglandins and leukotrienes, as well as proteolytic enzymes and phospholipases, which can lead to the production of other vasoactive and pain-producing molecules.[1811,2011,2012]

Mast cells also contain receptors for substance P, and it is presumed that part of the inflammatory effects produced by activation of trigeminal vascular fibers is caused by the action of released substance P on mast cells. This is a reasonable presumption because degranulation of dural mast cells, with release of the mast cell contents, is produced by antidromic activation of trigeminal afferents.[90,1091] Neither calcitonin gene-related peptide nor neurokinin A affect mast cells.[320,357,560,1593]

ARACHIDONIC ACID AND METABOLITES

Prostanoids (*prostaglandins, prostacyclin,* and *thromboxane A_2*) formed from arachidonic acid do not cause pain when applied to nociceptive nerve endings in modest concentrations—concentrations probably present in vivo at sites of inflammation. Rather, the primary role of PGE_2, PGI_2, and possibly other prostanoids, is to *lower the threshold* of the nociceptive endings of unmyelinated trigeminal fibers and to sensitize such endings to the effects of other chemical mediators such as bradykinin.[1625] These effects may reside in the ability of some prostanoids to increase the cyclic AMP content of nociceptive terminals.[650]

Most investigators have shown that the arachidonic acid metabolites called leukotrienes promote vascular permeability.[454] Leukotrienes have direct and potent actions on the endothelial lining of postcapillary venules, where they cause plasma leakage.[1594] Under normal conditions, but possibly not under conditions of neurogenic inflamma-

tion, increased formation of prostacyclin may prevent leukotriene-induced plasma leakage. Leukotrienes have also been implicated in the enhancement of nociceptor responsiveness, however.[1231,1622]

In contrast to the other major pathways of arachidonic acid metabolism, a possible role in nociception for products of the cytochrome P-450 epoxygenase pathway of the arachidonate cascade has not yet been formulated.

Despite our limited knowledge of the effects of arachidonic acid metabolites (*eicosanoids*) on neuronal membranes, these substances do appear central to many aspects of inflammation and nociception.[454]

BRADYKININ

Bradykinin has been implicated in the genesis of inflammation in a number of peripheral tissues. It is present at sites of inflammation at a very early stage of the process. The substance is, in fact, active in producing the signs of inflammation, namely dilatation of arterioles, increased vascular permeability, and activation of nociceptive neurons. In particular, bradykinin causes arterioles to relax through an endothelium-derived relaxing factor (EDRF)–mediated process. The peptide also has potent actions on vascular permeability, which, as a result, induces edema.[728,1075,1404] In addition, bradykinin produces pain in humans when administered intradermally or intra-arterially.[366,383] The pain presumably occurs because bradykinin excites and sensitizes nociceptive afferent terminals in peripheral somatic tissues and in viscera.[1562,1625] In experimental animals, bradykinin also excites intracranial vascular nociceptive endings.[457,530] B_2 receptors appear to be involved in the excitation of nociceptors—a conclusion inferred from observations that B_2 receptors are localized to sensory nerve terminals, and the pain caused by endogenous kinin release during inflammation is blocked by selective B_2 receptor antagonists.[832,1954,2138]

Bradykinin probably has dual actions on nociceptors: the direct action just described and an indirect one mediated by prostaglandins. Prostaglandins appear to be implicated in bradykinin-induced excitation of nociceptors for several reasons: cyclooxygenase inhibitors (which block the synthesis of prostaglandins) suppress bradykinin-induced responses, and PGE_2 and PGI_2 enhance the sensitizing effects of bradykinin on nociceptors.[338,1149,1397] In addition, bradykinin activates phospholipase A_2, which stimulates the synthesis and subsequent release of prostaglandins from cells.[1063,1066,1222] The peptide also causes the release of substance P from afferent nociceptive nerves.[288,751] Thus, not only does bradykinin excite nerve endings directly, but the peptide also has complex interactions with other inflammatory mediators.

SEROTONIN

Many inflammatory mediators— such as histamine, prostaglandins, leukotrienes, and bradykinin—formed at the site of inflammation or released from other cells participating in the inflammatory process are potent platelet receptor agonists. These mediators are responsible for the activation of platelets during an acute inflammatory response. Platelets play an important role in acute inflammation. Once activated, they secrete a number of important compounds—in particular, serotonin and the arachidonic acid metabolite thromboxane A_2—which contribute to the inflammatory response.[1442] When platelets aggregate at inflammatory sites, they liberate serotonin. The amine facilitates additional aggregation by binding to specific serotonin receptor sites on platelets. Although serotonin is rapidly cleared from the plasma by nonaggregating platelets and by endothelial cells, high levels of the free amine can still be attained at sites of endothelial lesions present at loci of inflammation where platelet aggregation occurs. Serotonin also enhances the actions of most other stimuli that can activate platelets.

SEROTONIN RECEPTORS

Our knowledge about serotonin receptors is incomplete and controversial. The current nomenclature is confusing and unsatisfactory. Nevertheless, there is substantial molecular, biochemical, and pharmacologic evidence for multiple serotonin receptor subtypes.[1565,1778] At first, three major categories of serotonin receptors were defined—$5\text{-}HT_1$, $5\text{-}HT_2$, and $5\text{-}HT_3$. When subsequently, multiple subtypes of 5-HT receptors were discovered, the classification of $5\text{-}HT_1$ receptors was modified, but not in ways that really elucidate their interrelationships. Recent studies based on the displacement of selective radioligands from homogenates of tissue have revealed that the $5\text{-}HT_1$ category is heterogeneous and appears comprised of perhaps four or more pharmacologically distinct subtypes. These have been designated $5\text{-}HT_{1A}$, $5\text{-}HT_{1B}$, $5\text{-}HT_{1D}$, and $5\text{-}HT_{1E}$.[1565] $5\text{-}HT_{1C}$ receptors are misleadingly named, for they clearly belong to the subfamily of $5\text{-}HT_2$ receptors if one considers the very close structural relationship between cloned $5\text{-}HT_{1C}$ and $5\text{-}HT_2$ receptors. In addition, these receptors share a substantial number of pharmacologic and biochemical features.

Previous pharmacologic data indicated that $5\text{-}HT_{1B}$ receptors were present in rat, hamster, mouse, and opossum, but not in humans. But recent molecular biologic data indicate that $5\text{-}HT_{1B}$ receptors also exist in humans.

Another designation in this group may be misleading. "$5\text{-}HT_1$-like" has been used to identify a particular serotonin receptor in blood vessels, even though this receptor appears similar, if not identical, to a subtype designated as $5\text{-}HT_{1D}$ in nervous tissue.* Activation of "$5\text{-}HT_1$-like" sites on cranial blood vessels is believed to cause constriction of

---

*References 1000, 1570, 1781, 1972, 2082

cerebral blood vessels. 5-HT_{1D} receptors are widespread and are the most common type of serotonin receptor subtype thus far observed in the human brain. Presynaptic terminals of peptide-containing trigeminal afferents innervate the cranial vessels. Although the issue is somewhat controversial, the prejunctional serotonin receptors located on these presynaptic terminals are also thought to be 5-HT_{1D} types. Activation of 5-HT_{1D} receptors located on the presynaptic terminals of trigeminovascular fibers appears to block the release of endogenous peptide transmitters from these fibers.

5-HT_2 receptors appear to produce effects that may have relevance to migraine. Thus, when activated, 5-HT_2 receptors cause smooth muscle in some cranial blood vessels to contract. In addition, the process increases capillary permeability, augments platelet aggregation, and depolarizes many types of central neurons.[1441] In vascular smooth muscle cells, 5-HT_2 receptors may also mediate production of prostacyclin and other products of arachidonic acid metabolism.[396,397]

Both the 5-HT_1 and 5-HT_2 families of serotonin receptors are linked to guanine nucleotide binding proteins (G-proteins). G-proteins play an intermediary role in transmembrane signaling and are responsible for the coupling of serotonin receptors to appropriate cellular effector systems that generate second messengers. In contrast to the G-protein–coupled 5-HT receptors, which modulate cell activities via second messengers, 5-HT_3 receptors consist of ligand-gated ion channels that, when activated directly, produce changes in membrane ionic permeability.

Serotonin is also a potent algesic substance that excites nociceptive C fibers when applied to nerve endings in skin, muscle, joints, and viscera.* It appears to cause the pain by activating peripheral 5-HT_3 receptors located on nocicep-

tive terminals.[528,873] In addition to activating nociceptors, serotonin also potentiates the nociceptive actions of other algesic agents such as bradykinin. Thus, in combination, bradykinin and serotonin induce vascular pain in human subjects.[1835] Unfortunately, no data are available concerning the effects of serotonin on intracranial nociceptors.

ACTIVATION OF THE TRIGEMINOVASCULAR SYSTEM

As the preceding sections have indicated, the pain of migraine appears to be caused in large measure, if not entirely, by an inflammatory process that involves the activation of the trigeminovascular system—i.e., the trigeminal and cervical dorsal root nociceptive afferent terminals that innervate cephalic arteries and venous sinuses. The nociceptive afferent fibers use neuropeptides such as substance P, neurokinin A, and calcitonin gene-related peptide as neurotransmitters. When these nociceptive afferent axons transmit pain messages orthodromically to the trigeminal complex and to the spinal cord, these neurotransmitter peptides are released both centrally and peripherally. The complex inflammatory process that follows—involving the trigeminovascular system and a number of inflammatory mediators—is hypothesized to cause the prolonged referred pain characteristic of migraine.

The trigeminovascular system may well be the final common pathway for the generation of migraine pain. But how the activation of trigeminovascular neurons is initiated is not known. In theory, trigeminovascular neurons could become activated at various points along their length from their axon terminals in the blood vessel wall to central terminations within the brain stem. The following sites may be involved:

1. *Trigeminal terminals in blood vessel walls.* There are several possible

---

*References 142, 187, 663, 666, 1149, 1365

explanations for the activation of these terminals. One is an insult to the blood vessel wall or to the surrounding dural or brain tissue. This insult is associated with the local synthesis or transport of algesic chemicals, and with the release of peptides from nerve endings. Another explanation involves a wave of spreading depolarization, such as that seen in spreading depression, that may possibly affect cerebral perivascular trigeminal fibers. During spreading depression, the concentration of K^+ may reach 60 mM. Such a concentration is sufficient to depolarize nerve fibers and terminals and to cause the local release of substance P and other peptides. As an alternative explanation, activation of trigeminovascular terminals could result from an alteration of the normal homeostatic processes involved in the relationships among platelets, plasma, endothelium, smooth muscle, and mast cells. It is also conceivable that substantially abnormal local vasodilatation could lead to increased transmural pressure and to activation of trigeminal terminals.[998]

2. *Trigeminal axons.* Under most circumstances, impulses in afferent nerve fibers are initiated near the peripheral sensory terminal. Other regions of nerve fibers are ordinarily resistant to the initiation of impulses unless they undergo rapid depolarization. In contrast, injured or demyelinated afferent fibers will discharge spontaneously (*ectopic discharges*). Such ectopic discharges could potentially explain how trigeminovascular neurons are activated. However, there is no data that afferent trigeminal or dorsal root fibers are abnormal in patients with migraine.

3. *Nucleus caudalis.* Laboratory experiments show that volleys from various types of afferent trigeminal and dorsal root fibers, and impulses in pathways descending from a number of supraspinal structures in the brain stem and cerebrum, have the capacity to depolarize the membrane of the central terminals of afferent trigeminal and dorsal root nociceptive fibers.[105,868] The depolarization is termed *primary afferent depolarization (PAD)*. PAD results from the release of the amino acid neurotransmitter gamma-aminobutyric acid (GABA) by interneurons located in the nucleus caudalis and in the dorsal horn. These interneurons, which make synaptic contacts (so-called axo-axonic synapses) in the nucleus caudalis and dorsal horn on the central terminals of trigeminal and dorsal root afferent fibers, release GABA when they are excited by afferent or descending inputs. If the amplitude of PAD is sufficient, antidromic primary afferent trigeminal root and dorsal root fiber discharges (*trigeminal root and dorsal root reflexes*) are produced. Such a process could result in the peripheral release of neuropeptides and result in migrainous head pain, but whether or not trigeminal and dorsal root reflexes can be produced by natural stimuli outside of the laboratory is not known.

Admittedly, we do not yet know the precise mechanism that activates trigeminovascular neurons and leads to the inflammatory process implicated in migrainous pain. There is, however, additional evidence to link the trigeminal nerve to a migraineur's suffering. Two pieces of clinical evidence suggest that hyperexcitability of the trigeminal system, or its reflex connections, is present between migraine attacks. First of all, a substantial number of migraineurs spontaneously develop discrete, jabbing, sharp pains—"ice-pick-like pains"—at the site of their customary headaches.[1641] These pains are postulated to result from spontaneous discharges of trigeminal afferent fibers. In addition, ice cream headaches—the transient head pain that develops when a cold stimulus contacts either the palate or the posterior pharyngeal wall—are frequent in patients with migraine.[538] For some migraineurs, the pain of ice cream headache is located in the same region of the head where their migraine attacks usually occur.[548] The pain is considered to involve a reflex mechanism that includes the trigeminal nerve.

It is a reasonable hypothesis that because migraine patients generally have an inherited lowered biologic threshold to a variety of external and internal stimuli, the appropriate combination of environmental and internal trigger factors may well be sufficient to initiate antidromic activity in the afferent fibers of the trigeminovascular system. If this is so, such neuronal activation may well give rise to the inflammatory process that causes migraine's well-known misery.

ENDOGENOUS ANTINOCICEPTIVE SYSTEMS

Among the hypotheses as to the cause of migraine is a proposal that migraine is a genetic disorder of the endogenous antinociceptive systems. These systems are comprised of CNS circuits responsible for the modulation of pain pathways.[1169,1830] The hypothesis grows out of much recent investigative work demonstrating that certain supraspinal structures exert potent effects on spinal cord and brain stem sensory function. In other words, transmission involving nociceptive trigeminal and spinal neurons is modulated and controlled by a number of CNS structures.[129,652,745,1035] Unquestionably several networks participate in the control of pain, but most is known about systems that have components in the mesencephalic periaqueductal gray matter (PAG) and adjacent pontine and medullary structures such as the raphe nuclei (particularly the nucleus raphe magnus, NRM) and the locus coeruleus. When activated by electrical stimulation, these structures can modify pain sensation and inhibit behavioral reactions evoked by noxious stimuli. The genetic abnormality underlying migraine is thought to result in a failure of these systems—the result of which is a

central hyperalgesia and an augmentation of the central perception of pain. The failure has been attributed to a deficiency of the neurotransmitters—endorphins and monoamines—involved in pain modulation.[1832] The following sections will review the anatomy of systems in the brain stem that participate in the modulation of pain transmission through the spinal and trigeminal pathways.

The pain-modulating networks in the brain are thought to be activated by nociceptive stimuli. The spinothalamic and trigeminothalamic tracts distribute collateral branches at various points in the brain stem as they ascend toward their destination in the thalamus. Both anatomic and electrophysiologic techniques have shown that neurons in the PAG and NRM receive substantial input from both trigeminal and spinal neurons conveying nociceptive information, and a substantial number of neurons in PAG and NRM respond to noxious stimuli.[151,2148] Interpretation of these data has led to development of an hypothesis involving the presence of *endogenous analgesic systems* to explain the functional significance of the descending brain stem systems. The PAG, NRM, and their spinal projections are thought to constitute a negative feedback loop activated by stimuli that cause pain. The negative feedback circuit produces an inhibition of the trigeminal and spinal transmission of nociceptive messages and analgesia.[129] It is presumed that these brain stem systems are active during migraine attacks.

Anatomy of Descending Pain-Modulating Pathways

The PAG is a major site capable of producing analgesia when appropriately stimulated. The connections of the PAG are widespread and complex. The major afferent input originates from rostral brain structures that include the hypothalamus, the frontal and insular cortex, and parts of the limbic system such as the amygdala (Fig. 7–6).[151] Ancillary, but significant, inputs to the PAG also directly come from the dorsal horn of the spinal cord and the trigeminal nuclear complex, or as collaterals of spinothalamic and trigeminothalamic axons. Activation of the PAG by electrical stimulation has several consequences: it diminishes spinal and trigeminal reflex responses, inhibits the firing of nociceptive neurons in the trigeminal nuclei and dorsal horn, and produces behavioral analgesia in animals and pain relief in humans.[148,988]

The PAG has only minor direct projections to the spinal cord and to the trigeminal nuclear complex. Descending influences from the PAG are for the most part relayed through synapses in several areas within the *rostral ventromedial medulla.* These medullary sites include the midline NRM and several nuclei in the adjacent ventral reticular formation.[1499] In turn, these nuclei project to the nulceus caudalis and to the dorsal horn of the spinal cord.[152,974,1317,1869] Therefore, it is not unexpected that electrical stimulation of sites in the rostral ventromedial medulla produces effects similar to those seen following stimulation of the PAG; namely, suppression of nociceptive responses and reflexes and reduction in firing of nociceptive neurons in the nucleus caudalis and dorsal horn.[339,531,1657,1964]

Although research emphasis has been placed on the mechanisms underlying inhibition of nociception and analgesia, recent data indicate that descending brain stem pathways appear to have two actions on nociceptive transmission—inhibitory effects and facilitatory effects—mediated by two physiologically distinct classes of cells in the rostral ventromedial medulla.[652]

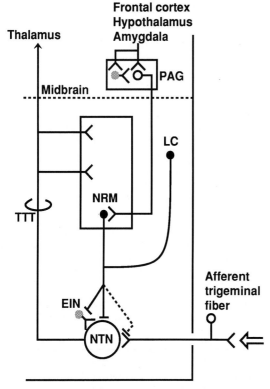

Figure 7–6. Schematic diagram of some of the circuitry involved in the descending modulation of nociceptive transmission. Anatomic studies have shown projections from the hypothalamus, the frontal cortex, and parts of the limbic system (such as the amygdala) to the midbrain periaqueductal gray matter (PAG). The PAG projects to the nucleus raphe magnus (NRM) in the rostroventral medulla. The NRM sends 5-HT–containing fibers, and the locus coeruleus (LC) sends norepinephrine-containing fibers, to make contact with: (*1*) nociceptive trigeminal neurons (NTN) in the nucleus caudalis, which project to the thalamus as trigeminothalamic tract (TTT) fibers, (*2*) enkephalin-containing interneurons (EIN), and (*3*) (possibly) the central terminals of primary afferent trigeminal fibers. Collateral branches of TTT fibers are distributed at various points in the brain stem.

Monoamines and Modulation of Nociception

That central monoaminergic pathways are involved in descending pain-modulating circuits is undoubted.[131,171,2159] Three major pieces of data support this conclusion. First, a large number of fibers containing serotonin, norepinephrine, and dopamine as neurotransmitters project from the brain stem to the trigeminal nuclei and to the dorsal horn of the spinal cord.

Second, a number of studies have established that activity in bulbospinal monoaminergic pathways is associated with a depression of nociceptive transmission. Finally, when monoaminergic neurons are destroyed or when CNS monoamines are depleted pharmacologically, analgesia produced by stimulation of the PAG and other brain stem sites is reduced.[18]

A major part of the endogenous antinociceptive system is comprised of serotonin-containing axons descending to the nucleus caudalis and to the spinal dorsal horn.[128,407] These serotonin-containing fibers, which originate in the NRM, are responsible for linking the PAG with the nucleus caudalis and spinal dorsal horn.[128] Serotonin's role in descending inhibition has been demonstrated in several ways. In particular, microapplication of serotonin inhibits spontaneous and synaptically induced firing of spinothalamic neurons; intrathecal administration of serotonin produces analgesia that can be suppressed by serotonin and antagonists.[2183] Several different serotonin receptor subtypes—including 5-HT_{1A}, 5-HT_{1B}, and 5-HT_3 types—may be involved in the modulation of central nociceptive responses.[769,2188,2209] The raphe nuclei are not, however, exclusively serotonergic. Cells containing peptides such as substance P or enkephalin and serotonin have been observed in several raphe nuclei.[240,1044]

Norepinephrine-containing neurons from the locus coeruleus, the subjacent nucleus subcoeruleus, and other pontine groups of norepinephrine-containing cells also project to the trigeminal nuclear complex and spinal cord.[1519,2137] Norepinephrine has a predominantely inhibitory effect on the discharge of spinal nociceptive cells and on spinal nociceptive reflexes.[1055,1056,1402] Intrathecal administration of selective α_2-agonists causes long-lasting analgesia, and α_2 binding sites are highly concentrated in the superficial layers of the dorsal horn.[1648] This strongly suggests that the analgesic effects are mediated by α_2-adrenoceptors.

Although investigations of brain stem control of nociception have emphasized descending serotonin and norepinephrine pathways, descending dopaminergic pathways may also be involved. The nucleus caudalis and spinal cord receive projections from dopamine-containing cell bodies located within the caudal diencephalon.[1244] Although the exact site of dopamine action in the trigeminal nucleus and in the spinal cord is unknown, there is evidence of its activity: a decrement of nociceptive neuron firing and an increase of the nociceptive threshold are produced by activity in the spinal dopaminergic system.[1036,1039] In addition, alterations in dopaminergic transmission attenuate the analgesic effects both of electrical stimulation of the PAG and of systemic morphine administration.[18,2063]

Endorphins

Endorphins—endogenous opioid peptides that share actions with the active stereoisomers of opiate alkaloids and are antagonized by pure opiate antagonists—have been linked to many of the modulatory effects brain stem structures have on nociceptive transmission.[162,1668] Midbrain and other brain stem nuclei connected with pathways descending to the spinal dorsal horn and to the nucleus caudalis are rich in certain endorphins and receive endorphin-containing fibers from other structures such as the basal hypothalamus. When injected into the PAG, morphine produces analgesia.[2181,2183] Opiate-sensitive regions have also been found in the NRM and surrounding regions in the medulla.[1211] The actions of opiates injected into these sites is prevented or partially blocked by opiate antagonists—an indication that opiates activate specific opiate receptors.[516,2183] In sum, brain stem areas are important for the clinical effects of opiates. Such a conclusion is reinforced by observations that lesions of the PAG or the raphe nuclei reduce the analgesia produced by systemic morphine administration.[2179]

Although multiple endogenous opioid ligands have been described, all endorphins appear to be derived from one of three precursors: pro-opiomelanocortin, pro-enkephalin, or dynorphin.

1. The precursor pro-opiomelanocortin gives rise to *β-endorphin*. This precursor is present in extremely high quantities in the intermediate lobe of the pituitary and in the corticotroph cells of the adenohypophysis. β-Endorphin–containing cell bodies are concentrated in the basal hypothalamus, which distributes axons to parts of the limbic system, to the PAG, and to the locus coeruleus.[654,1665] Thus, the β-endorphin system conforms well to loci believed to produce analgesia by means of electrical stimulation. It is not surprising that intraventricular administration of β-endorphin produces potent analgesia or that increases in cerebrospinal fluid (CSF) β-endorphin levels are seen after brain stimulation in humans. Current knowledge is also compatible with observations that bilateral destruction of β-endorphin–containing cell bodies in the hypothalamus diminishes the content of β-endorphin in the brain and lessens the analgesic actions of PAG stimulation.[988,1387,2117]

2. Pro-enkephalin gives rise to both *leu-enkephalin* and *met-enkephalin*. Cells and fibers containing enkephalins are widely distributed.[1103] Enkephalins are present in the neural lobe of the pituitary in fibers derived from the paraventricular and supraoptic nuclei of the hypothalamus. They are also present in the PAG, the raphe nuclei, and the nucleus caudalis and dorsal horn.[410,1104,1928] Several lines of evidence suggest that enkephalin-containing interneurons in the nucleus caudalis and dorsal horn play a role in the control of nociceptive information relayed in these structures.[1003] In particular, the cell bodies and proximal dendrites of spinothalamic cells receive synapses from these interneurons.[1709] Moreover, enkephalins applied in the vicinity of nociceptive neurons in the nucleus caudalis and spinal dorsal horn suppress the responses to noxious stimuli.[43,2208]

3. Prodynorphin is the precursor of *dynorphin.* Dynorphin is present in large quantities in the adenohypophysis, the PAG, and those layers of the nucleus caudalis and dorsal horn concerned with the processing of nociceptive information.[1105] Dynorphin, however, is not a potent analgesic substance; moreover, its role in nociceptive functioning is still a matter of dispute.

Endorphins and Migraine

Normally, the plasma and CSF contain measurable amounts of endogenous opioid substances. Based on findings that migraineurs have subnormal levels of *met*-enkephalin in the CSF, Sicuteri proposed an *endorphin theory of migraine.*[1829] He maintained that a deficiency of endogenous opioids was responsible for the pain of migraine headaches because the opioid-mediated endogenous pain control system was unable to inhibit pain inputs.[1829] Since then, a number of investigators have assayed the levels of various endogenous opioids in both plasma and CSF. Their results have been either inconsistent or not specific for migraine. In other words, both elevated and reduced CSF enkephalin levels have been reported.[56,1852]

The data for CSF β-endorphins are somewhat different. CSF β-endorphin levels are significantly reduced both between and during migraine headaches. Such reductions are not unique to migraineurs, however.[476,750,1447,1448,2066] They are also found in patients with chronic pain, whatever its cause or origin. In contrast, plasma β-endorphin levels are reported as normal between attacks of migraine.[95,104,622,1448,1988] Investigations by various groups of researchers have found higher, unchanged, and lower plasma levels of β-endorphin.[56,77,95,104] Patients with chronic daily headaches have consistently reduced levels. The meaning of all these data is unclear. A number of the studies suffer from methodologic shortcomings. It is difficult to draw inferences about the function of the endogenous endorphin system in migraine headaches from such inconsistent results.[621]

PRODROMES

As discussed in chapter 3, a large percentage of migraineurs have premonitory symptoms. Among them are irritability, depression and other alterations in mood, changes in behavior, fatigue, various gastrointestinal manifestations, changes in fluid balance, depression, and photophobia. These phenomena precede the aura and the headache phase of a migraine attack by hours or even days. Three major possibilities have been proposed for the genesis of prodromal symptoms:

1. *Hypothalamic dysfunction.* During the pre-headache phase, some migraineurs experience irritability, hunger, craving for food, difficulties with temperature control, and somnolence. Intriguing parallels have been described between the pre-headache phase of these patients and a similar catalog of symptoms produced by lesions of the ventromedial nucleus of the hypothalamus in experimental animals.[936]

2. *A dopaminergic mechanism.* When dopaminergic agents are administered to migraineurs, the compounds not only cause headaches, but also produce symptoms of drowsiness, nausea, and yawning.[33,310] Such observations have led some researchers to suggest that a dopaminergic mechanism gives rise to prodromal symptoms. Because administration of the dopamine receptor antagonist domperidone blocks the premonitory symptoms, and because domperidone does not cross the blood–brain barrier, dopaminergic receptors located in brain areas outside of the blood–brain barrier may be the ones involved.

3. *A serotonergic mechanism.* Involvement of serotonin in the production of prodromal symptoms is based on circumstantial evidence. In particular, via their wide distribution over the neuraxis, serotonin-containing neurons in the midbrain raphe system are hypothesized to play a key role in a number of behaviors such as mood, sleep, appetite, and cognitive function.[1362]

The complex changes in mood and behavior and the neurologic and autonomic symptoms manifested during the prodrome may conceivably involve complex interactions of all three: hypothalamic dysfunction combined with dopaminergic or serotonergic mechanisms.

NAUSEA AND VOMITING

Nausea and vomiting are common during migraine attacks. The so-called "vomiting center" in the brain stem is thought to be responsible for these symptoms. The vomiting center is activated by discharges in the trigeminovascular system. Emesis is a complex reflex event that has to integrate excitation and inhibition of both visceral and somatic musculature.[119,317] The reflex necessitates synchronized activity of a considerable number of motor nuclei, including those that innervate the abdominal musculature, the diaphragm, the intercostal muscles, and the muscles of the larynx, pharynx, and tongue. The process also involves the neurons and the intrinsic nerve cells that influence tone and peristalsis in the esophagus, stomach, and small intestine, as well as contraction of sphincteric muscles. In addition, the reflex interacts with autonomic functions responsible for pallor, salivation, cold sweats, pupillary dilatation, tachycardia, and hypotension.

Older studies indicated that vomiting in experimental animals could be induced by electrically stimulating the lateral medullary reticular formation of the brain stem.[2099] Lesions in this site rendered animals refractory to emetic agents. A standard textbook concept of the vomiting center evolved from these studies. This concept envisioned a variety of emetic stimuli converging on the vomiting center, whereupon the center coordinated all of the necessary somatic and autonomic activity. Recently, however, the concept of a discrete vomiting center has been revisited.[1388] Attempts to replicate older experiments have failed. Accordingly, it is now considered doubtful that a single anatomic site is responsible for all of the activity that occurs during vomiting.

Two alternative hypotheses have been proposed to explain how vomiting occurs. According to one theory, discharges in local reflex circuits activate each effector motor and autonomic nucleus involved in emesis.[455] The coordinated act of emesis is a consequence of these nuclei acting in sequence. This hypothesis clarifies observations that electrical stimulation of the medulla, rather than inducing the entire act of emesis, easily evokes particular components of it, such as salivation or retching.[1388]

Another theory has been offered to explain the process of vomiting. According to this view, the *nucleus tractus solitarius* is the "central pattern generator" for emesis.[317] The central pattern generator consists of an interneuronal network that coordinates and sequentially activates the various motor and autonomic nuclei. The nucleus tractus solitarius receives inputs from trigeminal primary afferents, including those from intracranial arterial structures.[78,144,377,1023] The area also receives inputs from baroreceptor, respiratory, gustatory, and gastrointestinal systems.[402,851,866,1766,2080] It is known to be involved in the integration of autonomic afferent inputs from many peripheral organs, and it also integrates other complex motor acts, such as swallowing, breathing, and chewing, that involve brain stem neurons. In sum, the central pattern generator is a site of convergence of afferent information, providing the trigger stimulus that generates the whole act of emesis.

Nausea and vomiting may also involve a chemoreceptor trigger zone located in the area postrema, a circumventricular structure located at the caudal aspect of the fourth ventricle. The area postrema lacks a blood–brain barrier, and, as a result, its neural structures are easily reached by chemical compounds and drugs circulating in the blood. The chemoreceptor trigger zone is stimulated by dopamine agonists, including L-dopa and apomorphine, and by opioids and ergots. Excitation of appropriate receptors in the chemoreceptor trigger zone results in stimulation of the groups of neurons that coordinate vomiting.

PHOTOPHOBIA

During a headache, almost all migraineurs develop an enhanced and generally disagreeable sensitivity to light. Light not only causes pain, but the patient also experiences an uncomfortable and exaggerated sense of brightness. After extirpation of the Gasserian ganglion, painful photophobia does not involve the eye on the side of the surgery, an observation indicating that the trigeminal nerve is necessary for the development of photophobia.[1212] Accordingly, it is believed that the pain associated with photophobia is carried through the ophthalmic division of the trigeminal nerve. The process appears to involve neurogenic inflammation of the eye.[1212] In contrast, the painless but disagreeable sense of excessive brightness may be caused by impaired central regulation of visual input.[539]

SUMMARY

The major loci of migraine pain consist of pial and dural blood vessels. Dilatation of the superficial temporal artery and its branches appears to be a major cause of migraine pain in only a minority of patients. Nociceptive afferent fibers from arteries and venous sinuses are carried in the trigeminal nerve (trigeminovascular system) and in the upper cervical nerve roots. Although the classical theory of the origin of migraine pain proposes that the pain results from vasodilatation with stretching of nociceptors located within the walls of blood vessels, documentation coupling intracranial vasodilatation and migrainous head pain is limited. Recent data indicate that neurogenic inflammation with vascular dilatation, edema formation in vessel walls, and a number of chemical and physiologic processes that excite and sensitize vascular afferent nociceptive terminals are more likely to produce the pain associated with migraine headaches.

Chapter 8

THE SEROTONIN HYPOTHESIS AND OTHER THEORIES

A unifying hypothesis of migraine must explain the complete, elaborate chain of events that takes place during a migraine attack. In particular, such an hypothesis must deal with the *cause of the migraine*, not just the mechanisms that give rise to putative changes in blood flow and to head pain. But despite a great deal of study and speculation, researchers are far from developing an adequate, unified hypothesis. There is even controversy about the mechanisms we understand best—namely, those that underlie the aura and pain of the migraine attack. Three major, competing hypotheses about those mechanisms were discussed in the previous two chapters: (1) spreading depression as the cause of the aura, (2) brain stem–aminergic control of cranial circulation, and (3) inflammatory trigeminovascular etiology of head pain. The present chapter will offer several other theories about the cause of migraine.

SEROTONIN AND THE INITIATION OF MIGRAINE ATTACKS

For three decades serotonin has been in the vanguard of speculation about migraine. There is a sizable collection of biochemical, pharmacologic, and anatomic evidence promoting roles for serotonin in the genesis of migraine.[684,685] One theory proposes that serotonin released from platelets sets off migraine attacks. Another school of thought claims that release of serotonin from perivascular terminals of putative serotonergic nerve fibers begins the attack. Systemic metabolic changes in serotonin metabolism are also suggested as the initiator of migraine headaches. These various proposals have given rise to what is called the *serotonin hypothesis of migraine.* Some aspects of serotonergic activity have been reviewed in previous chapters—namely, innervation of cerebral arteries by serotonergic fibers, inhibitory effects of raphe stimulation on the transmission of nociceptive information, and actions of serotonin both on cranial blood vessels and on nociceptive nerve endings. The ensuing sections will consider other aspects of serotoninergic activity that appear pertinent to the pathophysiology of migraine.

Location of Serotonin

The human body contains about 10 mg of serotonin, 90% in enterochromaffin cells in the mucosa of the gastrointestinal tract. Some of the remainder is present in the central nervous system and in a few peripheral nerves, but most of the remaining 10% is found in platelets. Serotonin is synthesized from dietary tryptophan both in enterochromaffin cells and in neurons. This is not the case in platelets. Accordingly, for all serotonin-containing cells except platelets, hydroxylation of tryptophan catalyzed by the enzyme tryptophan hydroxylase results in the formation of 5-hydroxytryptophan. 5-Hydroxytryptophan is then transformed into serotonin by the actions of the nonspecific enzyme, aromatic L-amino acid decarboxylase. A portion of the serotonin released by enterochromaffin cells overflows into the portal circulation. Most of it is removed from the blood by the liver or by pulmonary endothelial cells.[1967,2016] Platelets procure their supply of serotonin by avid uptake from plasma.[1249] As a result human blood contains about 0.1 to 0.3 μg/mL of serotonin—almost all of it stored in platelets. Significant concentrations of free serotonin are not present in peripheral plasma under normal circumstances.

The principal pathway involved in the metabolic degradation of serotonin is the oxidative deamination by monoamine oxidase resulting in the formation of 5-hydroxyindoleacetic acid (5-HIAA).

Normal Platelet Function

The behavior of platelets during and between migraine attacks has received considerable attention. Alterations in behavior have led Hanington to propose that migraine is a disease of platelets.[875,880] According to her hypothesis: (1) platelets are abnormal in migraineurs, (2) platelet behavior changes during migraine attacks, and (3) bouts of migraine occur because of changes in platelet function. This hypothesis has aroused considerable controversy, which remains unresolved.[878,1942] Although there is evidence that platelets may indeed be involved in the pathogenesis of migraine, their role is not at all clear.

Blood contains between 150,000 and 400,000 platelets/mL. Platelets are small, anuclear, ellipsoid cells with diameters of 1.5 to 3 μm.[2161] (Fig. 8–1). They have smooth surfaces with indentations into which the canalicular system opens. This system constitutes a network of channels leading from the interior of the platelet to the surface so that the extracellular space communicates with much of the interior. The cytoplasm of platelets accommodates two types of secretory granules. One group is comprised of dense bodies that contain calcium, serotonin, epinephrine, norepinephrine, dopamine, *met*-enkephalin (methionine-enkephalin), and nucleotides such as adenosine triphosphate (ATP), adenosine diphosphate (ADP), guanosine triphosphate (GTP), and guanosine diphosphate (GDP).[665,970] The other group is comprised of α-gran-

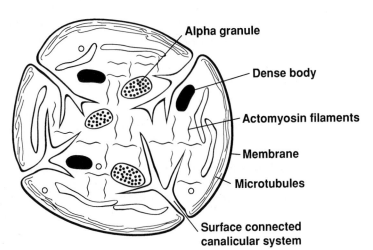

Figure 8–1. Diagram of an inactive platelet in the plane of the longest diameter. (Adapted from Winther, K and Hedman, C,[2161] p 302 with permission.)

Alpha granule

Dense body

Actomyosin filaments

Membrane

Microtubules

Surface connected canalicular system

ules that contain platelet factor 4 (PF$_4$) and β-thromboglobulin.[1081] When activated, platelets are believed to empty the substances stored in their secretory granules into the canalicular system that leads to the surrounding environment. In addition, activated platelets produce vasoactive prostanoids such as thromboxane A$_2$ (TXA$_2$), prostaglandin GH$_2$, and prostaglandin PGG$_2$.[467]

A wide variety of physiologic substances stimulate and activate platelets by acting at receptors located on the platelet surface: α-adrenoceptors, β-adrenoceptors, thrombin receptors, receptors for histamine, serotonin, ADP, and for the prostanoids prostacyclin and TXA$_2$.* The first responses in platelet activation are platelet adhesion and platelet shape change. Accordingly, in the presence of fibrin platelets stick together, establishing an irreversible aggregate. Next, normally discoid platelets are transformed into spheres, pseudopodia are extruded, and finally substances are released from granules through the surface-connected canalicular system (Fig. 8–2). In in vitro studies, when serotonin is the sole agonist, it induces nothing more than an insubstantial and reversible aggregation of platelets. In contrast, even low concentrations of serotonin strikingly enhance the platelet responses evoked by suboptimal concentrations of other agonists.[537,1803]

Platelet Activation, Serotonin, and Migraine

Interest in serotonin commenced following the observation that urinary levels of the main catabolic product of serotonin metabolism, 5-HIAA, are increased in some patients during bouts of migraine (Fig. 8–3).[1836] Although this observation has been confirmed, not all investigators have been able to find consistently increased urinary serotonin metabolite excre-

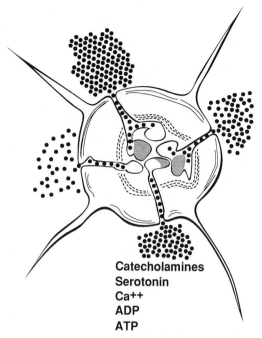

Catecholamines
Serotonin
Ca++
ADP
ATP

Figure 8–2. Diagram of an activated platelet. Different products are released through the canalicular system connected to the surface. ADP, adenosine diphosphate; ATP, adenosine triphosphate. (Adapted from Winther, K and Hedman, C,[2161] p 302, with permission.)

tion.[217,415,421,462,1078] As a result, serotonin's role in triggering or sustaining migraine attacks has intrigued many researchers. Despite the finding that the increments in urinary 5-HIAA excretion surpass the increases anticipated if the exclusive origin of the metabolite were the 5-HT released from platelets, interest in platelets as the source of the catabolized serotonin followed reports that the concentration of platelet-rich plasma serotonin can fall substantially (by about 30% to 45%) during bouts of migraine (Fig. 8–4).† In some individuals, the fall in plasma serotonin is preceded by a rise that ultimately leads to increased amounts of urinary free serotonin during attacks.[61] The change in serotonin levels is a systemic one, not confined to the cerebral circulation. Such reduced levels are

---

*References 260, 1070, 1121, 1391, 1596, 1837, 1932, 2162

†References 57, 63, 67, 170, 415, 447, 949, 1434, 1725, 1906

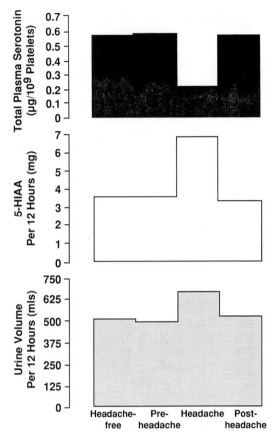

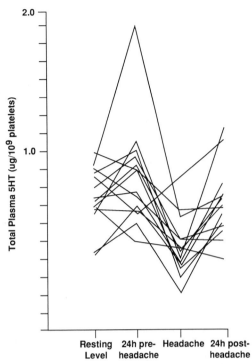

Figure 8–4. Mean values for plasma serotonin before, during and after migraine headache in a group of patients. The plasma levels reflect the serotonin content of platelet-enriched plasma. (Modified from Anthony, M et al,[63] p 41 (S Karger AG, Basel), with permission.)

Figure 8–3. Schematic representation of changes in total plasma serotonin (reflecting platelet serotonin), urinary excretion of 5-hydroxyindoleacetic acid (5-HIAA), and urine volume in migraine patients. Each column indicates a 12-hour period, first during a time of freedom from headache, then before, during, and after headache. (Modified from Curran, DA et al,[416] p 91 (S Karger AG, Basel), with permission.)

found in blood drawn both from the antecubital vein and from the external jugular vein. Curiously, a decrease in platelet serotonin is less likely to take place during attacks of migraine with aura[649] (Fig. 8–5). It is not known, however, whether the alterations in platelet serotonin levels are specific for, and causally associated with, the production of migraine attacks.

The reported declines of plasma serotonin during a migraine attack have been postulated to be caused by the liberation of serotonin from activated platelets and its subsequent catabo-

lism.[682] Other biochemical evidence for platelet activation and release of granule contents exists. For example, significantly elevated plasma levels of the platelet-specific products β-thromboglobulin and PF_4 are associated with the fall of serotonin in as many as 50% of migraine attacks.[447,741,1293]

What causes the changes in platelet serotonin activity in migraineurs is unclear. Under consideration are two possibilities: some kind of defect within the platelets themselves, and the presence of a serotonin-releasing factor circulating in plasma.

1. *A defect within the platelets.* Many studies have demonstrated that migraineurs have abnormal platelet function both during and between headache attacks, but whether or not that abnormal function is caused by platelet defects has not been suffi-

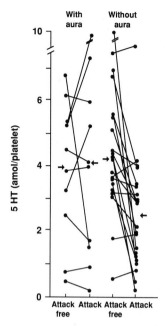

Figure 8–5. Serotonin content of individual platelets during migraine-free periods and during attacks; data taken from patients with aura and without aura. Arrows indicate group means, amol = 10^{-18} mol. (Modified from Ferrari, et al,[649] with permission.)

function in migraineurs.[322,880,1054,1214] Both normal and increased sensitivity to platelet-activating factor have been demonstrated in the platelets of migraineurs.[874,1061] Moreover, the relationship between migraine pathogenesis and platelet aggregation measured in vitro must remain suspect because serial investigation during acute bouts of migraine has failed to show a correlation between platelet aggregation and migraine-related neurologic symptoms.[391]

2. *A plasma-borne serotonin-releasing factor.* During bouts, the plasma of some migraineurs has been reported to contain a soluble factor capable of releasing serotonin from platelets taken either from migraine patients between attacks or from normal subjects.[557,1196,1434,1435] *Met*-enkephalin, which is co-stored with serotonin in platelet granules, is also released from platelets by plasma drawn during migraine attacks.[648] The evidence for the presence of a releasing factor is still equivocal, however, and some investigators deny its presence.

Regulation of the amount of serotonin contained in platelets is determined in large measure by the active transport of serotonin into platelets *(serotonin uptake).* Just as in other studies that consider some aspect of the relationship between serotonin and platelets in migraineurs, the data about serotonin uptake are equivocal. Thus, although normal serotonin uptake into the platelets of migraineurs has been reported, the literature includes both decreases and increases of uptake.[325,884,947,1292,2091] In particular, during and between migraine attacks, the maximal rate of uptake (V_{max}) has been reported to be either the same as control values, increased, or reduced.* Data also contradict with regard to the concentration of platelet serotonin during headache-free intervals. Most studies show that the serotonin content of platelets is nor-

ciently established. A number of reports indicate increased in vitro aggregatability of platelets in blood taken during and between attacks.* In addition, between migraine attacks, the proportion of circulating platelet microaggregates is greater than normal and is elevated still further during the prodromal period of an attack.[289,486,842,880] Unfortunately for our understanding of how platelet aggregation affects migraine, marked differences exist among various reports, and the hyperaggregatability of platelets is unrelated to the severity of the migraine. These discrepancies may be related in part to methodologic and technical differences and in part to how patients respond to different forms of treatment. ADP, for example, is reported to increase, decrease, and cause no change in platelet

---

*References 391, 486, 741, 875, 880, 948, 1134, 1214,

*References 380, 441, 1143, 1197, 1250, 1292, 1434, 1608, 1682

mal, but some reports show either increased or decreased serotonin levels.[441,447,1408,1434,2091]

There are several reasons the quantity of serotonin potentially available for release from platelets during migraine attacks may be trivial from a pharmocologic point of view. First, the quantity is exceedingly small and is thought to be insufficient to exert significant effects on the cerebral circulation.[1925] Even higher concentrations produced by slow infusions of the amine in humans produce only inconsequential reductions in cerebral blood flow (CBF).[1490] In addition, serotonin released from platelets is cleared from the plasma very rapidly; 95% is removed by one passage through the lungs.[2014] Finally, migraine attacks are not induced by intravenous administration of serotonin,[1109] so it seems unlikely that platelet-released serotonin by itself could be responsible for the changes in rCBF seen during migraine attacks. But platelet-derived serotonin may have additional actions. Serotonergic amplification mechanisms on platelet activation are presumably functioning during bouts of migraine. Serotonin is capable of inducing and facilitating the activation of platelets, and the local release of serotonin may lead to the enhanced release or biosynthesis of platelet prostanoids. In addition, synergism is manifest between serotonin and prostanoids such as TXA_2, both released from activated platelets. The significance of the serotonin amplification effects has never been thoroughly evaluated in migraine.

In sum, although abnormalities in platelet function have been reported in migraine sufferers, the role of these abnormalities in the genesis of migraine remains ambiguous. A consistent abnormality of platelet function in migraineurs has not been demonstrated.[1060] To accept the platelet disorder hypothesis, it would be necessary to show that activation of platelets specifically precipitates attacks of migraine. But platelet hyperaggregatability caused by platelet activation is not a finding limited to migraineurs. It has been seen in a number of other medical conditions, such as in patients with high levels of stress from any cause.[901] Moreover, it is still unclear if abnormal platelet activation and other derangements in platelet function are the cause of bouts of migraine or are only epiphenomena. In addition, changes in platelet function correlate poorly with the intensity of migraine in individual patients.[391]

Serotonin and Migraine

In addition to data describing possible relationships between platelet serotonin and migraine, a number of pieces of evidence have been used to support the serotonin hypothesis:

1. As decribed in chapter 6, a diversity of serotonin receptors exists on the extracranial and intracranial vasculature. Applied serotonin can produce both vasoconstriction and vasodilatation, but it is unclear whether nerve terminals containing serotonin innervate either large or small pial vessels.

2. Serotonin appears to be crucial in the regulation of the endogenous pain control pathways, as discussed in detail in chapter 7. Although the ways in which serotonin affects the rostral transmission of nociceptive information in the central nervous system is not completely understood, manipulation of serotonergic neurons has potent effects on both the behavioral responses to pain and on the responses of neurons in the spinal cord and the trigeminal nuclear complex to noxious stimuli. It is not known, however, if the endogenous pain control system is involved in either the genesis of migraine attacks or in the control of head pain caused by a bout of migraine.

3. As noted in chapter 7, serotonin excites peripheral nociceptive nerve endings by activating specific serotonin receptors located on the endings. Serotonin also potentiates the algesic actions of other compounds such as

bradykinin. Unfortunately, information is lacking concerning the actions of serotonin on trigeminovascular nociceptors.

4. The serotonin system in the brain has been implicated in the regulation of mood, appetite, and sleep, all of which are affected when patients develop an attack of migraine. But no evidence is available to implicate serotonin in the production of these symptoms during a migraine attack.

5. Several drugs that affect serotonin release and uptake cause headaches. Depletion of neural and platelet serotonin in migraineurs by reserpine provokes headaches that can duplicate the patients' usual bouts of migraine. Reserpine produces headaches only infrequently in control subjects.[419,667] The headaches are associated with a fall in platelet 5-HT and a rise in urinary 5-HIAA.[326,419] Headaches can also be induced in migraineurs by fenfluramine (m-trifluoromethyl-N-ethyl-amphetamine), a halogenated derivative of amphetamine.[1597] Like reserpine, it produces rapid serotonin release and depletes brain serotonin. It also selectively inhibits serotonin reuptake.[715,727] Treatment with the selective serotonin reuptake blockers zimelidine and femoxetine causes an increase in the frequency and severity of migraine attacks during the early stages of treatment.[1982]

These data suggest that an acute increase in serotonergic function, whether by release or by blockade of reuptake, can lead to the development of migraine in susceptible individuals. On the other hand, most of the drugs that have been used in these investigations are not selective with respect to their cellular targets of action, to the substances released, or to the compounds whose uptake is blocked. These drugs all have effects on aminergic systems other than the serotonin system. In other words, the migrainogenic effects seen after administration of these drugs are compatible with a role for serotonin in the genesis of migraine attacks, but it is equally possible that the function of neural or vascular systems that use

multiple amines must be affected to induce migraine attacks.

6. Activation of specific serotonin receptors may initiate migraine attacks. This idea is based on the effects of pharmacologic agents that are thought to act at specific serotonin receptors. Most efforts in this regard have involved study of the actions of m-chlorophenyl-piperazine (mCPP), the major metabolite of the antidepressant trazodone. This compound can induce severe headaches that resemble migraine without aura.[253] mCPP-induced headaches are more common in individuals with a personal or family history of migraine, but can also appear in individuals without such a history. Migraineurs have noted that mCPP provokes headaches that are indistinguishable from their naturally occurring headaches.

mCPP is a serotonin agonist with moderate affinity for both $5\text{-}HT_2$ and $5\text{-}HT_{1C}$ binding sites and a somewhat weaker affinity for $5\text{-}HT_{1D}$ sites.[864] Behavioral observations, however, suggest major agonist action at $5\text{-}HT_{1C}$ sites.[420] How activation of $5\text{-}HT_{1C}$ receptors initiates migraine is not known. Neither is the anatomic site of action of mCPP.[1239] $5\text{-}HT_{1C}$ binding sites are found in largest numbers on the choroid plexus, but the choroid plexus has not been implicated in the genesis of migraine. In contrast, $5\text{-}HT_{1C}$ binding sites are seen only in small numbers in the neocortex and the hippocampus. Moreover, other $5\text{-}HT_{1C}$ agonists such as ergotamine and dihydroergotamine—agonists more potent than mCPP at $5\text{-}HT_{1C}$ sites—are anti-migraine drugs.

7. Intravenous administration of serotonin can alleviate the symptoms of migraine.[62,1109] This effect is thought to result from a presynaptic inhibitory effect exerted by the amine on the terminals of trigeminovascular nociceptive afferents. This inhibitory effect is hypothesized to block the release of neuropeptides responsible for the initiation of the inflammatory process underlying the head pain of migraine. It is unusual

that a compound involved in the production of headaches would alleviate the symptoms of the clinical process.

8. As we shall see in chapters 9 and 10, many of the drugs used in migraine treatment—ergotamine, methysergide, cyproheptadine, propranolol, sumatriptan, and others—act at specific serotonin receptors. However, some act as agonists, some behave as antagonists, and others have mixed agonist–antagonist actions.

Thus, the involvement of serotonin in migraine is supported by a large amount and great variety of circumstantial evidence. But investigations have so far failed to specify a definitive locus or mechanism of action for the amine in the genesis of migraine headaches. For example, data supporting a role for the amine in migraine are not sufficient to distinguish between a vascular or a neurogenic site. The changes in serotonergic mechanisms reported to accompany migraine headaches may occur as a result of changes in the excitability of neurons in the raphe nuclei, from anomalies in the activation of platelets, or from altered mechanisms for uptake, storage, and release of the amine in neurons or platelets. Serotonin may have effects on cerebral neurons or cranial blood vessels, or it may work at both sites. But unambiguous data are lacking with regard to all of these points. It is even unclear whether an increase or a decrease of serotonergic function (i.e., a lack of serotonin or an augmented availability) is responsible for the development of a bout of migraine. In sum, sound, unambiguous proof that serotonin is the agent responsible for the genesis of migraine attacks is still lacking.

DOPAMINE AND MIGRAINE

Although emphasis has been placed on study of serotonin, a small body of suggestive evidence implicates dopamine in the pathogenesis of migraine. Functions involved in migraine attacks, such as pain perception, vomiting, and affect, are partially controlled by dopaminergic systems.[1572,2059] Migraineurs appear to be more sensitive than others to the effects of dopamine agonists. Thus, administration of low doses of dopaminergic agonists induces arterial hypotension more frequently in patients with migraine than in healthy controls.[224,1834] Headaches that are indistinguishable from spontaneous migraine attacks can be produced in some migraineurs, either by administration of small doses of apomorphine or by intravenous injection of dopamine.[310,755,1727] Moreover, in some migraineurs, when dopamine agonists such as apomorphine and bromocriptine are administered, signs and symptoms develop that are considered part of the migraine syndrome (or that are seen in some patients with migraine).[34] These signs and symptoms include anorexia, nausea, vomiting, pallor, sweating, and yawning. In addition, in some patients migraine attacks can be prevented by the peripheral dopamine antagonist domperidone, when administered during the premonitory phase.[2083] All of these findings suggest activation of dopamine receptors during bouts of migraine. Whether or not changes in dopamine metabolism occur during migraine attacks is not known.

THE SYMPATHETIC DYSFUNCTION THEORY

A number of the signs and symptoms associated with migraine headaches indicate peripheral autonomic nervous system dysfunction. No one questions the correlation between attacks of migraine and autonomic nervous system dysfunction such as cutaneous vasoconstriction, gastrointestinal complaints, sweating, nasal congestion, pupillary changes, and cardiac irregularities. At issue, however, is causation. Some authorities feel that dysfunction of the autonomic nervous system does not result from the migraine attack, but rather plays a central part in initiating it.[180,1047] In particular, abnormal activity in the sympathetic limb of the autonomic nervous system changes the tone of the cranial vasculature, thereby inaugurating a chain of events that produces both the aura and the pain of migraine attacks.[1336] According to this formulation, transient release of norepinephrine from sympathetic nerve endings produces vasoconstriction of cerebral blood vessels—a process that gives rise to the aura of classic migraine. The headache phase is associated with vasodilatation produced by a reflex hyperemia. Evidence used to support claims that sympathetic dysfunction is a major factor in the causation of migraine attacks includes the following:

1. Intracranial and extracranial arteries are well supplied with sympathetic nerve fibers.

2. Conditions that activate the sympathetic nervous system—such as emotional stress, exercise, orgasm, REM sleep, and hypoglycemia—can also trigger bouts of migraine.

3. Propranolol and some other β-adrenoceptor antagonists provide effective prophylaxis for many migraineurs.

Such evidence certainly implicates the sympathetic nervous system in attacks of migraine, but the data do not prove that sympathetic dysfunction causes the headache.

Migraineurs have been extensively studied with regard to the function of the peripheral sympathetic limb of their autonomic nervous systems.[1784] Impaired peripheral vasomotor reactivity, increased fluctuations in heart rate, defective cardiovascular reflexes, altered pupillary responses, and abnormal sweating function have been repeatedly demonstrated, but there is no unanimity of opinion as to whether migraineurs have hypoactive or hyperactive sympathetic nervous systems.* Moreover, biochemical investigations of peripheral sympathetic nervous system activity have yielded contradictory results.[59,1784] Thus, experimental sup-

port for the idea that dysfunction of the peripheral autonomic nervous system is responsible for initiating sieges of migraine is limited at best.

ARTERIOVENOUS ANASTOMOSES

More than three decades ago, Heyck proposed a model of migraine that some experts still find credible, although others reject it completely. Heyck's model depends on opening of arteriovenous anastomoses, or shunts, both in the brain and in extracerebral cranial structures.[942] Heyck's hypothesis grew from his unease with the then-current Wolff model of migraine, which asserted that dilatation of the extracerebral arteries caused migraine. Heyck proposed that unspecified processes caused carotid arteriovenous anastomoses in the head to open. This process diverted blood required for metabolic purposes from the capillaries, leading first to ischemia and then to aura symptoms. The vascular distension responsible for the migraine pain was thought to be produced by the surge of blood directly from arteries to veins through the opened anastomoses.

Experiments performed in nine patients provided the evidence to support Heyck's ideas. Blood from a peripheral artery and from the internal jugular vein (which samples cerebral blood) was drawn during migraine headaches from two patients with cerebral symptoms. Similarly, blood was drawn from the external jugular vein of seven patients with distinct hemicranial migraine; this provided blood samples from the noncerebral tissues of the head.[945] In the patients with cerebral symptoms, the arteriovenous oxygen difference was considerably lower than normal values, and in patients with hemicranial headache, the oxygen difference was significantly decreased on the side of the headache when compared to the other side. Heyck postulated that increased shunting of blood on the affected side could explain both

---

*References 73, 75, 223, 385, 533, 543, 624, 804, 808, 916, 1381, 1531, 1706, 1912

results. Although Heyck's theory remains intriguing, no direct data are available on the behavior of arteriovenous shunts during bouts of migraine. In addition, because the arteriovenous oxygen difference correlates inversely with the arterial blood flow, the decreased arteriovenous oxygen difference documented in Heyck's patients could be explained by a change in arterial blood flow.[1920]

SUMMARY

Fifty years ago a number of opinions existed about the etiology of migraine.[405] Most of these ideas—that migraine was caused by eye strain, hypophyseal strangulation by ossification about the sella turcica, periodic obstruction of the foramen of Monro, toxemia from some disorder of intestinal digestion, hepatobiliary upsets, allergy, or psychosomatic causes—do not fit in with our modern approaches to medicine. Most have been rightly discarded. Accordingly, enormous amounts of effort have gone into attempts to develop new hypotheses that could explain the symptoms of migraine headache. The dispute about whether migraine primarily represents dysfunction of the vascular or neurologic systems has been the focus of much recent debate.

Clearly, an either/or hypothesis is too simplistic, for both neural and vascular mechanisms are involved. Some research suggests that spreading depression—or a process akin to spreading depression—is responsible for producing the aura of classic migraine. Spreading depression, however, may not be the first step in the process. A mechanism involving vasospasm may cause changes in cerebral blood flow, changes that are the basis for the spreading depression. The picture grows even more complicated if one considers the extensive work done on aminergic brain stem nuclei. This research indicates that brain stem nuclei play several important roles in regulating cerebral blood flow, in controlling the excitability of cortical neurons, and in modulating endogenous pain control mechanisms. It may well be that a discharge from these nuclei initiates parts of the migrainous process; what activates the brain stem structures is not yet known.

Intriguing and convincing data point to the trigeminovascular system as the possible end-stage mechanism that mediates migraine pain. Neurogenic inflammation is associated both with the antidromic release of neuropeptides by trigeminal nerve endings and with the release of a number of other algesic substances from plasma, platelets, and mast cells. Such release of neuropeptides and algesic compounds causes vasodilatation and extravasation of plasma proteins and appears necessary for the sensitization of nociceptive nerve fibers. Another area of research has centered on serotonin. Much effort has been expended to implicate serotonin as the agent responsible for the genesis of migraine attacks. But no one has as yet found the locus for the changes in serotonin activity that could initiate the process. Where—blood vessels or neurons—does serotonin act if it is indeed responsible for migraine attacks? Finally, the roles played by the sympathetic nervous system, arteriovenous anastomoses, endorphins, and dopamine remain puzzling.

As we can see from the discussion in this chapter and in the two previous ones, the pathophysiology of migraine remains both enigmatic and poorly understood. No single hypothesis explains the process successfully. Thus, the causes of the symptoms of migraine headaches are still controversial. In part, this is so because a unifying explanation of migraine must account for the complete sequence of events in a typical attack of migraine; namely, prodrome, aura, headache pain, and postdrome. Moreover, the systemic, neurologic, cognitive, affective, gastrointestinal, and autonomic dysfunctions that are usually associated with bouts of migraine indicate altered function of the cerebrum, brain stem, hypothalamus, eye, intracranial and extracranial vasculature, and autonomic nervous system. A theory must account for dysfunction of all of these structures. A comprehensive and acceptable account of the mechanisms of symptoms must also encompass the modifications of cerebral blood flow, the role of platelets, the effectiveness of pharmacologic intervention, and the mechanism of action of migraine triggers. Such a comprehensive account is still beyond our ken.

Part III

TREATMENT OF PATIENTS WITH MIGRAINE

Chapter 9

TRIGGER FACTORS AND NON-PHARMACOLOGIC APPROACHES

AVOIDANCE OF TRIGGER FACTORS
NONPHARMACOLOGIC STRATEGIES
EXERCISE
PHYSICAL THERAPY
OPHTHALMOLOGIC TREATMENT
ACUPUNCTURE

At its mildest, migraine is an unpleasant disorder, but for many individuals migraine is a grim obstacle to normal life. Attacks can cause major disruptions in behavior, severely reducing the ability to work or to engage in family and social activities. For these reasons, patients with migraine must be taken seriously and treated with compassion and understanding. In fact, a satisfactory physician–patient relationship is crucial to effective control of migraine headaches. The physician who perseveres by spending adequate amounts of time with each patient and by combining this with judicious use of pharmacologic and nonpharmacologic approaches can frequently restore patients to worthwhile, reasonably pain-free lives.

Ideally, the treatment of a patient with migraine begins with an *empathetic* physician who takes a careful history and performs a physical examination in such a way that the patient is truly convinced of the diagnosis of migraine. Migraineurs are frequently anxious about the presence of organic and mental disease even though they often do not admit to such fears. Accordingly, it is the physician's duty to reassure them that potentially malignant causes of headache are not present. Once these anxieties are alleviated, the chief concern of a large number of patients is to understand the cause of the head pain and the various accompanying symptoms.[1517]

Patients need to be told what can be reasonably expected from working closely with their physicians. Some patients expect a complete "cure." Patients with this unrealistic expectation must be made to understand that only a minority of patients become absolutely headache-free even under optimal conditions, and that migraine differs from simple bacterial infections or surgically remediable conditions such as appendicitis. In contrast, migraineurs suffer from a chronic affliction that is probably inherited and that accordingly will require attention for the rest of their lives. Other patients expect that the condition can be ameliorated by simple measures such as changes in diet. In many cases, articles in the popular press or "self-help" books have led them to believe that treatment will not require much effort or responsibility on their part. This group of patients must be made to realize that simple measures

183

are useful and do constitute a valuable component of treatment, but are rarely sufficient for control of recurrent headaches. Some migraineurs expect that preventive medication will magically ameliorate their headaches. Many members of this group are unaware that antimigraine medications do not work in every individual and that many of the medications used for the therapy of migraine headaches have untoward side effects. Their preconceived ideas must be gently, but firmly, adjusted. Still other patients expect that narcotics and other analgesics, sedatives, and tranquilizers will be made readily available on demand. Again, these patients must be made aware of the dangers of these medications and taught that these drugs will frequently worsen their chronic problem.

Clarifying a patient's mistaken preconceptions or expectations about the treatment of migraine headaches is not the only problematic issue a physician faces. Patients frequently deviate from the recommendations given to them about medication regimens, diet, exercise, and changes in lifestyle.[618,830] The percentage of patients who make errors in taking prescribed drugs, or who are noncompliant, ranges between 29% and 59%.[1959] The percentage response to advice regarding diet and exercise is similar. Most troubling of all is the fact that many patients mishandle medication in ways that pose serious threats to their health.

Although physicians tend to blame the personality characteristics of the patient for noncompliance, a number of interconnected factors are usually at play. Compliance, for example, is affected by the patient's perceptions of physician's empathy and listening skills, by how acceptable the patient finds the treatment, and by the patient's beliefs regarding health matters in general. Patients who have some insight into the nature of their illness, who discern some benefits from their treatment, and who also perceive an association between the two, are more inclined to take medication properly than those who do not have this insight and who do not perceive the benefits.[668] In addition, some data indicate that noncompliant patients are more likely to be older and of lower socioeconomic status and educational attainment than patients who do comply.[459]

But the major determinant in compliance with therapy is the relationship between the physician and patient. Regular contact improves compliance.[1692] Effective communication between physician and patient is also crucial. Because much of what the physician tells the patient is forgotten, compliance can be improved if the patient is provided with written information about treatment regimens and with exact instructions regarding medications.[1238] Better compliance occurs when the physician is enthusiastic about treatment and optimistic about its outcome.

The management of patients with migraine headaches consists of several major components: (1) prevention of attacks by removal of known precipitants, (2) use of nonpharmacologic treatments, (3) treatment of acute attacks, and (4) long-term prophylactic medication to prevent recurring bouts.

This chapter will concentrate on the first two, especially the nonpharmacologic treatment of migraine headaches. Chapter 10 will focus on how best to deal with acute headaches; chapter 11 will discuss the role of prophylactic medications in preventing recurrent headaches. Finally, chapter 12 will take up other issues that need to be considered when caring for migraineurs.

AVOIDANCE OF TRIGGER FACTORS

The myriad of factors capable of provoking bouts of migraine were discussed in chapter 2. Approximately 85% of migraineurs recognize definite trigger factors.[2056] But although the majority of patients identify some precipitants, only a limited number are cognizant of all of them. Accordingly, once a diagnosis of migraine has been firmly established, the physician should systematically go through the list of potential triggers with each patient. When a migraineur becomes aware of how wide the range of possible triggers is, and how significant a role they may play in precipitating headaches, that individual will begin to see the need to keep a headache diary in an attempt to identify triggers for each headache. The common practice of simply giving patients a general list of trigger factors and foods to avoid is both insufficient and unsatisfactory; it is essential that the individual migraineur identify the triggering mechanisms that may be operative in the production of his or her own headaches. Then each patient must be made to realize that he or she confronts an option—to abstain from the provocative circumstance, or to chance an attack of migraine.

For many patients, identification of trigger factors is essential for successful headache management because removal of individual precipitants may produce a substantial reduction in the frequency of their attacks.[219] Identification and modification (or even removal) of these factors may be crucial components in the treatment of individual migraine patients. For example, many headaches may be prevented if a migraineur sensitive to alcohol or chocolate refrains from them. Similarly, headache frequency or severity may be substantially reduced if a migraineur stops using oral contraceptives if headaches seem to be worsened by them. Other patients improve if they receive appropriate amounts of sleep, do not oversleep on weekends, and eat meals on a regular schedule each day. In other words, elimination of triggers must be tailored to each patient. In contrast, narrow-minded insistence that everyone stick to a very restricted diet before it is known whether or not a particular patient is sensitive to specific foods or food additives may create formidable difficulties for the patient, and is often counterproductive to successful treatment. The roots of noncompliance often sprout from unappealing lifestyle changes that yield no fruitful results.

Patients often feel frustrated when they are asked to furnish accurate reports on the nature, severity, and frequency of their headaches. In part, the wide variability of migraine attacks in an individual is responsible for this frustration. Systematic daily recording is, however, necessary for the identification of trigger factors and will also serve to monitor medication and to evaluate other kinds of treatment. The systematic daily recording is commonly known as a *headache diary*.[1717] A number of variables can be recorded, but the most important aspects of the attack include the time of onset, the duration, the severity, any medication taken for the headache and its associated symptoms, and any identifiable precipitating factors. A $3'' \times 5''$ spiral-bound notebook is adequate for the task and can be routinely kept at hand.

Dietary Changes

Although as many as 45% of migraineurs contend that some or all bouts are linked to ingestion of specific foods, manipulation of a patient's diet alone will rarely produce dramatic results.[773,1550,1806,2056] Nonetheless, many physicians automatically place patients on an extremely restricted diet without taking the effort to determine beforehand if particular foods are typically followed by migraine attacks in these patients. Patient compliance with restricted, unappealing diets is notoriously poor. Furthermore, the stress of trying to stay on the diet—or of cheating—may itself induce migraine. Patients dislike being deprived of favorite foods for extended periods unless they are really convinced these foods are triggers. And if the patient does not fully comply with the dietary restriction, who is to say which foodstuffs, if any, in combination with new dietary stresses, might trigger an attack of migraine in a particular patient? There is no choice but to spend time and effort to distinguish the particular food sensitivities of individual patients and to remove only those foods that cause the individual patient's headaches.

Occasionally the association between food and the onset of head pain is unmistakable; more often it is not. Most patients have difficulty recognizing dietary factors, especially since some foods do not trigger headaches unless other precipitants are also present. In addition, a food's capacity to trigger a migraine attack is often dose-related. Maintenance of a food log or diary is a simple procedure to establish which foods are related to headaches. The patient can either jot down all foods and drinks ingested every day or retrospectively list the foods eaten the day before and the day of a headache. Using these aids, an intelligent person can determine which, if any, components of his or her diet are consistently reponsible for bouts of migraine.

Alternatively, a patient can be placed on an *elimination diet* to determine whether or not an allergic component contributes to the individual's migraine. The use of such diets is controversial; some studies show the merit of elimination diets, others demonstrate little benefit.[1357,1407] Such a diet should be free of foods (such as milk and other dairy products, eggs, corn, pork, wheat, soybeans, shellfish, onions, yeast-containing products, and citrus fruits) that are thought to cause migraine by allergic mechanisms. In some children, food dyes and colorings are the culprits, and should be eliminated. In most cases the diet must be adhered to for at least a month to 6 weeks to ascertain if a change in the frequency of migraine attacks has occurred. If a patient does have a dramatic response to an elimination diet, excluded foods can be reintroduced one at a time at weekly intervals to evaluate their individual effect.

Although very few patients state that their headaches are related to consumption of coffee or other caffeine-containing beverages, caffeine-withdrawal headaches may be responsible for weekend headaches and for headaches experienced on awakening. The consumption of caffeine should be limited in patients with migraine.

Sleep and Eating Patterns

A majority of migraineurs suffer less if they follow a consistent routine from day to day, including weekends. This can be a significant factor in circumventing headaches. For example, changes in sleep patterns are known to trigger migraines. Migraineurs should accordingly be counseled to refrain from oversleeping, undersleeping, or napping (unless napping is part of their regular schedule). Delayed awakening on weekends, holidays, and vacations can lead to migraine attacks in many patients, but they are often reluctant to give up the luxury of "sleeping in." There is a potential solution for these patients. Suggest that they set their alarms for the usual time, eat a small breakfast, and then go back to sleep.

As indicated in chapter 2, the relationship between low blood sugar and migraine is complex. But there is little doubt that many migraineurs are sensitive to fasting and to hunger. Because many patients find themselves stricken by a headache when they have missed a meal, emphasis must be placed on eating breakfast and not skipping lunch or delaying dinner. Some patients need to carry around a substantial snack in case they find themselves faced with a significant delay in food intake from expected times. In view of this, it is not surprising that some few patients report improvement of their symptoms when they are placed on a frequent-feeding, low-carbohydrate, high-protein diet.[491]

Medications and Hormones

Some medications can increase the frequency and severity of migraine attacks. This group includes some histamine (H$_2$) blockers, some calcium channel blockers, some nonsteroidal anti-inflammatory drugs (NSAIDs), a number of antihypertensive drugs, nitroglycerin, and some hormonal preparations (see Table 2–4). Substitutions of comparable medications by the patient's primary care physician can sometimes alleviate the situation.

Whether or not oral contraceptives should be discontinued depends in part on social factors. But even if these preparations do not appear to affect the frequency or severity of attacks, every patient must be fully informed of her increased risk factors so that she can make a rational decision about their use (see chapter 2). On the other hand, oral contraceptives *must be discontinued* if focal neurologic symptoms are present.

Physical and Environmental Factors

Many migraineurs are troubled by certain conditions of light, noise, smells, and temperature. Some environmental factors are unavoidable, but others can be modified if they precipitate bouts of migraine. In particular, patients should pay attention to lighting conditions at home and at work. Fluorescent lighting should be eliminated if it is a factor in the provocation of attacks. For some patients, tinted eyeglasses may be of value both indoors and outdoors. Migraineurs need to become aware that some trigger factors are beyond their control—hormonal variations in the menstrual cycle, barometric fluctuations, other people's choice of perfume or smoke. Being conscious of what may set off an attack may help each individual make decisions about how to deal with potential triggers. They may change seats in a restaurant, go home, leave a stressful task for another day, and so forth. From a psychological point of view, patients benefit from becoming aware of the extent to which they can intervene in preventing or mitigating an attack. There is comfort in knowing that one is not simply a hapless victim of a painful, disruptive condition.

NONPHARMACOLOGIC STRATEGIES

Clinicians have long realized that psychological phenomena can play a pivotal role in the genesis and maintenance of migraine headaches. In particular, a migraineur's psychological makeup may influence the triggering of some attacks. Psychological phenomena also determine the methods chosen to cope with repeated episodes of head pain, and the consequences of chronic head pain on personality, behavior and lifestyle. To address such factors in patients with migraine, a number of self-regulatory, noninvasive behavioral techniques such as biofeedback (both thermal and electromyographic), simple relaxation therapy/autogenetic training, hypnosis, and programs teaching cognitive stress-coping skills have been used.* All of these noninvasive treatment modalities reportedly reduce the frequency, and sometimes the intensity, of migraine headaches, although no one behavioral treatment has been proven substantially more effective than any other.[53,1158,1656,1890,1908] Reviews, however, have consistently concluded that 35%–50% of treated individuals report at least a 50% decrement in headache activity.[196,346,971,1041]

Biofeedback and other behavioral therapies are therefore widely accepted for patients with migraine headaches, even though studies that have examined their effectiveness can be criticized for their small sample sizes, absence of adequate control groups, intermingling of several different behavioral treatments in the same patient, and lack of satisfactory criteria to assess outcome.[968] No one has ascer-

---

*References 7, 49, 192, 194, 510, 706, 1123, 1392, 1881

tained the extent to which nonspecific factors and placebo effects may account for improvement. And, in addition, strict criteria to determine which behavioral method is most appropriate for an individual patient are unavailable. Most choices are based on accessibility of competent practitioners in the clinician's locale. When therapists of all sorts are available, many patients are taught biofeedback techniques and relaxation exercises as components of a comprehensive behavioral approach that includes cognitive restructuring, stress management techniques, and patient education.

A considerable obstacle to widespread use of behavioral therapies is their cost and availability. Behavioral interventions for migraine frequently necessitate 10 to 20 hours of professional contact.

Biofeedback

Biofeedback is the best known and most widely used nonpharmacologic procedure for the treatment of migraine headaches. The technique enables individuals to control skin temperature or muscle tension—functions of their nervous system—that were previously regarded as beyond volitional or conscious control. Biophysiologic instruments that measure these functions are used to teach patients how to control them. In general, the biofeedback training paradigm follows an operant conditioning framework.

Thermal biofeedback gained popularity many years ago when it was believed that an increase in peripheral blood flow would decrease cranial vascular activity. Although this is no longer thought to account for its efficacy, thermal biofeedback is still the most widely used type of feedback for patients with migraine headaches. Patients are taught to increase hand or finger temperature by means of electronic feedback, coupled with instruction by a trained therapist. A lightweight thermistor or a thermocouple is attached to a finger and information about skin temperature is immediately displayed either on a meter or a numerical display, or else it is converted to a tone. Subjects are instructed to try to make their hands grow warm; they are given simple instructions such as "warm your hands," "warm your hands and make the needle on the meter move." There may also be suggestions on the use of warmth-related imagery, or the repetitive use of autogenetic phrases such as "my hands are warm" or "I can feel the blood rushing into my fingers." By trial and error, each individual discerns the subjective state and subtle internal cues related to the changes in skin temperature. The intended effect of biofeedback is to enable patients to demonstrate voluntary control over their skin temperature both inside and outside of the biofeedback laboratory.

Electromyographic (EMG) biofeedback attempts to enhance voluntary control over the striated muscles of the head, face, and neck. For this purpose, surface electrodes are placed on the skin over selected muscle sites. The frontalis muscle, the trapezius, and the masseter muscles are typically selected.[100,1161] As with thermal biofeedback, the electrodes are connected to a visual or auditory display, and the patients are counseled to use imagery, autogenetic phrases ("my muscles are relaxed"), or whatever works to decrease electrical activity in the muscles.

The available data hold no exclusive status for *thermal* biofeedback in the management of migraineurs. In fact, EMG and thermal biofeedback are statistically equivalent with regard to their ability to reduce migraine activity.[367] Moreover, clinical evidence suggests the usefulness of combining finger temperature biofeedback with EMG biofeedback.[509,510,697,1359]

Biofeedback is frequently combined with a number of other behavioral techniques such as relaxation training (see below).[195] This mixture of treatments is believed to produce a better result than either treatment element by itself.[194]

Counseling and psychotherapy have also been combined with biofeedback, but the value of their concomitant use has not been determined.

A number of empirical investigations and reviews support observations that biofeedback therapy is an effective method of diminishing migraine activity.* In this regard, the major parameter of headache activity affected by biofeedback therapy appears to be frequency of headaches. Follow-up investigations of patients who have undertaken biofeedback training have shown that improvement is maintained for a year or longer.[192,509,510,1848,1890]

Although the factors that determine responsiveness to biofeedback have not been systematically investigated, the process seems to work better in young patients.[197,510,2133] Older patients typically take longer periods of time to learn the technique, and increased age has been correlated with a reduced response to it.[510] In contrast, children and adolescents seem to do particularly well with biofeedback. Data conflict regarding gender differences in response to biofeedback therapy.[510,1656] In addition, biofeedback may be more effective in the treatment of patients with classic migraine than common migraine.[740] Ingestion of large quantities of analgesic medications appears to obstruct biofeedback therapy, and patients who are not habituated to drugs seem to do better.[346,1380]

Although some data disagree regarding the relative efficacy of biofeedback and the most commonly used prophylactic therapy, propranolol, both forms of therapy demonstrate similar short-term improvements in headache activity.[972,1323,1913] Whether both are equally effective in the long-term management of migraine is unknown. Finally, it should be noted that several reviews have been critical of the efficacy of biofeedback in the treatment of migraine.[968,1042,2047,2048]

---

*References 6, 7, 49, 194, 195, 198, 199, 346, 510, 739, 1656, 1881, 2158

POSSIBLE MECHANISMS

At present, the mechanisms whereby biofeedback produces improvement in migraine are obscure. There are three major hypotheses: (1) that biofeedback enables patients to reduce sympathetic outflow, (2) that biofeedback gives patients some control over their responses to the headache attacks, and (3) that biofeedback gives rise to nonspecific therapeutic benefits.

1. *Biofeedback improves migraine because patients learn how to reduce excessive sympathetic outflow.* As discussed in chapter 7, some investigators have felt that dysfunction of the autonomic nervous system plays an important role in causing bouts of migraine.[180,1047] One corollary would be that control of sympathetic activity should improve a patient's condition. We do know that the peripheral vasculature in the fingers is primarily mediated by activity of the sympathetic nervous system and that significant parasympathetic innervation of the digital arterial bed is not present. As a result, in order for peripheral vasodilatation and ensuing hand warming to occur, decreased sympathetic nervous system activity is believed necessary. In other words, peripheral vasodilatation is postulated to result exclusively from reduced sympathetic (α-adrenergic) activity.

Doubt, however, must be cast on the idea that conscious ability to reduce sympathetic nervous system activity is by itself the important factor in determining the therapeutic outcome of biofeedback. Individuals who are taught to cool their hands by biofeedback training respond as well as patients who are taught to warm their hands.[738,1102,1189] Furthermore, being able to change sympathetic nervous system function (that is, to control digital or hand temperature) is not firmly correlated with reports of successful headache reduction.[346] The converse is also true: headaches have been successfully treated with thermal biofeedback in subjects who could not maintain the thermal responses. Most studies find no statistical relationship between headache improvement and the degree of control over hand warming.* Moreover, similar clinical results can be obtained with EMG biofeedback, which does not involve a learned autonomic change.[346]

Learned alterations in sympathetic activity may, in fact, be relatively unimportant in determining the therapeutic outcome of biofeedback. As noted below, relaxation training does not provide the patient with physiologic feedback information, yet it is as effective as some biofeedback procedures in the treatment of migraine headache.[200,1848] Perhaps, before a subject is able to achieve an adequate response to biofeedback, that subject must first relax. In other words, relaxation may be unknowingly combined with biofeedback to cause a generalized reduction in cutaneous sympathetic outflow that is not limited to the digits.

2. *Biofeedback is a method by which individuals can modify important cognitive, emotional, and behavioral responses.*[346] Biofeedback may derive its therapeutic potential by demonstrating to individuals that they can control bodily functions. The increase in awareness and perceived control of physiologic events is thought to be a critical component of the biofeedback process.[686,1672] Some investigators also feel that biofeedback serves to allow migraineurs to become more aware of the role that emotions and stresses play in the genesis of their headaches.[2048]

3. *Biofeedback-induced improvement in headache activity is caused by nonspecific therapeutic effects.* Controversy exists about the extent to which the treatment effects of biofeedback are caused by placebo effects produced by expectations of improvement, association with professionals concerned with migraine, and detailed record keeping.[367,1102,1508] Some studies, however, report that biofeedback results in greater headache reduction than a credible placebo control condi-

tion.[401] In contrast, other investigations found that similar reductions in headache intensity occurred whether patients were given true or false temperature feedback.[1437]

Relaxation Training

The rationale for *relaxation techniques* is based on the idea that physical tension contributes to head pain. And indeed, learning to relax by any one of the various methods is demonstrably beneficial for many patients with migraine. No attempt is made to determine why a patient's muscles become tense in particular situations or circumstances. Accordingly, these techniques may be especially valuable in the therapy of migraineurs who tighten up physically in response to emotional stress, especially if they are disinclined to identify and address the feelings openly.

Relaxation training is a less complicated and elaborate treatment than biofeedback. No equipment is needed, and little expertise is required. Relaxation training is thus much easier than biofeedback for a therapist to employ. Two of the best-known techniques are *progressive relaxation* and *autogenetic training:*

1. *Progressive relaxation.* A widely used relaxation method—the Jacobson technique—has the patient employ an orderly succession of muscle tensing and releasing exercises.[1020] Attention is focused on various major muscle groups in order to consciously relax them. Subjects sequentially tense and hold, and then relax, muscles throughout the body.[169] Focus is placed on the sensations associated with muscular contraction and its absence. Patients practice often, until they can relax their bodies easily without needing overt instructions.

The results of a number of investigations have indicated that progressive relaxation alone may be as efficacious as thermal biofeedback for the treatment of patients with migraine.[200,1848]

---

*References 1102, 1161, 1189, 1437, 2133

But the two procedures—relaxation and biofeedback—may not be clinically interchangeable. Some patients who fail to improve with relaxation training may improve after biofeedback. Whether this flows from physiologic or personality differences among patients is not known.

2. *Autogenetic training.* Autogenetic training stresses the silent repetition of, and concentration on, a series of brief phrases. Such phrases include autosuggestions that the extremities are heavy and warm, that respiration is even, and that the forehead is cool. Emphasis is placed on verbal methods rather than on directions regarding the conscious production of physiologic change.[1796] Regular practice over a period of many months is necessary. Repetition of the phrases is said to induce calmness, relaxation, and specific bodily and mental changes. In many instances autogenetic training is combined with thermal biofeedback.

Each technique educates the individual to be aware of muscle tightness and tenseness. An overall relaxed state can be developed. Other techniques that may produce the same types of effects include yoga and transcendental meditation.[163] The mechanisms through which relaxation reduces pain are still under debate.

Hypnosis

Hypnosis is used by trained psychologists to produce relaxation and to diminish patients' perceptions of pain.[1924] Hypnosis offers a less comprehensive approach than cognitive therapy, but shares many elements with it, including an emphasis on the role of mental events in pain production and the use of suggestion and imagery. While hypnotized, a patient has an increased receptivity to suggestion, the potential for revision of perception and memory, and the capacity for voluntary control of a variety of usually involuntary physiological functions. All of these features can be worthwhile in the control of

head pain. Hypnotherapy appears to provide results equivalent to other behavioral treatments, but it is impossible to perform a "blinded" study of hypnotherapy. Moreover, many patients cannot be hypnotized.

Cognitive Therapy

Cognitive therapy for headaches *(cognitive stress coping training, cognitive behavior therapy)* is based on the hypothetical notion that an individual's affect and behavior (including headache and headache behavior) are mainly determined by a process of cognitive appraisal whereby the individual comprehends events in terms of their perceived significance.[1313] Cognitive interventions undertake to furnish patients with a battery of problem-solving or coping skills that can be used to handle an extended spectrum of circumstances and problems (stressors) that give rise to a bout of migraine.[2046] Cognitive therapy is intended to provide patients with the ability to recognize, evaluate, and modify maladaptive thinking patterns and learned dysfunctional beliefs. The therapist usually endeavors to train the patient to control headaches by means of procedures intended to change a person's "cognitions"—that is, the manner with which he or she analyzes, assesses, and conceives of events. The idea is to cope more effectively with stresses that are considered to be causative factors in migraine pain. The therapist works from the premise that patients must be actively involved in learning to manage their problems.

Research in this field is difficult to assess. Obviously, the sensitivity and skills of the therapist are more critical than those needed to teach biofeedback or relaxation. Similarly, the relationship between patient and therapist must be good. Few published studies are available, and most involve small numbers of subjects. Among these studies, few have investigated their subjects in a controlled manner, and even then the investigatory techniques have varied widely among researchers.[266,1161,1123,1396] To date, this work has not established that cognitive techniques are superior to alternative behavioral techniques.[193]

Psychotherapy

Psychodynamic psychotherapy and psychoanalysis presuppose that headache pain is derived from strong and unresolved difficulties in the patient's unconscious.[10] As indicated in previous chapters, anger, anxiety, depression, and maladaptive reactions to stress may indeed be both important factors in the development of headaches and substantial determinants of how each migraineur responds to his or her affliction. Although formal psychotherapy and psychoanalysis for patients with migraine enjoyed a vogue in the past, however, no controlled studies have shown the efficacy of psychotherapy in the treatment of headache. Most clinicians have concluded that the results with regard to head pain are disappointing.[699]

Patients with migraine may, however, also have concurrent psychiatric disorders. For example, depression is often seen in patients with headaches, especially in persons with intense or disabling headaches.[733,1368–1370] In addition, many individuals with a history of migraine and major depression also have an anxiety disorder.[251] These disorders frequently warrant psychiatric consultation and may require individual psychotherapy.

EXERCISE

Excessively strenuous or physically stressful exercise may actually precipitate an attack of migraine. Moreover, exercise usually exacerbates an ongoing migraine, and most patients automatically restrict their activity level in the prodromal period or during an attack. But in some migraineurs, exercise can abort attacks.[449] In addition, aerobic exercise has been reported to be valuable as part of a program of migraine management.[660,859,1631,1853] Some data support the idea that a maintained program of regular aerobic exercise will decrease the frequency of migraine headaches.[449] Much research is still required, however, before a firm statement can be made regarding the connection between the management of migraine and exercise.

PHYSICAL THERAPY

As discussed in chapter 2, pain in the cervical or cranial region can act as a trigger for migraine attacks. For example, the pain resulting from a myofascial trigger point located in cranial, neck, or shoulder musculature may precipitate bouts of migraine. Whiplash and similar trauma to the cervical spine can exacerbate existing migraine. Treatment of the underlying myofascial and cervical problems, especially when combined with appropriate pharmacologic therapy, may be necessary to offer the patient as complete relief as possible from migraine.

Treatment of myofascial pain is accomplished by determining the perpetuating factors and using postural stretching and strengthening exercises. The perpetuating factors include physical factors such as poor posture and work-related stresses on muscles. In addition, spraying with a vasocoolant, followed by stretching the muscle bands or trigger points of a patient with a myofascial syndrome, is considered effective. Cooling and stretching is reported to deactivate the irritable points in the muscle. Several sweeps of the vasocoolant spray are sprayed on the involved muscle at a 30-degree angle in a direction away from its origin. The muscle is then stretched.[2032] Alternatively, many clinicians inject a local anesthetic into the trigger point. The inclusion of steroids in the injection has also been advocated, but is not universally accepted as beneficial. Treatment following these measures includes deep heat, massage, and exercise. Daily stretching exercises are also valuable. If the patient suffers from abnormal posture or occupational stresses such as awkward positions at the workplace, they must be identified and remedied, or the condition will recur.

OPHTHALMOLOGIC TREATMENT

Although controversy exists concerning the relationship between eyestrain caused by uncorrected refractive errors or disturbances of ocular alignment and migraine, no firm data indicate either that eyestrain is responsible for migraine headaches or that correction of ocular problems eliminates migraine headaches.

ACUPUNCTURE

Few systematic, controlled investigations discuss the value of acupuncture in the treatment of migraine headaches.[334,534,933,1107,1267] Most of the anecdotal evidence indicates some therapeutic gain, but research standards in this area have frequently been inadequate. Only one controlled study has been performed, and its results are not auspicious.[534] Moreover, any efficacy seems to decrease rapidly after the end of treatment.[1598] The treatment is painful for some patients, and requires repeated visits. Before it can be recom-mended, further controlled trials will be needed to compare acupuncture with standard drug and nondrug therapies.

SUMMARY

The management of patients who are afflicted with migraine is a complex affair. It always starts with the initial interview, which must be structured to provide the patient with an idea of what can and cannot be achieved from appropriate treatment. The crux of effective management of headache is to individualize therapy as much as possible to the patient's needs. As we shall see in the next three chapters, the mainstay of management is the prudent employment of one or more of the many medications that are comparatively specific for migraine. But medications alone—without support, counseling, and advice about behavior and lifestyle—are inadequate. Thus, in large measure, management of patients with migraine consists of a process of patient education so that the affected individual may make intelligent decisions about the removal or alteration of precipitating elements and about changes of lifestyle. Behavioral techniques—such as biofeedback and simple relaxation therapy—often lead to an impressive decrease in the frequency and intensity of the headaches. Wide clinical acceptance of behavioral techniques as treatment modalities for migraine has been gained, and one should not hesitate to use these procedures in appropriately selected patients.

Chapter 10

TREATMENT OF THE ACUTE ATTACK

SIMPLE ANTIPYRETIC ANALGESICS
ANALGESIC–SEDATIVE
   COMBINATION DRUGS
NONSTEROIDAL ANTI-
   INFLAMMATORY DRUGS
ISOMETHEPTENE MUCATE
ANTIEMETICS
ERGOTAMINE
DIHYDROERGOTAMINE
NARCOTICS
SUMATRIPTAN
CORTICOSTEROIDS
OTHER MEDICATIONS
EMERGENCY ROOM TREATMENT
MECHANISMS OF ACTION OF
   MEDICATIONS USED FOR ACUTE
   MIGRAINE ATTACKS

Fortunately, a substantial number of migraineurs have only mild or moderate headaches.[1279] As a consequence, the majority of migraine headaches are either disregarded or treated with simple over-the-counter (OTC) analgesics. Those afflicted with migraine will usually confer with a physician only if their attacks are intense, prolonged, or resistant to simple medications. They seek medical care especially when the frequency or severity of their headaches interferes with daily living.

For a great many migraineurs who need a physician's help, prophylactic medication and nonpharmacologic approaches (such as biofeedback and relaxation therapy) have undoubtedly diminished the frequency of migraine attacks. Only rarely, however, will such treatment prevent all attacks. Consequently, most migraineurs receiving prophylactic treatment will also require abortive or symptomatic therapy for their acute migraine attacks. Moreover, patients whose infrequent bouts do not justify daily prophylaxis will continue to need treatment for their acute attacks.

The objective in treating an acute attack is to reduce the severity of the pain, to lessen the nausea and vomiting, and to curtail the duration. Some patients' head pain and associated symptoms can be completely eliminated by abortive or symptomatic treatment. For others, the symptoms can only be reduced and made more bearable. Innumerable remedies and techniques aim at alleviating misery. Some have proven to be very effective, others are of little value but are still used because of convention. The remarkable variation in treatment strategies described by different authorities is an indication that no one particular therapy is unambiguously superior. Moreover, the response of acute bouts of migraine to various medications is difficult to assess because any agent administered for acute head pain has a large placebo effect.

Medications used for the abortive or symptomatic treatment of migraine generally need to be taken at the first sign that a headache is developing. Unfortunately many migraineurs are hesitant to take medications prior to the onset of severe pain, even though oral medications, when administered late in an attack, are poorly absorbed and thus may be ineffective. The need for early treatment must be emphasized during the initial consultation with a patient. Equally important, an adequate dosage of medication is necessary. Repeated ingestion of inadequate quantities of an agent can actually result in a protracted headache that might have been successfully treated if a sufficient amount of medication had been taken at the inception of the attack. Ironically, many of the medications that may effectively treat acute migraine headaches if given early enough in sufficiently high doses also have great potential to induce headache. All of these agents, such as simple analgesics, analgesic–sedative combination drugs, ergotamine, and opiates, have the capacity to cause chronic headaches, and some can produce addiction. Accordingly, their use must be carefully monitored and controlled. This applies equally to some OTC medications that television commercials have led the general population to view as "benign" capsules or tablets that may be taken at will.

The situation, then, is rather complicated. Physicians commonly find themselves facing patients who come to them with preconceived notions. Patients may not wish to take potent medications because they perceive this as a sign of "weakness." Such patients are inclined to wait to see how bad the headache is going to get before they "succumb" to taking pills. In trying to "tough it out," they may allow headaches that could have been controlled by early medication to develop into ones that are far less effectively treated. In addition, the same patients who are reluctant to take prescription drugs may not hesitate at all before taking frequent, even daily, OTC analgesics. In doing this, they may bring on themselves the so-called *chronic daily headache syndrome* (see chapters 3 and 12). Accordingly, the importance of the physician–patient discussion of medication can never be stressed too much.

Medications alone are frequently insufficient to treat an ongoing migraine attack. Many patients find it necessary to lie down in a darkened room, apply cold packs to their heads or necks, and attempt to sleep.[2154] Placing an ice pack on the scalp or neck lessens the pain intensity substantially in about one third to one half of migraineurs, especially if the headache is of mild-to-moderate intensity.[501,1170,1675] For some patients, the pain may be eliminated by even a short period of sleep, but for others, deep sleep lasting several hours is essential for relief.[204,207] Patients who are able to sleep recover better than those who only rest or doze. A short-acting sedative such as diazepam (10 mg) may be very helpful in this regard. "Walk-in clinics" in some countries provide the migraineur with a simple analgesic, an antiemetic, a sedative or tranquilizer, and a place to sleep for a few hours.[1494,2151] They are said to be remarkably successful. Solitude and sleep are, however, unrealistic for some patients, especially if attacks develop at work, away from home, or at a time and place where the migraineur must continue to act responsibly. In that situation, treatment that does not cause somnolence is necessary.

SIMPLE ANTIPYRETIC ANALGESICS

Simple antipyretic analgesics such as aspirin and acetaminophen (Tylenol) (and increasingly, OTC strength ibuprofen [Motrin, Advil]) form the mainstay of abortive antimigraine treatment. The value of these drugs is beyond question. They are probably the first medications tried by most who suffer from migraine. Rapid ingestion of one of these simple analgesics may be all that is required to treat a mild bout of migraine, although the therapeutic response is frequently incomplete, so that considerable residual discomfort remains.[1551,1698,2003] Whether or not there is a difference in efficacy among simple analgesics is difficult to determine objectively, however, because the methodology of most early published analgesic studies did not recognize the need to establish either adequate assay sensitivity or statistical power to distinguish among treatments. In addition, the difference among oral analgesics is much less than the difference between a therapeutic dose of any oral analgesic and a placebo. Evaluating efficacy is further complicated by the lack of any satisfactory measure of a patient's pain other than the patient's own reports of this subjective experience. The predilection of patients for certain medications is based, at least in part, on tradition and advertising. In the United States brand-name acetaminophen products (especially Tylenol) are the most widely advertised—and most widely used—painkillers, whereas in some European countries aspirin-containing products are more typically ingested.

In spite of the high-volume advertising for acetaminophen, data indicate that approximately 35%–45% of patients consider aspirin an effective medication for acute migraine attacks of mild or moderate intensity.[1698,2003] A dose of 650–975 mg should be administered as soon as possible after onset. The effects of aspirin are dose-related.[810] If the headache continues or returns, the same dosage of aspirin can be repeated in 4–6 hours. Acetaminophen, administered in a dose of 1000 mg, is considered to be similar in efficacy to 650 mg of aspirin.[1576] It should be used by migraineurs who cannot tolerate aspirin.

In individuals not having an attack of migraine, salicylates taken by mouth are absorbed relatively slowly. A peak value requires at least 2 hours, although substantial plasma levels occur in less than 30 minutes.[1227] The rate of absorption is, however, determined by two major factors—the rate of disintegration and dissolution of the aspirin tablets, and the gastric emptying time. The gastric emptying time is important because, although absorption does occur in part in the stomach, the process of absorption of aspirin (as well as of other antimigraine medications such as nonsteroidal anti-inflammatory drugs [NSAIDs] and Cafergot) takes

place largely in the upper small intestine. Unfortunately, reduced motility of the gastrointestinal tract is usually present during bouts of migraine, impairing absorption.[2075] Both delay of gastric emptying and gastric stasis occur even in those patients who do not complain of nausea.[241,1440] Nausea and vomiting associated with the attack itself are also prominent delaying factors. Drug-induced gastric irritation (which is frequently caused by aspirin) augments this effect. Furthermore, patients who vomit must not only endure the discomfort of it, but must also face the confusion of not knowing whether or not they have thrown up their medication, and if so, what part of the dose?

Gastric emptying and peristalsis during bouts of migraine can be promoted by the use of metoclopramide (Reglan). If adequate blood levels are attained, metoclopramide enhances the motility of smooth muscle from the esophagus through the proximal small bowel. In oral doses of 10 mg, metoclopramide is widely recommended as an adjunct to simple analgesics (and other medications) in the therapy of acute migraine.[1698,2003,2024] Although metoclopramide is believed to promote the absorption of aspirin during a bout of migraine, the compound is effective only when it has been given before the analgesic.[2075,2088] In one double-blind trial, concomitantly administered metoclopramide was not found to promote the efficacy of aspirin as a treatment for acute migraine attacks.[2003] Intramuscular or intravenous administration of metoclopramide is very efficacious, with more than 85% of patients reporting a significant reduction in nausea and vomiting.[995,1993] Some skepticism has been voiced about the efficacy of orally administered metoclopramide.[133] Wide variability in the bioavailability of the drug has been reported in healthy volunteers after they ingested 10 mg.[134] Accordingly, 10 mg of oral metoclopramide may not produce blood levels sufficient to stimulate the stomach in all individuals.

Effervescent aspirin is said to produce higher blood levels within a shorter period of time than do solid tablets and, as a result, effervescent aspirin preparations are often recommended by physicians.[1227,1228] Television commercials also urge its use for headaches accompanied by "upset stomach." One double-blind placebo-controlled investigation, however, showed that effervescent aspirin alleviated headaches in only 37% of patients.[2003] Absent further evidence, effervescent aspirin may be considered no better than ordinary tablets.

Serious adverse reactions are infrequent with the usual analgesic doses of aspirin, but continued use of aspirin may cause some people to experience epigastric discomfort or pain, heartburn, dyspepsia, or nausea. Although occult gastrointestinal bleeding occurs in many patients, the amount of blood lost is usually insignificant. The drug can, however, cause gastric ulceration if used excessively or for prolonged periods. In addition, patients who are extremely susceptible to its effects may develop gastric ulceration even when taking modest doses of the drug. This latter effect is rare; nevertheless, aspirin should not be used for patients with a recent history of peptic ulcer or gastrointestinal bleeding. Aspirin is also contraindicated for patients with bleeding disorders. And for the very small percentage of patients who are hypersensitive to aspirin, even small doses may result in development of a rash, or of a severe urticarial or asthmatic type of anaphylactic reaction.

ANALGESIC–SEDATIVE COMBINATION DRUGS

A large number and variety of compound preparations are prescribed for migraine attacks. These products, consisting of a simple analgesic combined with caffeine or a sedative–hypnotic, have a definite, but limited, place in migraine therapy for the treatment of patients with infrequent bouts (Table 10–1). Although extensive anecdotal evidence attests to the value of analgesic–sedative combination drugs in acute migraine attacks, they have not been evaluated in suitable double-blind trials.[676] Very few of these combination drugs have been subjected to appropriate scientific assessment; nor have barbiturate-containing preparations been approved by the Food and Drug Administration (FDA) as a treatment for migraine headaches.

The commonly used preparations combine butalbital, a short-acting barbiturate, which is presumably capable of reducing anxiety related to bouts of migraine, with either aspirin or acetaminophen. There are a number of caveats regarding their use, however. Frequent or daily dosage of these drugs can produce disastrous effects. Patients

Table 10–1 ANALGESIC–SEDATIVE COMBINATION DRUGS

Agent	Brand Name	Dosage
Aspirin 325 mg, butalbital 50 mg, caffeine 50 mg	Fiorinal	1–2 tablets q 4 h (maximum 6 tablets/d)
Acetaminophen 325 mg, butalbital 50 mg, caffeine 40 mg	Esgic, Fioricet	1–2 tablets q 4 h (maximum 6 tablets/d)
Acetaminophen 500 mg, butalbital 50 mg, caffeine 40 mg	Esgic Plus	1 tablet q 4 h (maximum 6 tablets/d)
Acetaminophen 325, butalbital 50 mg	Phrenilin	1–2 tablets q 4 h (maximum 6 tablets/d)
Acetaminophen 500 mg, butalbital 50 mg	Phrenilin Forte	1–2 tablets q 4 h (maximum 6 tablets/d)

who use these drugs to excess risk the consequence of developing rebound headaches *(drug-induced headaches)* (see chapter 12). Accordingly, all patients must be specifically warned of this particular risk, and their physicians must carefully monitor the quantities that are prescribed. Drugs containing barbiturates should never be prescribed for patients with depression, especially if there is any suspicion of suicidal tendencies. Furthermore, barbiturates impair mental and physical functioning, and patients must be warned against taking them if there is any possibility they will need to drive or operate machinery in the next several hours. In addition, drugs containing barbiturates should be used with extreme caution in elderly or debilitated patients, who may respond to ingestion of barbiturates with obvious excitement, depression, or confusion.

Caffeine

Caffeine has long been a constituent of OTC and of prescription analgesics. Caffeine combined with aspirin, acetaminophen, or salicylamide (with or without butalbital) is available. In addition to commercial products, many migraineurs discover by themselves that a caffeine-containing beverage will help abort their migraine attacks. Caffeine has several properties that may be of benefit in the treatment of migraine headaches. Concurrent oral administration of caffeine with aspirin increases the peak plasma concentration of aspirin. This effect presumably results from abilities of caffeine to increase gastric acidity and enhance gastric perfusion. Caffeine has independent analgesic effects that are equivalent to acetaminophen.[2100] It has mood-altering properties such that the increased mental alertness, lessened fatigue, and feeling of well-being that follow caffeine ingestion counterbalance some of the symptoms of migraine.[795,1953] In addition, caffeine causes cerebral vasoconstriction and

may also have anti-inflammatory properties.[1769] But restraint must be practiced to prevent overconsumption of caffeine-containing drinks and medications, because of the danger of producing caffeine-withdrawal headaches.

Whether or not caffeine increases the efficacy of analgesics has been a subject of debate. Some authorities find little evidence to support the supposition that caffeine is an analgesic adjuvant.[30,139,140] But the combination of caffeine—in a dosage greater than 65 mg—and a simple analgesic does appear to be more effective than a simple analgesic alone for treating a variety of painful states, such as tension-type headaches and dental and episiotomy pain.[1195] This same conclusion is also assumed to be true of migraine pain, even though insufficient data are available to draw any firm conclusion.

NONSTEROIDAL ANTI-INFLAMMATORY DRUGS

A number of NSAIDs are capable of producing pain reduction for patients suffering from acute migraine attacks (Table 10–2).* Most double-blind studies have found NSAIDs superior to placebos in the treatment of acute migraine attacks. NSAIDs diminish both the severity of attacks and their duration. The need for additional drugs is also reduced.[913,1607] In addition, NSAIDs have an advantage over most other medications used to treat acute migraine attacks in that they do not cause chemical dependence or interdose withdrawal symptoms. Use of NSAIDs is, however, restricted in acute attacks by their slow onset of action and their modest analgesic potency.

Although as a group NSAIDs are reported to be similar in efficacy, individual patients vary markedly in their responses to one NSAID or another. There is no way to predict which patients

_____

*References 502, 863, 1048, 1082, 1243, 1453, 1454, 1578, 1609

Table 10–2 SOME NSAIDs USED FOR ACUTE MIGRAINE ATTACKS

Agent	Brand Name	Dosage
Naproxen	Naprosyn	750–1000 mg at onset; if needed, 250–500 mg in 1 h (maximum 1500 mg/d)
Naproxen sodium	Anaprox	825 mg at onset; if needed, 275–550 mg in 1 h (maximum 1375 mg/d)
Ibuprofen	Motrin	400–800 mg at onset; if needed, 400–800 mg in 4 h (maximum 3200 mg/d)
Mefenamic acid	Ponstel	500 mg at onset; if needed, 250 mg in 4 h (maximum 1250 mg/d)
Diclofenac sodium	Voltaren	50–75 mg at onset; if needed, 50 mg in 1 h (maximum 200 mg/d)
Ketorolac	Toradol	60 mg IM at onset; if needed, 60 mg in 4 h (maximum 180 mg/d)

IM = intramuscular administration

might develop side effects to which NSAID. Prescribing these drugs, thus, is a matter of trial and error. If a particular NSAID is unsuccessful, an alternative drug in the same class of NSAIDs, or a drug from another class, should be tried. Because it may take several attempts to find the right "match" between patient and medication, each NSAID should be prescribed with an optimistic expectation that it will be helpful. Along with hopeful optimism, however, the patient can be told that if this medication is not fully effective, there are others that may be more compatible with his or her makeup.

Large doses (750–1000 mg) of naproxen (Naprosyn), in particular, appear to be effective therapy for acute migraine attacks.[1454,1760,2035] Several investigations have also found naproxen to be as effective as, or superior to, ergotamine.* Naproxen sodium (Anaprox), marketed separately, is reported to have the same pharmacologic profile as the parent compound, but has the additional advantage of being more rapidly absorbed than naproxen, and

therefore may have a faster onset of action. Doses between 825 and 1375 mg should be used. The mean time to reach peak plasma concentrations is about 1 hour for naproxen sodium and about 2 hours for naproxen, when administered to normal fasting individuals.[1433] Both naproxen and naproxen sodium appear to be more effective in patients with migraine when administered after an appropriate dose of metoclopramide.

Ibuprofen (Motrin) is also effective in treating bouts of migraine.[1120,1538] When administered in dosages of 400–800 mg, ibuprofen has been shown to produce a modest, but significant, reduction in headache pain and to be significantly more effective than placebo.[500,913] Ibuprofen is rapidly absorbed after oral administration in normal individuals. A peak plasma concentration is seen after 1–2 hours. Other NSAIDs, such as mefenamic acid (Ponstel) and diclofenac sodium (Voltaren), have been shown to have efficacy in reducing the severity and duration of migraine attacks.[471,1320,1394]

Ketorolac (Toradol) is the only parenteral NSAID available in the United States. It has an advantage compared to oral NSAIDs in that its onset of action is rapid—45 minutes to peak blood lev-

*References 1607, 1609, 1760, 2034, 2035

els. Nor does a full stomach or decreased gastric motility interfere with this time frame. When administered in a dose of 60 mg intramuscularly, it is reported to have a modest effect against acute migraine.[895]

Most patients tolerate NSAIDs well when these medications are prescribed for acute bouts of migraine. The most common adverse effects are gastrointestinal reactions, ranging from mild dyspepsia, epigastric pain, and heartburn to nausea, vomiting, and gastric bleeding. These side effects occur less frequently than with aspirin. Gastroduodenal ulcers have developed in only a few patients treated for migraine with NSAIDs. Most of the serious gastrointestinal side effects occur in patients who take NSAIDs on a chronic basis. One should be aware, however, that medications—such as antacids and H_2-antagonists—commonly used for the treatment of ulcers are not effective for the prevention of NSAID-induced gastric problems.[708] Drowsiness, headache, dizziness, fatigue, depression, and ototoxicity have been reported. Rare instances of jaundice, impairment of renal function, angioneurotic edema, skin rashes, thrombocytopenia, and agranulocytosis have also been seen. A few patients complain of fluid retention and edema. Contraindications to the prescription of NSAIDs include a history of ulcer disease or gastritis, kidney disease, and a bleeding diathesis.

Isometheptene Mucate

Isometheptene mucate is marketed in combination with acetaminophen and dichloralphenazone (Midrin). Isometheptene mucate is a sympathomimetic agent that acts as an α- and β-adrenoceptor agonist and as a vasoconstrictor; dichloralphenazone is a mild, nonbarbiturate sedative. Data demonstrate that this combination of medications is more effective than placebos for mild-to-moderate bouts of migraine.[498,1719,2191] Isometheptene mucate is not, however, a very potent medication, and it is

therefore not very effective for the treatment of severe headaches. Some patients find it quite satisfactory; others consider it useless. For patients with histories of attacks that are not terribly severe, it is worth trying.

Two or three capsules should be taken at the first sign of a headache and two capsules 45 minutes later if the head pain has not begun to regress. A total of five capsules can be taken in 1 day. The drug should not be administered more than two or three times a week, to avoid "rebound" effects. Isometheptene mucate is generally well tolerated, although drowsiness and nausea are possible side effects. Because of its adrenegic properties, it should not be prescribed for patients with severe hypertension, glaucoma, hepatic dysfunction, renal disease, or for patients taking monoamine oxidase inhibitors.

ANTIEMETICS

Because most acute bouts of migraine are associated with nausea or vomiting, the need for antiemetic medication is often very great. For some patients these symptoms can be as disturbing as the head pain itself. Although most patients are not completely overcome by vomiting, there are cases in which severe repetitive emesis, if left uncontrolled, leads to dehydration that requires hospitalization. Nausea may occur in the prodromal phase or very early in the headache phase. Antiemetic medications should accordingly be given as soon as possible. Early treatment is important, not just to allay troublesome symptoms, but also because some of the remedies administered for acute attacks of migraine can cause nausea, and it is helpful to have had antiemetic medication before these drugs are used.

Mention has already been made of the efficacy of metoclopramide in promoting the absorption of orally administered analgesics; in this regard, the case for metoclopramide as the drug of choice in acute bouts of migraine is convincing. As an antiemetic—as well as a gastric stimulant—metoclopramide is a relatively innocuous drug with few substantial side effects. It can, however, produce some uncomfortable central nervous system effects such as drowsiness, dizziness, and anxiety. The compound can also cause extrapyramidal symptoms, particularly when administered in high doses or when given intravenously. Dystonic reactions are more common in children and young adults.[485] In rare individuals, tardive dyskinesia has been reported to develop after relatively brief periods of treatment at low doses.

Other antiemetics will work effectively against the nausea and vomiting, although none have the same gastrokinetic actions as metoclopramide. In fact, some phenothiazine antiemetics actually delay the absorption of aspirin and other medications, and may therefore retard clinical recovery.[2088] Phenothiazines used for the treatment of nausea and vomiting accompanying migraine attacks include those in (1) the aliphatic group: chlorpromazine (Thorazine), promazine (Sparine), and promethazine (Phenergan) and (2) the piperazine group: prochlorperazine (Compazine) (Table 10–3). Drowsiness is the most common adverse reaction to all phenothiazines. Those in the piperazine group are less likely to cause drowsiness than those of the aliphatic group. Cholestatic jaundice, granulocytopenia, thrombocytopenia, urticaria, dermatitis, and gastroenteritis have occurred after administration of all phenothiazines. The frequency of these reactions in migraineurs is very small because the length of administration is limited and the dosage comparatively low. Extrapyramidal reactions, including akathisia, parkinsonism, and dystonia, have been described, especially with phenothiazines in the piperazine group. Extrapyramidal side effects are more common when high doses of antiemetic drugs are administered parenterally.

In addition to metoclopramide and the phenothiazines, trimethobenzamide hydrochloride (Tigan) can be used to control the nausea and vomiting of an acute migraine attack. With usual doses, the incidence of adverse effects is low; with larger doses, drowsiness, vertigo, diarrhea, and cutaneous hypersensitivity reactions may occur.

ERGOTAMINE

Ergotamine has been the drug of choice for the treatment of acute mi-

Table 10–3 ANTIEMETIC DRUGS USED FOR MIGRAINE

Agent	Brand Name	Dosage
Metoclopramide	Reglan	oral: 5–20 mg q 6–8 h IM: 10 mg
Chlorpromazine	Thorazine	oral: 10–25 mg q 4–6 h suppository: 50–100 mg q 6–8 h IM: 25–50 mg q 3–4 h
Promazine	Sparine	oral: 25–50 mg q 4–6 h IM: 50 mg
Promethazine	Phenergan	oral: 12.5–25 q 4–6 h suppository: 12.5–25 mg q 4–6 h IM: 12.5–25 mg q 4–6 h
Prochlorperazine	Compazine	oral: 5–10 mg q 6–8 h suppository: 25 mg q 12 h IM: 5–10 mg q 3–4 h
Trimethobenzamide	Tigan	oral: 250 mg q 6–8 h suppository: 200 mg q 6–8 h IM: 200 mg q 6–8 h

IM = intramuscular administration.

graine for many years. It is still one of the most effective medications available to abort migraine attacks, producing beneficial responses in 50%–90% of patients.[1574] The higher rates of response are mostly reports of older, uncontrolled trials. Ergotamine is, however, not an ideal drug. Its use is limited by the necessity for early administration, patient dissatisfaction with its side effects, incomplete and unreliable absorption, a small margin of safety, and ease of overuse, with ensuing toxicity or the development of rebound headaches.[1758,2001] Because of these factors, some authorities contend that it ought to be reserved as a remedy for only the most severe bouts of migraine.[365,2152] Nevertheless, the drug remains valuable and effective for patients who suffer from infrequent, but intense, attacks.

A response to ergotamine is used by some clinicians as a pharmacologic "test" to discriminate between different types of headaches. If a patient responds to ergotamine, a diagnosis of migraine is made by these physicians. Such use of ergotamine for diagnostic purposes is very ill-advised and should be discontinued. The response to ergotamine is far from infallible: positive therapeutic responses to ergots also occur among patients for whom the diagnosis of tension-type headache has been established on clinical grounds, and 10%–50% of patients who appear to be definitely migraineurs fail to respond positively to ergots.[123,984,1178]

Clinical Use of Ergotamine

Ergotamine is available in oral, sublingual, and rectal suppository formulations. Table 10–4 shows the common ergot preparations now marketed in the United States. In the past, ergotamine

Table 10–4 ERGOT PREPARATIONS AVAILABLE IN THE UNITED STATES

Agent	Brand Name	Dosage
ORAL		
Ergotamine 1.0 mg, caffeine 100 mg	Cafergot, Wigraine	2 tablets at onset; may repeat in 30 min (maximum 6/d)
Ergotamine 0.3 mg, belladonna 0.2 mg, phenobarbital 40 mg	Bellergal-S	1 tablet at onset; may repeat in 8 h (maximum 2/d)
RECTAL		
Ergotamine 2.0 mg, caffeine 100 mg	Cafergot Suppositories, Wigraine Suppositories	½ to 1 suppository *per rectum* at onset; may repeat in 1 h (maximum 2/d)
SUBLINGUAL		
Ergotamine 2.0 mg	Ergostat, Ergomar	1 tablet under tongue at onset; may repeat at 30-min intervals (maximum 3/d)
PARENTERAL		
Dihydroergotamine 1.0 mg/ml	DHE 45	1 ml SC, IM, or IV; may repeat in 30–60 min (maximum 3 mL/d)

SC = subcutaneous administration; IM = intramuscular administration; IV = intravenous administration.

was prescribed as an inhalant, but this formulation is no longer available. Parenteral ergotamine (Gynergen) is also not available. Because ergotamine is poorly and erratically absorbed when administered by some routes, plasma levels vary markedly depending on how the drug is used.[559] The bioavailability of ergotamine not only changes with the mode of administration, but also varies widely among patients when it is administered by the same method.[20,814] The unpredictable absorption renders constant achievement of adequate blood levels difficult and may account for the surprisingly wide variations in the clinical response to ergotamine among patients, and even in the same patient during different attacks.[23,406,863]

To be maximally effective, ergotamine must be administered in adequate doses. Data indicate that unless a peak plasma concentration of 0.20 ng/mL or higher is achieved within 1 hour, treatment with the drug is usually ineffective.[23] Peak concentrations measured after oral administration of 2 mg of ergotamine vary from 0.21 to 0.36 ng/mL in different investigations; although this is within the therapeutic range, the peak is often not reached quickly enough to be of benefit.[20,1746] Thus, oral ergotamine is absorbed slowly, so that plasma levels do not peak before 1–3 hours.[14,23,1746] Following sublingual administration, ergotamine has been reported to be undetectable in plasma.[2005] In contrast, after rectal administration of ergotamine suppositories, peak plasma concentrations are reached in approximately 1 hour. The plasma levels after rectal administration are higher than after oral administration, in one study 20 times higher (Fig. 10–1).[1008,1746] In general, peak values of approximately 0.45 ng/mL are seen at 1 hour after rectal administration of 2.0 mg.[20,1746]

The bioavailability of ergotamine taken orally is approximately 5%.[1746] The bioavailability after rectal administration is much greater than when taken orally.[814,1574] The bioavailability after sublingual administration is frequently insufficient for therapeutic purposes. Moreover, this route of administration of ergotamine has been found unsuccessful in two double-blind clinical trials.[406,1975]

The molecular properties of ergotamine have a bearing on the drug's clinical use. Each ergotamine molecule consists of a combination of peptide and lysergic acid moieties. For therapeutic uses two ergotamine molecules are combined with tartaric acid. Considering that ergotamine has such a fragile molecular structure, it is not unexpected that the compound is rapidly metabolized. When administered orally, ergotamine is absorbed from the upper gastrointestinal tract. It traverses the portal circulation to the liver before it reaches the systemic circulation.[1462] Because much of this metabolism occurs in the liver, ergotamine is subject to degradation there ("first-pass effect"). The lack of a first-pass effect accounts for the higher plasma levels of drug after administration per rectum compared to the levels reached when the same dose is administered per os. Rectally absorbed ergotamine avoids the splanchnic and portal circulation, passing to a large degree directly into the systemic circulation.

The metabolic breakdown of ergotamine is reported to proceed in two phases: the α phase has a plasma half-life of approximately 1.5–2.5 hours; the plasma half-life in the β phase is 20–30 hours.[14,1361,1509,1695] Even though peak plasma levels of ergotamine rapidly decline, the drug produces peripheral arterial vasoconstriction that prevails for 24 hours or even longer.[2004] The dissociation between the levels of ergotamine in plasma, and the compound's ability to maintain peripheral vasoconstriction, is largely unexplained. Possibly one or more of ergotamine's metabolites remains active and is responsible for the prolonged peripheral vasoconstrictions. An alternative hypothesis is that the drug dissociates from receptor sites extremely slowly.

Because of the considerable variation among individuals with regard to phar-

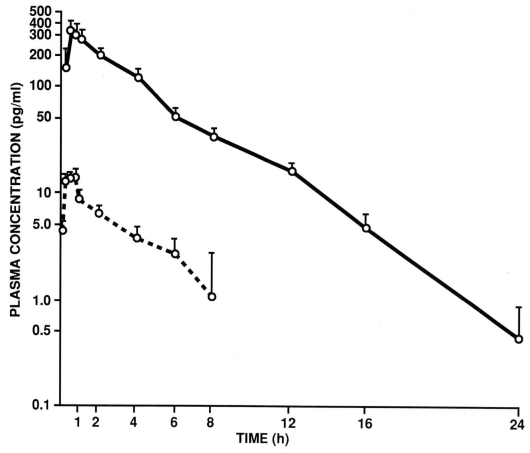

Figure 10–1. Mean plasma concentrations of ergotamine determined following single 2.0 mg oral (---) and rectal (————) doses in healthy volunteers. Vertical bars represent standard errors of the mean. (Adapted from Sanders,[1746] p 332, with permission).

macokinetics and pharmacodynamics, it is desirable to establish a suitable dose of ergotamine for each patient by means of practical trial. Attempts should be made to determine an appropriate, subnauseating dose either when the patient is free of headache or by titrating the dose during several headaches. This is necessary because administration of ergotamine in a dose that causes significant nausea and vomiting may worsen the intensity of the head pain. Therapeutic doses for different individuals range considerably—from 0.5–6.0 mg per attack.[2152] Most physicians are in agreement that the maximum total dose for any one attack should not exceed 6.0 mg orally or

4.0 mg per rectum. An adequate dose must be taken as soon as possible, but it is usually stated that increments can be added in half-hourly or hourly supplements. If the initial dose is without any effect at all, however, subsequent doses are frequently disappointing also. For this reason, some clinicians prefer to prescribe a single dose of ergotamine—usually 2–3 mg (provided that this is a subnauseating dose for the particular patient)—rather than divided doses. Experience with ergotamine use during several attacks allows an individual to establish the amount of the compound required to produce relief of head pain. During subsequent bouts, the total dose can be taken at the onset.

If the ergotamine dose that alleviates symptoms is established individually, a majority of patients can be expected to improve from treatment with this substance.[242]

Most pharmaceutical manufacturers' instructions for the use of ergotamine recommend a maximum dosage of 10 mg/week. If taken every week, however, this dosage is unfortunately well within the range found to cause chronic ergotism.[23,522,964] Moreover, a substantial risk of developing chronic headaches exists if ergotamine is used in the maximal recommended doses, or in lower doses more than twice a week. To prevent these problems, it has been suggested that the amount of ergotamine should be restricted to no more than 2 mg/week.[1783] This is, however, clearly too low a dose to be of benefit for many patients.

The slow absorption of ergotamine from the upper gastrointestinal tract, and the high incidence of vomiting associated with bouts of migraine, substantially limits the efficacy of oral ergotamine. Because of greater absorption with resulting higher serum levels, administration of ergotamine by suppository (Cafergot, Wigraine) appears to be the best method for personal use. Suppositories contain 2 mg of ergotamine and 100 mg of caffeine; some patients find that they can only tolerate one half or one third of a suppository. The use of suppositories is limited, however, by the necessity to store them in the refrigerator if the ambient temperature is high enough to soften them. Most individuals who use ergotamine suppositories also require prescription of an oral or sublingual ergotamine preparation that can be used when away from home. Oral ergotamine tablets (Cafergot, Wigraine) contain 1 mg of ergotamine and 100 mg of caffeine. The usual initial dose is two tablets, but some patients require as many as five tablets. Sublingual ergotamine (Ergomar, Ergostat) is supplied in uncoated tablets containing 2 mg of ergotamine. The usual dose is one tablet. The disagreeable taste of the sublingual tablets is objectionable to many patients. An occasional patient responds well to Bellergal-S—a combination of ergotamine (0.3 mg), phenobarbital (40 mg), and belladonna (0.2 mg).

Ergotamine's effect in terminating bouts of migraine is notably improved by the concurrent intake of caffeine, although it is not known why this is so. Caffeine is said to augment the rate of absorption of oral ergotamine, but the combination of caffeine and ergotamine does not produce higher peak levels.[20,21,1779] Administering ergotamine together with metoclopramide is also superior to the use of each alone for acute migraine.[862] Metoclopramide not only alleviates the nausea of migraine, but is also thought to optimize the absorption of oral ergotamine by increasing the rate of its passage through the stomach.

Ergotamine and Classic and Complicated Migraine

Some physicians hesitate to use ergotamine in patients who have attacks of migraine with aura, and many are understandably reluctant to prescribe it for hemiplegic or basilar migraine, in which vasoconstriction is tacitly assumed to be important in the pathogenesis of the neurologic symptoms. The hesitation stems from a fear of causing increased intracranial vasoconstriction that could lead to permanent neurologic deficits. Ergotamine, however, primarily constricts the external carotid artery and its branches.[1181,1767] The drug does not significantly reduce cerebral blood flow in normal individuals.[42,566,855,1736,2006] But it is conceivable that migraineurs have a cerebrovascular reactivity to ergots that is different from non-migraineurs—a possibility that has not been studied in depth. A few isolated case reports do attribute the development of neurologic deficits and occlusion or spasm of arteries in the carotid system to the use of ergotamine. Despite these isolated examples, as a rule, ergotamine can be used with relative impunity for patients with classic migraine who are still in the aura phase of the attack. In contrast, most physicians hesitate to use ergotamine for patients who have attacks characterized by prolonged aura or for those who suffer from complicated migraine.[1999]

Adverse Reactions

Although side effects do occur with considerable frequency, ordinarily the untoward effects are not alarming and do not require discontinuance of the drug. Nausea and vomiting are considered the most common adverse effects, reportedly occurring with a frequency ranging from 10% to 75%. The frequency depends on the dose and the route of administration, but all estimates of the frequency of ergotamine-induced nausea and vomiting are unreliable because these same symptoms are so regularly a part of the migraine attack itself.[1226,1514,1973,2191] One or more of the following symptoms are estimated to be induced by ergotamine in 5%–10% of patients: abdominal cramps, diarrhea, dizziness, muscle cramps in the thigh and calf muscles, and paresthesias involving the fingers and toes. Other side effects such as syncopal episodes, dyspnea, chest pain, limb claudication, and tremor are less common. Drowsiness may occur in some patients.

Ergotamine is, however, highly toxic when taken in large or frequently repeated doses. In addition, a small number of patients have an idiosyncratically great sensitivity to ergotamine.[902] In either situation, patients may develop the more serious picture of clinical *ergotism*. The manifestations of this syndrome are caused either by vasoconstriction of peripheral arteries or other vascular beds, or by development of an encephalopathy. Individuals with hypersensitivity to the drug are particularly susceptible to ergotamine's vasoconstrictive effects and can develop toxic symptoms after taking recommended doses for brief periods of time. Vascular effects may also occur after modest doses of the drug and after relatively brief exposures. These phenomena are, however, much more frequent in patients who take the drug daily.

The circulatory changes produced by hypersensitivity to ergot or by chronic use of immoderate amounts of ergots can be impressive. Ergots can produce profound peripheral vasospasm that especially affects the lower extremities. Secondary occlusion and thrombosis of medium and small arteries may be superimposed on the vasospasm. The vasospastic segment of the artery typically develops in the lower one third of the leg; fortunately some collateral circulation is usually present around it. Intermittent paresthesias of the distal extremities, coolness of the digits, and claudication of the legs and arms are followed by loss of arterial pulses in the affected limbs. Although these phenomena are at times reversible, the end result may be gangrene of the toes and sometimes the fingers. Because misuse of ergots can lead to such severe sequelae, patients must be clearly (and perhaps repeatedly) warned of the dangers of overuse.

Ergotamine has the potential to constrict many vascular beds, including the coronary, renal, cerebral, mesenteric, and ophthalmic.[636,640] Ergotamine taken in standard amounts has caused myocardial ischemia, myocardial infarction, recurrent angina, cardiac arrest, and even sudden death.* Reports of renal arterial spasm have appeared.[636,1518] Peroneal nerve palsies have also occurred, probably caused by constriction of the vasa nervorum.[1366,1561] Ergotamine also constricts veins.[13,262] As a result of this property, varicose veins can become painful. Thrombophlebitis has developed, occasionally after only a single administration of the drug.

Excessive amounts of ergotamine can produce encephalopathy with altered

---

*References 160, 319, 712, 720, 793, 1118, 1884, 2189

mentation, focal motor or sensory symptoms, seizures, and even coma.[992,1366,1809] The cause of the diffuse cerebral dysfunction is uncertain. Both direct toxic effects on the brain and severe cerebral vasoconstriction with ischemia have been postulated as the mechanisms. In several cases, arteriography has demonstrated occlusion or spasm of the internal carotid artery, or segmental narrowing of intracranial arteries.[261,934,1671,1809] Cerebral atrophy has also been described in chronic users of ergotamine.[654]

Ergotism with vasospasm is treated by immediate and complete withdrawal of the drug, and by efforts to preserve an effective circulation in the affected parts by the use of pharmacologic agents such as anticoagulants, low molecular weight dextran, and potent vasodilator drugs such as intravenous sodium nitroprusside.[313] Epidural and sympathetic blocks have also been tried with some success.

In addition to causing ergotism, overuse of ergots can lead to fibrosis that involves the pleura, pericardium, and retroperitoneum. This has been reported in a few patients after long-term daily use of ergotamine.[1676,1931,1990] Rare individuals develop cardiac murmurs, which are thought to be indicative of aortic or mitral valve disease.[1649,1921] Anorectal ulcers from the frequent use of suppositories have also been seen.[600,1062]

Contraindications to Use of Ergotamine

Preexisting coronary artery or peripheral vascular disease such as atherosclerosis, Raynaud's phenomenon, thromboangiitis obliterans (Buerger's disease), and thrombophlebitis constitute absolute contraindications to the prescription of ergotamine because serious vasoconstrictive side effects are more likely to occur in patients with these conditions (Table 10–5). Most physicians hesitate to prescribe ergotamine for patients with hypertension

Table 10–5 CONTRAINDICATIONS TO USE OF ERGOTS

Peripheral vascular disease
Coronary artery disease
Thrombophlebitis
Marked hypertension
Bradycardia
High doses of β-blockers
Impaired hepatic function
Hyperthyroidism
Malnutrition
Pregnancy and nursing
Infection and fever
Age greater than 60 years*

*Relative contraindication

for fear that the drug will produce an excessive elevation of blood pressure. It is uncertain if hypertensive individuals respond excessively to ergotamine, but in normotensive persons documented increases in systolic and diastolic pressure of up to 20 mm Hg, lasting up to an hour occur following parenteral administration of between 0.25 and 0.5 mg of the compound.[1224,2004] Ergotamine should be also used with caution in individuals who are taking high doses of β-blockers because of the potential for prominent vasoconstriction and excessive bradycardia.[201]

Because ergotamine is metabolized by the liver and excreted by the kidney, diseases of these organs may facilitate accumulation of ergotamine, producing toxic effects following administration of normal doses. A tendency to excessive vasoconstriction seems to be a consequence of certain medical conditions such as hyperthyroidism, malnutrition, pregnancy, and infection, particularly when associated with sepsis. The concurrent use of troleandomycin (triacetyloleandomycin) or erythromycin may also predispose to the development of peripheral vasoconstrictive side effects.[835,1159] Patients who have used ergots safely and feel comfortable with the drug may forget over time that when it was originally prescribed they were warned not to take it concurrently with these antibiotics or when they have an infectious process. Accordingly, physicians should make it a habit to remind their patients of this danger. To be safe, migraineurs must be told to limit their use of ergotamine when they are suffering from any infectious process. Ergotamine should not be prescribed for pregnant women, although, in general, doses much larger than those required to treat an attack of migraine are needed to produce uterine contractions and abortion. Ergotamine may produce symptoms of ergotism in infants exposed through breast feeding; accordingly, this is not a drug that nursing mothers should take.[32]

DIHYDROERGOTAMINE

Dihydroergotamine (DHE) has close chemical similarities to ergotamine, but differs significantly in that its arterial vasoconstrictive properties are much less substantial than those of ergotamine. This makes it a considerably safer drug to use. It also produces little, if any, physical dependence. Moreover, in contrast to ergotamine, which is usually ineffective unless administered early, DHE has the potential to reduce or eliminate head pain well into the course of a headache—or even at its peak. DHE thus constitutes a safe and effective treatment for severe bouts of migraine.*

DHE is currently only available for parenteral use. The best results are obtained when DHE is administered intravenously following parenteral premedication with an antiemetic (Figure 10–2). DHE should not be administered alone because of a high incidence of nausea and vomiting.[1726] More than 85% of patients with acute migraine attacks are reported to respond to intravenous administration of DHE combined with appropriate antiemetic medication.[304,1635] An intravenous infusion of normal saline solution should be started. An injection of an antiemetic such as metoclopramide (10 mg intramuscularly or intravenously) or prochlorperazine (3.5–5.0 mg intrave-

nously) should be given.[571,1637,1726] Intravenous undiluted DHE is administered by slow (over 3–4 minutes) injection in a 0.5- to 1.0-mg dose. If the headache is unaffected by DHE, or if it is attenuated but returns, DHE in a dosage of 0.5–1.0 mg may be administered a second time, provided that at least 30–60 minutes have elapsed since it was first given. If repetitive (every 8 hours) intravenous administration of DHE is required, the patient must be hospitalized. The latter regimen is usually reserved for the treatment of status migrainosus or of drug-induced headaches (see below and chapter 12).

DHE may also be administered intramuscularly in doses of 0.5–1.0 mg, which can be repeated at 1-hour intervals to a total of 3.0 mg.[707,721,907,1726] It can also be given subcutaneously, but plasma levels after subcutaneous administration are 40% lower than after intramuscular dosing. Its use should be preceded by administration of an antiemetic. DHE can be prescribed for home intramuscular or subcutaneous injection. Patients need to be taught self-injection. Self-injection may prevent a visit to the emergency room or to a physician's office. Peak levels are rapidly attained after parenteral administration: 2–11 minutes following intravenous injection and 30 minutes after intramuscular.[946,1079]

DHE may be administered as a nasal spray. Such a product is not yet available in the United States, but some pharmacies are able to make DHE in spray form. The nasal spray formulation has been shown to deliver this compound effectively. It is already available in several European countries and a New Drug Application has been filed with the FDA in the United States. Data from controlled studies are only available in abstract form, but the agent is said to be effective in between 34% and 52% of patients.[1800]

Nausea is the most distressing side effect of DHE, but sedation, anxiety, diarrhea, abdominal discomfort, muscle pain, fatigue, and body aches have also been reported.[304,1635] Some patients become restless and anxious.[153] Worsen-

_____

*References 153, 304, 707, 1635, 1841, 2019

DIHYDROERGOTAMINE PROTOCOL

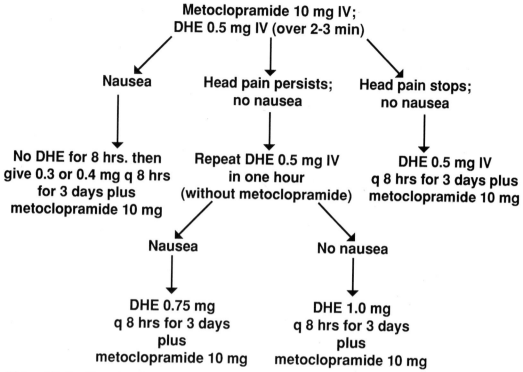

Figure 10–2. Algorithm for the determination of the appropriate dosage of DHE for patients with intractable migraine. (Adapted from Raskin,[1637] p 551, with permission.)

ing of the headache is seen in a small number of patients.[304] DHE generally causes only minimal amounts of peripheral arterial constriction.[42,478] Idiosyncratic hypersensitivity to the drug takes place on occasion, and isolated instances of severe peripheral arterial and coronary spasm have been reported.[1770,1794,2057] Patients with Prinzmetal's angina, ischemic heart disease, uncontrolled hypertension, or infections should not receive DHE because of the potential for ergot hypersensitivity with coronary vasoconstriction. DHE should not be used in pregnant patients.

NARCOTICS

Although the use of narcotics in the treatment of acute migraine attacks is the subject of intense debate, they nevertheless have a place in the care of certain patients. Some authorities have stated that narcotics are ill-advised for treating acute bouts of migraine because of the risk of addiction.[76,1493] In a Danish study, approximately 13 persons per 1 million inhabitants per year were estimated to become dependent on narcotics originally prescribed for migraine.[1184] Not everyone would agree that such an addiction rate is a serious problem. But even if one does agree that a substantial risk for addiction does exist, the infrequent use of small oral doses of narcotics in patients who cannot tolerate the side effects of ergots, or who obtain no relief from other medications, is still far better than unnecessary and prolonged distress. Prescribing very limited amounts is the key to preventing addiction. In addition, the physician must know the patient well and maintain regular follow-up appointments. A physician's abstract fear of the potential for addiction should never condemn a particular patient to suffering unless that patient has a history of self-overmedication.

The combination of a simple analgesic with codeine (such as the mixture of acetaminophen or aspirin and codeine) or the combination of aspirin, caffeine, and butalbital with codeine may be used if more potent analgesics than aspirin or NSAIDs are required. Propoxyphene (Darvon) has been favored by some clinicians, perhaps because it was originally thought that propoxyphene did not have the dependence liability of codeine. Clinical experience, however, has indicated that propoxyphene has the potential for abuse and addiction, giving it no advantage over codeine in this regard. Several clinical trials have shown that 90–120 mg of propoxyphene orally is equipotent to 60 mg of codeine. Propoxyphene has a substantially longer half-life than codeine, however, and will accumulate to a greater degree. More potent narcotic analgesics such as oxycodone combined with aspirin (Percodan) or acetaminophen (Percocet, Tylox) or hydrocodone and acetaminophen (Vicodin) may be used, but their use should be restricted to the most severe cases. Finally, because it is poorly absorbed, meperidine (Demerol) is not very effective as an oral medication. The analgesic effects of the combination of an opioid and an antipyretic analgesic appear substantially greater than increasing the dose of either drug administered by itself.[141]

In contrast to the narcotics just discussed—which are all pure opiate agonists—some clinicians advocate the use of mixed agonist–antagonist opioid analgesics for the treatment of acute migraine because of a supposed lower potential for abuse. Drugs of this kind include butorphanol (Stadol, Dorphanol), nalbuphine (Nubain), and pentazocine (Talwin). Mixed agonist–antagonist opioid analgesics behave as partial agonists and antagonists at different opioid receptors. Analgesics that are partial agonists bind to opiate receptors, but have only a low intrinsic activity. As a result their dose-response curves exhibit a "ceiling effect" with regard to analgesia at less than the maximal effect produced by a full agonist. Most mixed agonist–antagonist opioid analgesics do not have significant advantages over the established full agonist analgesics, and have been shown to have potential for abuse and addiction.[987] Moreover, their antagonist activity makes the possibility of supplementation with a pure agonist problematical.[556]

The mixed agonist–antagonist butorphanol is available in a nasal spray (Stadol NS). The medication has been reported to be safe and effective for the treatment of acute bouts of migraine, but many patients have adverse reactions.[503] These include dizziness and extreme drowsiness. Hallucinations have been reported. Although the preparation is not labeled as a controlled substance, it has potential for abuse and addiction, particularly because it is dispensed in a vial that contains approximately 15 doses. Patients must be warned about the ability of the drug to induce dependency when abused.

Euphoria develops at times in some patients receiving opiates; this sensation may be advantageous for the patient with an acute migraine attack. Some patients, however, suffer unpleasant dysphoria. Considerable sedation, drowsiness, confusion, dizziness, and unsteadiness may also occur. Pruritus (mostly limited to the face, palate, and torso) can occur and is sometimes very distressing. This side effect can often be controlled with a low dose of an antihistamine such as diphenhydramine (Benadryl). And of course constipation is the most common side effect of all opiates. Nausea and vomiting are also frequently seen.

SUMATRIPTAN

The parenteral form of sumatriptan (Imitrex) has recently been released in the United States by the FDA. After being tested in appropriately controlled studies in an extensive series of international trials, sumatriptan has been found to be an effective antimigraine drug.* Sumatriptan may substantially diminish the need to administer potent analgesics and parenteral ergots for intense or prolonged migraine attacks in many patients. The response to this drug is not determined by the type of migraine—classic or common—or by the duration of the symptoms. Sumatriptan's actions on aura symptoms are still unknown. Remarkably, it is said to be effective when given late in bouts of migraine.

Moreover, its efficacy is sustained despite repeated injections over months in the same individual. Sumatriptan is not only significantly more effective in reducing the severity and duration of moderate-to-severe head pain than is a placebo, but oral sumatriptan is superior to either oral Cafergot or aspirin combined with metoclopramide in decreasing head pain.[1506] Sumatriptan renders nearly twice as many patients free of pain than does Cafergot.

Sumatriptan can be administered orally (100 mg) or subcutaneously (6 mg).[2009] Depending on the report, response rates for individual attacks vary from 51% to 84%, but all agree that the drug is more effective administered subcutaneously rather than orally. Even among responders, however, not all respond to every treatment course.

The drug usually acts within 1 hour; in fact, approximately 45% of patients are able to function normally 1 hour after a subcutaneous injection. A second dose can be given 1 hour later if complete relief of the headache has not been achieved, but most patients who do not improve significantly with a 6.0-mg subcutaneous dose will usually not benefit following a second 6.0-mg dose. The maximum recommended dose that may be given in a 24-hour period is two 6-mg injections separated by at least 1 hour. In addition to relieving head pain, sumatriptan also reduces the accompanying symptoms of nausea, vomiting, photophobia, and phonophobia. Despite its ability to relieve nausea and vomiting during migraine attacks, gastric emptying is delayed by sumatriptan. The efficacy of sumatriptan is unaffected by the concomitant use of common migraine prophylactic drugs.

The drug is well absorbed after both oral administration and subcutaneous injection.[436,681,998] Peak plasma levels are found approximately 15 minutes after subcutaneous injection and within 1 hour after oral administration. Circulating sumatriptan is cleared rapidly and predominantly by metabolism. The major metabolite is the indoleacetic acid analog, which is inactive at serotonergic receptors. It has a short half-life of approximately 2 hours.[680,2000] Small reductions of approximatey 20% in the oral absorption of sumatriptan during migraine attacks have been demonstrated,[681] presumably a reflection of gastric stasis. Food does not affect the absorption of oral sumatriptan.

Unfortunately, patients receiving sumatriptan have a high headache recurrence rate. About one third of patients will suffer a recurrence of their headache within 24 hours.[789] The median time to recurrence is about 10–14 hours. This is so whether the drug is administered orally or subcutaneously. The rate of recurrence of headache at 48 hours is higher following administration of sumatriptan than following administration of Cafergot.[2008] This phenomenon is presumably related to the long duration of many migraine attacks compared with the short plasma half-life of sumatriptan (2 hours). The recurrence of migraine symptoms responds well to a second dose of sumatriptan.

Adverse Effects

In general, the treatment of acute migraine with sumatriptan is well toler-

---

*References 294, 295, 430, 431, 646, 788, 1330, 2010

ated. Adverse reactions are usually mild and transient, consisting of paresthesias, dizziness, or light-headedness, drowsiness, sensations of warmth or heat, flushing, feelings of heaviness or pressure in the head or other body parts, weakness, and nausea or vomiting.[265] Some of these symptoms resemble those caused by the migrainous process itself. Following parenteral administration, adverse symptoms last for only a few minutes, but after oral administration the duration may be up to 1 hour. When they inject sumatriptan, most patients feel a mild pain or stinging or burning sensations lasting 30 seconds at the injection site. Transient elevations of blood pressure are seen in some individuals, but the elevations are generally small—approximately 10 mm Hg—and without clinically significant effect.

Approximately 5% of individuals report vague chest discomfort—mainly a feeling of tightness or pressure in the chest. Other patients report chest discomfort radiating into the shoulders, arms, neck, or throat and sometimes accompanied by dyspnea. These latter symptoms are short-lasting and appear to be dose-related. Although a very small percentage of patients experience minor electrocardiographic (ECG) changes such as prolongation of the PR interval, isolated ventricular extrasystoles, P-wave shifts, and T-wave changes, the same types of changes have been seen after administration of placebo. A very few patients have severe chest pain accompanied by widespread ECG changes (marked ST elevations) consistent with myocardial ischemia. In other words, the drug has the potential to cause coronary vasospasm and cardiac ischemia in patients with and without a history of coronary artery disease.[2156] Prudence would dictate that patients with a history of coronary artery disease or Prinzmetal's angina should not be treated with subcutaneous sumatriptan, or that at the very least they should use the drug under medical supervision for the first

two or three migraine attacks. The manufacturer recommends that patients in whom unrecognized coronary artery disease is possible (post-menopausal women, men over age 40 years, patients with risk factors such as hypertension, hypercholesterolemia, obesity, diabetes, history of smoking, or a strong family history of coronary artery disease) should have the first dose of sumatriptan administered in a physician's office. Rare reports have appeared indicating that sumatriptan may cause serious arrhythmias, including atrial fibrillation, ventricular fibrillation, and ventricular tachycardia.[418]

Sumatriptan—in contrast to ergots—has little or no effect on the resistance to blood flow in a number of major vascular trees.[643,1574] Nor does sumatriptan alter total peripheral resistance when administered to experimental animals in therapeutic doses.[643] The drug has been shown to have minimal effects on peripheral arteries in humans. In other words, sumatriptan's peripheral vasoconstrictive effects are negligible.

Concomitant use of migraine prophylactic preparations has not been shown to have any effect on either the efficacy or untoward effects of sumatriptan.

Contraindications to the Use of Sumatriptan

Parenteral sumatriptan is not to be used in patients with hemiplegic or basilar migraine. It can give rise to elevations of blood pressure and so should not be given to patients with uncontrolled hypertension. Sumatriptan should probably not be administered concomitantly with ergotamine-containing medications because of the theoretical possibility of additive vasoconstrictive effects. As indicated above, subcutaneous sumatriptan should not be prescribed for patients with the potential for coronary artery disease or with Prinzmetal's angina because of the possibility of coronary vasospasm.

The safety of sumatriptan has yet to be established in children.

CORTICOSTEROIDS

Few objective data are available regarding the use of corticosteroids in acute migraine. Theoretically, oral steroids should not act quickly, requiring at least 12–24 hours to terminate an attack. Despite this, some recommend short courses of corticosteroids such as prednisone or dexamethasone for the symptomatic treatment of migraine.[721,1795] Corticosteroids, however, can lead to osteonecrosis even if they are used for short periods of time, or intermittently such as for 3–4 days per month. In view of the seriousness of osteonecrosis, steroids should probably not be used for the usual migraine attack.

OTHER MEDICATIONS

A number of other medications have been tried in an attempt to abort or symptomatically treat acute migraine attacks. A few uncontrolled studies have yielded conflicting data regarding the efficacy of propranolol for this purpose.[632,2023] One controlled trial indicated that propranolol had no significant effect in aborting acute attacks of migraine when compared to placebo.[111] The literature is equally confusing with regard to both intravenous and sublingual administration of calcium channel blockers. Both satisfactory and negative results have been reported.*

EMERGENCY ROOM TREATMENT

Migraineurs come to emergency rooms when a particular headache is intense or prolonged, and either the

headache does not respond to the usual self-administered medications or the patient has used up all of his or her prescription medications. Many of these patients have simply been struck by an unusually severe headache. Others, however, have been suffering from the headache for weeks or even months. Individuals in this latter group characteristically find that their headaches have been increasing in severity for a substantial period of time, and they have had progressively poorer responses to their regular medication. Frequently they are suffering from drug-induced headaches as a result of rebound cycles involving narcotics, ergotamine, or barbiturates (see chapter 12). They are commonly emotionally exhausted ("last-straw syndrome").[571] A few patients with migraine come to the emergency room because of physical or emotional dependence on narcotics.

One must consider differential diagnoses of meningitis, encephalitis, subarachnoid hemorrhage, or a brain tumor if a patient thought to be having an acute migraine attack has significant fever, rigidity of the neck or signs of meningeal irritation (Kernig's and Brudzinki's signs), substantial alteration of consciousness or cognition, oculomotor pareses, papilledema or fundal hemorrhages, or a cranial bruit. The physician in the emergency room must be especially concerned if the headache is described as the "worst" headache the patient has ever endured. Appropriate diagnostic tests such as a computerized tomography or magnetic resonance imaging scan or a lumbar puncture must be rapidly obtained under these circumstances.

All patients who seek help at emergency rooms are desperate for immediate relief of pain, nausea, and vomiting. Traditionally, parenteral administration of narcotic analgesics combined with antinausea medication has been *the* emergency room treatment for severe migraine attacks. In fact, patients often insist on an injection of a narcotic and an antiemetic. This regimen does indeed provide relief to some patients,

---

*References 234, 962, 1033, 1403, 1581, 1914, 2042

enabling them to fall asleep and awaken much improved. Many clinicians, however, have significant reservations about the use of parenteral opiates. Significant potential for iatrogenic drug addiction exists, and because many emergency room physicians see increasing numbers of narcotic-seeking patients, genuine migraineurs with substantial headaches may receive inadequate doses of medication if they go to an emergency room where the staff is apprehensive about gratifying drug-seeking behavior.

Narcotic injections are of little benefit and may produce only ephemeral relief for a significant number of patients. In fact, they may be effective in less than one third of patients.[721] Their headaches either continue or recur in spite of the treatment. On occasion, this failure can be attributed to administration of an insufficient dose of a narcotic or to its administration in a bustling, noisy, brightly illuminated room. All too often, emergency rooms are too frenetically busy to provide appropriate—and necessary—ancillary anemities such as rest in a quiet, darkened room. But at other times, even a substantial dose of a narcotic injected in an appropriate setting will do no more than sedate the patient for an hour or two; the headache then returns unabated. As a consequence of these limitations, in the emergency room treatment of acute migraine narcotics should give way whenever possible to other modes of treatment (Table 10–6).

Ergotamine is frequently of no help in the emergency room treatment of migraine because once a patient has come to an emergency room, it is usually too late for ergotamine to be of much benefit. If used at this stage of a headache, instead of improving the patient's condition, ergotamine typically does nothing but increase nausea and vomiting. In contrast, intravenous DHE is exceedingly helpful in this type of situation, because it can lessen or eradicate migrainous head pain well into the headache, or even at its peak. It is more effective than narcotics such as meperidine (Demerol).[153] Based on clinical experience, DHE may compete well with sumatriptan in effectiveness, although a comparative study has yet to be done. Even so, sumatriptan may well change the emergency room treatment of acute migraine attacks. As indicated above, sumatriptan appears to be extremely effective in severe migraine attacks, even when given late in the attack.

Chlorpromazine (Thorazine) has become a frequently administered drug for acute bouts of migraine. A number of both controlled and uncontrolled studies attest to its efficacy.* The compound has even been reported to be more efficacious than DHE.[154] Chlorpromazine can be given intramuscularly in a dose of 1 mg/kg or intravenously in doses of 5–50 mg.[1014,1182] When administered intravenously, it should be injected slowly into the tubing of a normal saline infusion, or diluted in normal saline solution for administration as a drip. As many as 75% of patients report complete relief from intravenous chlorpromazine.[1182] Chlorpromazine can cause orthostatic hypotension; this is its major drawback in an emergency room setting. It is advisable to keep all patients who have received parenteral chlorpromazine supine for 2–4 hours, and to record their blood pressure at frequent intervals. Some patients may require intravenous fluids (250–500 mL) for postural hypotension. Prochlorperazine (10 mg intravenously) is also reported to act quickly to relieve migraine headaches.[1053] Prochlorperazine is less sedating than chlorpromazine, and easier to administer intravenously. Finally, it should be noted that the adverse effects of the phenothiazines include seizures and dystonic reactions.

Some authorities recommend the addition of parenteral corticosteroids such as dexamethasone (Decadron, 8–20 mg) to other medications in an emergency room setting.[721,1151,1168,1327] In a limited study, patients receiving dexa-

---

*References 154, 1014, 1182, 1183, 1351

Table 10–6 EMERGENCY ROOM TREATMENT OF MIGRAINE

Agent	Dosage
Dihydroergotamine (DHE 45)	0.5–1 mg IV (after metoclopramide [Reglan] 10 mg IV or IM or prochlorperazine 3.5–5 mg IV)
Sumatriptan (Imitrex)	6.0 mg SC
Chlorpromazine (Thorazine)	1.0 mg/kg IM; 5–50 mg IV
Prochlorperazine (Compazine)	10 mg IV
Meperidine (Demerol)	100 mg IM (with promethazine [Phenergan] 25 mg or hydroxyzine]Vistaril] 25–50 mg IM)
Dexamethasone (Decadron)	8–20 mg IM

IV = intravenous administration; IM = intramuscular administration; SC = subcutaneous administration.

methasone in combination with other treatments such as meperidine or DHE were reported to have a better outcome than patients who did not receive steroids.[721]

MECHANISMS OF ACTION OF MEDICATIONS USED FOR ACUTE MIGRAINE ATTACKS

Antimigraine drugs could work in a number of possible ways; in particular, they could have anti-inflammatory action, they could block the release of neuropeptides from trigeminovascular fibers, or they could cause vasoconstriction of intracranial vessels. As the following section will demonstrate, we know a lot about the mechanisms of action of some antimigraine drugs; others are not as well understood.

Aspirin, Aspirin-like Drugs, and NSAIDs

NSAIDs have a potent effect on pain induced by inflammatory conditions, but only a limited effect on pain provoked by an acute, high-intensity stimulus. The analgesic effects of NSAIDs are therefore thought to result primarily from their anti-inflammatory properties. The anti-inflammatory actions of NSAIDs are attributed to their inhibitory actions on the synthesis of prostanoids.[2062] By inhibiting the enzyme cyclooxygenase, NSAIDs reduce the conversion of arachidonic acid to the unstable endoperoxide intermediate PGG_2—and thus reduce the levels of prostaglandins, prostacyclin (PGI_2), and thromboxane A_2 (TXA_2). The hypothesis of action is that NSAIDs prevent the sensitization of peripheral nerve terminals by prostanoids. But NSAIDs differ in their relative potencies to reduce inflammation, and their abilities to reduce prostaglandin synthesis do not always correlate with their anti-inflammatory effects.

Individual anti-inflammatory agents inhibit cyclooxygenase by differing mechanisms. Some are competitive inhibitors. Others, such as acetaminophen, can block the action of the enzyme only in an environment that is low in peroxides, such as in the hypothalamus. Acetaminophen has little, if any, ability to inhibit the formation of prostanoids in peripheral tissues. It may have some anti-inflammatory actions, but the mechanism for its effect on pain is unknown.

The effectiveness of aspirin, aspirin-like drugs, and NSAIDs in the treatment of migraine has buttressed the idea that an inflammatory reaction in the cranial vasculature features prominently in causing migraine pain. And indeed, aspirin's ability to selectively block neurogenic inflammation in dural tissue has been demonstrated. Electrical stimulation of the trigeminal ganglion induces plasma extravasation in both intracranial (dura mater) and extracranial (eyelid, lip, conjunctiva) cephalic tissues.[293] The leakage in the dura, but not in extracranial tissues, is attenuated by aspirin.

In addition to their beneficial anti-inflammatory actions, it is speculated that NSAIDs are helpful, at least in part, because they disturb platelet function. NSAIDs do indeed prevent the formation by platelets of TXA_2, and as a result, they reduce the ability of platelets to aggregate. This phenomenon, however, is probably not of major importance in migraine treatment because much larger doses are needed to diminish head pain than to inhibit platelet aggregation.

Aspirin-like drugs and NSAIDs are also reported to exert actions on the central nervous system (CNS). For example, several investigators have noted that central pain signals in the thalamus can be inhibited by systemic administration of NSAIDs.[316,1069] In addition, modulation of inflammation via actions on the brain has been demonstrated.[332] The mechanism of these central actions is unclear.

Antiemetics

As reviewed in chapter 7, the chemoreceptor trigger zone located in the area postrema of the fourth ventricle is involved in production of nausea and vomiting. The area postrema is abundantly supplied with receptors for dopamine, histamine, and acetylcholine. This presumably accounts for the finding that dopaminergic, histaminergic, and muscarinic antagonists are antiemetic to varying degrees.[1572] To be more specific, the chemoreceptor trigger zone has a high density of dopamine receptors (D_2) receptors, histamine (H_1), and muscarinic cholinergic receptors.[1572] No single antiemetic drug binds to all three neurotransmitter receptors, but all bind to at least one of the three. In particular, a number of drugs with significant dopaminergic antagonist properties are beneficial in the treatment of nausea and vomiting.

Metoclopramide's antinausea effects have traditionally been thought to be the result of its blocking action at D_2-receptors in the chemoreceptor trigger zone.[318,683,1030] Its action on gastric emptying is imperfectly understood. Metoclopramide stimulates smooth muscle tone in the gastrointestinal tract.[448,1106,1677] Because the actions of metoclopramide are inhibited by anticholinergic drugs and potentiated by cholinergic agonists, the drug may work in part through a peripheral muscarinic action and an increased release of acetylcholine from cholinergic nerves. More recent investigations have demonstrated that enhancement of gastric emptying occurs following injection of metoclopramide into the hypothalamus of experimental animals.[387,388] If this observation is extrapolated to humans, it may be that metoclopramide acts not only peripherally, but also centrally to enhance gastrointestinal activity.

Ergots

For many years it was presumed that ergots alleviated migraine attacks through potent and selective constriction of painful, dilated, and stretched arterial vessels of the external carotid vasculature.[822] Evidence that ergotamine constricts branches of the external carotid artery dates back more than 50 years to the early plethysmographic experiments performed by Harold G. Wolff and his colleagues. These investigators not only reported that ergotamine reduced the amplitude of the pulsations of scalp arteries, but they also correlated the changes with a lessening of head pain. However, no correlation was possible in some of their subjects. Moreover, as discussed in chapter 7, branches of the external carotid artery are the principal site of migraine pain in only a minority of migraineurs. Extracranial arterial vasoconstriction is thus unlikely to be the basis for the therapeutic action of ergots in most patients with migraine headache.

Whether or not ergots cause significant intracranial vasoconstriction is still unclear. As noted above, ergots do not significantly alter cerebral blood flow (CBF) in healthy, non-migrainous volunteers.[42,855,2006] CBF measurements are largely a function of arteriolar diameter, whereas the vasoconstrictor action of ergots seems to be focused on large arteries. Moreover, the results of studies that used transcranial Doppler (TCD) techniques to measure blood flow velocity in large arteries have been conflicting. Ergots have been reported to increase velocity in healthy volunteers, but to cause no change in velocity in migraineurs both in interictal periods and during events.[521,2006] In addition, TCD does not detect changes in the diameter of the dural arteries—and these may be an important locus of migraine pain.

Ergotamine and DHE penetrate the blood–brain barrier poorly, but small amounts penetrate the brain and enter the cerebrospinal fluid.[21,561] Ergot alkaloids thus have the potential to affect the excitability of CNS neurons directly. Radiolabeled DHE, injected intravenously in cats, marks those nuclei in the brain stem and spinal cord—the nucleus caudalis and the dorsal horn—that are involved in the transmission of nociceptive information.[779] A high density of specific binding sites can be seen in the midbrain, with clear delineation of the raphe nuclei and the periaqueductal gray matter (PAG). Moreover, the population of cells in the nucleus caudalis that is excited by stimulation of pain-sensitive intracranial structures is inhibited by ergotamine and DHE administered in doses equivalent to those used to treat migraine attacks.[787,1164] DHE and ergotamine may affect the initial central synapses of trigeminovascular afferents and inhibit the transmission of nociceptive impulses in the trigeminal system.

The exact molecular site of action of ergot compounds is difficult to pinpoint because these substances have diverse and complex pharmacologic effects. Ergots are nonselective pharmacologic agents, interacting with a number of neurotransmitter receptors.[1348] At the very least, ergotamine and DHE are known to have high or moderate affinity binding at the following biogenic amine receptor sites: 5-HT_{1A}, 5-HT_{1C}, 5-HT_{1D} ("5-HT_1-like"), 5-HT_2, dopamine$_2$, and α_1-, α_2-, and β-adrenergic receptors.[264,474,1348,1570] Although the multiple sites of possible ergot activity confuse the picture, evidence suggests that the adverse peripheral vasoconstrictive effects of ergots result from stimulation of α_2-adrenergic receptors.[1685]

As just indicated, ergot alkaloids can bind to the subpopulation of serotonin receptors designated "5-HT_1-like" in the vasculature, and 5-HT_{1D} in nervous tissue.* Binding to this type of receptor is presumed to account for why ergots—in concentrations similar to those used to treat acute migraine headaches—block neurogenic inflammation of the dura. Experimental data have shown that ergot alkaloids reduce plasma extravasation produced either by electrical stimulation of the trigeminal ganglion or by administration of capsaicin, a compound that depolarizes unmyelinated nociceptive afferent nerves and causes the release of neuropeptides from nerve endings.[1304,1734] The data also suggest that inhibition of plasma extravasation occurs at a prejunctional site of action. Thus, ergots do not inhibit plasma extravasation induced by the administration of substance P or neurokinin A, the peptide neurotransmitters putatively released directly from trigeminovascular fibers. Activation of prejunctional 5-HT_{1D} receptors located on afferent nociceptive fiber terminals that control the release of endogenous peptide transmitters is believed to be the basis for the ability of ergots to reduce neurogenic inflammation.[290]

The anti-inflammatory property of ergots is not thought to result from their

---

*References 1000, 1570, 1781, 1972, 2082

vasoconstrictive actions, because other vasoconstrictor agents do not have anti-inflammatory properties. Thus, the therapeutic effects of ergots in patients with migraine headaches probably do not require changes in the caliber of blood vessels. On the other hand, by diminishing the pressure in edematous, pain-sensitive intracranial blood vessels, vasoconstriction might raise the threshold for activation of perivascular nociceptive afferents. Stimulation of "5-HT$_1$-like" receptors induces constriction in the cranial blood vessels in a number of species, including man.[373,1000,1528]

Sumatriptan

In contrast to ergots, which bind in differing degrees to a wide variety of receptors, sumatriptan is a remarkably selective pharmacologic agent. But like ergots, sumatriptan does possess high (nanomolar) affinity for those serotonin receptors designated "5-HT$_1$-like" in blood vessels, and 5-HT$_{1D}$ in nervous tissue; the compound also displays some affinity for 5-HT$_{1A}$ receptors.[1570,1781,2082] Sumatriptan is essentially inactive at all other serotonin receptor sites and has negligible affinity at various other neurotransmitter binding sites.[1570] Sumatriptan is presumed to derive its antimigraine efficacy from its ability to activate 5-HT$_{1D}$/"5-HT$_1$-like" receptors.

Even though the selectivity of its molecular sites of action is known, it is still unclear how sumatriptan works. Two major hypotheses have been offered to explain the antimigraine actions of sumatriptan.

1. *Sumatriptan acts on prejunctional neuronal receptors on trigeminovascular fibers.* Sumatriptan selectively reduces neurogenically mediated inflammatory responses in the dura mater. Sumatriptan reduces dural plasma extravasation produced by trigeminal nerve stimulation; the compound also diminishes the release of the trigeminovascular peptide neurotransmitter calcitonin-gene-related peptide produced by trigeminal ganglion stimulation.[290,292] These effects are similar to those produced by ergots, and as with ergots, are thought to result from activation of prejunctional 5-HT$_{1D}$ receptors on the peripheral ends of trigeminovascular fibers. A prejunctional action is postulated because sumatriptan does not block the dural plasma leakage produced by exogenous substance P or neurokinin A. These results cannot be accounted for by vasoconstriction alone.[292,1734]

2. *Sumatriptan acts at intracranial vascular receptor sites, causing intracranial vasoconstriction.* Sumatriptan is said to constrict intracranial vessels selectively, without affecting the blood flow to other organs. As evidence of this, when sumatriptan is administered to experimental animals, the carotid arterial resistance increases and the carotid artery blood flow decreases.[643,1000,1573] This increased carotid arterial resistance has been attributed to vasoconstriction that is limited to carotid arteriovenous anastomoses or shunts.[479,1573] The vasoconstrictor effect on arteriovenous anastomoses is assumed to redirect the blood flow to the capillary bed. Because of the limitation of sumatriptan's vasoconstrictor activity to arteriovenous shunts, the drug does not cause significant changes in blood flow to the brain and extracerebral capillary beds.[1574,1801] It is difficult to see how constriction of arteriovenous shunts in the carotid circulation can be responsible for sumatriptan's antimigraine actions unless one subscribes to Heyck's model of migraine, in which opening of arteriovenous anastomoses both in the brain and the extracerebral cranial structures is responsible for the symptoms of migraine (see chapter 8).[942]

Sumatriptan, when administered perivascularly to experimental animals in vivo, causes constriction of pial vessels.[373,1000,1529] But because of its low lipophilicity, sumatriptan does not readily cross the blood–brain barrier.[998,1001] As a result, pial arteries do not constrict if sumatriptan is administered parenterally.[374,999] Presumably sumatriptan cannot cross the intimal barrier of pial vessels to obtain access to the smooth muscle serotonin receptors. As a result, systemic administration of sumatriptan does not affect rCBF.

Only limited data are available concerning the actions of sumatriptan on human cranial vessels. Blood velocity in patients with migraine, measured by means of TCD, is increased in the internal carotid and middle cerebral arteries, an indication that sumatriptan causes constriction of large cranial arteries.[296,521,694] A possible relationship between the changes in blood velocity in large vessels and sumatriptan's antimigraine activity has been postulated, but the changes in blood velocity are short lived.[521]

Finally, a constrictive effect of sumatriptan can be observed in the perfused isolated meningeal circulation of human dura removed postmortem, and in biopsied human middle meningeal arteries.[1001,1027] It is possible that vasoconstriction of distended dural blood vessels is implicated in sumatriptan's antimigraine actions, but human in vivo studies are lacking.

Despite a great deal of scientific effort, no one has resolved whether the antimigraine actions of sumatriptan relate to its vascular (vasoconstrictive) effects or to its neuronal actions. The weight of evidence, however, would appear to favor a prejunctional action of sumatriptan on trigeminovascular nerve terminals.[1423]

Opiates

The effects of opioid analgesics (narcotics, opiates) are mediated by specific binding sites—or receptors—located on cell membranes. Such receptors can be found both on presynaptic terminals and cell bodies, and on dendrites of CNS neurons. Opiate binding studies have resulted in the identification of as many as five opioid receptors—μ, κ, δ, ϵ, and σ.[1133]

The clinical relevance of some of these receptor sites is, however, open to question. For example, the identity of what has been called the "ϵ receptor" is currently in question.[1133] σ Receptor agonists, it turns out, are also potent noncompetitive antagonists at certain excitatory amino acid receptors, and activation of σ receptors produces dysphoria, hallucinations, and stimulation of respiratory and vasomotor centers. These data suggest that σ receptors may not function as opioid receptors.

The most important opioid receptors from the clinical point of view appear to be the μ receptors. Activation of μ receptors produces analgesia that is mediated by effects mainly in supraspinal structures. This activation also appears responsible for many of the other clinical effects caused by opiates, such as euphoria, respiratory depression, constipation, pruritus, nausea and vomiting, and physical dependence. Although the mediation of analgesia at a spinal level seems to involve both δ and receptors, κ receptors are also believed responsible for miosis and sedation. Extensive cross-binding of drugs active at κ receptors has, however, hindered investigation of these sites. Different clinically used opiates activate different opioid receptors to different degrees. For example, morphine exerts much of its action at μ receptors with less effects at δ binding sites, but nalbuphine and pentazocine activate κ sites and have some action at σ receptors. Both electrophysiologic and behavioral studies have shown that the analgesic effect of opiates results from actions at both spinal and supraspinal sites.[553]

Systemically administered opiates act both within the dorsal horn and nucleus caudalis, where opioid receptors are concentrated in the more superficial layers.[361,2180] High levels of receptors are located in the substantia gelatinosa in the vicinity of the terminals of small primary afferent fibers. A significant proportion of these opioid receptors are located on the presynaptic terminals of unmyelinated primary afferent fibers.[651,725] These fibers secrete neuropeptides such as substance P as neurotransmitters. The presynaptic opioid receptors are inhibitory receptors. They prevent the release of neuropeptides, thereby blocking the transmission of information from peripheral nociceptors to second-order projection neurons located in the dorsal horn and in the nucleus caudalis.[1220,1221] Convincing data also support a direct action of opiates on second-order neurons.[2178]

Opiates also have supraspinal actions that activate the descending antinociceptive systems reviewed in chapter 7.[130,872,2177] These descending antinociceptive systems are activated by opioid receptors located mainly in the PAG, the locus coeruleus, and the raphe nuclei. Data now indicate that receptors in these supraspinal sites are activated by a much lower concentration of opiates than needed to activate spinal receptors. In therapeutic doses, opiates may act predominantly via descending antinociceptive systems.

Recently, systemically administered opiates have been found to have peripheral actions.[1935] These effects, which involve μ, κ, and δ receptors, are presumably exerted on the peripheral terminals of primary afferent fibers. The result is an inhibition of neurogenic inflammation in peripheral tissues.[1220,1221] It is not known yet whether or not such anti-inflammatory effects occur intracranially.

SUMMARY

Although countless treatments have been used in the past to manage acute migraine headaches, the clinician now has available a number of effective agents that can substantially lessen the severity and the duration of attacks, and in some cases even eradicate the symptoms. But it is also clear that no unanimity exists as to the best treatment for acute migraine attacks, that many of the medications require subtlety in their use, and that many drugs have the potential to cause unpleasant adverse effects. It is also obvious that some of the agents used for the treatment of acute migraine attacks have serious potential for abuse, and if used in an injudicious manner by the clinician, will only succeed in making patients much worse in the long run. When a suitable combination of medications is used carefully, legions of headache sufferers can be helped. All that is necessary is that the clinician remain vigilant to possible difficulties.

Chapter 11

PROPHYLACTIC MEDICATION

β-ADRENOCEPTOR BLOCKING
   AGENTS
CALCIUM CHANNEL BLOCKERS
ANTIDEPRESSANTS
METHYSERGIDE
NONSTEROIDAL ANTI-
   INFLAMMATORY DRUGS
CYPROHEPTADINE
PIZOTIFEN
LITHIUM
VALPROIC ACID
MISCELLANEOUS AGENTS
MECHANISMS OF ACTION OF
   PROPHYLACTIC MEDICATIONS

Many patients with severe or frequent attacks of migraine require daily prophylactic medication for control of their headache symptoms. Extensive clinical experience and a variety of controlled trials have established that prophylactic drugs can lessen the frequency and severity of migraine attacks. All preventive drugs have side effects, however, and they should be prescribed with circumspection. Moreover, finding the proper medication in its effective dose for a particular patient is not always an easy task.

Authorities disagree about guidelines for administering preventive medication. Some physicians prescribe prophylactic drugs for patients who have more than one headache each month. Others feel that daily medication is warranted only if the frequency is greater than one headache per week.* Simple

calendar accountings like this, I think, beg the question. Aspects of an individual's headache problem other than frequency must enter into the decision. For example, one would not hesitate to prescribe preventive medication for patients who have relatively infrequent attacks if the headaches were long-lasting or they were sufficiently incapacitating to disrupt the patient's life, causing recurrent absences from work and interfering with family responsibilities and pleasures. Prophylaxis for infrequent attacks would also be warranted if the bouts were not readily controlled by symptomatic or abortive medication, or if each episode was characteristically accompanied by frightening neurologic signs or symptoms.

Quite a few individuals, however, are reluctant to use daily medication. The concept of preventive medication may be foreign to some patients, particularly if they have been treated only with analgesic medication for many years. As a result, physicians must patiently explain the plan of therapy and the rationale for the use of prophylactic medication. Compliance with daily prophylaxis may be difficult unless the patient understands the purpose of the medication, comprehends the idea that a prophylactic agent usually does not work immediately, and accepts the possibility that the medications will have some side effects. Migraineurs with long-standing headaches have often seen many physicians in the quest for relief from suffering. If they are in a physician's office, that is *prima facie* evidence that they have not found successful treatment. (But it is also evi-

---

*References 208, 605, 1114, 1493, 1636, 1755, 1805

221

dence that they are still hoping to find help.) Their hope may carry considerable skepticism, however, for previous physicians may not have taken the necessary time or effort to enlighten them appropriately regarding drugs and side effects. As a consequence, these individuals may distrust all physicians and all medications. The absolute necessity of educating patients becomes even clearer when one adds in the fact that approximately half of all patients who go to a physician for whatever reason either will not take the prescribed drug at all, will not take it as prescribed, or will stop treatment as soon as they are feeling better.[618,830]

Patients who come for treatment not infrequently have had previous trials of a number of preventive medications without success. Many so-called "nonresponders," however, have never been given an adequate dosage of preventive medication or they have not had medication administered for a sufficient period of time. Before stating that a patient has not responded to a previously prescribed medication, attempts must be made to obtain all old records—including physician's and pharmacist's records—to assure that it was given in adequate doses and for an adequate trial period. In addition, many patients have been tried on medications at a time when they were taking daily analgesics, excessive amounts of ergots, or immoderate quantities of caffeine. Patients abusing drugs in this manner will not respond to prophylactic treatment until withdrawal of the other medication(s) has been accomplished.

Determination of how well a specific medication is working is important because only rarely do prophylactic agents completely eliminate headaches in a migraineur. Objective evaluation of the efficacy of preventive medication is sometimes very difficult, but it must be attempted. A headache diary is often very valuable in this regard, for several reasons:

1. The beneficial effects of most preventive agents increase with time. Accordingly, prophylactic agents often must be tried for substantial periods before the treating physician can be sure whether or not the medication is working.

2. The natural history of migraine may be exceedingly erratic. Patients with the disorder are prone to suffer from relapses and to enjoy remissions. The time course of these events may be exceptionally variable.

3. Drugs prescribed for migraine can have an impressive, and often intense, placebo effect.[389] Migraineurs are particularly prone to report therapeutic effects of a drug when the physician demonstrates personal interest in the efficacy of the agent. These effects may be very dramatic in first few weeks of therapy, although they often diminish with time.

A headache diary, conscientiously kept, can document the actual condition of the patient. This is especially useful when one drug is abandoned as unsuccessful and another is tried.

Several prophylactic agents have been shown to be superior to placebo in well-controlled clinical trials. No published policies, however, provide an absolute basis for deciding which is the most rational prophylactic agent for a particular patient. The treating physician must individualize therapy based on a number of factors. These include the presence of existing medical disorders (Table 11–1), potential interactions with medications prescribed for other purposes, potential side effects, high or low blood pressure, obesity, a documented history of depression or of difficulties with sleep, or untoward previous experiences with the medication under consideration. Some generalizations can be made. β-Blockers should be avoided in patients with bronchospastic conditions such as asthma and in individuals with depression. Methysergide should not be prescribed for patients with angina pectoris or peripheral vascular disease. Tricyclic antidepressants should not be administered to patients with epilepsy, obesity, or

Table 11–1 ANTIMIGRAINE DRUGS AND CONCOMITANT MEDICAL CONDITIONS

Medical Disorder	Contraindicated Antimigraine Drugs
Hypotension	β-Blockers, calcium channel blockers
Gastrointestinal disease	NSAIDs
Asthma	β-Blockers
Arteriosclerotic heart disease	Ergots, methysergide
Epilepsy	Tricyclics
Hypertension	MAO inhibitors
Depression	β-Blockers
Obesity	β-Blockers, tricyclic antidepressants, valproic acid, cyproheptadine, pizotifen

Adapted from Klapper[1114] with permission.

cardiac conduction difficulties. Monoamine oxidase (MAO) inhibitors should not be given to patients with hypertension. Nonsteroidal anti-inflammatory drugs (NSAIDs) should be restricted in patients with peptic ulcer (see Table 11–1).[1114] Migraineurs who are pregnant or who are trying to conceive should not be taking most anti-migraine drugs.

β-Blockers are generally considered the "first-line" prophylactic drugs by most authorities. This opinion is supported by extensive clinical experience. Calcium channel blockers are worthwhile options and should be tried in patients who have contraindications to the use of, or intolerable side effects from, β-blockers. Hypertensive individuals may respond well to either β-blockers or calcium channel blockers. Cyclic antidepressants are often of value in patients who have depressive features, who are clinically depressed, or who have sleep disturbances accompanying their migraine. They are most often beneficial in patients with chronic daily headaches. Methysergide, MAO inhibitors, and lithium are usually prescribed only for patients unresponsive to other therapies. These, and several other options, are discussed below.

If a given medication is ineffectual in preventing attacks of migraine, or if it is causing intolerable adverse effects, a different preventive agent should be tried. Sometimes a different member of the same class will work; other times,

another type of medication will have to be tried. Some patients with refractory headaches may only respond on the third or fourth attempt. Sometimes a combination of two medications is efficacious. For example, a synergistic effect between propranolol and amitriptyline has been described.[492,1323]

A number of medications effective in the prevention of migraine have not been approved for this purpose by the Food and Drug Administration (FDA). In general, the manufacturer has not performed the necessary investigations required for FDA approval. Any approved medication may, however, be used for an unapproved condition.[631]

β-ADRENOCEPTOR BLOCKING AGENTS

β-Blockers are the substances most widely prescribed for the prevention of recurrent bouts of migraine. Propranolol (Inderal), timolol (Blocadren), nadolol (Corgard), metoprolol (Lopressor), and atenolol (Tenormin) have all been reported to diminish the frequency of migraine attacks in patients with either common or classic migraine.* The effects of these agents on the duration and the intensity of bouts of migraine is

---

*References 47, 257, 508, 674, 675, 689, 1045, 1724, 1929, 1947, 1949, 1952, 2114, 2149

clear-cut, as will be discussed in the ensuing paragraphs.

Adrenoceptors

Researchers divide adrenergic receptors into two different types—α and β—based on the specificity of chemical agents capable of activating or blocking the respective receptors. By definition, all β-adrenoceptor blockers demonstrate an antagonistic action at β-adrenergic receptors. β-blockers may, however, be categorized into selective and nonselective types, depending on their relative abilities to antagonize the actions of norepinephrine and sympathomimetic amines at the two major classes of β-receptors—β_1 and β_2. At low concentrations, β_1-selective antagonists inhibit β_1-receptors, which are predominantly located in cardiac and adipose tissue, and have less action at β_2-receptors, which prevail in the bronchi and vascular smooth muscle. At high doses, selectivity may be lost and both β_1- and β_2-receptors may be blocked. Nonselective β-blockers antagonize both β_1- and β_2-adrenoceptors. Blockade of β_2-adrenoceptors is responsible for some of the adverse effects of β-antagonists, such as bronchospasm, hypoglycemia, and increased peripheral vascular insufficiency, but many of the side effects are related to β_1-adrenoceptor antagonism. These include bradycardia, postural dizziness, and cold extremities.

Propranolol, timolol, and nadolol are nonselective β-blockers; atenolol and metoprolol are β_1-selective agents. β_1-selective drugs are preferable for the treatment of patients who suffer from asthma and other respiratory problems, in patients who are liable to develop hypoglycemia, and perhaps in patients with peripheral vascular disease. Moreover, β_1-selective drugs do not reduce the physical tolerance of healthy individuals to the same degree as do the nonselective β-adrenoceptor antagonists.

Clinical Use of Propranolol

The optimal dose of propranolol must be determined for each individual patient (see Table 11–2). To achieve a therapeutic effect without undue delay, propranolol can be administered in an initial dose of 60–80 mg/day, preferably in a long-acting preparation (Inderal LA). If there are no side effects, or if the drug has not produced a substantial fall in blood pressure and pulse, the dose can be incrementally increased at a rate that depends on the patient's response. Some clinicians raise the dose every third or fourth day; others prefer to do it at weekly or biweekly intervals. Long-acting propranolol is best administered twice a day when higher doses are used. The latter regimen is more likely to prevent headaches that occur on awakening or that develop in the early morning. Some individuals with migraine do very well when they take doses of propranolol as low as 40 mg daily.[386,1530] But a number of clinical observations and experimental data indi-

Table 11–2 β-BLOCKERS USED FOR MIGRAINE PROPHYLAXIS

β-Blocker	Brand Name	Starting Dose	Maximum Dose
Propranolol	Inderal	60–80 mg/d	240–320 mg/d
Timolol	Blocadren	20 mg/d	60 mg/d
Nadolol	Corgard	40 mg/d	240 mg/d
Metoprolol	Lopressor	100 mg/d	250 mg/d
Atenolol	Tenormin	100 mg/d	200 mg/d

cate that the amount of improvement in most patients is proportional to dose.*

If efficacy is not seen at low or moderate dosages, doses as high as 240–320 mg/day should be administered—provided the individual can tolerate these dosages—before deciding that propranolol is an ineffective agent in a particular patient.[1443] Some authorities even suggest trying 480 mg/day.[1946] Many migraineurs are, however, sensitive to the cardiovascular effects of the drug and cannot tolerate high doses. A pulse of less than 50 bpm or a systolic blood pressure of less than 100 mm Hg indicates that a higher dose should not be used. Some patients have an unexpected sensitivity, and develop dramatic bradycardia and hypotension even when they are taking modest doses.

Although in a typical patient the plasma levels of propranolol usually vary directly with the dose, the plasma levels vary up to 20-fold when the same oral doses of the drug are given to a number of subjects.[1459,2132] Furthermore, the plasma levels of the drug do not correlate well with the clinical responses.[386,1077,1154,1787] This would suggest that the clinical response is contingent in large measure on an individual's sensitivity to propranolol, rather than to the dosage or the amount of β-blockade produced.

Improvement may be seen in some migraineurs immediately, but the number of patients responding to the medication increases with time.[1688] An effect of treatment is usually seen within 4 weeks, but a 3-month trial at maximum doses of propranolol should be given before considering that the patient is a nonresponder. Before treatment is instituted, patients must understand that relief may not come until a prolonged course of propranolol has been tried. Otherwise they may become too discouraged by a lack of immediate efficacy to continue taking the medication faithfully. On occasion, patients indi-

cate that their headaches have worsened after starting propranolol. In most instances, continued administration will ultimately produce a therapeutic effect. Some people for whom the drug has provided relief notice a loss of efficacy after a period of time. For them, an increase in the dosage usually remedies the situation. Once a therapeutic effect has been attained, high doses of propranolol may be reduced slowly in some patients for maintenance purposes.

If propranolol is effective, the drug can be administered indefinitely. For some migraineurs, however, a 6-month or longer period of treatment is sometimes sufficient to eliminate migraine for an extended period of time. One long-term investigation of patients who had taken propranolol for 8–16 months demonstrated that 46% of migraineurs maintained their improvement when a placebo was substituted for the drug.[507] But another investigation showed that the positive effect of successful prophylaxis lasted only an average of 6 months (range: 1 to 28 months) after discontinuation of treatment.[2164]

If for any reason propranolol is to be discontinued, the dosage should be tapered over a period of 10 days to 2 weeks. Abrupt termination may cause a "rebound" headache or may precipitate angina pectoris in patients with preexisting coronary artery disease. Severe consequences of rapid withdrawal are, however, infrequent in healthy individuals, as witnessed by the fact that many migraineurs suspend their use of propranolol precipitously without deleterious effects.[709]

Effectiveness of Propranolol

A number of appropriately controlled trials of propranolol indicate that propranolol is more efficacious than placebo.* But there is a substantial range in these reports. The results of a num-

---

*References 603, 1722, 1724, 1943, 1971

*References 237, 507, 508, 674, 965, 1283, 2114, 2149

ber of investigations indicate that between 55% and 93% of patients with common or classic migraine respond well.[1547] These figures may, however, be overly optimistic, and the frequency of response to propranolol may be much lower. In point of fact, a few studies have failed to demonstrate a significant difference between propranolol and a placebo.[965,1952] Most studies have commented that, although propranolol reduces the frequency of bouts of migraine, reductions in severity and duration of headaches by the drug are less common.[328]

A new type of statistical evaluation, meta-analysis, allows findings from multiple studies to be aggregated and subjected to statistical analysis as a whole. Meta-analysis has shown that when daily headache recordings are used to assess treatment outcomes, only a 44% reduction in migraine activity is produced by propranolol.[972,973] In comparison, placebo caused on average about a 14% decrement in migraine activity.

Investigations comparing the effectiveness of propranolol with other prophylactic agents such as other β-blockers, calcium channel blockers, NSAIDs, amitriptyline, and methysergide have not found an invariable benefit of one prophylactic medication over another.* It still remains for the physician and patient to work together to find the best agent in each case. Nevertheless propranolol will probably remain the agent first selected for prophylactic treatment of most migraineurs.

Use of Other β-Blockers

Timolol, metoprolol, and atenolol have all been shown to be superior to placebo in double-blind studies.† The same is probably also true for nadolol.[1724] Various studies have compared the

effects of two different β-blockers,[1488,1502,2007] and only one demonstrated an advantage of one over another. Nadolol, in a dose of 160 mg daily, was found to be better than the same daily dose of propranolol.[1971] Some β-blockers are not efficacious in the prevention of migraine attacks. These include pindolol (Visken) and acebutolol (Sectral).[603,1446,1867]

Pharmacokinetics

Hydrophilic β-blockers such as nadolol and atenolol are not as readily absorbed from the gastrointestinal tract as lipophilic β-blockers such as propranolol and metoprolol. The former agents are also not as extensively metabolized as the lipophilic drugs and therefore have comparatively long plasma half-lives.[409] Propranolol is rapidly metabolized in humans, with a plasma elimination half-life of 3–5 hours. Conventional propranolol tablets produce a high initial peak plasma level followed by a swift fall. This means that the drug has to be administered two to four times a day to achieve any stability of plasma levels. In contrast, long-acting propranolol preparations show prolonged absorption and lower peak levels. Long-acting propranolol produces sustained blood levels with much smaller variations over a 24-hour period than does a conventional form of the drug.[1207] The half-life after a dose of long-acting propranolol is between 10 and 20 hours—three to four times that of conventional propranolol. The long-acting form of propranolol is therefore favored because the necessity for multiple dosing is eliminated and patient compliance is enhanced.

Side Effects of β-Blockers

Although many patients complain of side effects, the β-blockers as a group have a considerable safety margin. In general, tolerance to adverse effects is acquired over a period of weeks. β-

---

*References 24, 146, 841, 1487, 1502, 1763, 1893, 1971, 2007
†References 47, 257, 675, 1045, 1076, 1949

Blockers do not have to be immediately discontinued if some side effects such as fatigue, cold extremities, or diarrhea appear. These effects usually decrease substantially with time.

Fatigue appears to be the most ubiquitous side effect following administration of all β-blockers and may occur even with low doses. It tends to diminish in the course of a few weeks. Many patients complain of not feeling well while taking β-blockers. This feeling may reflect sluggishness, decreased alertness, or fatigue.[1689] Gastrointestinal side effects include nausea, vomiting, diarrhea, and flatulence. Sexual dysfunction with impotence has been reported; so has alopecia.

β-Blockers are capable of causing a number of unwanted central nervous system (CNS) and behavioral effects. These include sedation, drowsiness, lethargy, sleep disorders, nightmares, and hallucinations. On rare occasions, delirious states and paranoid psychosis have been reported.[1128] Some patients complain of major memory problems. Depression, often of a serious nature, has been seen during administration of β-blockers.[92,1600] The depression may consist of both mood disturbances and neurovegetative symptoms. It may be unresponsive to therapeutic doses of tricyclic antidepressants and usually requires discontinuation of β-blockers.[1354]

Although the commonly used β-blockers do penetrate the CNS to some extent, attempts have been made to correlate the CNS side effects with the lipid solubility of various β-blockers. Lipophilic blockers such as propranolol, which readily cross the blood–brain barrier, have been postulated to cause more CNS side effects than hydrophilic β-adrenoceptor antagonists such as atenolol, which do not cross the blood–brain barrier with ease.[1128] The hypothesis has been difficult to prove, however; CNS disturbances with hydrophilic β-blockers has been reported.[535]

A few case reports have maintained that strokes occurred as a consequence of administering propranolol to patients with migraine.[115,763,1612] Some of the patients appear to have had other risk factors that have complicated analysis of the possible linkage between propranolol and the development of their strokes. If propranolol does predispose to the development of cerebrovascular symptoms, it must do so only very rarely.

Contraindications of the Use of β-Blockers

β-Blockers should not be administered to patients with inadequate cardiac reserve because such drugs could precipitate heart failure. They should also not be prescribed for individuals with significant atrioventricular (AV) conduction disturbances (greater than first-degree AV block) and should be administered with caution to migraineurs with slow sinus rates. The concomitant use of calcium channel blockers and β-blockers is contraindicated because of the increased propensity for both AV block and severe depression of ventricular function.

β-Blockers may cause peripheral vasoconstriction. Accordingly, they should be avoided by patients who suffer from significant occlusive problems in peripheral arteries. For similar reasons, ergotamine or methysergide should be used with extreme caution in patients on high doses of β-blockers, because of the increased potential for significant vasoconstriction.[201]

Because these drugs increase airway resistance, individuals with asthma, chronic obstructive pulmonary disease, or chronic bronchitis should probably not receive β-blockers. Although β_1-selective agents have been reported to have a lower incidence of untoward pulmonary effects than similar doses of nonselective drugs, β_1-selective agents are only comparatively selective and do have antagonistic actions at β_2-adrenoceptors, particularly at higher doses.[1616] Selective β_1-blockers may therefore induce bronchospasm in some sensitive patients with pulmonary problems.

Diabetics who take insulin or oral hypoglycemic agents may also experience difficulty with β-blockers because the clinical manifestations of hypoglycemia can be concealed by blockade of β-receptors. β-Blockers can, on rare occasions, even induce hypoglycemia.[1872] The use of propranolol and other β-blockers by migraineurs with mild diabetes mellitus who do not need insulin or oral hypoglycemic agents is usually safe.[2175] β-Blockers also mask many of the signs and symptoms of hyperthyroidism, and should not be prescribed for individuals with this condition.

CALCIUM CHANNEL BLOCKERS

Calcium channel blockers (calcium channel antagonists) are a chemically heterogeneous group of agents that act at calcium channels (Table 11–3). Calcium channel blockers of four different classes are used for the prevention of migraine headaches: (1) phenylalkylamines (verapamil), (2) dihydropyridines (nifedipine, nimodipine), (3) benzothiazepines (diltiazem), and (4) piperazine derivatives (flunarizine).

Some calcium channel blockers are extremely successful in inhibiting migraine attacks.* Most of the positive effects are related to headache frequency; less dramatic effects are reported with regard to headache severity and duration. But the number of participating

---

*References 35, 285, 337, 914, 915, 1033, 1058, 1364, 1377, 1568, 1634, 1887

patients in most controlled studies of the efficacy of calcium channel blockers has been low, many of the studies suffer from design deficiencies, and the dropout rate has been high. As a result, the published data showing that they are effective antimigraine drugs are much less convincing than data available for propranolol and other β-blockers. In addition, calcium channel blockers have a slow onset of action in many patients. The debut of a clinical response is frequently deferred for 2–8 weeks, which may cause difficulties with patient compliance. Calcium channel blocking agents with disparate chemical structures vary in their effects on cells. As a result, there are differences both in their clinical effects as antimigraine drugs and in their side effects. Despite these confusing details, for some patients a calcium channel blocker can be an effective preventive medication.

Side Effects

The side effects of various calcium channel blockers differ, but in general, their untoward effects are dose-dependent. Side effects are primarily produced by unwanted extensions of their calcium blocking effects on the smooth muscle of peripheral blood vessels and bowel, the CNS, and the heart. The most common side effects are due to extensive vasodilatation, which can lead to dizziness, hypotension, and flushing. Hypotension, usually modest and well tolerated, can also occur.

Table 11–3 CALCIUM CHANNEL BLOCKERS USED FOR MIGRAINE PROPHYLAXIS

Calcium Channel Blocker	Brand Name	Starting Dose	Maximal Dose
Verapamil	Calan, Isoptin	120–240 mg/d	480 mg/d
Nifedipine	Procardia, Adalat	30 mg/d	90 mg/d
Nimodipine	Nimotop	90 mg/d	180 mg/d
Diltiazem	Cardizem	120 mg/d	360 mg/d
Flunarazine	Sibelium	10 mg/d	10 mg/d

Contraindications

Calcium channel blockers exert a negative inotropic effect on cardiac muscle. This effect is rarely evident clinically in individuals with normal hearts, but these agents should not be used as antimigraine agents in patients with evidence of ventricular dysfunction. They are also contraindicated in patients with sinoatrial (SA) or AV nodal conduction disturbances because calcium is involved in the genesis of action potentials in the specialized conducting cells of the heart. AV block and bradycardia may result. These agents also reduce arterial blood pressure at rest by dilating peripheral arterioles and reducing the total peripheral resistance. They should not be administered to individuals with low systolic blood pressures (less than 90 mm Hg). Significant decreases in blood pressure and cardiac output may occur in patients who are also receiving β-blockers. In general, the two agents should not be administered concomitantly for migraine prophylaxis.

Verapamil

Both open and controlled studies and contemporary clinical experience indicate that verapamil (Calan, Isoptin) is a very effective antimigraine drug.* Unfortunately the controlled studies have been small and characterized by high dropout rates. Data from all types of sources indicate that, as for β-blockers, the primary improvement with verapamil treatment occurs with regard to migraine frequency. Little change in the intensity of head pain has been noted. In most investigations, the drug has been shown to work equally well in patients with common and classic migraine. Administration of higher doses of verapamil (320 mg/day) seems to be more effective than lower doses (240

mg/day).[1896] Many patients tolerate 480 mg a day without difficulty.

Side effects are seen in approximately 40% of patients, but they are usually either modest or impermanent.[1058] Verapamil is among the most constipating of the calcium channel blockers, with constipation being the most commonly reported untoward effect of the drug. Vascular changes such as edema of the hands and feet, flushing, and lightheadedness, and cardiac abnormalities such as bradycardia, hypotension, and AV conduction defects are less commonly seen. If slight hand tremor develops, the drug can be administered at night to minimize daytime symptoms.

Nifedipine

The results of a number of drug trials leave the status of nifedipine (Procardia, Adalat) as an antimigraine medication ambiguous at the present time. In open studies it has been reported to be effective in decreasing the frequency of migraine attacks in a majority of patients with both common and classic migraine.[1058,1071,1374] Other investigations have reported that it is of little utility in migraine prevention.[24,1344] Moreover, the high frequency of side effects indicates that other calcium channel blockers should be used first before resorting to nifedipine. In a controlled study, propranolol (180 mg/day) has been demonstrated to be superior to nifedipine (90 mg/day).[24]

Nifedipine has a higher incidence of side effects than other calcium channel blockers.[24,1344,1375] As many as 50%–70% of patients report untoward effects. This incidence of side effects among migraineurs appears to be higher than the incidence in patients receiving the drug for cardiac conditions. The most common adverse effect is postural hypotension with dizziness, but vascular complaints such as edema or flushing are also seen frequently. Other patients report gastrointestinal symptoms such as nausea and vomiting, mental changes including diffi-

*References 1058, 1302, 1374, 1617, 1896, 1899

culty in concentration, weight gain, non-migrainous headaches, and fatigue.

Nimodipine

Published trials present unclear data as to whether or not nimodipine (Nimotop) is effective in preventing migraine attacks. Open, uncontrolled studies have shown that nimodipine has antimigraine actions, but the results of controlled studies are conflicting; the agent has been shown to be both better than, and no different from, placebo.* The small sample sizes of these trials may account for the varying results. A large, multicenter, double-blind investigation in Europe concluded, however, that nimodipine has no, or at most a very slight, prophylactic effect in migraine. The statistical power of that study was reduced by a very high rate of placebo response.[1384,1385]

Nimodipine is very well tolerated by most patients. Small numbers of patients may develop side effects that include myalgia, muscle cramps, postural hypotension, gastrointestinal and vascular complaints, headache, fatigue, menstrual discomfort, and some behavioral alterations such as irritability.

Diltiazem

Pilot studies of the antimigraine actions of diltiazem (Cardizem) have demonstrated positive results.[1673,1880] These preliminary results are encouraging, but need to be corroborated in appropriately controlled investigations before the efficacy of the drug can be determined. Diltiazem is well tolerated, with unwanted symptoms reported by fewer than 3% of patients. The most common side effects are headache, nausea, edema, and rash.

Flunarazine

Flunarazine (Sibelium, available in Europe) is the most widely studied antimigraine calcium channel blocker. A number of controlled clinical trials have determined that flunarazine is efficacious in migraine prevention.† The percentages of patients who have shown improvement have ranged from 30% to 66% in different investigations The antimigraine effect is primarily expressed as a decreased number of attacks. Flunarazine is equally effective in both migraine with aura and migraine without aura. The onset of action is slow, but it increases progressively over a period of 3 months, Several studies have reported that flunarazine (10 mg/day) is equivalent to propranolol (120–160 mg/day), other β-blockers, and methysergide.[743,841,1282,1822,1930] In other words, flunarazine is one of the most impressive migraine prophylactic medications currently available.

Adverse reactions are usually mild. The most substantial side effects include daytime drowsiness and sedation, gastrointestinal symptoms, mild vertigo, anxiety, dry mouth, sleep disturbances, vivid dreams, muscle fatigability, and paresthesias. Weight gain is sometimes a prominent complaint. The most serious unwanted effects—depression, parkinsonism, and tardive dyskinesia—are fortunately rare.[356,1373]

ANTIDEPRESSANTS

Antidepressants form an important part of the therapy for many patients with migraine. Several types of antidepressants—the cyclic antidepressants, MAO inhibitors, and fluoxetine—have all been used for the treatment of migraine, but with varying degrees of success.

---

*References 55, 671, 749, 914, 1058, 1375, 1956

†References 690, 1272, 1364, 1887, 1910, 1911

Cyclic Antidepressants

There are two classes of cyclic antidepressants—the tricyclics and the heterocyclics. Both tricyclic and heterocyclic antidepressants have proved beneficial in the treatment of migraineurs who suffer from frequent attacks of common or classic migraine or from the chronic daily headache syndrome. These drugs are also of value in migraine sufferers who are depressed or who have sleep disturbances. They are much less useful in patients with infrequent attacks of migraine.

Considering the wide use of cyclic antidepressants as antimigraine drugs, it is surprising that only amitriptyline (Elavil, Endep) and doxepin (Sinequan, Adapin) have been subjected to the scrutiny of controlled studies.[392,802,1416] Such trials have shown that amitriptyline decreases the frequency, duration, and severity of migraine attacks, and that doxepin is efficacious in the therapy of what some call mixed tension–vascular headaches. Amitriptyline is reported to be as effective a prophylactic agent as propranolol, but the incidence of side effects is higher.[2204] Moreover, as noted above, propranolol and amitriptyline appear to act synergistically when administered concomitantly.[492,1323] A number of other cyclic antidepressants have been found in clinical practice to be clearly efficacious as antimigraine drugs. Indeed, some antidepressants have distinct advantages compared to amitriptyline and doxepin. Such data, however, are anecdotal because the drugs have unfortunately never been subjected to controlled studies (Table 11–4).

Which antidepressant to try first depends on how well the pharmacologic characteristics of a particular agent correspond to the individual patient's clinical problems. For example, a migraineur who is afflicted with insomnia (as well as headaches) will frequently receive benefit from a tricyclic agent with sedative properties, such as amitriptyline or doxepin. Agents with significant sedative action may also be useful in the treatment of depressed migraineurs whose depression is associated with anxiety. In contrast, desipramine (Norpramin, Pertofrane), nortriptyline (Pamelor, Aventyl), and protriptyline (Vivactil) are less sedating or nonsedating, and may be administered to patients without sleep problems or to patients who complain of persistent fatigue. The low incidence of anticholinergic and cardiovascular effects during treatment with trazodone (Desyrel) makes this agent particularly useful in elderly patients, patients with cardiovascular disease, and patients intolerant to other antidepressants.

Table 11–4 CYCLIC ANTIDEPRESSANTS: PHARMACOLOGIC FEATURES

Antidepressant	Brand Name	Anticholinergic	Sedation	Orthostatic Hypotension	Dose Range
Amitriptyline	Elavil, Endep	+ + + +	+ + +	+ +	50–150 mg/d
Doxepin	Sinequan, Adapin	+ +	+ + +	+ +	50–150 mg/d
Imipramine	Tofranil	+ +	+ +	+ +	50–150 mg/d
Nortriptyline	Pamelor, Aventyl	+ +	+ +	+	50–100 mg/d
Desipramine	Norpramin, Pertofrane	+	+	+	50–150 mg/d
Protriptyline	Vivactil	+ + +	+	+	15–40 mg/d
Maprotiline	Ludiomil	+	+ +	+	75–150 mg/d
Trazodone	Desyrel	+	+ +	+	50–300 mg/d

+ = slight; + + = moderate; + + + = high; + + + + = very high.

Because the effects of most cyclic antidepressants are prolonged and cumulative, a single daily dose is effective in most cases. Administration at bedtime is convenient and will minimize sedation and anticholinergic side effects during the daytime. Protriptyline and desipramine may, however, have mild-to-moderate stimulant effects in some patients, and are therefore not generally prescribed as a single bedtime dose. They may be given either in the morning or in divided daytime doses.

How individual patients respond to tricyclic and heterocyclic antidepressants varies widely. Some migraineurs, for example, cannot abide as little as 10 mg of amitriptyline given as a nocturnal dose, because of intolerable drowsiness, sedation, and fatigue in the morning; other patients perceive only modest adverse effects when 150–200 mg a day are administered. To minimize side effects, starting doses should be low. Slow augmentation of the dose, by small weekly or biweekly increments, may also help to lessen the intensity of the side effects.

Generally, the plasma concentration of some tricyclic compounds—imipramine, desipramine, and nortriptyline—is correlated with antidepressant efficacy. But a large interpatient variability of plasma levels for a given dose of an antidepressant has been well documented.[2207] This variation is mainly determined by genetic factors, and is the result of disparate rates of drug metabolism by the liver in different people. No data are available concerning the relationship between plasma levels and therapeutic efficacy in migraine patients. Monitoring of plasma levels may be useful in some treatment-resistant patients, but, in general, changes in signs and symptoms should be relied on to regulate dosage.

Most migraine sufferers who are going to improve on antidepressants derive some benefit within a week or 10 days.[392,395] Maximum effects, however, may not develop until 4–8 weeks have elapsed at the dose appropriate for each patient.

Side Effects of Cyclic Antidepressants

Almost all individuals treated with tricyclic and heterocyclic antidepressants experience some type of side effect. Side effects are customarily mild in the doses used for antimigraine therapy but can be severe enough to warrant discontinuation of treatment in some patients. Untoward effects occur more often when cyclic antidepressants are administered with other medications or when the individual has coexisting medical disorders. These compounds should be used with caution in elderly patients because these patients develop a much higher incidence of side effects than do younger individuals. The unwanted effects of cyclic antidepressants are usually most pronounced at the beginning of therapy and discourage many patients from continuing with treatment. Patients should be reassured that some side effects will decrease over time.

Common adverse responses to cyclic antidepressants result from actions on the CNS. Some patients become excessively sedated, particularly if they are taking amitriptyline, doxepin, or trazodone. Administration of a single dose at bedtime usually allows the major sedative effects to occur during sleep. Because tolerance to the sedative properties of the cyclic antidepressants frequently evolves, these drugs can usually be administered so as to circumvent excessive sedation. Treatment is initiated with a low dose at night. As soon as the morning "hangover" sedation has lessened and is tolerable, the dose is increased a bit. The procedure is repeated until that person's therapeutic dose has been reached.

In contrast, some patients become anxious and agitated when given cyclic antidepressants. Visual and auditory hallucinations as well as delirium have been reported. Hallucinations are usually of the hypnagogic variety. They may be alleviated by dividing the daily dose rather than administering the dose entirely at bedtime. A fine, high-frequency tremor of the upper extremities sometimes accompanies therapy, occurring in about 10% of patients who receive these medications. It is usually a postural tremor, more easily observed when the arms are outstretched. The incidence of tremor is much higher in elderly patients, especially when large doses are prescribed. Myoclonus, either when conscious or asleep, is also an occasional side effect of tricyclic antidepressants. Rare patients develop signs of cerebellar dysfunction with ataxia, dysarthria, and nystagmus.

All cyclic antidepressants appear to lower the seizure threshold. Seizures are most often observed in patients treated with high doses of cyclic antidepressants for long periods of time or in patients who have had their dosage rapidly increased. Infrequently, patients will experience their first seizure while taking these drugs. In patients with preexisting epilepsy, doses should be kept low and increments in dosage made slowly. Maprotiline has a higher risk for producing seizures than other cyclic agents.

All cyclic agents, particularly amitriptyline, have substantial anticholinergic (atropine-like) effects. These include dry mouth, constipation, ileus, delayed micturition, and urinary retention. Anticholinergic effects may interfere with memory. If intolerable, the dose may have to be reduced or the drug replaced with another that has a lower incidence of anticholinergic side effects. Another common complaint is blurred vision caused by a failure of accommodation. The difficulty with accommodation results from relaxation of the ciliary muscle. Vision for distant objects is usually not disturbed. Tolerance sometimes develops after a few weeks of treatment. As a paradox, excessive sweating is a rather common complaint.

The anticholinergic actions of cyclic antidepressants promote pupillary dilatation, which can potentially precipitate glaucoma. But clinically this is a rare occurrence. The threat is probably highest in elderly patients with narrow-angle glaucoma. Tricyclic and heterocyclic antidepressants can be used in individuals with open-angle glaucoma, provided that they continue to take pilocarpine or other eyedrops.

In healthy adults, cyclic antidepressants are usually free of substantial untoward cardiovascular effects except for postural hypotension. These agents should, however, be used with extreme caution in patients with cardiovascular problems. One of the most common adverse effects is tachycardia. Tricyclic and heterocyclic antidepressants produce this by blocking cholinergic vagal inhibition of the SA node. The tachycardia may be extreme, but in most patients so affected, the rate increases by only 10–15 bpm.[277,767] Because of its substantial anticholinergic actions, amitriptyline is the antidepressant most likely to cause tachycardia.[330]

Significant cardiac conduction abnormalities are not common complications of therapy with tricyclic and heterocyclic antidepressants, although they can slow both atrial and ventricular depolarization in some patients.[1710] These compounds exert their major action on intraventricular conduction. The electrocardiographic (ECG) indications of this consist of an increase in PR and QRS intervals and a decrease in T-wave amplitude.[767] Cyclic antidepressants can also produce nodal and bundle branch blocks. Some antidepressants increase the risk of arrhythmias in patients with preexisting conduction abnormalities or heart block.[758] A baseline ECG will distinguish those patients with cardiac conduction disease in whom further slowing of conduction would be undesirable. A pretreatment ECG should be obtained in any patient older than age 50 or in any patient suspected of having cardiac disease.

Orthostatic (postural) hypotension is a common adverse reaction of cyclic antidepressant therapy. It may be severe enough to require discontinuation of therapy. Orthostatic hypotension is thought to occur because cyclic antidepressants are able to block α-adrenoreceptor sites on arteries. It may cause patients to become dizzy or light-headed, or to have syncopal episodes when they rise from a recumbent position. Nortriptyline has much less potential than other tricyclic antidepressants to cause orthostatic hypotension. Amitriptyline—and particularly imipramine—tends to cause more severe hypotensive actions than other agents. The problem is greater in older patients and in patients who are taking other drugs, such as β-blockers and calcium channel blockers, capable of causing hypotension. The objective fall in blood pressure produced by tricyclic antidepressants will not usually diminish, but the related, subjective complaints of dizziness or light-headedness frequently decrease during the first few months of treatment.[768]

Increased appetite, craving for sweets, and concomitant weight gain develop frequently enough that patients should be warned of this problem before starting treatment. In some patients weight gain may be substantial, reaching levels of 3–5 pounds per month.[908,1804] Ironically, concern over weight gain may cause enough stress to aggravate the headaches the cyclic antidepressants were meant to treat. Weight gain is often a cause for discontinuation of treatment.

Cyclic antidepressants may disrupt sexual desire and function. Decreased libido, delay of orgasm, and orgasmic impotence have been described in both men and women. Men may have difficulty achieving or maintaining penile erection. Endocrine problems such as amenorrhea and galactorrhea have been described in women. Trazodone, unlike any of the other antidepressants, can cause priapism and permanent impotence.[1186] Priapism requires emergency urological treatment.

Allergic reactions, blood dyscrasias, and jaundice are infrequent side effects. Although somewhat elevated levels of alkaline phosphatase and transaminases are common, antidepressant therapy does not have to be discontinued unless symptoms or signs of hepatic dysfunction appear.

Amoxapine (Asendin) has activity at dopamine receptors. This means that it can cause a full range of extrapyramidal side effects. These include acute dystonic reactions, akathisia, parkinsonian signs and symptoms, and tardive dyskinesia, as well as neuroendocrine actions such as hyperprolactinemia, galactorrhea, and amenorrhea. Even though amoxapine has had excellent prophylactic effects in some patients, its potential to do permanent harm should give pause to anyone considering its use.

Contraindications to the Use of Cyclic Antidepressants

Cyclic antidepressants are best avoided in patients with defects in bundle-branch conduction, second-degree heart block, or when other cardiac depressants are being administered to treat heart disease. The presence of cardiac arrhythmias does not constitute an absolute contraindication. Most clinicians, however, will not prescribe these agents in patients predisposed to arrhythmias, despite findings that the antiarrhythmic effects of some of the agents may be desirable in some cardiac patients. Trazodone does not appear to slow cardiac conduction. Uncontrolled seizures and severe prostatism are additional contraindications to the use of tricyclic and heterocyclic antidepressants. Caution is needed when heterocyclic antidepressants are used in patients with severely impaired hepatic function or renal failure.

Monoamine Oxidase Inhibitors

Investigation of the use of MAO inhibitors in the prophylaxis of migraine has been limited and largely uncontrolled.[65,221,1109] Nonetheless, many clinicians depend on MAO inhibitors for the treatment of individuals refractory to other measures and agents. In particular, MAO inhibitors are helpful in patients with chronic daily headaches who have features of both migraine and tension-type headaches. Their usefulness is limited by the frequency of side effects, the necessity to remain on a tyramine-free diet, and the potentially serious interactions with other medications.

Phenelzine (Nardil) is the MAO inhibitor most frequently used for the treatment of migraine. The drug should only be prescribed for patients who can be trusted to restrict their diet and to refrain from taking other agents that have the potential to interact with phenelzine. Close and regular oversight of the patient is essential. The usual dose of phenelzine is 15 mg three or four times a day. It is best to begin with 15 mg/day for several days, and then to increase the dose gradually until either a therapeutic effect or a dosage of 60 mg is attained. In some patients, the dosage may then be slowly decreased to a lower maintenance level.

The combined use of tricyclic antidepressants and MAO inhibitors has customarily been contraindicated because of the supposed potential for dangerous adverse reactions. Physicians have long been warned to wait 2 weeks or more between ceasing treatment with tricyclic antidepressants and initiating MAO inhibitors. Combined therapy has been safe, however, when both agents were used in conservative dosages and when patients have been carefully supervised. Such combination is thought to be effective in some patients whose migraine is refractory to treatment, but the usefulness of this treatment has not been reported. If the drugs are given properly, the occurrence of adverse effects is unlikely.[1793,1813,2141] The tricyclic antidepressant should be started first in low dosages, with the MAO inhibitor added a few days later.[37] The dosage of both drugs can be increased slowly over a period of time. An MAO inhibitor can be administered to a patient taking tricyclic antidepressants, but the reverse should probably not be done.

MAO inhibitors produce a wide range of distinctive adverse reactions. These include drowsiness, headaches, changes in behavior, tremor, muscle twitching, convulsions, weakness, fatigue, constipation and other anticholinergic effects, and weight gain. Insomnia is often a major problem, but can often be controlled by taking all of the medication before 3:00 P.M. Approximately 10% of men develop sexual dysfunction, either impotence or inability to ejaculate. Women may lose sexual desire or the ability to reach orgasm.

The most prominent cardiovascular effect of MAO inhibitors is orthostatic hypotension. This may or may not be associated with modest elevations of basal diastolic and systolic pressures. The orthostatic hypotension is rarely severe enough to require discontinuation of therapy. In contrast, dramatic and often life-threatening hypertensive crises can develop in patients taking MAO inhibitors. Hypertensive crises may develop spontaneously or as a result of the ingestion of vasoactive amines or administration of sympathomimetic substances.

Because of the potential for stroke or death from hypertensive crises, patients using MAO inhibitors must follow a restricted diet very carefully to avoid ingesting exogenous vasoactive amines. MAO inhibition in the intestines, blood vessels, and liver allows vasoactive amines to gain unrestricted entry to the systemic circulation. These substances can then cause the excessive release of norepinephrine and other catecholamines both from sympathetic nerve endings and from the adrenal medulla. This excessive release can produce a substantial hypertensive reaction with palpitations, vomiting, sweating, chest pain, stiff or sore neck, and throbbing headache. Hypertensive crises are the most hazardous toxic effect of MAO inhibitors, and in some patients have resulted in intracranial bleeding. In the most severe cases, death has ensued.

Patients must eliminate foods that contain p-tyramine, which occurs naturally in some foods and develops in others as the products ripen, ferment, or even warm to room temperature (see chapter 2 for a more complete discussion). Matured and ripened cheeses, unrefrigerated or fermented meats and fish, sauerkraut, raspberries, avocados, some brands of beers and ales, Chiantis, and meat and yeast extracts are common foods in which p-tyramine occurs naturally. Other amines are also potentially dangerous: L-dopa in fava beans; serotonin, dopamine, and norepinephrine in bananas; β-phenylethylamine in chocolate; and methylxanthines in coffee and tea. These foods should be excluded from the patient's diet. Patients should be provided with a wallet-size card containing the list of foods to be avoided. Such a card can easily be consulted before eating.

Patients taking MAO inhibitors must be warned about possible drug interactions. They must not use proprietary medications that contain sympathomimetics (phenylephrine, pseudoephedrine, phenylpropanolamine), such as nasal decongestants and cold, sinus, allergy, asthma, or diet medications.[903] Their dentists should be aware of the dangers of injecting sympathomimetic vasoconstrictors in conjunction with local anesthesia. Stimulants such as amphetamines and related drugs are contraindicated. So is cocaine, a substance the patient may avoid discussing. It is incumbent that the physician tactfully, but pointedly, tell patients of the danger of even one-time use.

A serious and potentially life-threatening reaction can occur after concomitant administration of the narcotic meperidine. The reaction is characterized by restlessness, agitation, seizures, coma, profound hyperthermia, and hypotension or hypertension. Other narcotics should also be administered with extreme caution. The antitussive dextromethorphan, contained in many over-the-counter cold and cough remedies, may also cause such a reaction. In addition, MAO inhibitors noticeably potentiate the nervous-system symptoms of alcohol and anesthetics. Patients should carry a card in their wallets so that the anesthesiologist will be forewarned in the event emergency surgery is needed. The medication should be withdrawn several weeks before elective surgery. Fluoxetine is another compound that should not be administered to patients taking MAO inhibitors. In addition, simultaneous administration of MAO inhibitors and either β-blockers or calcium channel blockers must be performed with caution because severe orthostatic hypotension—which is sometimes a side effect of MAO inhibitor therapy—can become apparent when these drugs are combined.

Because of the potential for serious hypertensive crises, MAO inhibitors should not be used in patients with hypertension, or cardiovascular or cerebrovascular disease. They are also contraindicated in patients with liver disease, advanced renal disease, asthma, and chronic bronchitis.

Fluoxetine

Fluoxetine (Prozac) has been reported in one open and in one controlled study to produce improvement in migraine patients.[11,189] Patients should be started on 20 mg/day or every other day, taken in the morning. Some patients may require a higher dosage. It can be increased to 40 mg after 3–6 weeks. The maximum dosage of fluoxetine is 80 mg/day. A month of treatment may be necessary for the appearance of optimal effects.

Fluoxetine is well tolerated by many patients. In contrast to cyclic antidepressants, fluoxetine has few anticholinergic effects and produces little orthostatic hypotension or drowsiness. In fact, some patients feel more energetic, which provides the rationale for morning administration. The agent may, however, cause restlessness, anxiety, agitation, insomnia, heartburn, diarrhea, headache, and nausea. Fluoxetine should be taken after food to minimize the nausea. It may produce a decreased appetite with weight loss.

Some patients have complained of impotence and a decreased libido. Patients, having heard the controversy surrounding Prozac's psychological side effects and potential for causing behavioral changes (including suicide), may be unwilling to try the drug unless these matters are openly discussed.

METHYSERGIDE

Methysergide (Sansert) is a very effective agent for the prevention of migraine attacks, having been approved by the FDA for this purpose. It also has potential for serious side effects, and this has led to its unwarranted avoidance by many physicians. This is unfortunate because some patients respond to methysergide but not to any other prophylactic medications. The most serious complication—retroperitoneal fibrosis—is an exceedingly rare result of methysergide therapy today; the drug should therefore be used more frequently than it is.

Methysergide is exceptionally valuable for patients with intense, recurrent bouts of migraine that have not responded to "first-string" medications such as propranolol, calcium channel blockers, and cyclic antidepressants. The agent appears particularly useful for prophylaxis when attacks are frequent.[417] A number of open studies have shown that, when used properly, more than 60% of migraineurs have positive responses to methysergide.[416,417,815,1941] It is said to suppress migraine completely in more than 25% of patients.[417]

Patients should be started on methysergide gradually—one tablet a day at first, with the addition of one tablet every 3 or 4 days until a total has been reached of one tablet three or four times a day. Gradual buildup of dosage limits the appearance of some side effects, particularly those related to the gastrointestinal tract. Once benefit has been attained, some patients can reduce the daily dose to less than three or four tablets. Methysergide must be administered in divided doses because it has a relatively short half-life of only about 2 hours. Methysergide frequently causes nausea and indigestion; for this reason, it should be taken with meals and with some food if taken at bedtime. The efficacy of methysergide usually becomes apparent within 2 or 3 days, but, on occasion, beneficial effects are not seen before 3 or 4 weeks have elapsed.

Side Effects

As indicated above, numerous side effects limit the usefulness of methysergide. Most patients develop them on the first or second day of therapy. Most side effects are minor in terms of danger to the patient. Adverse gastrointestinal effects such as nausea, vomiting, abdominal pain, diarrhea, and constipation are frequent. The drug can affect the CNS, causing drowsiness, vertigo, giddiness, ataxia, insomnia, vivid dreams, anxiety, poor concentration and difficulty thinking, confusion, a sense of unreality, feelings of depersonalization, and depression. It is not uncommon for the first dose of methysergide to bring on frightening hallucinatory experiences comparable to those that develop during recreational use of lysergic acid diethylamide (LSD). Cardiovascular side effects with vasoconstrictor actions may occur. These can induce pain, pallor, coldness, numbness, and paresthesias of the extremities. Rarely, the vasoconstriction can cause arterial insufficiency of the lower extremities, with claudication of the legs and constriction of the coronary arteries with angina-like pain.[71,932,1096,1938] Peripheral pulses may be diminished or absent. Musculoskeletal symptoms such as muscle cramps, myalgia, arthralgia, and joint stiffness may appear. A number of miscellaneous side effects also can develop, including hair loss, weight gain, pedal edema, nasal congestion, flushing, and sweating. Approximately 40% of migraineurs taking methysergide have at least one minor side effect, such as abdominal discomfort or muscle cramps. But many minor adverse reactions are usually temporary and may abate with maintained use of the agent.

Fibrotic Disorders

Long-term uninterrupted usage of methysergide can provoke the development of extra connective tissue in the retroperitoneal space, the lungs, and the endocardium.* Infrequent instances of constrictive pericarditis, constriction of the great vessels, and rectosigmoid strictures have also been reported.[746,1507,1652]

The overall incidence of fibrotic complications has been estimated to be as low as 1 in 5000 patients.[816,941] Many of the patients who developed fibrosis when the drug was first used in the 1960s took more than the recommended maximal dose of 8 mg daily, and did so for many months to years. Today, the fibrotic complications of chronic methysergide therapy are very infrequent.[276,1960] This reduction is presumably attributable to the current practice of intermittent use. Methysergide is now usually administered for no longer than 4–6 months at a time to prevent the buildup of connective tissue. It is then discontinued for 4–8 weeks and reinstituted if necessary. Because many of the fibrotic changes are partly, or even largely, reversible when treatment with methysergide is discontinued, the "drug holiday" presumably provides time for regression of fibrotic lesions that have formed.[816] The drug should be gradually withdrawn to avoid rebound effects.

Physical findings attributable to excessive growth of fibrous tissue are usually nonspecific. Retroperitoneal fibrosis typically does not produce clinical symptoms or signs early in its course. Later, when it produces ureteral obstruction and hydronephrosis, it may be associated with fatigue, weight loss, fever, and dysuria. The most frequent complaint is dull, noncolicky pain localized to the back, flank, or abdomen. Retroperitoneal fibrosis may also cause constipation if it involves the bowel and claudication, edema, and muscular atrophy if it affects the aorta, vena cava, and common iliac vessels.

Pleuropulmonary fibrosis may cause symptoms of chest pain, dyspnea, and fever. Physical examination may reveal signs of pleural effusion with a friction rub. Endocardial fibrosis of the aortic valve, mitral valve, or root of the aorta can produce systolic or diastolic cardiac murmurs.

To monitor the possible development of fibrotic complications, patients being treated with methysergide should be evaluated once a year by means of careful cardiac auscultation, a chest x-ray, and either an intravenous pyelogram or abdominal magnetic resonance imaging scan.

Contraindications to the Use of Methysergide

Methysergide should not be used in patients in whom vasoconstriction may prove to be a problem. Thus, the drug should not be prescribed for individuals with peripheral vascular disease, coronary artery disease, or marked hypertension. Many patients take ergotamine during methysergide therapy but probably should not do so because of methysergide's predilection to potentiate the action of vasoconstrictive agents. Methysergide is also a potent venoconstrictor; therefore, patients with a history of thrombophlebitis should best avoid the medication.[12] Because it can increase gastric acid secretion, methysergide may activate peptic ulcer. It should not be given to patients with either active ulcer disease or a history of peptic ulcer.[301,416] In view of its propensity to cause fibrotic reactions, methysergide should not be administered to patients with valvular heart disease, chronic pulmonary disease, collagen diseases, or fibrotic conditions. Renal and liver impairment also limit its use.

---

*References 371, 606, 628, 746, 747, 816, 821, 1553

NONSTEROIDAL ANTI-INFLAMMATORY DRUGS

NSAIDs are safe and reasonably effective agents for migraine prophylaxis. Most controlled investigations that have compared NSAIDs and placebo for the prevention of migraine have indicated that NSAIDs are significantly superior to placebo.* Trials of fenoprofen (Nalfon), naproxen (Naprosyn), mefenamic acid (Ponstel), tolfenamic acid (available in Europe), and ketoprofen (Orudis) have all demonstrated variable levels of efficacy in reducing the frequency of migraine attacks.

The side effects of NSAIDs have been discussed in chapter 10. The chronic use of NSAIDs is, however, associated with a higher incidence of adverse reactions than when these compounds are used occasionally for acute attacks of migraine. Adverse renal effects, for example, have been reported during continual use. These include glomerular nephritis, interstitial nephritis, the nephrotic syndrome, and renal papillary necrosis. Because the untoward renal effects of NSAIDs are more likely to occur in patients with preexisting renal dysfunction, patients taking NSAIDs for long-term migraine prophylaxis must have normal renal function before starting treatment. There is also a higher risk of gastrointestinal side effects with chronic use of NSAIDs.

Aspirin, either by itself or combined with dipyridamole (Persantine), has been used for migraine prophylaxis. Most trials have shown a small, but significant, benefit of low-dose aspirin in reducing the frequency, and sometimes the intensity, of migraine attacks.† The largest trials have, however, been performed in men; convincing data showing efficacy in women are not available. Aspirin is not as potent as more frequently used therapeutic agents such as β-blockers.[840] Moreover, patients may develop a chronic daily headache by consuming aspirin on a daily basis.

Indomethacin is of little use in the prophylaxis of ordinary cases of migraine.[64,625] It is, however, effective in the treatment of exertional migraine, benign orgasmic cephalgia, and ice-pick headaches. The accepted dosage is 25–50 mg three times a day with meals or with antacids.

Cyproheptadine

Cyproheptadine (Periactin) is of restricted usefulness in the prophylactic treatment of migraine.[417,1176,1642] Controlled studies of its efficacy are lacking, but clinical experience indicates that it may help a few patients. In particular, it is said to be beneficial for preventing migraine in children. But despite its widespread use for this purpose, convincing data are lacking.

The medication is frequently given in divided doses because of its tendency to cause drowsiness. The usual dosage is 4 mg three or four times a day. An occasional migraineur can tolerate a total dosage of 32 mg/day. Because of its prolonged duration of action, cyproheptadine can also be given once daily at bedtime. Stimulation of appetite with subsequent weight gain can occur during extended, or even acute, administration of the drug. Other side effects result from its anticholinergic properties and include urinary retention and dry mouth.

PIZOTIFEN

Pizotifen (Sandomigran, available in Europe and Canada) is structurally similar to cyproheptadine and to the tricyclic antidepressants. Data concerning the efficacy of pizotifen are conflicting.‡ Different controlled studies have shown it to be either no better than, or

---

*References 145, 157, 504, 511, 1049, 1243, 1386, 1763, 1950, 2128, 2199
†References 279, 1072, 1314, 1504, 1579

‡References 82, 96, 327, 919, 997, 1718, 1833, 1866

superior to, placebo. Pizotifen (0.5 mg) can be taken three times a day or administered as a single nocturnal 1.5-mg dose. The dose can be increased to 3 mg per night if necessary. The drug enhances appetite in almost all patients, and weight gain is therefore exceedingly common. It may also cause drowsiness.

LITHIUM

Although the overall effectiveness of lithium in the treatment of migraine is unclear, both open studies and clinical experience have demonstrated efficacy.[349,1458] Patients whose attacks have a cyclical pattern are said to respond well to lithium.[1358] This cyclical pattern can be identified when a patient reports having intervals of almost daily headaches for a few weeks that alternate with intervals during which he or she is free, or relatively free, of headaches. In contrast, for some patients with ordinary migraine, lithium has been reported to exacerbate headaches.[1546]

Because of its small margin of safety and its short half-life, lithium carbonate or citrate is administered in divided doses. Even the slow-release preparations of lithium are given two to three times a day. The initial dose is usually 300 mg twice a day. The amount may be increased by 300 mg every 4 or 5 days, after checking blood levels. Because safe blood levels are crucial, lithium is suitable only for patients who are willing and able to have blood drawn repeatedly on a fixed schedule. To compare blood levels from one test to the next, each venipuncture must be made at approximately the same number of hours after the last dose of lithium. Patients who cannot or will not comply with such a regimen should not be considered as candidates for a trial of lithium therapy.

The concentration of the cation in the blood needs monitoring because levels must stay within a definite, narrow range. Adverse reactions may occur at levels that are close to therapeutic levels. Between 0.75 and 1.25 mEq/L is thought to be the optimal serum concentration. These are levels obtained 12 hours after the last oral dose of lithium. A constant interval must be used because lithium levels fluctuate between doses. The dosage needed to maintain a safe level varies among different individuals, but usually ranges between 750 mg and 2.25 g per day of lithium carbonate.

Pharmacokinetic data indicate that several days are required to achieve a steady state after initiating therapy or changing the dose.[379] Accordingly, until therapeutic levels are obtained, lithium levels should be drawn every 4 or 5 days. Dosage adjustment based on serum levels obtained before a steady state has been reached can be both deceptive and harmful unless the physician is aware of the pharmacokinetics of lithium. After a dose schedule that produces therapeutic levels has been established, blood levels should continue to be monitored every month for the first 6 months, and every 2 or 3 months afterward.

Lithium therapy is attended by a number of side effects. Many occur initially and are generally not serious. They include nausea, loose but not frequent stools, fine tremor of the hands, lethargy, muscular weakness, memory problems, weakness, polyuria, and polydipsia. The tremor is made worse by sustained posture of the extremities or by the performance of purposeful movements. Although the tremor usually appears when therapy is initiated and decreases over time, it may persist from the beginning of treatment, appear at any time, or recur.[1029] Polyuria and polydipsia, although typically mild and transient, are occasionally a major problem and may persist throughout treatment. Some of these side effects may be reduced by giving lithium after meals and by further dividing doses.

More serious side effects occur when lithium levels are too high. Gastrointestinal symptoms—abdominal pain, marked vomiting, and diarrhea—may be prodromal; they sometimes herald impending toxicity. Serious side effects affect the central nervous and neuromuscular systems. These include drowsiness, generalized coarse tremors, ataxia, nystagmus, dysarthria, hyperactive tendon jerks, mental confusion, seizures, and coma.

Some side effects that develop during therapy are not related to dose or blood level. For example, some patients develop diffuse and nontender enlargement of the thyroid gland. Most patients typically remain euthyroid, but obvious hypothyroidism can be observed. For this reason, thyroid function tests should be obtained in all patients receiving long-term lithium treatment. Headache, peripheral edema, alopecia, and rashes have also been seen. Weight gain—often of 20 or more pounds—is reported to occur in many patients on lithium therapy.[2071]

Because lithium is eliminated mainly by the kidneys, the cation should not be given to patients with renal or cardiac disease whenever interference with excretion is possible. Patients should not receive diuretics or be on a salt-restricted diet, because sodium depletion augments the reabsorption of the cation by the renal tubules so that lithium may accumulate to toxic levels. Similar elevations of blood lithium levels may occur during bouts of diarrhea or in the presence of excessive sweating.

VALPROIC ACID

Recently both open and controlled investigations have shown that sodium valproate has potential for the prophylaxis of migraine.[938,1328,1412,1909] Valproate is unusual among antimigraine agents in that it is reportedly most effective in reducing the frequency and duration of severe attacks, and much less effective against mild attacks.[938]

Valproic acid (Depakene) is available in 250-mg capsules and in a syrup containing the sodium salt (equivalent to 250 mg of valproic acid per 5 mL). Divalproex sodium (Depakote), a mixture of equal proportions of valproic acid and sodium valproate, is available in 125-, 250-, and 500-mg tablets. The recommended initial dosage is 15 mg/kg of body weight per day in divided doses. The dose may be increased at weekly intervals by 5–10 mg/kg/day until headaches are under control or side effects occur. The dose is adjusted to keep a blood level between 75 and 100 μg/mL. It is unclear whether or not the concentration in the blood is correlated with antimigraine efficacy,[938,1328,1909] but blood levels should be checked to avoid toxicity.

Ingestion of valproate may be accompanied by a number of side effects—drowsiness, sedation, ataxia, anorexia, nausea, and vomiting. A lower incidence of gastrointestinal side effects is seen when divalproex sodium is administered. The CNS side effects develop infrequently and, as a rule, respond to a decrease in dosage. A dose-related hand tremor affects approximately 10% of patients taking valproate but is rarely severe enough to limit treatment. Appetite stimulation leading to weight gain, as well as rash and alopecia, have been observed occasionally.

Valproate may affect hepatic function. In particular, elevation of transaminase enzymes in the plasma occurs in up to 40% of patients. This can be seen during the first several months of therapy and is not accompanied by any symptom of hepatic dysfunction or other abnormalities in liver function. An uncommon complication mainly seen in chldren is a fulminant hepatitis that is frequently fatal.[536] For this reason, the drug should not be prescribed as an antimigraine medication in any patient with a history of hepatitis or other liver disease. Serious hepatotoxicity may be preceded by nonspecific symptoms, such as malaise, weakness, lethargy, anorexia, and vomiting. Patients should have their liver function and blood ammonia levels determined before initiating treatment, and liver function should be subsequently monitored at frequent intervals, particularly during the first 6 months.

MISCELLANEOUS AGENTS

A number of medications were in vogue for the prophylaxis of migraine in the past. Some of these agents are still used by some clinicians but probably should be discarded for use in most patients with migraine.

Anticonvulsants

The anticonvulsants phenytoin (Dilantin) and carbamazepine (Tegretol) have been used for migraine prophylaxis. Anecdotal reports suggest that phenytoin may be effective in the preventive treatment of migraine in some children.[1390] One controlled study of the use of carbamazepine as an antimigraine drug showed that it was more effective than placebo, but these results could not be corroborated.[68,1683] These drugs have little place in the current management of migraine.

Clonidine

The usefulness of clonidine as an antimigraine drug has been extensively investigated.[1073,1723] Early uncontrolled trials suggested that it was an effective prophylactic drug. Later investigations indicated that clonidine is no better than placebo and certainly inferior to more established agents such as the β-blockers.* At present, most physicians regard clonidine as having limited merit for the prevention of migraine. Clonidine, however, may have a role in the treatment of patients who require help in withdrawing from opiates, alcohol, nicotine, and perhaps benzodiazepines.[137,790]

Benzodiazepines

Benzodiazepines have been extensively used as migraine preventatives

---

*References 232, 1083, 1405, 1847, 1951

because of the assumption that many migraine attacks are precipitated by anxiety. Difficulties with dependency and withdrawal substantially restrict their use for a chronic and recurring problem. They should not be used for migraine prevention.

MECHANISMS OF ACTION OF PROPHYLACTIC MEDICATIONS

As indicated above, several classes of drugs with different, but overlapping pharmacologic effects can be successfully used to prevent migraine attacks. No single action is shared by all of the many drugs that are efficacious in the prophylactic treatment of migraine. Two major general hypotheses have been proposed to explain the therapeutic actions of some of these agents.

One of these maintains that the clinical efficacy of prophylactic antimigraine medications is related to serotonin receptors. This hypothesis is based largely on data showing that a number of antimigraine drugs have high affinity for the $5\text{-}HT_2$ serotonin receptor subtype in human brain (Table 11–5).[951,1240,1566] Thus, methysergide, cyproheptadine, and pizotifen display nanomolar affinity for $5\text{-}HT_2$ receptor subtypes, and amitriptyline and funarazine are only slightly less potent. Moreover, verapamil and nifedipine exhibit moderate affinities for the same receptors.[15] The antimigraine efficacy of these medications is thought to result from inhibition of $5\text{-}HT_2$ receptor-mediated actions such as cranial vasoconstriction platelet aggregation, and smooth muscle cell production of prostacyclin. Implicit in this formulation is an assumption that serotonin is responsible for initiating the migrainous process.

Inhibition of $5\text{-}HT_2$ receptor activation may not be the only mechanism by which antimigraine drugs affect $5\text{-}HT_2$ receptors. Chronic administration of both cyclic antidepressants and MAO inhibitors decreases the number of 5-

Table 11-5 EFFECTS OF PROPHYLACTIC DRUGS ON BRAIN NEUROTRANSMITTER RECEPTORS

Drug	Receptor				
	α_1	α_2	β	5-HT$_2$	5-HT$_{1A}$
Propranolol	−	−	+++	+	++
Amitriptyline	+++	−	−	+++	
Methysergide	+	+	−	++++	++
Cyproheptadine	++	+	−	++++	++
Pizotifen	++	+	−	++++	++
Flunarazine	++	−	−	+++	
Verapamil				++	
Nifedipine				+	
Diltiazem				+	
Nimodipine	−	−	−	−	

Symbols represent *in vitro* binding affinities (K_i values). ++++ = 0.3–3 nM; +++ = 3–30 nM; ++ = 30–300 nM; + = 300–3,000 nM; − = >3,000 nM.

Data from Leysen et al,[1240] Hiner et al,[951] and Peroutka.[1566] Modified from Greenberg.[829]

HT$_2$ binding sites (down-regulation) (see below). Such a decrease in the apparent density of 5-HT$_2$ receptors would be expected to cause changes similar to those seen when receptors are inhibited. In addition, although some compounds that antagonize serotonin receptors or cause their density to diminish are antimigraine agents, not all 5-HT$_2$ receptor antagonists are effective in preventing migraine. This finding suggests that additional actions at other receptors may well be necessary for antimigraine activity.[1441] And, indeed, some agents that bind to 5-HT$_2$ receptor sites also bind to other sites (see Table 11–5). Moreover, because a number of antimigraine drugs—in particular, propranolol and other β-adrenoreceptor antagonists—are largely inactive at 5-HT$_2$ receptors, it may be that for some patients relief comes from something other than inhibition of 5-HT$_2$ receptors, whereas other patients benefit from actions of 5-HT$_2$ sites in combination with other phenomena.

The second general hypothesis holds that the beneficial effects of antimigraine drugs result from actions at calcium channels. Some, but not all, calcium channel blockers are effective antimigraine drugs. Cyproheptadine, amitriptyline, and pizotifen, which are not considered to be calcium channel blockers, possess properties antagonistic to calcium channel activation (Table 11–6).[1276,1567–1569]

A number of different types of calcium channels are located in the membranes of all excitable cells, including neurons and smooth muscle cells. Calcium channels are large membrane-spanning glycoprotein molecules that allow the controlled entry of ionic calcium from the extracellular fluid into cells. Such channels can be opened either by changes in membrane potential (voltage-gated channels, voltage-dependent channels) or by the action of specific transmitter substances or of intracellular second messengers that activate channel-associated receptor molecules (ligand-gated channels). Calcium channel blockers such as verapamil, nifedipine, diltiazem, and nimodipine prevent the passage of calcium through both types of channels. In addition, the contraction of the smooth muscle of cerebral arteries is more sensitive to calcium antagonists than the smooth muscle of peripheral arteries.

Cerebral vasoconstriction is thought by some to be responsible for the migraine aura.[2186] Calcium channel blockers (and other agents with calcium-channel–antagonist properties) are hy-

Table 11–6 INHIBITION OF AGONIST-INDUCED CONTRACTION OF CANINE BASILAR ARTERIES*

Drug	Serotonin	Norepinephrine
Nimodipine	0.20	0.19
Nifedipine	6.2	
Cyproheptadine	55	45
Methysergide	330	1,400
Amitriptyline	1,200	1,100
Flunarazine	2,400	
Propranolol	>10,000	>10,000

*Concentrations of inhibitory compounds (IC_{50} values in nM) required to produce a 50% decrease in the amount of contraction produced in canine basilar artery segments by 100 nM serotonin or 1 μM norepinephrine.
Data from Peroutka and Allen[1567] and Peroutka et al.[1568]

pothesized to work as antimigraine drugs by preventing the initial vasoconstriction. Such vasoconstriction requires the intracellular entry of calcium ions via specific voltage-dependent channels located on smooth muscle cell membranes. Calcium channel blockers inhibit cerebral vasoconstriction by antagonizing the entrance of extracellular calcium into vascular smooth muscle cells. As a result, calcium channel blockers are capable of selectively inhibiting the action of vasoactive substances and transmitters on the intracerebral vasculature.[1564] Calcium channel blockers could thus suppress the putative cerebral vasospasm postulated by some to be the causative mechanism in migraine.

If a vascular locus of action is in fact responsible for the antimigraine effects of calcium antagonists, one would expect the most vasoactive calcium channel blockers to be the most effective antimigraine agents. But this does not seem to be the case. Nimodipine, which has potent actions on cranial blood vessels, is either not at all effective, or only marginally effective as an antimigraine drug. In contrast, flunarazine, which has little or no vascular activity, is very effective therapeutically.

Spreading depression of cortical electrical activity may play a role in classic migraine. If so, calcium channel blockers might affect the process directly, or else affect the small blood vessel vaso-

constriction that accompanies spreading depression. Flunarazine does inhibit spreading depression of electrical activity in experimental animals, but high doses are required.[2090] The mechanism of this action has not been explored nor have the effects on spreading depression of other calcium antagonists been reported.

β-Blockers

No one really knows what mechanisms and loci of action enable β-blockers to prevent migraine. Because propranolol blocks β-receptors necessary for peripheral vasodilatation, it has been assumed that the drug also prevents the cranial vasodilatation believed by some to be the cause of migrainous head pain. But propranolol has little effect on cerebral blood flow.[1491] A number of investigations have shown that blockade of β-adrenoceptors is not sufficient to prevent migraine headaches nor is blockade of β-receptors necessary for antimigraine activity. D-Propranolol, for example, which lacks β-blocking activity, appears as effective clinically as the racemic mixture of D- and L-propranolol used commercially.[1951] L-Propranolol is an effective β-blocker. Reports correlating the ability of propranolol to reduce the frequency of headaches with its ability to produce peripheral β-blockade as manifested by reduced heart rate are inconsistent.[386,1154] Moreover, a number of potent β-blockers such as pindolol, alprenolol, oxprenolol, and acebutolol have shown no efficacy as antimigraine agents.[601,603,604,1446,1867] These latter compounds apparently exert intrinsic sympathomimetic activity (i.e., they are partial agonists at β-receptors). This property is claimed to render them ineffective in migraine prophylaxis.[623,2115]

Some β-blockers stabilize the membranes of peripheral nerve cells and heart. This property was once thought to be important in explaining antimigraine efficacy, but the membrane-stabilizing effects of β-blockers probably have little clinical relevance because they are only seen at plasma levels 50- to 100-fold higher than those necessary to produce β-blockade. As further evidence against this theory, propranolol and metoprolol have membrane-stabilizing activity, whereas nadolol and atenolol do not. Even so, all four agents have therapeutic actions in patients with migraine.

Affinity for 5-HT receptors has also been thought to have relevance to the antimigraine action of β-blockers. This is another untenable assertion. Clinical efficacy does not correlate with the actions of β-adrenoceptor antagonists at 5-HT$_1$ binding sites; moreover, β-blockers have negligible affinity for 5-HT$_2$ sites.[1382,1445] Pindolol, alprenolol, and oxprenolol all interact with 5-HT binding sites at low concentrations, yet are of no value in migraine.[1383] One is forced to conclude that the therapeutic antimigraine actions of β-adrenergic antagonists cannot be ascribed solely to antagonism of serotonin receptors.

Antidepressants

Antidepressants affect various aspects of neurotransmission involving biogenic amines. Most hypotheses about the mechanisms of action of antidepressants relate to changes in receptor responses to those transmitters. Several different actions have been described. These involve interference with the transport or metabolism of biogenic amines; changes in the up- or down-regulation of receptors; receptor antagonism; and changes in firing rates of certain neurons.

1. *Interference with the transport or metabolism of biogenic amines.* Uptake of biogenic amines by the presynaptic terminals from which they were released is the major way by which the amines are inactivated. All cyclic antidepressants and fluoxetine potentiate the actions of biogenic amine neurotransmitters in the CNS by inhibiting their uptake at presynaptic nerve terminals. Remarkable differences have been observed among the cyclic compounds with regard to their potency and selectivity in inhibiting the neuronal transport of norephinephrine and serotonin. For example, desipramine and nortriptyline are more potent blockers of norepinephrine uptake than are imipramine and amitriptyline. The two former drugs also more effectively inhibit the uptake of norepinephrine than of serotonin. In contrast, amitriptyline inhibits the uptake of norepinephrine and serotonin equally well. Fluoxetine is a serotonin uptake blocker with minimal effect on other neurotransmitter uptake systems.[1669]

In contrast to cyclic antidepressants, MAO inhibitors work by blocking the oxidative deamination of monoamines by the enzyme MAO. The nonspecific MAO inhibitors used for the treatment of migraine block MAO located in the intestines, liver, brain, platelets, and blood vessels.

Preventing the neuronal uptake of biogenic amines, or reducing metabolic breakdown of them, prolongs their effects at synapses and is believed to enhance postsynaptic responses to the amines. It is unclear, however, whether or not uptake or block of metabolism of amines has much to do with how these drugs function as antimigraine agents. Blockade of amine uptake occurs promptly after administration of cyclic antidepressants, but the appearance of antidepressive and antimigraine effects usually takes several weeks. Similar observations have been made with regard to MAO inhibitors. In experimental animals, peak tissue increases in the concentrations of norepinephrine, serotonin, and dopamine usually occur within the first week of treatment. Levels then decline over a 6-week period even though the degree of MAO inhibition is maintained.[308,1679] Thus, the degree of transport or enzyme inhibition, as well as the transmitter concentrations, does not appear to correlate with the clinical effects of these agents. These findings lend support to the hypothesis that secondary adaptive changes (such as changes in the regulation of receptors) plays a significant—and possibly critical—role in the effects of antidepressants.

2. *Up- or down-regulation of receptors.* Antimigraine and antidepressant actions of cyclic antidepressants, MAO inhibitors, and serotonin uptake blockers may be related to indirectly mediated actions on receptors for biogenic amines. For example, long-term administration of tricyclic antidepressants causes augmented central neuronal responsiveness to α_1-adrenergic agonists in experimental animals. This may be a consequence of an increase in the apparent concentration of adrenergic α_1-binding sites (*up-regulation.*)[2072] Long-term administration of cyclic antidepressants or MAO inhibitors may also increase neuronal sensitivity to serotonin, even though a decrease in the number of 5-HT_2 receptors and the number of β-adrenergic binding sites (*down-regulation*) has been documented.[166,220,1571] With regard to fluoxetine, down-regulation of the number of 5-HT_1 receptors is the most frequently reported neuronal effect of chronic exposure.[138] Data about how antidepressants affect other types of neurotransmitter receptors is contradictory. Nevertheless, although the association between adaptive changes in receptors and the emergence of therapeutic antimigraine responses is not yet understood, it is considered a prerequisite for antidepressant effects.[51]

3. *Receptor antagonism.* Cyclic antidepressants may not only produce changes in regulation of some receptor sites, but also may act as antagonists at various neurotransmitter receptors. This group of drugs possesses moderate-to-high affinity for muscarinic cholinergic, α_1-adrenergic, and both H_1 and H_2 histaminergic receptors. Actions at these receptors are, however, most likely responsible for untoward side effects rather than for therapeutic actions.

4. *Changes in firing rates of central noradrenergic and serotonergic neurons.* Electrophysiologic studies have shown that administration of both cyclic antidepressants and MAO inhibitors reduces the firing rate of neurons in the locus coeruleus and the nuclei of experimental animals.[220,1469,1620,1819] In view of the various hypotheses that implicate altered activity in the locus coeruleus and raphe nuclei in the initiation of migraine attacks, these changes in firing rates may be the basis for the antimigraine actions of antidepressants.[1169,2126] Unfortunately, no data supporting this view are available.

In sum, current evidence from animal experimentation suggests that all antidepressants produce some kinds of delayed changes in receptor sensitivity. These changes appear to form the basis of their clinical antidepressant actions. What is not clear, however, is whether antidepressants exert their antimigraine prophylactic effects in the same way.

Cyclic antidepressants also have analgesic properties, which may play a role in their antimigraine actions. Tricyclic drugs appear more efficient in this regard than do heterocyclic drugs.[1505] Several speculative ideas about the processes involved in the analgesic effect of antidepressants have been proposed:

1. *Alleviation of an accompanying depression.*[81,428,2064,2095] Because depression makes pain all the more distressing, alleviating depression could very well also alleviate pain. Antidepressants, however, can decrease pain

both for patients without any signs of depression and for depressed patients, in the absence of antidepressive actions. Antidepressants also have analgesic properties when administered in doses smaller than those usually effective for treating depression.

2. *Modulation of the endogenous antinociceptive systems.*[638] Central descending monoaminergic pathways—particularly those that use serotonin and norepinephrine as neurotransmitters—are involved in the rostral transmission of pain impulses (see chapter 7). The inhibition of synaptic serotonin and norepinephrine uptake, as discussed above, potentiates the action of these descending pathways, producing an inhibition of the trigeminal and spinal transmission of nociceptive impulses. These actions may account for analgesic properties that make tricyclic antidepressants even more useful as antimigraine agents.

Methysergide

Although most authorities agree that the ability of methysergide to block 5-HT_2 receptors is responsible for the prophylactic value of the drug, methysergide has other actions as well. For example, methysergide reportedly functions as a partial agonist, binding to 5-HT_{1A} sites.[1565] Methysergide also has weak vasoconstrictor effects, but it is not known whether or not these are a reflection of its 5-HT_{1A} agonist actions.[1926]

Lithium

Which molecular mechanisms of lithium are related to its therapeutic actions is not known.[1340] The cation does have a number of effects on neurotransmitter systems, second messengers, and ion channels. In particular, lithium produces changes in the sero-tonin system. Lithium has been reported to affect several serotonergic processes, including synthesis, release, and uptake of serotonin.[954,1085,1122] Both long- and short-term treatment with lithium has been shown to increase brain serotonin turnover, although some investigations have indicated a decreased concentration of serotonin. Chronic lithium treatment decreases the number of serotonin receptor sites in the hippocampus and striatum but not in the cortex or hypothalamus.[2033] It is unclear which, if any, of these effects are pertinent to the antimigraine actions of lithium.

SUMMARY

Prophylactic medication can alleviate the burden of living with migraine. The preceding discussion about the mechanisms of action by which these drugs work, however, should leave no doubt that researchers have only just begun to learn what effects prophylaxis has at the molecular level. But although we may not be clear about how various compounds work, there is a wealth of empirical data about which drugs to try on which patients. Physicians can now select from a considerable number of pharmaceutical agents for the prevention of migraine. Both uncontrolled and controlled trials, and many years of clinical experience, have shown that prophylactic drugs, if used appropriately, are effective in lessening the frequency and severity of migraine in the majority of patients with recurrent migraine attacks. No guidelines exist to ascertain the "appropriate" preventive drug for a given patient. It remains unclear why patients with virtually equivalent clinical headache syndromes react so differently to prophylactic medications. As a result, the physician must learn to individualize therapy.

Chapter 12

SPECIAL SITUATIONS

DRUG-INDUCED HEADACHE
STATUS MIGRAINOSUS
TREATMENT OF MIGRAINE IN
   CHILDREN
TREATMENT OF MENSTRUAL
   MIGRAINE
THE PREGNANT AND POSTPARTUM
   MIGRAINEUR
THE POSTMENOPAUSAL
   MIGRAINEUR
MIGRAINE IN THE ELDERLY

The preceding chapters have discussed approaches to acute bouts of migraine and strategies to prevent headaches. These treatments are appropriate for migraineurs in general, although the approach must be tailored to each individual patient. Some migraineurs, however, need additional consideration—perhaps because they are pregnant, very young, or very old. Even more often, extra attention is needed because their long search for relief has caught them up in the cycle of daily headache induced by the very drugs meant to help them. It is to these patients, who may need even more empathy than usual from their physicians, that this chapter turns.

DRUG-INDUCED HEADACHE

One of the most difficult therapeutic challenges facing those who treat patients with recurrent migraine headaches is migraine complicated by chronic daily headache. This type of headache, which all too frequently re-sults from excessive intake of antimigraine medication, has been variously designated as *drug-induced headache, analgesic rebound headache, analgesic abuse headache,* or *ergotamine headache.* The clinical characteristics of patients with the chronic daily headache syndrome are described in detail in chapter 3. Many patients with this problem complain of a constant, diffuse, dull discomfort in their head, upon which are superimposed recurrent episodes of throbbing pain more typical of migraine. Most of these patients are caught up in a vicious cycle of headache and medication abuse. The cycle is characterized by daily headache for which the patient ingests, on a daily or more or less daily "schedule," one or a combination of over-the-counter (OTC) antipyretic analgesics (such as aspirin or acetaminophen), or prescription analgesic–sedative combination drugs containing butalbital, narcotic medications, or ergotamine (Table 12–1).[823,1335,1753] Excessive caffeine intake may complicate the picture. Not only do many of the medications contain caffeine, but additionally, many patients with this syndrome drink substantial quantities of coffee.[753]

Analgesic drugs, ergots, or caffeine taken in excessive amounts for prolonged periods of time can both cause and sustain headache.[287,514] Some patients use only one kind of drug, but a substantial number use two or more. Nicotine and alcohol are also used by considerable numbers of patients with this syndrome.[753] Other medication, including nasal sprays, sinus medications, antihistamines, and tranquiliz-

Table 12–1 MEDICATIONS THAT CAN LEAD TO DRUG-INDUCED HEADACHES

- Aspirin and aspirin-containing medications
- Acetaminophen and acetaminophen-containing medications
- Butalbital-containing compounds
- Ergotamine tartrate
- Dihydroergotamine
- Narcotics
- Caffeine
- Isometheptene mucate
- Sedative–hypnotics and tranquilizers

ers, are often used to excess or even daily by the headache sufferer. A period of at least 3 months of excessive medication use is probably necessary before a daily headache develops; most of these problems evolve over a period of several years. Many patients have been using analgesics and other medications since childhood or adolescence.[753]

Migraineurs frequently practice self-medication without medical control or supervision, taking excessive amounts of both prescribed and OTC medications for headache. Some patients make a distinction between prescription and OTC medications. They mistakenly believe that they are following doctor's orders because they perceive OTC medications as harmless.

Sufferers of chronic daily headache frequently ingest medication at the onset of the slightest symptoms. This often provides a rhythm not only to the patient's daily life, but frequently to that of persons around the patient. In contrast, many patients hide their drug-taking behavior. Countless patients who anticipate and dread an impending headache premedicate themselves every day in an attempt to ward off a bout of head pain. Apprehension of losing one's job because of absence caused by headaches is another factor in the prophylactic intake of analgesics and antimigraine drugs.[753] Most patients have significant emotional and physical dependence on analgesics and ergots, and have developed tolerance to the therapeutic effects of the drugs. Because of the development of tolerance to

analgesics and ergots, these patients ingest larger and larger quantities in a futile endeavor to salvage a constantly diminishing therapeutic effect.

For most patients, antimigraine drugs are first prescribed by well-meaning primary care physicians and nonheadache specialists who are unfortunately unaware of the dangers of worsening migraine through the overuse of analgesics, narcotics, and ergots. Physicians prescribing these medications often do not set limits on their use. As a result, these agents are used in progressively larger quantities and ultimately in unmistakable excess. Most headache sufferers and their physicians tacitly assume that substantial daily use of analgesics, narcotics, and ergots results from severe, unremitting daily head pain. It is now widely conceded, however, that the daily use of analgesics, narcotics, and ergots worsens and maintains head pain, thereby playing an important role in the transformation of episodic headache to daily headache.[46,1015,1146,1252,1630] In other words, the headaches are believed to be "drug-induced headaches." These headaches are ameliorated, often dramatically, after drug intake is stopped, supporting the argument that this type of headache is produced by excessive amounts of drugs.

Butalbital-containing preparations are the most regularly abused compounds.[1630] It is not unusual for patients to take 30 tablets per week, and some ingest 85 or more.[1332] Patients may also develop a chronic daily headache by consuming only aspirin or acetaminophen.[1015,1184,1335,1632] Many patients ingest substantial quantities of OTC medications—6 to 10 tablets or more may be taken in a day. The critical threshold dosage at which acetaminophen or aspirin induces daily headache is estimated to be approximately 1000 mg/day.[1796] Aspirin and acetaminophen are equally effective in their capacity to stimulate chronic headaches, but for some unknown reason nonsteroidal anti-inflammatory drugs (NSAIDs) are said not to induce chronic headaches.[1223,1234] This picture may change as OTC NSAIDs are more and more heavily marketed.

Ergotamine abuse with subsequent physical dependence and chronic headache evolves at an inconstant pace in migraine patients. Ergotamine abuse frequently worsens headaches, shortens the duration of headache relief produced by ergotamine, and renders ineffective previously effective migraine prophylaxis.* Ergotamine abuse is generally seen in migraineurs who use the compound more than two or three times a week.[1756,1758] The weekly dose is greater than 10 mg in most cases, and some patients take as much as 10–15 mg *per day.*[1758] Some susceptible individuals may develop drug-induced daily headaches while ingesting only 0.5–1.0 mg of ergotamine several times a week.[23,1758] Very few patients who use ergots excessively show clinical evidence of significant peripheral ischemia. But findings of subclinical ergotism—alterations of the peripheral circulation and changes in the cardiovascular system and in the electroencephalogram—may follow the continuous use of ergotamine in weekly doses of more than 7–10 mg.[522,964] Of interest are reports that the intensity of withdrawal symptoms does not appear to equate with either the dose of ergotamine or the length of ergotamine abuse.[23,1705] When administered for extended periods of time, dihydroergotamine (DHE) can also induce chronic headaches in some patients.[1786] Thus, even though it reduces the number of acute bouts of migraine, daily intake of DHE is capable of producing chronic headache.

Because excessive ingestion of caffeine can be a factor in the production of chronic daily headaches, care must be taken to avoid overconsumption of coffee and caffeine-containing soft drinks and medications. Many migraineurs drink excessive amounts of caffeine because the substance improves performance and mood, and relieves fatigue

and irritability. Moreover, the psychostimulating effects of caffeine can offset the lethargy produced by excessive doses of analgesic, narcotic, and sedative drugs. Many chronic headache patients ingest an amount of caffeine equivalent to more than 3 to 4 cups of strong coffee per day; some, an amount found in 6 to 10 cups.[1786] Cessation of caffeine intake produces a caffeine withdrawal headache. When this occurs, rapid relief can be obtained through further ingestion of caffeine. Thus, a vicious cycle may be perpetuated. Caffeine-withdrawal headaches may well contribute to the abuse of combination drugs that contain caffeine.[515]

Abrupt cessation of butalbital-containing medications, ergotamine, caffeine, or narcotics consistently results in an increase in the severity of head pain. The headache is usually disabling and is accompanied by nausea. Withdrawal headache ordinarily begins within 24–48 hours following discontinuation of the drug and may last for 72 or more hours. At times, vomiting, abdominal cramps, and diarrhea accompany the headache. Restlessness and insomnia are common complaints, as are tremors and muscle cramps. Seizures have been reported to follow abrupt withdrawal of butalbital in patients taking very large daily doses.

Prevention of Drug-Induced Headache

To limit the development of drug-induced headaches, not only patients, but doctors too must understand the dangers of prescribing excessive amounts of certain headache remedies. The quantity and frequency of use of medications must be plainly specified to every patient. Patients must be clearly warned about the dangers of medication overuse and must comprehend that this warning extends to OTC products. The phenomenon of analgesic rebound needs to be explained in detail to all patients. Patients must accept the

---

*References 23, 46, 964, 1543, 1577, 1705, 2001

fact that overuse of analgesics, narcotics, ergots, and caffeine not only may lead to daily headache, but will also prevent potentially beneficial preventive medications from functioning effectively.

To err on the side of caution, analgesics should probably not be used more often than 4 days a month, and limited to two unit doses per week.[1015,1783] Ergotamine should probably be confined to one unit dose per week.[1783] Unfortunately no clear-cut guidelines as to the limits of drug administration have been agreed upon by all authorities.

Treatment of Drug-Induced Headache

The initial step in treating drug-induced headache consists of withdrawing the offending drug or drugs.[1146,1334,1756] Before this can happen, the individual patient has to be convinced that detoxification is necessary for alleviation of the daily headache problem. This usually requires much effort and time on the part of the physician, who must be persuasive and convincing. Treatment for this type of problem will not be successful unless the patient desires the treatment and is willing to stay with it despite considerable discomfort. The patient must realize that effective prevention of migraine is not possible until analgesics and ergotamine have been eliminated.

The procedures used for withdrawal vary among different authorities and different centers. Medications can be withdrawn suddenly or gradually over a period of weeks. Whatever method is used, all analgesics and ergots must ultimately be eliminated if the program is to be successful. A reduction in dosage is insufficient and will not alleviate the headache symptoms. Depending on the amount and type of drug overuse—and the patient's psychological and social circumstances—the withdrawal can be managed in an outpatient or an inpatient situation. Outpatient treatment is far less expensive, but poor patient compliance may be a problem. Hospitalization ensures compliance. When the individual has been taking large amounts of abortive medication, drug withdrawal may be difficult, if not impossible, on an outpatient basis because of the severity of the withdrawal symptoms. In those cases, hospitalization is necessary to provide supportive measures such as intravenous fluids to control the alterations in fluid and electrolyte balance resulting from vomiting. On the other hand, abrupt withdrawal may be effective in an outpatient setting if sufficient explanation is provided for patients as to what to expect and how to deal with the discomfort.[939] Some patients may, in fact, benefit from outpatient withdrawal, in that the misery of detoxification can give rise to a sense of mastery and self-control.

Every patient, no matter how enthusiastic over achieving detoxification, must face continuing problems of psychologic as well as physiologic dependence on drugs. Any program, whether inpatient or outpatient, ought to be integrated with behavioral therapy and psychologic support to aid patients in the complete management of their headache problems.

A number of drugs have been used successfully to ease the pain of withdrawal: NSAIDs, phenothiazines, corticosteroids, DHE, and isometheptene.* Sedatives may also be valuable to counteract the withdrawal symptoms. The short-term use of parenteral narcotics may be necessary. Antinausea remedies are essential if detoxificiation is accomplished rapidly. The Raskin DHE protocol (see Fig. 10–2) is usually of great benefit during the early stages of withdrawal, but it requires hospitalization.[1637] Sumatriptan is reported to be effective during the withdrawal phase.[520] A single subcutaneous dose (2.0 mg) may alleviate the headache for as long as 6–10 hours.

During the period of withdrawal, or once the withdrawal headache has di-

---

*References 22, 1252, 1325, 1637, 1820, 2001

minished, effective prophylactic medication such as β-blockers or tricyclic antidepressants must be administered to prevent the recommencement of self-medication with analgesics and ergots.[1146] Effective prevention is generally possible after detoxification and removal of analgesics and ergots has occurred, even though the same medications were ineffective in the presence of daily symptomatic medication.

The rate of success of withdrawal from analgesics and ergots varies between 40% and 100% in different series of patients. These reported differences largely reflect both the duration of the follow-up period and the particular drugs from which the patients under study were withdrawn. The mean rate appears to be approximately 70%.* After the initial withdrawal period, the improvement in headache frequency and severity is usually maintained. Moreover, irritability and insomnia are frequently reduced, apathy and depression are typically alleviated, and general health usually improves.

Following detoxification, patients must be warned against returning to their former medication practices. They must also understand that acute migraine attacks are to be treated with care and circumspection. NSAIDs, aspirin, or acetaminophen, in combination with metoclopramide, should be the mainstay of treatment. Sumatriptan may be of great help in many of these patients. Use of ergotamine should be very much curtailed, restricted to those who persist in having severe migraine attacks despite appropriate prophylactic therapy. Medications containing barbiturates or narcotics should either be severely limited or prohibited.[519]

STATUS MIGRAINOSUS

Status migrainosus is the designation applied to severe, unrelenting bouts of migraine that persist for more than 72 hours. The same abuse of medication that gives rise to the chronic daily headache syndrome is considered to be an important factor in many cases of status migrainosus. Some attacks of prolonged migraine headaches, however, develop without any cause; others follow head trauma, systemic illness, high fever, or aseptic meningitis.[390] These prolonged attacks typically include intense nausea and persistent vomiting, prostration, dehydration, electrolyte imbalance, and significant emotional distress. The pain, nausea, and vomiting of these sieges do not respond to the usual analgesic medications or to appropriate parenteral medication administered in a physician's office. Many of these patients have made multiple trips to emergency rooms.

In general, patients in status migrainosus require hospitalization to treat the problem. The patients should be put to rest in a darkened, quiet room. Intravenous fluids are necessary to correct the alterations of fluid and electrolyte balance that result from vomiting and excessive sweating. Antiemetics should be used in appropriate doses. Most patients with status migrainosus do not obtain much relief from narcotic analgesics even when they are administered parenterally in adequate doses.[571] Ergotamine is usually of no help because of the duration of the symptoms.

The repetitive injection of intravenous DHE every 8 hours has transformed the treatment of status migrainosus.[1635,1637] More than 90% of patients are free of headaches within 48 hours of treatment.[1635] Figure 10–2 shows how the dose of DHE is determined. A dose of 0.5 mg of DHE is administered following a 10-mg intravenous dose of metoclopramide. If nausea occurs, no more DHE is given for 8 hours. After 8 hours, depending on the intensity and duration of the nausea following the initial dose of DHE, the next DHE dose ought to be 0.3 or 0.4 mg given with metoclopramide. For those patients whose head

---

*References 23, 46, 136, 515, 983, 1015, 1146, 1280, 1705, 2001

pain vanishes and in whom nausea does not develop, the dose is continued at 0.5 mg every 8 hours with metoclopramide. If, on the other hand, the headache is not substantially reduced after the first 0.5-mg dose of DHE, another 0.5-mg dose is administered 1 hour later without metoclopramide. If nausea occurs after this second 0.5-mg dose, 0.75 mg is selected to be the final 8-hourly dose. If nausea does not occur after the second 0.5-mg dose, the final dose is 1.0 mg given with 10 mg metoclopramide. Electrocardiographic monitoring should be performed during the first two injections of DHE in patients who are older than age 60 years. Most patients become headache-free within 8–16 hours.

Repetitive DHE causes few serious side effects. Diarrhea occurs in about half of the patients. The diarrhea usually responds to administration of diphenoxylate and atropine (Lomotil). Pain in the leg muscles and abdominal discomfort may appear, but are usually eliminated by reducing the dose of DHE.

Some clinicians recommend the addition of parenteral corticosteroids to other treatments.[324,565,721] No consensus about the dose or method of administration has been reached.[571] Some use 100–250 mg of hydrocortisone administered by injection over about 10 minutes into the intravenous tubing of a normal saline drip. Others inject dexamethasone in a dosage of 12–20 mg either intramuscularly or intravenously. A repeat parenteral dose, or its oral equivalent, may be necessary in 8–12 hours, but, in general, if corticosteroids have not ended status migrainosus within 24 hours, it is improbable that they will do so, and they should be discontinued.

The preceding pages of this book have dealt exclusively with the migraineur in general—that is to say, a composite person of no particular age or gender. But migraine does change its course over the decades. For many people, the symptoms of childhood migraine are totally unlike those of mid-life or old age.

Appropriate methods of treatment need to reflect these differences. A woman's migraine is often affected by hormonal changes during menstrual cycles, pregnancy, and menopause. These factors too require consideration when decisions are made about how to care for a particular patient. The following sections of this chapter take up the special considerations of migraine in children, menstrual migraine, migraine during pregnancy and lactation, migraine during and after menopause, and migraine in the elderly.

TREATMENT OF MIGRAINE IN CHILDREN

Migraine attacks may include symptoms that are frightening to children and their parents. Because most families are unaware that migraine occurs in childhood, parents often come to physicians terrified that their child is suffering from serious organic disease. Reassuring both parent and child is crucial. Once other causes of headache have been excluded, the family must be persuaded that no serious medical or neurologic disease is present, and that no further specialized diagnostic tests are necessary. Once they are reassured, the cause of the head pain and other symptoms can be explained to them.

After the parents are convinced that their youngster is not gravely ill, they can begin to be educated about how to help their child minimize the number and intensity of migraine attacks. Parents must be informed about general measures that affect migraine: diet, sleep, and trigger factors. For the most part, the same approach to these factors can be used in children as is used in adults. But, in addition, children often consume far more junk food (full of chemical additives and colorings) than do adults. Elimination of these products may be very helpful in individual cases. The parent may have to provide "competing snacks"—either homemade or purchased from a health food store—or it may be impossible to keep the child away from potential precipitants. Emphasis should be placed on determining and eliminating areas of stress at school and at home. Stress is frequently a problem in childhood migraine. If it is not recognized and dealt with, medications will often be of little value.

Many symptomatic and preventive medications have been recommended for the treatment of childhood migraine. But clinical decisions as to what type of therapy to use are difficult to make because most commonly used medications have not been properly investigated in children. Data are lacking about the effectiveness of most medications against childhood migraine. Moreover, a number of useful drugs have not been approved for children under age 12 years. The adolescent, on the other hand, can be treated as an adult with regard to the doses of most medications used for acute migraine. In addition, difficulty is experienced in the evaluation of antimigraine therapy in children because many children show a progressive reduction in headache frequency regardless of the form or type of treatment.[183] Between 30% and 40% of children appear to grow out of their affliction.[183,370,1613]

Acute Attacks of Migraine

The pharmacologic treatment of acute attacks of migraine in children is complicated by a number of factors. Although abortive drugs should be used early in a bout of migraine, it is frequently difficult for young children to recognize this early phase of the attack. In addition, they are usually not allowed to carry medicine to school and to take it by themselves in an unsupervised manner in a school situation. Nor will most schools administer medications. And even when the situation enables them to have their medication with them, young children are unable to take the responsibility for administering it safely and properly. Thus, abortive medication is frequently unavailable

when needed at the very onset of an attack.

Once an attack is underway, simple antipyretic analgesics are frequently capable of reducing the pain of mild to moderate headaches in children (Table 12–2). If at all possible, treatment should be limited to the administration of such analgesics. Although aspirin may be useful against childhood migraine, it should not be ingested by children under age 12 because of the possibility of Reye's syndrome should the child be suffering from an unnoticed, subclinical virus infection. Reye's syndrome, which consists of severe hepatic dysfunction and encephalopathy, is a rare, but frequently fatal, consequence of infection with various viruses, particularly the influenza virus. The use of salicylates has been strongly implicated in the development of Reye's syndrome in children. Controversy regarding the age at which risk factors for the development of Reye's syndrome exist. Some authorities recommend that aspirin be withheld until age 16 or even age 18.

Isometheptene mucate is useful for treating older children and adolescents (see chapter 9). The older child (over age 8 or 10 years) can take an adult dose of two capsules at the first sign of a headache and two capsules 45 minutes later if the headache is still present. A total of five capsules can be taken in 1 day.

If nausea and vomiting are conspicuous components of the bout of migraine, antiemetics can be given. Prochlorperazine and metoclopramide are widely used for this purpose. When metoclopramide is given to children, however, intense and unpleasant dystonic reactions occasionally occur. These include oculogyric crises and muscle spasms. Prochlorperazine may also cause extrapyramidal symptoms. The lowest effective dosage should be administered.

Ergotamine preparations should be used in low doses and are best avoided altogether for very young children (under age 6 years). In older children the drug should be reserved for those

**Table 12–2 MEDICATIONS FOR ACUTE MIGRAINE
ATTACKS IN CHILDREN**

Agent	Brand Name	Dose	Pediatric Form
Aspirin*		7–10 mg/kg (maximum 30–65 mg/kg/d)	Chewable tablets
Acetaminophen	Tylenol, Tempra	5–7 mg/kg; may repeat in 2 h (maximum 30–40 mg/kg/d)	Elixir, suspension, chewable tablets
Ibuprofen	Motrin, Advil, Pedia-Profen	5–10 mg/kg; may repeat in 4–6 h (maximum 40 mg/kg/d)	Suspension
Acetaminophen with codeine	Tylenol with Codeine Elixir	5–10 ml; may repeat in 4–6 h (maximum 30 mL/day)	Elixir
Propoxyphene	Darvon-N	0.5–0.75 mg/kg; may repeat in 4–6 h (maximum 2–3 mg/kg/d)	Suspension
Metoclopramide	Reglan	2–10 mg (maximum 10–15 mg/d)	Syrup
Prochlorperazine	Compazine	2.5–5.0 mg (maximum 7.5–15 mg/d)	Suppository, syrup
Isometheptene mucate	Midrin	65–130 mg (maximum 260–520 mg/d)	None
Ergotamine		1.0 mg (maximum 6 mg/d)	None

*May be contraindicated because of danger of developing Reye's syndrome.

uncommon patients with infrequent, exceptionally severe, long-lasting bouts of migraine. Unfortunately, the recommended dose of ergotamine has not been determined for children. Intravenously administered DHE is now being used successfully by some pediatric neurologists to treat acute attacks in children as young as age 6 years.[1838]

The effectiveness and toxicity of sumatriptan in children is unknown. Presumably the drug can be used in older children, but until scientific data are available, it should not be used in younger children.

Even more so than in adults, children require rest for an acute attack of migraine. Sleep seems to be the most efficient treatment for childhood attacks.

The fact that a variety of symptomatic treatments are available for the treatment of acute migraine attacks in children is confirmation of the fact that management of acute attacks in children is sometimes unsatisfactory. No preparation is efficacious in all chil-

dren, and some patients may be refractory to all agents.

Prophylactic Therapy

A smaller percentage of children are treated prophylactically than adults because of the ingrained hesitancy of physicians to treat growing children with medication for a prolonged period. Happily, behavioral therapy appears valuable for use in childhood migraineurs, particularly if the parents and physicians are disinclined to use medications or if pharmacotherapy has been tried and found to be ineffective.[550,2134] Although some of the reports are uncontrolled studies and have involved only small numbers of children, their results indicate that children may respond to behavioral therapy better than adults.[644,1156] If behavioral therapy is not an option, as with adults the primary element when advising prophylactic therapy is the frequency and severity of the attacks. Children should not receive continuous prophylactic medication unless the bouts of migraine are severe and frequent and interfere with school or relations with other children. Among the drugs in use for childhood prophylaxis against migraine are cyproheptadine, anticonvulsants, β-blockers, and some antidepressants, as well as other medications known to be effective for adult migraineurs.

Cyproheptadine (Periactin) is extensively used for the therapy of childhood migraine. In fact, it may be the most frequently prescribed medication for this condition, despite a dearth of published information regarding its effectiveness. Only one controlled pilot study has reported efficacy.[185] The usual dosage is 2–4 mg two or three times a day. As in adults, drowsiness, appetite stimulation, and anticholinergic effects can be produced.

In years past, anticonvulsant agents, particularly phenobarbital and phenytoin, were preferred for the preventive treatment of childhood migraine. Some practitioners still find them useful in those patients who do not respond to propranolol.[118,1390,1613] But neither phenobarbital nor phenytoin has been exposed to thorough testing for effectiveness against migraine. Moreover, the use of these drugs is limited by their subtle effects on attention, learning, and behavior. When a choice is made to use phenytoin, it is usually administered in one of two ways: 50 mg administered three times a day, or 50 mg given in the morning and 100 mg at bedtime to children up to age 10 or 12 years.[118] Adolescent patients usually require larger doses of 200–300 mg/day. Phenobarbital is still used in very young patients (under age 5 years) who suffer from severe or frequent migraine. The recommended dosage is 30 mg twice or three times a day, or 30 mg given in the morning and 60 mg at night. The use of phenobarbital may be restricted by the appearance of either sedation or hyperactivity.

Although the value of propranolol and other β-blockers has not been established in children, its use has been recommended, and it is considered to be the most important prophylactic drug for the therapy of childhood migraine.[1614] Three controlled studies of propranolol in children are available. The frequency of attacks was reduced in one study, but two other studies showed no differences between treatment and control.[677,1283,1500] Timolol has been reported to be no more effective than control in children.[1465] Pediatric patients should be started on 1–2 mg/kg of propranolol per day, and the dose gradually increased to 5 mg/kg/day unless a therapeutic effect is reached at a lower dose. See chapter 9 for a discussion of the side effects of propranolol.

All of the drugs for the preventive treatment of migraine in adults can potentially be used for patients with childhood migraine. Little data exist with regard to the efficacy of calcium channel blockers. Flunarazine showed a significant reduction of headache frequency and duration.[1910,1911] One controlled trial of nimodipine in children demonstrated it to be ineffective.[135] Methysergide is not recommended because of the high incidence of side effects. Tricyclic antidepressants have a role in the treatment of children who are both clinically depressed and have migraine.

Because migraine in children has a high remission rate, attempts should be made to discontinue prophylactic medication at the end of 6 months or at the end of the school year. Therapy can be recommended if headaches recur.

TREATMENT OF MENSTRUAL MIGRAINE

As noted in chapter 2, approximately 60% of women patients are conscious of some association between menstruation and their migraine attacks.* Fewer

---

*References 831, 1172, 1450, 1806, 2056, 2173

than 15% of women patients, however, indicate that their headaches are limited to the time of menstruation.[616] Many women remark that standard prophylactic medications such as propranolol are efficacious in eliminating their headaches—except for the one headache a month they suffer from just before or during their menses and, indeed, migraine occurring at the time of menstruation is frequently very difficult to manage. At the present time, no universally effective treatment for menstrual migraine is available (Table 12–3).

Symptomatic approaches to acute menstrual migraine are the same as the treatment for any other acute attack of migraine. Antiemetics, NSAIDs, analgesics, and ergots are used. Patients who are afflicted with migraine that occurs exclusively at the time of their menses may be treated freely with analgesics because use of analgesics at only one time of the month does not appear to cause analgesic rebound headaches. For this small group of menstrual migraineurs, compound preparations consisting of a simple analgesic combined with caffeine, barbiturate, or narcotic may be very effective.

Because migraine limited to menstruation occurs at approximately the same time in each menstrual cycle, preventive medications can be used perimenstrually and may not have to be used all month. But perimenstrual administration of prophylactic agents may be complicated by the inexactness of the timing of menstrual cycles. Most menstrual cycles during the middle reproductive years are between 25 and 30 days—the distribution of cycle length is skewed toward the longer length. But the interval between cycles can vary both in each individual woman and among women. The greatest variability is found in the years shortly after menarche and immediately preceding menopause, when it is difficult to predict when menstruation will occur. This irregularity increases the difficulties of prescribing perimenstrual medication for some women.

For women whose cycles are reasonably predictable, premenstrual medication is worth trying. NSAIDs are often very effective when administered in adequate doses on a regular basis about the time of vulnerability. Naproxen sodium (550 mg twice a day from the seventh day before the expected menses through the third day of menstrual flow) is reported to be effective in reducing headache intensity and duration.[1744] Fenoprofen (Nalfon) and mefenamic acid have also been shown to be of value in menstrual migraine.[1395] Variability in responsiveness among different women make it imperative to try different classes of NSAIDs if the first NSAID is ineffective.

Women who are not already taking daily prophylactic medication throughout the month may also use β-blockers, calcium channel blockers, or methysergide perimenstrually.[562] The medication is usually begun 3–5 days before menstruation and continued through menstruation, and the dosage is then tapered.

Ergot dependence does not appear to pose a problem if the medication is given prophylactically on a daily basis *only* during the vulnerable period of the menstrual cycle. A Cafergot tablet twice a day or half a suppository at bedtime may be prescribed for the days at risk. Alternatively, Bellergal-S, a sustained-release tablet containing ergotamine

Table 12–3 TREATMENT OPTIONS FOR MENSTRUAL MIGRAINE

- NSAIDs
- Perimenstrual use of standard prophylactic drugs
- Ergotamine and its derivatives
- Biofeedback
- Hormonal therapy
  Estrogens (with or without androgens or progesterone)
  Synthetic androgens (danazol)
  Antiestrogens (tamoxifen)
  Prolactin release inhibitors (bromocriptine)

Adapted from Silberstein,[1839] p 789 with permission.

(0.3 mg), phenobarbital (40 mg), and belladonna (0.2 mg), is useful in some patients with menstrual migraine. The dose of Bellergal-S is one tablet twice a day.

Only a few investigations have explored the value of biofeedback and other behavioral methods for the treatment of menstrual migraine.[739,1108,1891,1989] Although there is conflict among results, most studies show that biofeedback has efficacy.

Hormonal therapy may be required for menstrual migraine if all simpler treatments are of no avail. A number of different strategies have been tried with varying degrees of success. Because the physiologic withdrawal of estrogen in the premenstrual phase of the cycle is thought to be the causative event leading to menstrual attacks of migraine, numerous attempts have been made to artificially elevate estrogen levels. Efforts to prevent catamenial migraine by raising estrogen levels, however, have generated contradictory data as to efficacy.* Moreover, in the past, estrogens have usually produced serious menstrual irregularities as side effects. A large part of the variability among reports stems from the use of different methods of estrogen administration that produce different levels of the hormone. A stable plasma level throughout each full day may be necessary to induce a therapeutic effect without disturbing the menstrual cycle.[475] The poor beneficial results of most studies of oral estrogens may be attributed to failure to maintain such stable levels. Percutaneous estradiol appears effective when used daily for the 7 days that encompass both the anticipated migraine attack and menstruation.[475,481] Estradiol implants may also have promise.[1291] This method of administration suppresses ovulation and prevents any alterations in estrogen levels related to the cycle. Cyclic oral progesterone is then added to induce menses. The risks of long-term treatment with estrogen should be considered before this type of therapy can be encouraged for a comparatively benign, if painful, condition.

Although some older, and mostly anecdotal, studies did show that progesterone preparations suppressed menstrual migraine attacks, the results have been largely inconsistent.[443,827,1285,1858] At the present time there is little enthusiasm for this form of treatment.

Danazol (Danocrine), tamoxifen (Nolvadex), and bromocriptine (Parlodel) have been reported to be efficacious in preventing catamenial migraine attacks, but have not been subjected to large controlled clinical trials. They cannot be recommended yet for common practice. Danazol is an ethyltestosterone derivative that suppresses the enzymatic synthesis of sex steroids and binds competitively to both androgen and progestin receptors. It prevents the elevation of both estrogen and progesterone levels in the ovulatory and midluteal phases of the menstrual cycle and, as a result, maintains a constant low level of estrogen.[927,1948] An unacceptable rate of adverse effects—weight gain, fluid retention, acne, hot flashes, hair loss, decreased breast size—occurs when danazol is administered in doses of 800 mg/day. But a recent uncontrolled investigation reported that 400 mg administered daily for 25 days each month was effective in the treatment of menstrual migraine.[1241] Only a small number of patients developed severe side effects—joint pain and acne.

Tamoxifen given in doses of 10–20 mg/day for the 7 to 14 days preceding menstruation, followed by 5–10 mg/day for 3 days during menses, has been reported to be effective against menstrual migraine in an open trial.[1478] Tamoxifen is a nonsteroidal triphenylethylene derivative that has antiestrogenic properties. The most frequent adverse effects include hot flashes, nausea, and vomiting.

There is one other medication, not part of the usual armamentarium of an-

---

*References 475, 480, 481, 1280, 1291, 1901–1905

timigraine therapy, that can be considered for perimenstrual use. Bromocriptine, an inhibitor of prolactin release, may limit the symptoms of the premenstrual syndrome and headache in dosages of 2.5 mg twice a day from the time of expected ovulation to the start of menstruation.[39,40,159]

Finally, it should be pointed out that a number of generally ineffective treatments are widely prescribed for patients with menstrual migraine. Because bouts of migraine are often accompanied by fluid retention, practitioners hypothesize that premenstrual fluid retention is somehow connected to the monthly headaches. Diuretics can reduce the fluid retention associated with menses, but the fluid reduction does not prevent menstrually related migraine.[1658] Nor has the efficacy of pyridoxine (vitamin B_6) been established in controlled studies.[860]

THE PREGNANT AND POSTPARTUM MIGRAINEUR

Management of migraine in a pregnant woman is especially difficult because of the potential teratogenicity of drug treatment. The vast majority of antimigraine drugs should not be administered either to pregnant patients or to patients who are trying to conceive. Many of the drugs used to treat migraine have been shown to cross the placental barrier and to produce pharmacologic effects in the fetus. Fortunately, for 75% of women, migraine ameliorates during pregnancy and may even stop, particularly during the second and third trimester.*

Acute Migraine Attacks during Pregnancy

Acetaminophen appears benign enough to administer to women with acute attacks of migraine who are preg-

*References 303, 616, 1172, 1285, 1450, 1903

nant or attempting to become pregnant. Acetaminophen crosses the placenta but has not been found to cause problems. The frequency of congenital abnormalities is not increased following maternal acetaminophen ingestion.[83]

All of the opioid analgesics cross the placenta and have the potential to cause dependence and withdrawal symptoms in the fetus and newborn if used regularly or abused.[36] Meperidine, provided its administration is rigidly controlled by the physician and it is prescribed in only limited amounts, appears relatively safe.[1636] There have been no large prospective studies of a possible association of limited use of meperidine and teratogenic changes in fetuses. But neither are there reports of any increased risk of malformations in the offspring of women who took the narcotic during the first trimester.[1043] Meperidine, however, has poor oral potency. A 50-mg oral dose is only equivalent to 650 mg of aspirin. An infrequent injection of meperidine is probably safe for acute attacks of migraine, but meperidine's use should be limited close to term because it causes neonatal depression.

Almost all other drugs have potential side effects for the fetus. In particular, the use of NSAIDs and aspirin can lead to premature closure of the ductus arteriosus, which is ordinarily maintained in the dilated state by prostaglandins. Aspirin can also increase intrapartum blood loss and impair neonatal hemostasis. The latter can lead to neonatal bleeding disorders and to intracranial hemorrhage in premature infants.[1968] Occasional use of asprin is not contraindicated, but regular use of aspirin should be avoided.

Ergot preparations are not recommended for use during pregnancy because the drug can cross the placenta.[994] Although doses much larger than those required to treat an attack of migraine are needed to produce uterine contractions and abortion, pregnancy constitutes a contraindication to its use.[1626]

The analgesic–sedative combination drugs contain barbiturates. Sporadic administration is presumably safe, but the repetitive administration of barbiturates during pregnancy may cause neonatal withdrawal symptoms, hypotonia, reduced responsiveness, and feeding problems.[2040]

Prophylactic Medication during Pregnancy

Propranolol has been recommended for migraine prophylaxis during pregnancy, even though the untoward effects of β-blockers in pregnant migraineurs have not been adequately investigated.[434] From their use in the treatment of hypertension and other cardiac-related conditions during pregnancy, one can infer that they are usually safe.[1707] Propranolol may, however, be associated with intrauterine fetal growth retardation, prematurity, prolonged labor, respiratory depression, hypoglycemia, and hyperbilirubinemia.[1018,1618] The incidence of retardation of uterine growth is low—probably less than 5%.[1650,1707] And no one really knows to what extent these unfortunate effects may be a consequence of the development of fetal distress in high-risk obstetric patients. Propranolol may cause neonatal bradycardia, hypoglycemia, and apnea, but these symptoms can be circumvented by discontinuing the drug at least 2 weeks before the estimated date of delivery.[1618]

Amitriptyline may be a safe drug to administer for migraine prevention in late pregnancy. No association between the use of tricyclic antidepressants and birth defects has been established, although the possibility of teratogenesis is still a matter of dispute.[1132] Neonatal dyspnea, cyanosis, tachypnea, irritability, tachycardia, and feeding difficulties have been seen in cases where the mother took tricyclic antidepressants until the time of birth.

The Nursing Migraineur

Treating a lactating woman with medication is problematical. A number of antimigraine drugs pass into mother's milk from the plasma and therefore have the potential to affect the nursing infant. Aspirin has been reported to produce metabolic acidosis in infants.[360] One case report has documented symptoms of ergotism in an infant exposed to ergotamine through breast feeding. On the basis of this case report, the American Academy of Pediatrics states that the use of ergots is contraindicated in nursing mothers.[32] Metoclopramide is also concentrated in human milk, but its effects in infants are not known. And although the effect of antidepressant drugs on nursing infants is unexplored, these agents do appear in human milk; they probably should not be prescribed. In contrast, some medications may be compatible with breast feeding because of a low milk-to-plasma ratio.[255] These drugs include acetaminophen, NSAIDs, codeine, β-blockers, and verapamil. They have not been reported to produce untoward signs and symptoms in infants or to have effects on lactation. Even so, consultation between the physician taking care of the mother and the baby's pediatrician is probably prudent in most cases. Nursing may have to be discontinued if the mother is crippled by migraine that cannot be treated effectively out of concern for her infant.

THE POSTMENOPAUSAL MIGRAINEUR

As reviewed in chapter 2, migraine is frequent in menopausal and postmenopausal women. In fact, some women develop migraine for the first time during this period of their lives. The problem is complicated by the hormonal changes that characterize the menopause and succeeding years, and by the changes in hormonal levels when estrogen is administered.

Hormonal replacement therapy is given widely to postmenopausal women not only to relieve menopausal symptoms, but also because of the value of estrogens in retarding osteoporosis and coronary artery disease. Some investigators who have treated postmenopausal women with estrogens report a reduction in the frequency of migraine headaches; others report increased frequency.[93,309,347,452,1144] The dose, type, and route of administration of hormone are presumably critical factors in determining outcome. To reduce the increased risk of endometrial cancer correlated with the administration of estrogens, these agents are typically prescribed in a cyclical fashion—taken for 21 days and then stopped for 7 days. In general, this type of cyclic estrogen therapy instituted at menopause has been shown to worsen headaches. The headaches are especially prominent during days in which estrogen is not administered. In contrast, daily administration of the hormone—with or without progesterone—may benefit migraineurs.[1144] The augmented risk of developing endometrial cancer associated with daily estrogen therapy can be offset to an extent by coupling the estrogen with a small, daily amount of progestin.

The frequency of migraine headaches appears to be inversely correlated with the dosage of estrogen used for replacement therapy.[480] The amount of estrogen should be reduced to the minimal dose that controls menopausal symptoms. Some women who are having problems with migraine benefit by changing the type of estrogen preparation. Thus, most women take equine-derived conjugated estrogen preparations combined with the androgen methyltestosterone (Premarin). Substitution of a simpler form of estrogen such as pure estradiol (Estrace), synthetic ethinyl estradiol (Estinyl), or estrone (Ogen) may alleviate migraine symptoms. Estrogen implants and transdermal patches may keep the concentration of estrogen more uniform,

and this may be beneficial in reducing the frequency of headache.

Discontinuation of replacement estrogens can result in a marked improvement in many migraineurs, although the improvement may take months to become apparent.[445,480,1144] Recommendations to terminate estrogen replacement are difficult to make, however, when many studies have shown that estrogen reduces by about 50% the risk of a coronary event in postmenopausal women.[122] In view of its benefits for the heart and the bones, as well as its ability to obviate severe menopausal symptoms, estrogen replacement therapy may be necessary for a migraineur. When such a decision is made, if possible, estrogens should be prescribed in a low dose in an uninterrupted manner.

MIGRAINE IN THE ELDERLY

Although the prevalence of migraine may decline with advancing age, migraine headaches are not uncommon in elderly patients.[2107] The treatment of migraine in elderly patients is, however, complicated by a variety of factors. As people age, they need smaller doses of medication; unless practitioners take account of age, there is danger of overmedication. The elderly also have a greater potential for the development of drug side effects. The overall incidence of adverse drug reactions is two to three times that found in young adults.[1464] Migraine treatment may also be complicated by the frequency of concomitant medical illnesses, the use of multiple medications, and a longer list of contraindictions to various medications. Some of these obstacles to treatment can be reduced if all an elderly patient's medical problems are identified, a careful drug history is taken, medications are prescribed one at a time in limited starting doses, and the dosages are raised very carefully and very slowly.[572] Effective and safe use of drugs in elderly patients is a matter of careful individualization of the therapeutic regimen and of constant vigilance.

The physiologic changes associated with aging may have pharmacologic consequences.[2157] For example, hepatic blood flow, renal function, serum albumin, lean muscle mass, and total body water decrease in the elderly, while body fat and plasma α_1-acid glycoprotein increase. The pharmacokinetics, binding, and excretion of drugs will be affected in various ways in geriatric migraineurs. Thus, decreased hepatic blood causes a modest increment in the bioavailability of propranolol.[2069] In contrast, the free concentration of weak bases such as propranolol that bind to α_1-acid glycoprotein in plasma may decrease because of the increased concentration of α_1-acid glycoprotein.[3] The sensitivity of cardiac β-receptors appears to decline with age, but whether similar effects occur in cranial blood vessels or neurons is not known.[2070]

A number of medications used for the symptomatic relief of migraine headaches may cause a great deal of difficulty in elderly patients (Table 12–4).

Ergotamine, for example, can cause vasoconstriction sufficient to produce signs and symptoms of vascular insufficiency in the extremities, heart, and brain. Problems of this type are rare in younger people. In older individuals, who may have preexistent—but asymptomatic—vascular disease, ergot derivatives may cause vascular insufficiency. In general, ergots should not be prescribed for patients older than age 60 years. Similarly, barbiturates, such as butalbital included in analgesic–sedative combination drugs, usually have no acute deleterious actions in younger patients, whereas in elderly individuals they may produce depression, confusion, and sometimes paradoxical excitement. These medications should not be used to treat migraine in the elderly. Care must be taken when administering sumatriptan to individuals who may have coronary artery disease. NSAIDs have an augmented chance of causing hyperkalemia, renal failure, or gastrointestinal hemorrhage in patients of advanced age.[190,833] Small elderly women seem to be most susceptible to the development

Table 12–4 CONTRAINDICATIONS TO ANTIMIGRAINE MEDICATION IN THE ELDERLY

Medication	Contraindication
ABORTIVE DRUGS	
Aspirin	Peptic ulcer
Acetaminophen	Renal or liver disease
Codeine	Constipation
Barbiturates	Mental slowing and confusion
Ergotamine, dihydroergotamine	Hypertension, peripheral atherosclerotic vascular disease, Raynaud's disease, coronary heart disease, cerebrovascular disease
Sumatriptan	Coronary artery disease
PROPHYLACTICS	
Tricyclic antidepressants	Glaucoma, prostatism, cardiac arrhythmias
β-Blockers	Heart block, bronchospasm, hypotension, heart failure, depression
Calcium channel blockers	Heart block, heart failure, peripheral edema, hypotension, constipation
Methysergide	Retroperitoneal and pleuropulmonary fibrosis, peripheral vascular disease, renal disease, ischemic cardiac disease, cardiac valvular disease

Adapted from Edmeads,[572] page 184, by courtesy of Marcel Dekker, Inc.

of gastritis and ulcer formation, with its attendant risk of hemorrhage. NSAIDs can also produce confusion and disorientation in the elderly. In contrast, isometheptene mucate appears to be tolerated by elderly migraineurs and does not bear many of the risks associated with ergots. It should be used with caution, however, in patients with cardiovascular or peripheral vascular disease.

Similar cautions attend the prescription of preventive medications. Adverse effects of β-blockers are more common in elderly migraineurs, but these agents still may be used with appropriate monitoring. The calcium channel blockers are useful agents. Anticholinergic side effects of cyclic antidepressants are especially troublesome in elderly patients. These side effects may be central (causing confusion, delirium, and cognitive impairment) or peripheral (causing dry mouth, blurred vision, tachycardia, urinary retention, and constipation). Older individuals are also more prone to develop cardiovascular complications, such as postural hypotension. Adverse reactions to cyclic antidepressants result in part from age-related alterations in hepatic demethylation pathways.[2] These changes limit the metabolism of such drugs as amitriptyline and imipramine. Accordingly, cyclic antidepressants should be started in very small dosages—no more than 10 mg/day. Moreover, they should not be administered as a single nightly dose because of an increased incidence of side effects when the entire dose is given at one time. The low frequency of anticholinergic and cardiovascular effects makes trazodone especially practical for use in the elderly.

SUMMARY

No one knows how many migraineurs are so mildly affected that they find self-medication with OTC products adequate. Other patients—whose attacks vary in frequency and range from miserable to excruciating—present themselves in great numbers to a variety of medical practitioners. Too many of them fail to receive a regimen of care individually suited to their needs. The chapters that deal with treatment address this failure. They aim at providing strategies for reducing migraine attacks through lifestyle changes or prophylactic medication. But no matter how successful these strategies may be, it is a rare migraineur who becomes totally headache-free. The chapter on treating the acute attack addresses this problem. As this book goes to press, many patients need emergency room care for acute attacks. As sumatriptan and other drugs grow in availability and acceptance, physicians may need to spend far less time on acute attacks. Many individuals may find it possible to treat themselves with great success. Headaches induced by the excessive use of analgesic medication, however, will probably continue to concern the physician. As long as commercials for analgesics encourage those with pounding heads and upset stomachs to use particular products, individuals with frequent headaches will continue to transform themselves into victims of the chronic daily headache syndrome. Physicians will continue to face individuals who need relief from suffering. And always, as a careful physician attempts to help a migraineur, attention must be given to the stage of life and the circumstances in which the patient lives.

IN CONCLUSION

This book has been devoted to discussion of migraine's clinical presentations and epidemiology, the basic aspects of its pathophysiology, a compassionate approach to the management of patients with migraine, and a modern discussion of the various pharmaceutical preparations used in the treatment of the disorder. However, despite much progress in our understanding of migraine in recent decades, a great deal about the diagnosis, definition, pathogenesis, and treatment of migraine remains unclear. I have concentrated on topics that seem to be of fundamental significance or that have important implications for future developments. Certain points bear repetition.

Reasonable diagnostic criteria have recently been formulated by the International Headache Society that offer more precise definitions of various migraine syndromes. The criteria reflect an effort toward making migraine diagnosis more objective despite a lack of either specific pathology or definitive diagnostic tests. Despite these advances in classification, skepticism is still voiced concerning the capacity to discriminate between migraine and tension-type headaches. Some epidemiologists and clinicians who have focused on the severity of head pain have indicated that a discrete classification and separation of tension-type and migraine headaches may not be possible. The head pain, however, is just one attribute of a complex affliction. Attacks of migraine can be divided into five stages—prodrome, aura, headache, resolution, and postdrome—each with its own characteristic spectrum of clinical phenomena and accompanying symptoms. In particular, it is now realized that premonitory or prodromal phenomena—often vague symptoms, poorly recognized by both patients and physicians—occur in many patients hours to days before the headache. The prodrome should be recognized by clinicians as part and parcel of the migraine attack. The clinician must also be cognizant that the aura of classic migraine can consist of poorly recognized cognitive and psychologic symptoms as well as the commonly recognized visual, sensory, and motor symptoms. In addition, the treating physician should realize that migraine is frequently accompanied by metabolic, autonomic, and systemic disturbances.

Advances have been made in understanding the complicated interactions between genetic substrate, external irritants and triggers, lifestyle practices, and medical conditions in the genesis of migraine attacks. Both internal and environmental elements are presumed to act on a susceptible nervous system predisposed to develop the malady by an inherited alteration in the biologic threshold to certain stimuli. Although neither the pattern of inheritance nor the intrinsic central defect is known, the management of patients with migraine headaches must include identification of trigger factors and removal of known precipitants. Different patients find their attacks triggered by different agents or processes. Practicing physicians should be able to educate their patients on how to circumvent these provocative factors.

Far too much effort has been expended in an effort to identify personality traits shared by the majority of patients with migraine and to assign the cause of migraine to a defect in character or psychologic makeup. Much evidence indicates that no one personality type is characteristic of migraineurs. Patients with migraine must be treated as individuals because different migraineurs vary considerably in the ways in which they deal both with the stresses that cause headaches and with the recurrent torment of migraine attacks.

Despite attempts to find an objective test that can be used to either make or confirm the diagnosis of migraine, no biologic marker for the affliction is presently available. In a similar vein, laboratory tests are not needed to make the diagnosis in the vast majority of patients with migraine. Although nonspecific abnormalities are seen with considerable frequency in computed tomographic scans, magnetic resonance imaging, electroencephalograms, visual evoked potentials, and thermograms, the abnormalities are rarely significant or diagnostic. Far too many examinations are performed on migraineurs simply because the tests are available.

The two principal, and seemingly competing, hypotheses of the causation of migraine—the vascular and neurogenic theories—are now conditionally integrated. A consensus has been evolving that the migraine process begins in the brain and then progresses to implicate extracerebral blood vessels. The mechanisms involved are, however, still the subject of debate.

Much work has focused on the decreases in cerebral blood flow observed during attacks of migraine with aura. The seemingly modest nature of the changes, the anterior expansion of the areas of low blood flow as attacks progress (so-called spreading oligemia), and the apparent failure of the expansion of the region of reduced blood flow to respect major cerebral arterial boundaries has led to much speculation that the alterations in blood flow are secondary to neuronal changes possibly caused by the process of spreading depression. But because of inherent inaccuracies in blood flow measurements caused by Compton scatter, alternative hypotheses are possible. Progressive ischemia in the territory of a major cerebral artery may be responsible for the data putatively demonstrating spread of an oligemic process.

Modifications in the firing pattern of monoamine-containing neurons in the brain stem have been causally implicated in the changes in blood flow accompanying bouts of migraine. Thus, stimulation of adrenergic neurons in the locus coeruleus and possibly adjacent areas of the brain stem in experimental animals has the capacity to reduce cerebral blood flow and to augment extracranial blood flow in ways that resemble those seen during blood flow examinations in humans during bouts of migraine. Activation of the serotonergic neurons in the raphe nuclei can induce vasodilatation. These monoaminergic nuclei are also involved in control of the endogenous pain-control system. A discharge of the neurons in brain stem nuclei may very well initiate parts of the migrainous process, but we do not yet know what activates the brain stem structures.

Important progress has been made in understanding the nociceptive mechanisms operating during migraine attacks. Much new evidence favors the idea that the final common link in the migrainous process involves the trigeminovascular system—the trigeminal nerve and its connections with the intracranial and extracranial vasculature. A process of neurogenic inflammation associated with vasodilatation and an increase in vascular permeability appears to follow activation of trigeminal sensory fibers and the subsequent release of vasoactive neuropeptides such as substance P, neurokinin A, and calcitonin gene-related peptide. The inflammatory process—initiated by peptide release and generated by the release or formation of multiple inflammatory mediators from mast cells, blood vessels, and tissue cells—is believed to sensitize trigeminal nociceptors and to produce and maintain the pain of migraine headache. Good evidence favors the idea that some effective medications used for the acute treatment of migraine (such as ergotamine, dihydroergotamine, and sumatriptan) block this process by preventing the release of neuropeptides, whereas other medications (such as nonsteroidal anti-inflammatory drugs [NSAIDs]) reduce inflammation by inhibiting the synthesis of prostanoids.

The association between serotonin and migraine has been buttressed by a substantial aggregate of circumstantial biochemical, pharmacologic, and anatomic evidence. Early efforts concentrated on changes in concentrations of platelet serotonin and urinary 5-hydroxyindoleacetic acid during a migraine attack. More recent work has focused on the actions of a number of agents that can either precipitate or relieve migraine attacks by effects variously believed to be exerted on serotonergic neurons or on serotonergic receptors located on trigeminovascular fibers, blood vessels, and platelets. The precise role of serotonin in migraine remains enigmatic, however, because both the locus of the alterations in serotonin activity that inaugurate the migrainous process and the exact site of action of serotonin is unknown.

Physicians treating patients with migraine must be aware of the disruptive consequences bouts of headache have on the individual's behavior. Family interactions, work, social activities, and leisure projects may all be curtailed. As a result, the management of patients afflicted with migraine requires much time, persistence, and understanding. Simply prescribing medications is insufficient. Adequate treatment requires support, counseling, and advice about behavior and lifestyle. The patient must be guided to make reasoned judgments about the elimination or alteration of precipitating factors and about changes of lifestyle. In large measure, however, the mainstay of migraine management consists of the judicious administration of appropriate medications. Ergots and NSAIDs are still the major drugs used for abortive or symptomatic treatment, but the use of sumatriptan will presumably modify that role in the future. The emergency room treatment of migraine should de-emphasize the traditional administration of parenteral narcotics and stress the use of dihydroergotamine, phenothiazines, and sumatriptan.

Recent emphasis has been appropriately placed on the complications and hazards of the excessive use of symptomatic antimigraine therapy. Treatment of recurrent migraine headaches is often complicated by the production of drug dependence and the development of a chronic daily headache. A headache–medication abuse cycle with daily headache and daily employment of OTC analgesics, prescribed analgesic–sedative preparations (containing butalbital), narcotics, or ergotamine can develop unless both physicians and patients understand the dangers of medication overuse.

A large number of effective medications—β-blockers, calcium channel blockers, antidepressants, antiserotonergics, and others—are now available for the prevention of migraine and should be used for all patients with frequent bouts of migraine or with headaches sufficiently incapacitating to disrupt the patient's life. Choice of medication is determined in large part by the presence of existing medical conditions and by potential side effects. Prophylactic drugs, when used appropriately in patients with frequent or disabling headaches, are capable of decreasing the frequency and severity of migraine in most migraineurs. Prophylactic drugs may be used alone or with behavioral techniques. Behavioral techniques, including biofeedback and relaxation therapy, are often exceedingly helpful in decreasing the frequency and intensity of bouts of migraine.

REFERENCES

1. Abdel-Halim MS, Ekstedt T, and Anggard E: Determination of prostaglandin $F_{2\alpha}$, E_2, D_2 and 6-keto F_1 alpha in human cerebrospinal fluid. Prostaglandins 17:405–409, 1979.

2. Abernethy DR, Greenblat DJ, and Shader RI: Imipramine and desipramine disposition in the elderly. J Pharmacol Exp Ther 232:183–188, 1985.

3. Abernethy DR and Kerznel L: Age effects on alpha-1-acid glycoprotein concentrations and imipramine plasma protein binding. J Am Geriatr Soc 32:705–708, 1984.

4. Abramson JH, Hopp C, and Epstein LM: Migraine and non-migrainous headaches: A community survey in Jerusalem. J Epidemiol Community Health 34:188–193, 1980.

5. Ad Hoc Committee on Classification of Headache. Classification of headache. JAMA 179:717–718, 1962.

6. Adams HE, Feuerstein M, and Fowler JL: Migraine headache: Review of parameters, etiology and intervention. Psychol Bull 87:217–237, 1980.

7. Adler CS and Adler SM: Biofeedback therapy for the treatment of headaches: A five-year follow-up. Headache 16:189–191, 1975.

8. Adler CS and Adler SM: Evaluating the psychological factors in headache. In Adler CS, Adler SM, and Packard RC (eds): Psychiatric Aspects of Headache. Williams & Wilkins, Baltimore, 1987, pp 70–83.

9. Adler CS and Adler SM: The migraine patient: Descriptive studies. In Adler CS, Adler SM, and Packard RC (eds): Psychiatric Aspects of Headache. Williams & Wilkins, Baltimore, 1987, pp 131–141.

10. Adler CS and Adler SM: Psychotherapy and the headache patient. In Adler CS, Adler SM, and Packard RC (eds): Psychiatric Aspects of Headache. Williams & Wilkins, Baltimore, 1987, pp 313–331.

11. Adly S, Straumanis J, and Chesson A: Fluoxetine prophylaxis of migraine. Headache 32:101–104, 1992.

12. Aellig WH: Influence of ergot compounds on compliance of superficial hand veins in man. Postgrad Med J 52 (Suppl 1):21–23, 1976.

13. Aellig WH: Influence of pizotifen and ergotamine on the venoconstrictor effect of 5-hydroxytryptamine and noradrenaline in man. Eur J Clin Pharmacol 25:759–762, 1983.

14. Aellig WH and Nüesch E: Comparative pharmacokinetic investigations with tritium-labelled ergot alkaloids after oral and intravenous administration in man. Int J Clin Pharmacol 15:106–112, 1977.

15. Affolter H, Burkard WP, and Pletscher A: Verapamil, an antagonist at 5-hydroxytryptamine receptors of human blood platelets. Eur J Pharmacol 108:157–167, 1985.

16. Ahles TA, Sikora TL, Sturgis ET, and Schaefer CA: The effect of postural variation on the electromyographic evaluation of tension headache and nonheadache control participants. Headache 26:353–355, 1986.

17. Aicardi J and Newton R: Clinical findings in children with occipital spike wave complexes suppressed by eye opening. In Andermann F and

Lugaresi E (eds): Migraine and Epilepsy. Butterworth, Boston, 1987, pp 111–124.

18. Akil H and Liebeskind JC: Monoaminergic mechanisms of stimulation-produced analgesia. Brain Res 94:279–296, 1975.

19. Alafaci C, Dhital KK, and Burnstock G: Purinergic mechanisms in cerebral circulation. In Olesen J and Edvinsson L (eds): Basic Mechanisms of Headache. Elsevier, Amsterdam, 1988, pp 163–176.

20. Ala-Hurula V, Myllylä V, Arvela P, Heikkilä J, Kärki N, and Hokkanen E: Systemic availability of ergotamine tartrate after oral, rectal and intramuscular administration. Eur J Clin Pharmacol 15:51–55, 1979.

21. Ala-Hurula V, Myllylä V, Arvela P, Heikkilä J, Kärki N, and Hokkanen E: Systemic availability of ergotamine tartrate after three successive doses and during continuous medication. Eur J Clin Pharmacol 16:355–360, 1979.

22. Ala-Hurula V, Myllylä V, Hokkanen E, and Tokola O: Tolfenamic acid and ergotamine abuse. Headache 21:240–242, 1981.

23. Ala-Hurula V, Myllylä V, and Hokkanen E: Ergotamine abuse: Results of ergotamine discontinuation, with special reference to the plasma concentrations. Cephalalgia 2:189–195, 1982.

24. Albers GW, Simon LT, Hamik A, and Peroutka SJ: Nifedipine versus propranolol for the initial prophylaxis of migraine. Headache 29:214–217, 1989.

25. Allan W: The inheritance of migraine. Arch Intern Med 13:590–599, 1928.

26. Allen JM, Todd N, Crockard HA, Schon F, Yeats JC, and Bloom SR: Presence of neuropeptide Y in human circle of Willis and its possible role in cerebral vasospasm. Lancet ii:550–552, 1984.

27. Alvarez WC: Can one cure migraine in women by inducing menopause? Report on forty-two cases. Mayo Clin Proc 15:380–382, 1940.

28. Alvarez WC: The migrainous personality and constitution; the essential features of the disease: A study of 500 cases. Am J Med Sci 213:1–8, 1947.

29. Alvarez WC: The migrainous scotoma as studied in 618 persons. Am J Ophthalmol 49:489–504, 1960.

30. AMA Drug Evaluations, 5th ed. American Medical Association, Chicago, 1983, pp. 67–167.

31. Amat G, Louis PJ, Loisy C, Centonze V, and Pelage S: Migraine and the mitral valve prolapse syndrome. Adv Neurol 33:27–29, 1982.

32. American Academy of Pediatrics Committee on Drugs: Transfer of drugs and other chemicals into human milk. Pediatrics 84:924, 1989.

33. Amery WK, Waelkens J, and Caers I: Dopaminergic mechanisms in premonitory phenomena. In Amery WK and Wauquier A (eds): The Prelude to the Migraine Attack. Baillière Tindall, London, 1986, pp 64–77.

34. Amery WK, Waelkens J, and Van den Bergh V: Migraine warnings. Headache 26:60–66, 1986.

35. Amery WK, Wauquier A, Van Nueten JM, De Clerch F, Van Reempts JV, and Janssen PAJ: The anti-migrainous pharmacology of flunarizine (r-14-950), a calcium antagonist. Drugs Expt Clin Res 7:1–10, 1981.

36. Amon I: Alkaloids. In Kuemmerle HP and Brendel K (eds): Clinical Pharmacology in Pregnancy. Thieme-Stratton, New York, 1984.

37. Ananth J and Luchins D: A review of combined tricyclic and MAOI therapy. Comprehensive Psychiatry 18:221–229, 1977.

38. Andermann F: Migraine–epilepsy relationships. Epilepsy Res 1:213–226, 1987.

39. Andersch B, Hahn L, Wendestam C, Ohman R, and Abrahamsson L: Treatment of premenstrual tension syndrome with bromocriptine. Acta Endocrinol 88:165–177, 1978.

40. Andersen AN, Larsen JF, Steenstrup OR, Svendstrup B, and Nielsen J: Effect of bromocriptine on the pre-

menstrual syndrome: A double-blind clinical trial. Br J Obstet Gynecol 84:370–374, 1977.

41. Andersen AR, Friberg L, Skyhøj Olsen TS, and Olesen J: Delayed hyperemia following hypoperfusion in classic migraine. Single photon emission computed tomographic demonstration. Arch Neurol 45:154–159, 1988.

42. Andersen AR, Tfelt-Hansen P, and Lassen NA: The effect of ergotamine and dihydroergotamine on cerebral blood flow in man. Stroke 18:120–123, 1987.

43. Andersen RK, Lund JP, and Puil E: Enkephalin and substance P effects related to trigeminal pain. Can J Physiol Pharmacol 56:216–222, 1978.

44. Anderson B, Heyman A, Whalen RE, and Saltzman HA: Migraine-like phenomena after decompression from hyperbaric environment. Neurology 15:1035–1040, 1965.

45. Anderson CD and Franks RD: Migraine and tension headache: Is there a physiological difference? Headache 21:63–71, 1981.

46. Andersson PG: Ergotamine headache. Headache 15:118–121, 1975.

47. Andersson PG, Dahl S, Hansen JH, et al.: Prophylactic treatment of classic and non-classic migraine with metoprolol—a comparison with placebo. Cephalalgia 3:207–212, 1983.

48. Andrasik F: Psychologic and behavioral aspects of chronic headache. Neurol Clin 8:961–976, 1990.

49. Andrasik F, Blanchard EB, Neff DF, and Rodichok LD: Biofeedback and relaxation training for chronic headache: A controlled comparison of booster treatments and regular contacts for long term maintenance. J Consult Clin Psych 52:609–615, 1984.

50. Andrasik F, Kabela E, Quinn S, Attanasio V, Blanchard EB, and Rosenblum EL: Psychological functioning of children who have recurrent migraine. Pain 34:43–52, 1988.

51. Andree TH, Mikuni M, and Meltzer HY: Effect of subchronic treatment with neuroleptics, imipramine, and the combination on serotonin receptor binding in rat cerebral cortex. Psychopharmacol Bull 20:349–353, 1984.

52. Andres KH, von During M, Muszynski K, and Schmidt RF: Nerve fibers and their terminals of the dura mater encephali of the rat. Anat Embryol 175:289–301, 1987.

53. Andreychuk T and Skriver C: Hypnosis and biofeedback in the treatment of migraine headache. Int J Clin Exp Hypn 23:172–183, 1975.

54. Angus-Leppan H, Lambert GA, Boers P, Zagami AS, and Olausson B: Craniovascular nociceptive pathways relay in the upper cervical spinal cord in the cat. Neuroscience Lett 137:203–206, 1992.

55. Ansell E, Fazzone T, Festenstein R, Johanson ES, Thavapalan M, and Wilkinson M: Nimodipine in migraine prophylaxis. Cephalalgia 8:269–272, 1988.

56. Anselmi B, Baldi E, Casacci F, and Salmon S: Endogenous opioids in cerebrospinal fluid and blood in idiopathic headache sufferers. Headache 20:294–299, 1980.

57. Anthony M: The mechanisms underlying migraine. Med J Aust (Suppl) 2:11–15, 1972.

58. Anthony M: Plasma free fatty acids and prostaglandin E_1 in migraine and stress. Headache 16:58–63, 1976.

59. Anthony M: Biochemical indices of sympathetic activity in migraine. Cephalalgia 1:83–89, 1981.

60. Anthony M: Unilateral migraine or occipital neuralgia? In Clifford Rose F (ed): New Advances in Headache Research. Smith-Gordon, London, 1989, pp 39–43.

61. Anthony M and Hinterberger H: Amine turnover in migraine. Proc Aust Assoc Neurologists 12:43–47, 1975.

62. Anthony M, Hinterberger H, and Lance JW: Plasma serotonin in migraine and stress. Arch Neurol 16:544–552, 1967.

63. Anthony M, Hinterberger H, and

Lance JW: The possible relationship of serotonin to the migraine syndrome. Res Clin Stud Headache 2:29–59, 1969.

64. Anthony M and Lance JW: Indomethacin in migraine. Med J Aust 1:56–57, 1968.

65. Anthony M and Lance JW: Monoamine oxidase inhibitors in the treatment of migraine. Arch Neurol 21:263–268, 1969.

66. Anthony M and Lance JW: Histamine and serotonin in cluster headache. Arch Neurol 25:225–231, 1971.

67. Anthony M and Lance JW: The role of serotonin in migraine. In Pearce J (ed): Modern Topics in Migraine. Heinemann, London, 1975, pp 107–123.

68. Anthony M, Lance JW, and Somerville B: A comparative trial of pindolol, clonidine and carbamazepine in the interval therapy of migraine. Med J Aust 1:1343–1346, 1972.

69. Anthony M, Lord GDA, and Lance JW: Controlled trials of cimetidine in migraine and cluster headache. Headache 18:261–264, 1978.

70. Antonaci F and Sjaastad O: Chronic paroxysmal hemicrania (CPH): A review of clinical manifestations. Headache 29:648–656, 1989.

71. Apesos J and Foise R: Lower extremity arterial insufficiency after long-term methysergide maleate therapy. Arch Surg 114:964–967, 1979.

72. Apley J and Hale B: Children with recurrent abdominal pain: How do they grow up? Br Med J iii:7–9, 1973.

73. Appel S, Kuritzky A, Zahavi I, Zigelman M, and Akselrod S: Evidence for instability of the autonomic nervous system in patients with migraine headache. Headache 32:10–17, 1992.

74. Appenzeller O: Barogenic headache. In Clifford Rose F (ed): Handbook of Clinical Neurology, Vol 4. Elsevier, Amsterdam, 1986, pp 395–404.

75. Appenzeller O: Reflex vasomotor function: Clinical and experimental studies in migraine. Res Clin Stud Headache 6:160–166, 1978.

76. Appenzeller O: Migraine and cluster headache. In Johnson RT (ed): Current Therapy in Neurologic Disease. Decker, Toronto, 1987, pp 59–61.

77. Appenzeller O, Atkinson RA, and Standefer JC: Serum β-endorphin in cluster headache and common migraine. In Clifford Rose F and Zilkha KJ (eds): Progress in Migraine Research. Pitman, London, 1981, pp 106–109.

78. Arbab MAR, Delgado T, Wiklund L, and Svendgaard NA: Brain stem terminations of the trigeminal and upper spinal ganglia innervation of the cerebrovascular system: WGA-HRP transganglionic study. J Cereb Blood Flow Metab 8:54–63, 1988.

79. Arbab MAR, Wiklund L, and Svendgaard NA: Origin and distribution of cerebral vascular innervation from superior cervical, trigeminal and spinal ganglia investigated with retrograde and anterograde WGA-HRP tracing in the rat. Neuroscience 19:695–708, 1986.

80. Aring CD: The migrainous scintillating scotoma. JAMA 220:519–522, 1972.

81. Aronoff GM and Evans WO: Doxepin as an adjunct in the treatment of chronic pain. J Clin Psychiat 43:42–47, 1982.

82. Arthur GP and Hornabrook RW: The treatment of migraine with BC-105 (pizotifen). A double-blind trial. NZ Med J 73:5–9, 1971.

83. Aselton P, Jick H, Milunsky A, Hunter JR, and Stergachis A: First trimester drug use and congenital disorders. Obstet Gynecol 65:451–455, 1985.

84. Asherson RA: Anti-phospholipid antibodies: Clinical complications reported in the medical literature. In Harris EN, Exner TRR, Hughes GRV, and Asherson RA (eds): Phospholipid Binding Antibodies. CRC, Boca Raton, FL, 1991, pp 387–402.

85. Askmark H, Lundberg PO, and Olesson S: Drug-related headache. Headache 29:441–444, 1989.

86. Aston-Jones G and Bloom FE: Activity of norepinephrine-containing locus coeruleus neurons in behaving

rats anticipates fluctuations in the sleep-waking cycle. J Neuroscience 1:876–886, 1981.

87. Aston-Jones G, Ennis M, Pieribone VA, Nickell WT, and Shipley MT: The brain nucleus locus coeruleus: Restricted afferent control of a broad efferent network. Science 234:734–737, 1986.

88. Aston-Jones G, Shipley MT, Chouvet G, et al.: Afferent regulation of locus coeruleus neurons: Anatomy, physiology and pharmacology. Prog Brain Res 88:47–75, 1991.

89. Atkinson RA and Appenzeller O: Headache in small vessel disease of the brain: A study of patients with systemic lupus erythematosus. Headache 15:198–201, 1975.

90. Aubineau P, Henry F, Reynier-Rebuffel AM, Callebert J, Issertial O, and Seylaz J: Mast cell degranulation and 5-HT secretion are induced by neuropeptides in rat dura matter [sic] and in rabbit cerebral vessels. Cephalalgia 11 (Suppl 11):11, 1991.

91. Aubineau P, Sercombe R, and Seylaz J: Parasympathomimetic influence of carbachol on local cerebral blood flow in the rabbit by a direct vasodilator action and an inhibition of the sympathetic-mediated vasoconstriction. Br J Pharmacol 68:449–459, 1980.

92. Avorn J, Everitt DE, and Weiss S: Increased antidepressant use in patients prescribed beta blockers. JAMA 255:357–360, 1986.

93. Aylward M, Holly F, and Parker RJ: An evaluation of clinical response to piperazine oestrone sulphate (Harmogen) in menopausal patients. Curr Med Res Opin 2:417–423, 1974.

94. Babb RR and Eckman PB: Abdominal epilepsy. JAMA 222:65–66, 1972.

95. Bach FW, Jensen K, Blegvad N, Fenger M, Jordal R, and Olesen J: β-endorphin and ACTH in plasma during attacks of common and classic migraine. Cephalalgia 5:177–182, 1985.

96. Bademosi O and Osuntokun BO: Pizotifen in the management of migraine. Practitioner 220:325–326, 1978.

97. Badran RH, Weir RJ, and McGuiness JB: Hypertension and headache. Scott Med J 15:48–51, 1970.

98. Baier WK: Genetics of migraine and migraine accompagnée: A study of eighty-one children and their families. Neuropediatrics 16:84–91, 1985.

99. Bakal DA: The Psychobiology of Chronic Headache. Springer, New York, 1982.

100. Bakal DA and Kaganov JA: Muscle contraction and migraine headache: Psychophysiologic comparison. Headache 17:208–215, 1977.

101. Bakal DA and Kaganov JA: Symptom characteristics of chronic and non-chronic headache sufferers. Headache 19:285–289, 1979.

102. Baker HL: Computerized transaxial tomography (EMI scan) in the diagnosis of cerebral vascular disease. Experience at the Mayo Clinic. In Whisnat JP (ed): Cerebral Vascular Diseases. Grune & Stratton, New York, 1975, pp 195–215.

103. Bakke M, Tfelt-Hansen P, Olesen J, and Møller E: Action of some pericranial muscles during provoked attacks of common migraine. Pain 14:121–135, 1982.

104. Baldi E, Salmon S, Anselmi B, et al.: Intermittent hypoendorphinemia in migraine attack. Cephalalgia 2:77–81, 1982.

105. Baldissera F, Broggi G, and Mancia M: Primary afferent depolarization of trigeminal fibers induced by stimulation of brain stem and peripheral nerves. Experientia 23:398, 1967.

106. Baldrati A, Bini L, D'Alessandro R, et al.: Analysis of outcome predictors of migraine towards chronicity. Cephalalgia 5 (Suppl 2):195–199, 1985.

107. Balla JI: The late whiplash syndrome. Aust NZ J Surg 50:610–614, 1980.

108. Balla J and Iansek R: Headaches arising from disorders of the cervical spine. In Hopkins A (ed): Headache: Problems in Diagnosis and Treatment. WB Saunders, London, 1988, pp 241–267.

109. Bana DS and Graham JR: Observations on prodromes of classic migraine in a headache clinic population. Headache 26:216–219, 1986.

110. Bana DS, Yap AU, and Graham JR: Headache during hemodialysis. Headache 12:1–14, 1972.

111. Banerjee M and Findley L: Propranolol in the treatment of acute migraine attacks. Cephalalgia 11:193–196, 1991.

112. Barabas G, Ferrari M, and Matthews WS: Childhood migraine and somnambulism. Neurology 33:948–949, 1983.

113. Barbiroli B, Montagna P, Cortelli P, et al.: Complicated migraine studied by phosphorus magnetic resonance spectroscopy. Cephalalgia 10:263–272, 1990.

114. Barbiroli B, Montagna P, Cortelli P, et al.: Abnormal brain and muscle energy metabolism shown by ^{31}P magnetic resonance spectroscopy in patients affected by migraine with aura. Neurology 42:1209–1214, 1992.

115. Bardwell A and Trott JA: Stroke in migraine as a consequence of propranolol. Headache 27:381–383, 1987.

116. Barkley GL, Tepley N, Nagel-Leiby S, Moran JE, Simkins RT, and Welch KMA: Magnetoencephalographic studies of migraine. Headache 30:428–434, 1990.

117. Barlow CF: Migraine in childhood. Res Clin Stud Headache 5:34–46, 1978.

118. Barlow CF: Headaches and Migraine in Childhood. Lippincott, Philadelphia, 1984.

119. Barnes JH: The physiology and pharmacology of emesis. Mol Aspects Med 7:397–508, 1984.

120. Barolin GS: Migraine and epilepsies—A relationship? Epilepsia 7:53–66, 1966.

121. Barré N: Sur un syndrome sympathique cervical postérieur et sa cause fréquente: l'arthrite cervicale. Rev Neurol (Paris) 33:1246–1248, 1926.

122. Barrett-Connor E: Risks and benefits of replacement estrogen. Annu Rev Med 43:239–251, 1992.

123. Barrie MA, Fox WR, Weatherall M, and Wilkinson MIP: Analysis of symptoms of patients with headaches and their response to treatment with ergot derivatives. Q J Med 37:319–336, 1968.

124. Barrie M and Jowett A: A pharmacological investigation of cerebrospinal fluid from patients with migraine. Brain 90:785–794, 1967.

125. Bartleson JD: Transient and persistent neurologic manifestations of migraine. Stroke 15:383–386, 1984.

126. Bartleson JD, Swanson JW, and Whisnat JP: A migrainous syndrome with cerebrospinal fluid pleocytosis. Neurology 31:1257–1262, 1981.

127. Bartschi-Rochaix W: Headache of cervical origin. In Vinkin PJ and Bruyn GW (eds): Handbook of Clinical Neurology, Vol 5. North-Holland, Amsterdam, 1968, pp 192–203.

128. Basbaum AI, Clanton CH, and Fields HL: Three bulbospinal pathways from the rostral medulla of the cat: An autoradiographic study of pain-modulating systems. J Comp Neurol 178:209–224, 1978.

129. Basbaum AI and Fields HL: Endogenous pain control systems: Brainstem spinal pathways and endorphin circuitry. Annu Rev Neuroscience 7:309–338, 1984.

130. Basbaum AI, Marley NJE, O'Keefe J, and Clanton CH: Reversal of morphine and stimulus-produced analgesia by subtotal spinal cord lesions. Pain 3:43–56, 1977.

131. Basbaum AI, Moss MS, and Glazer EJ: Opiate and stimulation produced analgesia: The contribution of the monamines. Adv Pain Res Ther 5:323–329, 1983.

132. Basser LS: The relation of migraine and epilepsy. Brain 92:285–300, 1969.

133. Bateman DN, Khan, C and Davies DS: Concentration effect studies with oral metoclopramide. Br J Clin Pharmacol 8:179–182, 1980.

134. Bateman DN, Khan C, and Davies DS: The pharmacokinetics of metoclopramide in man with observations in the dog. J Clin Pharmacol 9:371–377, 1980.

135. Battistella PA, Ruffilli R, Moro R, et al.: A placebo-controlled crossover trial of nimodipine in pediatric migraine. Headache 30:264–268, 1990.

136. Baumgartner C, Wessely P, Bingöl C, Maly J, and Holzner F: Longterm prognosis of analgesic withdrawal in patients with drug-induced headaches. Headache 29:510–514, 1989.

137. Baumgartner G and Rowen R: Clonidine vs. chlordiazepoxide in the management of acute alcohol withdrawal syndrome. Arch Intern Med 147:1223–1226, 1987.

138. Beasley CM, Mascia DN, and Potvin JH: Fluoxetine: A review of receptor and functional effects and their clinical implications. Psychopharmacology 107:1–10, 1992.

139. Beaver WT: Analgesic combinations. In Lasagna L (ed): Combination Drugs: Their Use and Regulation. Stratton, New York, 1975, pp 52–72.

140. Beaver WT: Aspirin and acetaminophen as constituents of analgesic combinations. Arch Intern Med 141:293–300, 1981.

141. Beaver WT: Combination analgesics. Am J Med 77:38–53, 1984.

142. Beck PW and Handwerker HO: Bradykinin and serotonin effects on various types of cutaneous nerve fibers. Pfluegers Arch 347:209–222, 1974.

143. Beckham JC, Krug LM, Penzien DB, et al.: The relationship of ovarian steroids, headache activity and menstrual distress: A pilot study with female migraineurs. Headache 32:292–297, 1992.

144. Beckstead RM and Norgren R: An autoradiographic examination of the central distribution of the trigeminal, facial, glossopharyngeal, and vagal nerves in the monkey. J Comp Neurol 184:455–472, 1979.

145. Behan PO and Connelly K: Prophylaxis of migraine: A comparison between naproxen sodium and pizotifen. Headache 26:237–239, 1986.

146. Behan PO and Reid M: Propranolol in the treatment of migraine. Practitioner 224:201–204, 1980.

147. Behan WMH, Behan PO, and Durward WF: Complement studies in migraine. Headache 21:55–57, 1981.

148. Behbehani MM and Fields HL: Evidence that an excitatory connection between periaqueductal gray and the nucleus raphe magnus mediates stimulation-produced analgesia. Brain Res 170:85–93, 1979.

149. Behrens MM: Headache associated with disorders of the eye. Med Clin North Am 62:507–521, 1978.

150. Behrman S: Migraine as a sequela of blunt head trauma. Injury 9:74–76, 1977.

151. Beitz AJ: The organization of afferent projections to the midbrain periaqueductal gray of the rat. Neuroscience 7:133–159, 1982.

152. Beitz AJ, Wells WE, and Shepard RD: The location of brainstem neurons which project bilaterally to the spinal trigeminal nuclei as demonstrated by the double fluorescent retrograde tracer technique. Brain Res 258:305–312, 1983.

153. Belgrade MJ, Ling LJ, Schleevogt MB, Ettinger MG, and Ruiz E: Comparison of single-dose meperidine, butorphanol, and dihydroergotamine in the treatment of vascular headache. Neurology 39:590–592, 1989.

154. Bell R, Montoya D, Schuaib A, and Lee MA: A comparative trial of three agents in the treatment of acute migraine headache. Ann Emerg Med 19:1079–1082, 1990.

155. Bell WE: Orofacial Pains: Classification, Diagnosis, Management, 3rd ed. Year Book, Chicago, 1985.

156. Bell WE, Joynt RJ, and Sahs AL: Low spinal fluid pressure syndromes. Neurology 10:512–521, 1960.

157. Bellavance AJ and Meloche JP: A comparative study of naproxen sodium, pizotyline and placebo in migraine prophylaxis. Headache 30:710–715, 1990.

158. Belton CH: Migraine with facial oedema: Some general practitioner observations. NZ Med J 58:578–584, 1959.

159. Benedek-Jaszmann LJ and Hearn-Sturtevant MDH: Premenstrual tension and functional infertility. Aetiology and treatment. Lancet *i*:1095, 1976.

160. Benedict CR and Robertson D: Angina pectoris and sudden death in the absence of atherosclerosis following ergotamine therapy for migraine. Am J Med 67:177–178, 1979.

161. Benna P, Bianco C, Costa P, Piazza D, and Bergamasco B: Visual evoked potentials and brain-stem auditory evoked potentials in migraine and transient ischemic attacks. Cephalalgia 5 (Suppl 2):53–58, 1985.

162. Bennett GJ and Mayer DJ: Inhibition of spinal cord interneurons by narcotic microinjection and focal electrical stimulation in the periaqueductal central gray matter. Brain Res 172:243–257, 1979.

163. Benson H, Klemchuk HP, and Graham JR: The usefulness of the relaxation response in the therapy of headache. Headache 14:49–52, 1974.

164. Berger JR: Neurologic complications of human immunodeficiency virus infection. Postgrad Med J 81:72–79, 1987.

165. Bergeron RT and Wood EH: Oral contraceptives and cerebrovascular complications. Radiology 92:231–238, 1969.

166. Bergstrom DA and Kellar KJ: Adrenergic and serotonergic receptor binding in rat brain after chronic desmethylimipramine treatment. J Pharmacol Exp Ther 209:256–261, 1979.

167. Bergström S, Carlson LA, Ekelund LG, and Orö L: Cardiovascular and metabolic response to infusions of prostaglandin E_1 and to simultaneous infusions of noradrenaline and prostaglandin E_1 in man. Acta Physiol Scand 64:332–339, 1965.

168. Berne RM, Rubio R, and Curnish RR: Release of adenosine from ischemic brain: Effect on cerebral vascular resistance and incorporation into cerebral adenine nucleotides. Circ Res 35:262–271, 1974.

169. Bernstein DA and Borkovec TD: Progressive Relaxation Training: A Manual for the Helping Professions. Research Press, Champaign, IL, 1973.

170. Berstad JR: Total 5-hydroxyindoles in blood related to migraine attacks. Acta Neurol Scand 54:293–300, 1976.

171. Besson JM and Chaouch A: Peripheral and spinal mechanisms of nociception. Physiol Rev 67:67–186, 1987.

172. Bevan JA, Buga GM, Jope CA, Jope RS, and Moritoki H: Further evidence for a muscarinic component to the neural vasodilator innervation of cerebral and cranial extracerebral arteries of the cat. Circ Res 51:421–429, 1982.

173. Bickerstaff ER: Impairment of consciousness in migraine. Lancet *ii*:1057–1059, 1961.

174. Bickerstaff ER: The basilar artery and the migraine-epilepsy syndrome. Proc Roy Soc Med 55:167–169, 1962.

175. Bickerstaff ER: Ophthalmoplegic migraine. Rev Neurol (Paris) 110:582–588, 1964.

176. Bickerstaff ER: Neurological Complications of Oral Contraceptives. Clarendon Press, Oxford, 1975.

177. Bickerstaff ER: Basilar artery migraine. In Clifford Rose F (ed): Handbook of Clinical Neurology, Vol 4. Elsevier, Amsterdam, 1986, pp 135–140.

178. Bickerstaff ER: Migraine variants and complications. In Blau JN (ed): Migraine. Clinical and Research Aspects. Johns Hopkins University Press, Baltimore, 1987, pp 55–75.

179. Biesold D, Inanami O, Sato A, and Sato Y: Stimulation of the nucelus basalis of Meynert increases cerebral cortical blood flow in rats. Neuroscience Lett 98:39–44, 1989.

180. Biggs M and Johnson ES: The autonomic nervous system and migraine pathogenesis. In Amery WK, Van Neuten JM, and Wauquier A (eds):

The Pharmacological Basis of Migraine Therapy. Pitman, London, 1984, pp 99–107.

181. Bigley GK and Sharp FR: Reversible alexia without agraphia due to migraine. Arch Neurol 40:114–115, 1983.

182. Bill A and Linder J: Sympathetic control of cerebral blood flow in acute arterial hypertension. Acta Physiol Scand 96:114–121, 1976.

183. Bille B: Migraine in school children. Acta Pediatr Scand 51 (Suppl 136):3–151, 1962.

184. Bille B: Migraine in childhood and its prognosis. Cephalalgia 1:71–75, 1981.

185. Bille B, Ludvigsson J, and Sanner G: Prophylaxis of migraine in children. Headache 17:61–63, 1977.

186. Bird N, MacGregor A, and Wilkinson MIP: Ice cream headache—site, duration, and relationship to migraine. Headache 32:35–38, 1992.

187. Birrell GJ, McQueen DS, Iggo A, and Grubb BD: The effects of 5-HT on articular sensory receptors in normal and arthritic rats. Br J Pharmacol 101:715–721, 1990.

188. Birt D: Headaches and head pain associated with disease of the ear, nose and throat. Med Clin North Am 62:523–531, 1978.

189. Bittman B and Emanuele S: Fluoxetine: Side effects and efficacy in a headache population. Headache Quarterly, Current Treatment and Research 3:82–85, 1992.

190. Blackshear JL, Davidman M, and Stillman MT: Identification of risk for renal insufficiency for nonsteroidal anti-inflammatory drugs. Arch Intern Med 143:1130–1134, 1983.

191. Bladin PF: The association of benign rolandic epilepsy with migraine. In Andermann F and Lugaresi E (eds): Migraine and Epilepsy. Butterworth, Boston, 1987, pp 145–152.

192. Blanchard EB: Long-term effects of behavioral treatment of chronic headache. Behavior Therapy 18:375–385, 1987.

193. Blanchard EB: Psychological treatment of benign headache disorders. J Consult Clin Psychol 60:537–551, 1992.

194. Blanchard EB and Andrasik F: Psychological assessment and treatment of headache: Recent developments and emerging issues. J Consult Clin Psychol 50:859–879, 1982.

195. Blanchard EB and Andrasik F: Biofeedback treatment of vascular headache. In Hatch JP, Fisher JG, and Rugh JD (eds): Biofeedback Studies and Clinical Efficacy. Plenum, New York, 1987, pp 1–79.

196. Blanchard EB, Andrasik F, Ahles TA, Teders SJ, and O'Keefe DM: Migraine and tension headache: A meta-analytic review. Behavior Therapy 11:613–621, 1980.

197. Blanchard EB, Andrasik F, Evans DD, and Hillhouse J: Biofeedback and relaxation treatments for headache in the elderly: A caution and a challenge. Biofeedback and Self-Regulation 10:69–73, 1985.

198. Blanchard EB, Andrasik F, Neff DF, et al.: Biofeedback and relaxation training with three kinds of headache: Treatment effects and their prediction. J Consult Clin Psychol 50:562–575, 1982.

199. Blanchard EB, Applebaum KA, Guarnieri P, Morrill B, and Dentinger MP: Five year prospective follow-up on the treatment of chronic headache with biofeedback and/or relaxation. Headache 27:580–583, 1987.

200. Blanchard EB, Theobald DE, Williamson DA, Silver BV, and Bronn DA: Temperature biofeedback in the treatment of migraine headaches: A controlled evaluation. Arch Gen Psychiatry 35:581–588, 1978.

201. Blank NK and Rieder MJ: Paradoxical response to propranolol in migraine. Lancet ii:1336, 1973.

202. Blau JN: Migraine: A vasomotor instability of the meningeal circulation. Lancet ii:1136–1139, 1978.

203. Blau JN: Migraine prodromes separated from the aura: Complete migraine. Br Med J 281:658–660, 1980.

204. Blau JN: Resolution of migraine attacks: Sleep and the recovery phase. J Neurol Neurosurg Psychiatry 45:223–226, 1982.

205. Blau JN: Pathogenesis of migraine attack: Initiation. J R Coll Physicians Lond 19:166–168, 1985.

206. Blau JN: Headache: History, examination, differential diagnosis and special investigations. In Clifford Rose F (ed): Handbook of Clinical Neurology, Vol 4. Elsevier, Amsterdam, 1986, pp 43–58.

207. Blau JN: Adult migraine: The patient observed. In Blau JN (ed): Migraine. Clinical and Research Aspects. Johns Hopkins University Press, Baltimore, 1987, pp 3–30.

208. Blau JN: A clinicotherapeutic approach to migraine. In Blau JN (ed): Migraine. Clinical and Research Aspects. Johns Hopkins University Press, Baltimore, 1987, pp 185–213.

209. Blau JN: A note on migraine and the nose. Headache 28:495, 1988.

210. Blau JN: The nature of migraine: Do we need to invoke slow neurochemical processes? In Sandler M and Collins GM (eds): Migraine: A Spectrum of Ideas. Oxford University Press, Oxford, 1990, pp 4–17.

211. Blau JN: Migraine postdromes: Symptoms after attacks. Cephalalgia 11:229–231, 1991.

212. Blau JN and Cumings JN: Method of precipitating and preventing some migraine attacks. Br Med J ii:1242–1243, 1966.

213. Blau JN and Davis E: Small blood-vessels in migraine. Lancet ii:740–742, 1970.

214. Blau JN and Dexter SL: The site of pain origin during migraine attacks. Cephalalgia 1:143–147, 1981.

215. Blau JN and Diamond S: Dietary factors in migraine precipitation: The physician's view. Headache 25:184–187, 1985.

216. Blau JN and Engel H: Episodic paroxysmal hemicrania: A further case and review of the literature. J Neurol Neurosurg Psychiatry 53:343–344, 1990.

217. Blau JN, Horsfield D, Quick J, and Cumings JN: The production of migraine and biochemical changes in induced attacks. In Smith R (ed): Background to Migraine. Heinemann, London, 1967, pp 145–153.

218. Blau JN and Solomon F: Smell and other sensory disturbances in migraine. J Neurol 232:275–276, 1985.

219. Blau JN and Thavapalan M: Preventing migraine: A study of precipitating factors. Headache 28:481–483, 1988.

220. Blier P and de Montigny C: Serotonergic but not noradrenergic neurons in rat central nervous system adapt to long-term treatment with monoamine oxidase inhibitors. Neuroscience 16:949–955, 1985.

221. Blumenthal L and Fuchs M: Current therapy for headaches. Southern Med J 56:503–508, 1963.

222. Blumer D and Heilbronn M: Chronic pain as a variant of depressive disease: The pain-prone disorder. J Nerv Ment Dis 170:381–406, 1982.

223. Boccuni M, Alessandri M, Fusco BM, and Cangi F: The pressor hyperresponsiveness to phenylephrine unmasks sympathetic hypofunction in migraine. Cephalalgia 9:239–245, 1989.

224. Boccuni M, Fanciullacci M, Michelacci S, and Sicuteri F: Impairment of postural reflex in migraine: Possible role of dopamine receptors. In Corsini GU and Gessa GL (eds): Apomorphine and Other Dopamimetics. Raven, New York, 1981, pp 267–273.

225. Bodian M: Transient loss of vision following head trauma. NY J Med 64:916–920, 1964.

226. Bogduk N: The anatomy of occipital neuralgia. Clin Exp Neurol 17:167–184, 1981.

227. Bogduk N: The anatomical basis for cervicogenic headache. J Manipulative Physiol Ther 15:67–70, 1992.

228. Bogousslavsky J, Dizerens K, Regli F, and Despland PA: Opercular

cheiro-oral syndrome. Arch Neurol 48:658–661, 1991.

229. Bogousslavsky J and Regli F: Ischemic stroke in adults younger than 30 years of age. Cause and prognosis. Arch Neurol 44:479–482, 1987.

230. Bogousslavsky J, Regli F, Van Melle G, Payot M, and Uske A: Migraine stroke. Neurology 38:223–227, 1988.

231. Boisen E: Strokes in migraine: Report on seven strokes associated with severe migraine attacks. Dan Med Bull 22:100–106, 1975.

232. Boisen E, Deth S, Hubbe P, Jansen J, Klee A, and Leunbach G: Clonidine in the prophylaxis of migraine. Acta Neurol Scand 58:288–295, 1978.

233. Bolmsjö M; Hemisphere cross talk and signal overlapping in bilateral regional cerebral blood flow measurements using xenon 133. Eur J Nucl Med 9:1–5, 1984.

234. Bonuso S, DiStasio ED, Marano E, Sorge F, and Leo A: Sublingual flunarizine: A new effective management of the migraine attack. A comparison versus ergotamine. Headache 26:227–230, 1986.

235. Bonvento G, LaCombe P, and Seylaz J: Effects of electrical stimulation of the dorsal raphe nucleus on local cerebral blood flow in the rat. J Cereb Blood Flow Metab 9:251–255, 1989.

236. Book HE: Is empathy cost-efficient? Am J Psychother 45:21–30, 1991.

237. Borgensen SE, Nielsen JL, and Moller CE: Prophylactic treatment of migraine with propranolol. Acta Neurol Scand 50:651–656, 1974.

238. Borges LF and Moskowitz MA: Do intracranial and extracranial trigeminal afferents represent divergent axon collaterals? Neuroscience Lett 35:265–270, 1983.

239. Bousser MG and Conard J: TIAs, migraine and platelets. Headache 27:552, 1987.

240. Bowker RM, Steinbusch HWM, and Coulter JD: Serotonergic and peptidergic projections to the spinal cord demonstrated by a combined retrograde HRP histochemical and immunocytochemical staining method. Brain Res 211:412–417, 1981.

241. Boyle R, Behan PO, and Sutton JA: A correlation between severity of migraine and delayed gastric emptying measured by an epigastric impedance method. Br J Clin Pharmacol 30:405–409, 1990.

242. Bradfield JM: A new look at the use of ergotamine. Drugs 12:449–453, 1976.

243. Bradshaw P and Parsons M: Hemiplegic migraine, a clinical study. Q J Med 34:65–85, 1965.

244. Braff MM and Rosner S: Trauma of the cervical spine as cause of chronic headache. J Trauma 15:441–446, 1975.

245. Brandt KD and Lessell S: Migrainous phenomena in systemic lupus erythematosus. Arthritis Rheum 21:7–16, 1978.

246. Brant-Zawadzki M, Fein G, Van Dyke C, Kieman R, Davenport L, and de Groot J: MR imaging of the aging brain: Patchy white matter lesions and dementia. AJNR 6:675–682, 1985.

247. Brazil P and Friedman AP: Craniovascular studies in headache. A report and analysis of pulse volume tracings. Neurology 6:96–102, 1956.

248. Brenner C, Friedman AP, and Carter S: Psychologic factors in the etiology and treatment of chronic headache. Psychosom Med 11:53–56, 1949.

249. Breslau N: Migraine, suicidal ideation, and suicide attempts. Neurology 42:392–395, 1992.

250. Breslau N and Davis GC: Migraine, major depression and panic disorder: A prospective epidemiologic study of young adults. Cephalalgia 12:85–90, 1992.

251. Breslau N, Davis GC, and Andreski P: Migraine, psychiatric disorders, and suicide attempts: An epidemiologic study of young adults. Psychiatry Res 37:11–23, 1991.

252. Brewerton TD and George MS: A study of the seasonal variation of mi-

graine. Headache 30:511–513, 1990.

253. Brewerton TD, Murphy DL, Mueller EA, and Jimerson DC: Induction of migrainelike headaches by the serotonin agonist m-chlorophenylpiperazine. Clin Pharmacol Ther 43:605–609, 1988.

254. Brewis M, Poskanzer DC, Rolland C, and Miller H: Neurological disease in an English city. Acta Neurol Scand 42 (Suppl 24):1–89, 1966.

255. Briggs GR, Freeman RK, and Yaffe SJ: Drugs in Pregnancy and Lactation, 3rd ed. Williams & Wilkins, Baltimore, 1990.

256. Briggs JF and Belloms J: Precordial migraine. Dis Chest 21:635–640, 1952.

257. Briggs RS and Millac PA: Timolol in migraine prophylaxis. Headache 19:379–381, 1979.

258. Briley DP, Coull BM, and Goodnight SH: Neurological disease associated with antiphospholipid antibodies. Ann Neurol 25:221–227, 1989.

259. Broderick JP and Swanson JW: Migraine-related strokes. Clinical profile and prognosis in 20 patients. Arch Neurol 44:868–871, 1987.

260. Brodie GN, Baenziger NL, Chase LR, and Majerus PW: The effects of thrombin on adenyl cyclase activity and a membrane protein from human platelets. J Clin Invest 51:81–88, 1972.

261. Brohult J, Forsberg O, and Hellström R: A case of multiple arterial thromboses after oral contraceptives and ergotamine. Acta Med Scand 181:453–456, 1967.

262. Brooke OG and Robinson BF: Effect of ergotamine and ergometrine on forearm venous compliance in man. Br Med J i:139–142, 1970.

263. Brower KJ: Self-medication of migraine headaches with freebase cocaine. J Subst Abuse Treat 5:23–26, 1988.

264. Brown AM, Patch TL, and Kaufmann AJ: The antimigraine drugs ergotamine and dihydroergotamine are potent 5-HT$_{1C}$ receptor agonists in pig-

let choroid plexus. Br J Pharmacol 104:45–48, 1991.

265. Brown EG, Endersby CA, Smith RN, and Talbot JCC: The safety and tolerability of sumatriptan: An overview. Eur Neurol 31:339–344, 1989.

266. Brown JM: Imagery coping strategies in the treatment of migraine. Pain 18:157–167, 1984.

267. Bruyn GW: Cerebral cortex and migraine. Adv Neurol 33:151–172, 1982.

268. Bruyn GW: Epidemiology of migraine: 'A personal view.' Headache 23:127–133, 1983.

269. Bruyn GW: Intracranial arteriovenous malformations and migraine. Cephalalgia 4:191–207, 1984.

270. Bruyn GW: Migraine and epilepsy. Funct Neurol 1:315–329, 1986.

271. Bruyn GW: Migraine equivalents. In Clifford Rose F (ed): Handbook of Clinical Neurology, Vol 4. Elsevier, Amsterdam, 1986, pp 155–171.

272. Bruyn GW: Psychiatric and mental presentations of the migraine prodrome, aura, and attack. In Adler CS, Adler SM, and Packard RC (eds): Psychiatric Aspects of Headache. Williams & Wilkins, Baltimore, 1987, pp 181–191.

273. Bruyn GW and Weenink HR: Migraine accompagnee—a critical evaluation. Headache 6:1–22, 1966.

274. Bücking H and Baumgartner G: Klinik und Pathophysiologie der initialen neurologischen Symptome bei fokalen migränen (Migraine ophthalmique, Migraine accompagneé). Arch Psychiatr Nervenkr 219:37–52, 1974.

275. Buckle RM, du Boulay G, and Smith B: Death due to cerebal vasospasm. J Neurol Neurosurg Psychiatry 27:440–444, 1964.

276. Buff DD, Bogin MB, and Faltz LL: Retroperitoneal fibrosis. A report of selected cases and review of the literature. NY State J Med 89:511–516, 1989.

277. Burckhardt D, Raed E, Muller V, Imhof P, and Neubauer H: Cardiovascular effects of tricyclic and

tetracyclic antidepressants. JAMA 239:213–216, 1978.

278. Bures J, Buresova O, and Krivanek J: The Mechanism and Application of Leão's Spreading Depression of Electroencephalographic Activity, Academic, New York, 1974.

279. Buring JE, Peto R, and Hennekens CH: Low-dose aspirin for migraine prophylaxis. JAMA 264:1711–1713, 1990.

280. Burke EC and Peters GA: Migraine in childhood. Am J Dis Child 92:330–336, 1956.

281. Burnstock G: Neurogenic control of cerebral circulation. Cephalalgia 5 (Suppl 2):25–33, 1985.

282. Burnstock G: Local control of blood pressure by purines. Blood Vessels 24:156–160, 1987.

283. Busija DW and Heistad DD: Effects of cholinergic nerves on cerebral blood flow in cats. Circ Res 48:62–69, 1981.

284. Busija DW, Marcus ML, and Heistad DD: Pial artery diameter and blood flow velocity during sympathetic stimulation in cats. J Cereb Blood Flow Metab 2:363–367, 1982.

285. Bussone G, Baldini S, D'Andrea G, et al.: Nimodipine versus flunarizine in common migraine: A controlled pilot trial. Headache 27:76–79, 1987.

286. Bussone G, Giovannini P, Boiardi A, and Boeri R: A study of the activity of platelet monoamine oxidase in patients with migraine headache or with 'cluster headaches.' Eur Neurol 15:157–162, 1977.

287. Busto U, Sellers EM, Naranjo CA, Cappell H, Sanchez-Craig M, and Sykora K: Withdrawal reaction after long-term therapeutic use of benzodiazepines. N Engl J Med 315:854–859, 1986.

288. Butler JM and Hammond BR: The effects of sensory denervation on the responses of the rabbit eye to prostaglandin E_1, bradykinin, and substance P. Br J Pharmacol 69:495–502, 1980.

289. Buttinelli C, Lazzaro MP, Lenzi GL, Paolucci S, and Prencipe M: Correla-tion between migraine and circulating platelet aggregates. Cephalalgia 5 (Suppl 2):87–88, 1985.

290. Buzzi MG, Carter WB, Shimuzi T, Heath H, and Moskowitz MA: Dihydroergotamine and sumatriptan attenuate levels of CGRP in plasma in rat superior sagittal sinus during electrical stimulation of the trigeminal ganglion. Neuropharmacology 30:1193–1200, 1991.

291. Buzzi MG, Dimitriadou V, Theoharides TC, and Moskowitz MA: 5-Hydroxytryptamine receptor agonists for the abortive treatment of vascular headaches block mast cell, endothelial and platelet activation within the rat dura mater after trigeminal stimulation. Brain Res 583:137–149, 1992.

292. Buzzi MG and Moskowitz MA: The antimigraine drug sumatriptan (GR43175) selectively blocks neurogenic plasma extravasation from blood vessels in dura mater. Br J Pharmacol 99:202–206, 1990.

293. Buzzi MG, Sakas DE, and Moskowitz MA: Indomethacin and acetylsalicylic acid block neurogenic plasma protein extravasation in rat dura mater. Eur J Pharmacol 165:251–258, 1989.

294. Byer J, Gutterman DL, Plachetka JR, and Bhatacharyya H: Dose-response study for subcutaneous GR43175 in the treatment of acute migraine. Cephalalgia 9 (Suppl 10):349–350, 1989.

295. Cady RK, Wendt JK, Kirchner JR, Sargent JD, Rothrock JF, and Skaggs H: Treatment of acute migraine with subcutaneous sumatriptan. JAMA 265:2831–2835, 1991.

296. Caekebeke JFV, Ferrari MD, Zwetsloot CP, Jansen JC, and Saxena PR: Antimigraine drug sumatriptan increases blood flow velocity in large cerebral arteries during migraine attacks. Neurology 42:1522–1526, 1992.

297. Cahill GF and Soeldner JS: A non-editorial on non-hypoglycemia. N Engl J Med 291:905–906, 1974.

298. Cala LA and Mastaglia FL: Computerized axial tomography findings in patients with migrainous headaches. Br Med J ii:149–150, 1976.

299. Cala LA and Mastaglia FL: Computerized tomography in the detection of brain damage. 2. Epilepsy, migraine, and general medical disorders. Med J Aust 2:616–620, 1980.

300. Calamia KT and Hunder GG: Giant cell arteritis (temporal arteritis) presenting as fever of undetermined origin. Arthritis Rheum 24:1414–1418, 1981.

301. Caldara R, Ferrari C, Barbieri C, Rosmussi M, Rempini P, and Telloli P: Effect of two antiserotoninergic drugs, methysergide and metergoline, on gastric acid secretion and gastrin release in healthy man. Eur J Clin Pharmacol 17:13–18, 1980.

302. California Medical Association Scientific Board Task Force on Clinical Ecology: Clinical ecology—a critical appraisal. West J Med 144:239–245, 1986.

303. Callaghan N: The migraine syndrome in pregnancy. Neurology 18:197–201, 1968.

304. Callaham M and Raskin NH: A controlled study of dyhydroergotamine in the treatment of acute migraine headache. Headache 26:168–171, 1986.

305. Camfield PR, Metrakos K, and Andermann F: Basilar migraine, seizures and severe epileptiform EEG abnormalities. Neurology 28:584–588, 1978.

306. Camp WA and Wolff HG: Studies on headache: electroencephalographic abnormalities in patients with vascular headache of the migraine type. Arch Neurol 4:475–485, 1961.

307. Campbell DA, Hay KM, and Tonks EM: An investigation of the salt and water balance in migraine. Br Med J ii:1424–1429, 1951.

308. Campbell IC, Robinson DS, Lovenberg W, and Murphy DL: The effects of chronic regimens of clorgyline and pargyline on monoamine metabolism in the rat brain. J Neurochem 32:49–55, 1979.

309. Campbell S: Double-blind cross-over study of estrogen replacement therapy. In Campbell S (ed): The Management of the Menopause and Post-Menopausal Years. MTP Press, Lancaster, 1976, pp 149–158.

310. Cangi F, Fanciullacci M, Pietrini U, Boccuni M, and Sicuteri F: Emergence of pain and extra-pain phenomena from dopamimetics in migraine. In Pfaffenrath V, Lundberg PO, and Sjaastad O (eds): Updating in Headache. Springer-Verlag, Berlin, 1985, pp 276–280.

311. Caplan LR: Transient global amnesia. In Vinken PJ, Bruyn GW, and Klawans HL (eds): Handbook of Clinical Neurology. Vol 45. Elsevier, Amsterdam, 1985, pp 205–218.

312. Caplan LR, Chedru F, Lhermitte F, and Mayman C: Transient global amnesia and migraine. Neurology 31:1167–1170, 1981.

313. Carliner NH, Denune DP, Finch CS, and Goldberg LI: Sodium nitroprusside treatment of ergotamine induced peripheral ischemia. JAMA 227:308–309, 1974.

314. Carlson LA, Ekelund LG, and Oro L: Clinical and metabolic effects of different doses of prostaglandin E_1 in man. Acta Med Scand 183:423–430, 1968.

315. Carlsson J, Fahlkrantz A, and Augustinsson LE: Muscle tenderness in tension headache treated with acupuncture or physiotherapy. Cephalalgia 10:131–141, 1990.

316. Carlsson KH, Monzel W, and Jurna I: Depression by morphine and the non-opioid analgesic agents, metamizol (dipyrone), lysine acetylsalicylate, and paracetamol, of activity in rat thalamus neurones evoked by electrical stimulation of nociceptive afferents. Pain 32:313–326, 1988.

317. Carpenter DO: Neural mechanisms of emesis. Can J Physiol Pharmacol 68:230–236, 1990.

318. Carpenter DO, Briggs DB, and Strominger N: Responses of neurons of canine area postrema to neurotransmitters and peptides. Cell Molec Neurobiol 3:113–126, 1983.

319. Carr P: Self-induced myocardial infarction. Postgrad Med J 57:654–655, 1981.

320. Carraway RE, Cochrane DE, Granier C, Kitabgi P, Leeman E, and Singer EA: Parallel secretion of endogenous 5-hydroxytryptamine and histamine from mast cells stimulated by vasoactive peptides and compound 48/80. Br J Pharmacol 81:227–229, 1984.

321. Carrea GF, Gerson DE, Schnur J, and McNeil BJ: Computed tomography of the brain in patients with headache or temporal lobe epilepsy: Findings and cost-effectiveness. J Comput Assist Tomogr 1:200–203, 1977.

322. Carrieri P, Sorge F, Orefice G, and De Feo S: Platelet function in childhood migraine. Cephalalgia 5 (Suppl 2):99–101, 1985.

323. Carroll D: Retinal migraine. Headache 10:9–13, 1970.

324. Carroll JD: Migraine—general management. Br Med J ii:756–757, 1971.

325. Carroll JD, Coppen A, Swade CC, and Wood KM: Blood platelet 5-hydroxytryptamine accumulation and migraine. Ups J Med Sci (Suppl) 31:10–12, 1980.

326. Carroll JD and Hilton BP: The effects of reserpine injection on methysergide treated control and migrainous subjects. Headache 14:149–156, 1974.

327. Carroll JD and Maclay WP: Pizotifen (BC 105) in migraine prophylaxis. Curr Med Res Opin 3:68–71, 1975.

328. Carroll JD, Reidy M, Savundra PA, Cleave N, and McAinsh J: Long-acting propranolol in the prophylaxis of migraine: A comparative study of two doses. Cephalalgia 10:101–105, 1990.

329. Carvalho VC: Nerve cells in the human cavernous sinus. Anat Anz 159:29–32, 1985.

330. Cassem N: Cardiovascular effects of antidepressants. J Clin Psychiatry 43:22–28, 1982.

331. Castaldo JE, Anderson M, and Reeves AG: Middle cerebral artery occlusion with migraine. Stroke 13:308–311, 1982.

332. Catania A, Arnold J, Macaluso A, Hiltz ME, and Lipton JM: Inhibition of acute inflammation in the periphery by central action of salicylates. Proc Natl Acad Sci USA 88:8544–8547, 1991.

333. Catino D: Ten migraine equivalents. Headache 5:1–11, 1965.

334. Ceccerielli F, Ambrosio F, Avila M, Duse G, Munari A, and Giron GP: Acupuncture vs. placebo in the common migraine: A double-blind study. Cephalalgia 7:499–500, 1987.

335. Celentano DD, Linet MS, and Stewart WF: Gender differences in the experience of headache. Soc Sci Med 30:1289–1295, 1990.

336. Celentano DD, Stewart WF, and Linet MS: The relationship of headache symptoms with severity and duration of attacks. J Clin Epidemiol 43:983–994, 1990.

337. Cerbo R, Casacchia M, Formisano R, et al.: Flunarizine-pizotifen single-dose double-blind cross-over trial in migraine prophylaxis. Cephalalgia 6:15–18, 1986.

338. Chahl LA and Iggo A: The effects of bradykinin and prostaglandin E_1 on rat cutaneous afferent nerve activity. Br J Pharmacol 59:343–347, 1977.

339. Chan SH: Suppression of dental pulp-evoked trigeminal responses by nucleus reticularis gigantocellularis in the cat. Exp Neurol 66:356–364, 1979.

340. Chancellor AM, Cull RE, Kilpatrick DC, and Warlow CP: Neurological disease associated with anticardiolipin antibodies in patients with systemic lupus erythematosus: Clinical and immunological features. J Neurol 238:401–407, 1991.

341. Chancellor AM, Wroe SJ, and Cull RE: Migraine occurring for the first time in pregnancy. Headache 30:224–227, 1990.

342. Chang JY, Ekblad E, Kannisto P, and Owman C: Serotonin uptake into cerebrovascular nerve fibers of rat, visualization by immunohisto-

chemistry, disappearance following sympathectomy, and release during electrical stimulation. Brain Res 492:79–88, 1989.

343. Chao D, Sexton JA, and Davis SD: Convulsive equivalent syndrome of childhood. J Pediatr 64:499–508, 1964.

344. Chapman LF, Ramos AO, Goodell H, Silverman G, and Wolff HG: A humoral agent implicated in vascular headache of the migraine type. Arch Neurol 3:223–229, 1960.

345. Chapman LF and Wolff HG: Studies of proteolytic enzymes in cerebrospinal fluid: Capacity of incubated mixtures of cerebrospinal fluid and plasma proteins to form vasodilator substances that contract the isolated rat uterus. Arch Intern Med 103:86–94, 1959.

346. Chapman S: A review and clinical perspective on the use of EMG and thermal biofeedback for chronic headaches. Pain 27:1–43, 1986.

347. Chaudhuri TK and Chaudhuri ST: Estrogen therapy for migraine. Headache 15:139–142, 1975.

348. Chaytor JP, Crathorne B, and Saxby MJ: The identification and significance of 2-phenylethylamine in foods. J Sci Food Agric 26:593–598, 1975.

349. Chazot G, Chauplannaz G, Biron A, and Schott B: Migraines: traitement par lithium. Nouve Presse Méd 8:2836–2837, 1979.

350. Chen TC, Leviton A, Edelstein S, and Ellenberg JH: Migraine and other diseases in women of reproductive age. The influence of smoking on observed associations. Arch Neurol 44:1024–1028, 1987.

351. Cheng XM, Ziegler DK, Li SC, Dai QS, Chandra V and Schoenberg BS: A prevalence survey of "incapacitating headache" in the People's Republic of China. Neurology 36:831–834, 1986.

352. Cherry PD, Furchgott RF, Zawadzki JV, and Jothianandan D: Role of endothelial cells in relaxation of isolated arteries by bradykinin. Proc Natl Acad Sci USA 79:2106–2110, 1982.

353. Childs AJ and Sweetnam MT: A study of 104 cases of migraine. Br J Ind Med 18:234–236, 1961.

354. Chitwood DD: Patterns and consequences of cocaine use. NIDA Res Mongr Series 61:111–129, 1985.

355. Chorobski J and Penfield W: Cerebral vasodilator nerves and their pathway from the medulla oblongata. Arch Neurol Psychiatry 28:1257–1289, 1932.

356. Chouza C, Scaramelli A, Caamano JL, De Medina O, Alijanati R, and Romero S: Parkinsonism, tardive dyskinesia, akathisia and depression induced by flunarizine. Lancet i:1303–1304, 1986.

357. Church MK, Lowman MA, Rees PH, and Benyon RC: Mast cells, neuropeptides and inflammation. Agents Actions 27:8–16, 1989.

358. Chutorian AM: Benign paroxysmal torticollis, tortipelvis and retrocollis in infancy. Neurology 24:366–367, 1974.

359. Clark D, Hough H, and Wolff HG: Experimental studies on headache: Observations on headache produced by histamine. Arch Neurol Psychiatry 35:1054–1069, 1936.

360. Clark JH and Wilson WG: A 16-day-old breast-fed infant with metabolic acidosis caused by salicylate. Clin Pediatr 20:53–54, 1981.

361. Clark SL and Ryall RW: The antinociceptive action of etorphine in the dorsal horn is due to a direct spinal action and not to activation of descending inhibition. Br J Pharmacol 78:307–319, 1983.

362. Clarke GJR and Waters WE: Headache and migraine in a London general practice. In Waters WE (ed): The Epidemiology of Migraine. Boehringer Ingelheim, Bracknell-Berkshire, 1974, pp 14–22.

363. Clifford T, Lauritzen M, Bakke M, Olesen J, and Møller E: Electromyography of pericranial muscles during treatment of spontaneous common migraine attacks. Pain 14:137–147, 1982.

364. Clifford Rose F: The migraine clinic at Charing Cross Hospital. Hemicrania 7:2–5, 1976.

365. Clifford Rose F and Peatfield RC: Treatment of migraine and cluster headache. Practitioner 225:1321–1325, 1982.

366. Coffman JD: The effect of aspirin on pain and hand blood flow responses to intra-arterial injection of bradykinin in man. Clin Pharmacol Ther 7:26–37, 1966.

367. Cohen MJ, McArthur DL, and Rickles WH: Comparison of four biofeedback treatments for migraine headache: Physiological and headache variables. Psychosom Med 42:463–480, 1980.

368. Collaborative Group for the Study of Stroke in Young Women: Oral contraceptives and increased risk of cerebral ischemia or thrombosis. N Engl J Med 288:871–878, 1973.

369. Collaborative Group for the Study of Stroke in Young Women: Oral contraceptives and stroke in young women; associated risk factors. JAMA 231:718–722, 1975.

370. Congdon PJ and Forsythe WI: Migraine in childhood: A study of 300 children. Dev Med Child Neurol 21:209–216, 1979.

371. Conley JE, Boulanger WJ, and Mendeloff GL: Aortic obstruction associated with methysergide maleate therapy for headaches. JAMA 198:808–810, 1966.

372. Conn JW: The diagnosis and management of spontaneous hypoglycemia. JAMA 134:130–138, 1947.

373. Connor HE, Feniuk W, and Humphrey PPA: Characterization of 5-HT receptors mediating contraction of canine and primate basilar artery by use of GR43175, a selective 5-HT$_1$-like receptor agonist. Br J Pharmacol 96:379–387, 1989.

374. Connor HE, Stubbs CM, Feniuk W, and Humphrey PPA: Effect of sumatriptan, a selective 5-HT$_1$-like receptor agonist, on pial vessel diameter in anaesthetized cats. J Cereb Blood Flow Metab 12:514–519, 1992.

375. Connor RCR: Complicated migraine: A study of permanent neurological and visual defects caused by migraine. Lancet ii:1072–1075, 1962.

376. Constantinovici A, Constantinescu AI, and Constantinovici A: Hemicrania and migraine accompanying the course of endocranial tumors. Rev Roum Neurol Psychiatr 13:21–25, 1975.

377. Contreras RJ, Beckstead RM, and Norgren R: The central projections of the trigeminal, facial, glossolaryngeal and vagus nerves: An autoradiographic study in the rat. J Auton Nerv Syst 6:303–322, 1982.

378. Cooper PE, Fernstrom MH, Rorstad OP, Leeman SE, and Martin JB: The regional distribution of somatostatin, substance P and neurotensin in human brain. Brain Res 218:219–232, 1981.

379. Cooper TB: Pharmacokinetics of lithium. In Meltzer HY (ed): Psychopharmacology: The Third Generation of Progress. Raven, New York, 1987, pp 1365–1375.

380. Coppen A, Swade C, Wood K, and Carroll JD: Platelet 5-hydroxytryptamine accumulation and migraine. Lancet ii:914, 1979.

381. Corbett JJ: Neuro-ophthalmic complications of migraine and cluster headaches. Neurol Clin 1:973–995, 1983.

382. Corbett JJ: Ocular aspects of migraine. In Blau JN (ed): Migraine. Clinical and Research Aspects. Johns Hopkins University Press, Baltimore, 1987, pp 625–633.

383. Cormia FE and Dougherty JW: Proteolytic activity in development of pain and itching: Cutaneous reactions to bradykinin and kallikrein. J Invest Dermatol 35:21–26, 1960.

384. Correa FM, Innis RB, Uhl GR, and Snyder SH: Bradykinin-like immunoreactive neuronal systems localized histochemically in rat brain. Proc Natl Acad Sci USA 76:1489–1493, 1979.

385. Cortelli P, de Carolis P, Sturani A, et al.: Cardiovascular and biochemical assessment in migraine patients submitted to tilt test. Funct Neurol 1:285–290, 1986.

386. Cortelli P, Sacquegna T, Albani F, et al.: Propranolol plasma levels and relief of migraine. Arch Neurol 42:46–48, 1985.

387. Costall B, Gunning SJ, and Naylor RJ: An analysis of the hypothalamic sites at which substituted benzamide drugs act to facilitate gastric emptying in the guinea-pig. Neuropharmacology 24:869–875, 1985.

388. Costall B, Gunning SJ, Naylor RJ, and Simpson KH: A central site of action for benzamide facilitation of gastric emptying. Eur J Pharmacol 91:197–205, 1983.

389. Couch JR: Placebo effect and clinical trials in migraine therapy. Neuroepidemiology 6:178–185, 1987.

390. Couch JR and Diamond S: Status migrainosus: Causative and therapeutic aspects. Headache 23:94–101, 1982.

391. Couch JR and Hassanein RS: Platelet aggregability in migraine. Neurology 27:643–648, 1977.

392. Couch JR and Hassanein RS: Amitriptyline in migraine prophylaxis. Arch Neurol 36:695–699, 1979.

393. Couch JR and Hassanein RS: Headache as a risk factor in atherosclerosis-related diseases. Headache 29:49–54, 1989.

394. Couch JR, Ziegler DK, and Hassanein RS: Evaluation of the relationship between migraine headache and depression. Headache 15:41–50, 1975.

395. Couch JR, Zeigler DK, and Hassanein R: Amitriptyline in the prophylaxis of migraine. Neurology 26:121–127, 1976.

396. Coughlin SR, Moskowitz MA, Antoniades HN, and Levine L: Serotonin receptor-mediated stimulation of bovine smooth muscle cell prostacyclin synthesis and its modulation by platelet-derived growth factor. Proc Natl Acad Sci USA 78:7134–7138, 1981.

397. Coughlin SR, Moskowitz MA, and Levine L: Identification of a serotonin type 2 receptor linked to prostacyclin synthesis in vascular smooth muscle cells. Biochem Pharmacol 33:692–695, 1984.

398. Coulthard M: Recurrent abdominal pain: A psychogenic disorder? Arch Dis Child 59:189–190, 1984.

399. Couturier EGM, Hering R, and Steiner TJ: Weekend attacks in migraine patients: Caused by caffeine withdrawal? Cephalalgia 12:99–100, 1992.

400. Covelli V, Maffione AB, Munno I, and Jirillo E: Alterations of nonspecific immunity in patients with common migraine. J Clin Lab Analysis 4:9–15, 1990.

401. Cox DJ, Freundlich A, and Meyer RG: Differential effectiveness of electromyographic feedback, verbal relaxation instructions, and medication placebo. J Consult Clin Psychol 43:892–898, 1975.

402. Crill WE and Reis DJ: Distribution of carotid sinus and depressor nerves in cat brain stem. Am J Physiol 214:269–276, 1968.

403. Crisp AH, Kalucy RS, McGuinness B, Ralph PC, and Harris G: Some clinical, social and psychological characteristics of migraine subjects in the general population. Postgrad Med J 53:691–697, 1977.

404. Critchley M: The Parietal Lobes. Hafner, New York, 1969.

405. Critchley M and Ferguson FR: Migraine. Lancet i:123–126, 182–187, 1933.

406. Crooks J, Stephen SA, and Brass W: Clinical trial of inhaled ergotamine tartrate in migraine. Br Med J i:221, 1964.

407. Cropper EC, Eisenman JS, and Azmitia EC: 5-HT-immunoreactive fibers in the trigeminal nuclear complex of the rat. Exp Brain Res 55:515–522, 1984.

408. Crowell GF, Stump DA, Biller J, McHenry LC, and Toole JF: The transient global amnesia–migraine connection. Arch Neurol 41:75–79, 1984.

409. Cruickshank JM: The clinical importance of cardioselectivity and lipophilicity in beta blockers. Am Heart J 100:160–177, 1980.

410. Cruz L and Basbaum A: Multiple opioid peptides and the modulation of pain: Immuno-histochemical analysis of dynorphin and enkephalin in the trigeminal nucleus caudalis and

spinal cord of the cat. J Comp Neurol 240:331–348, 1985.

411. Cudennec A, Duverger D, and MacKenzie ET: Nature of the regional increases in cerebral blood flow induced by raphe stimulation. J Cerebral Blood Flow Metab 9 (Suppl 1):S375, 1989.

412. Cudennec A, Duverger D, Serrano A, Scatton B, and MacKenzie ET: Influence of ascending serotonergic pathways on glucose use in the conscious rat brain. II. Effects of electrical stimulation of the rostral raphé nuclei. Brain Res 444:227–246, 1988.

413. Cuetter AC and Aita JF: CT scanning in classic migraine. Headache 23:195, 1983.

414. Cugini P, Romit A, Di Palma L, and Giacovazzo M: Common migraine as a weekly and seasonal headache. Chronobiol Int 7:467–469, 1990.

415. Curran DA, Hinterberger H, and Lance JW: Total plasma serotonin, 5-hydroxyindoleacetic acid and *p*-hydroxy-*m*-methoxymandelic acid excretion in normal and migrainous subjects. Brain 88:997–1010, 1965.

416. Curran DA, Hinterberger H, and Lance JW: Methysergide. Res Clin Stud Headache 1:74–122, 1967.

417. Curran DA and Lance JW: Clinical trial of methysergide and other preparations in the management of migraine. J Neurol Neurosurg Psychiatry 27:463–469, 1964.

418. Curtin T, Brooks A, and Roberts, J: Cardiorespiratory distress after sumatriptan given by injection. Br Med J 305:713–714, 1992.

419. Curzon G, Barrie M, and Wilkinson MIP: Relationships between headache and amine changes after administration of reserpine to migrainous patients. J Neurol Neurosurg Psychiatry 32:555–561, 1969.

420. Curzon G, Kennett GA, Shah K, and Whitton P: Behavioral effects of *m*-chlorophenylpiperazine (*m*CPP), a reported migraine precipitant. In Sandler M and Collins G (eds): Migraine: A Spectrum of Ideas. Oxford University Press, London, 1990, pp 173–179.

421. Curzon G, Theaker P, and Phillips B: Excretion of 5-hydroxyindoleacetic acid (5HIAA) in migraine. J Neurol Neurosurg Psychiatry 29:85–90, 1966.

422. Cushing H: A method of total extirpation of the gasserian ganglion for trigeminal neuralgia. JAMA 34:1035–1041, 1900.

423. Cutrer FM and Baloh RW: Migraine-associated dizziness. Headache 32:300–304, 1992.

424. Dacey RG and Bassett JE: Histaminergic vasodilation of intracerebral arterioles in the rat. J Cereb Blood Flow Metab 7:327–331, 1987.

425. Dacey RG, Basset JE, and Takayasu M: Vasomotor responses of rat intracerebral arterioles to vasoactive intestinal peptide, substance P, neuropeptide Y, and bradykinin. J Cereb Blood Flow Metab 8:254–261, 1988.

426. Dahl E: The innervation of the cereberal arteries. J Anat 115:53–63, 1973.

427. Dahl E, Russell D, Nyberg-Hansen R, and Rootwelt K: Cephalalgia 10:87–94, 1990.

428. Dahl LE, Dencker SJ, and Lundlin L: A double-blind study of dothiepin hydrochloride (Prothiaden) and amitriptyline in out-patients with masked depression. J Int Med Res 9:103–107, 1981.

429. Dahlgren N, Lindvall O, Sakabe T, Stenevi U, and Siesjo BK: Cerebral blood flow and oxygen consumption in rat brain after lesions of the noradrenergic locus coeruleus system. Brain Res 209:11–23, 1981.

430. Dahlöf C, Edwards C, and Toth AL: Sumatriptan injection is superior to placebo in the acute treatment of migraine with regard to both efficacy and general well-being. Cephalalgia 12:214–220, 1992.

431. Dahlöf C, Winter P, and Ludlow S: Oral GR43175, a 5-HT$_1$-like agonist, for the treatment of an acute migraine attack: An international study—preliminary results. Cephalalgia 9 (Suppl 10):351–352, 1989.

432. D'Alecy LG and Rose CJ: Parasympathetic cholinergic control of cere-

bral blood flow in dogs. Circ Res 41:324–331, 1977.

433. D'Alessandro R, Benassi G, Lenzi PL, et al.: Epidemiology of headache in the Republic of San Marino. J Neurol Neurosurg Psychiatry 51:21–27, 1988.

434. Dalessio DJ: Classification and treatment of headache during pregnancy. Clin Neuropharmacol 9:121–131, 1986.

435. Dalgaard P, Kronborg D, and Lauritzen M: Migraine with aura, cerebral ischemia, spreading depression, and Compton scatter. Headache 31:49–51, 1991.

436. Dallas FAA, Dixon CM, McCulloch RJ, and Saynor DA: The kinetics of ^{14}C-GR43175 in rat and dog. Cephalalgia 9 (Suppl 9):53–56, 1989.

437. Dalsgaard-Nielsen T: Migraine diagnostics with special reference to pharmacological tests. Int Arch Allergy 7:312–322, 1955.

438. Dalsgaard-Nielsen T: Migraine and heredity. Acta Neurol Scand 41:287–300, 1965.

439. Dalsgaard-Nielsen T: Some aspects of the epidemiology of migraine in Denmark. Headache 10:14–23, 1970.

440. Dalsgaard-Nielsen T, Engberg-Pedersen H, and Holm HE: Clinical and statistical investigations of the epidemiology of migraine. Dan Med Bull 17:138–148, 1970.

441. Dalsgaard-Nielsen T and Genefke IK: Serotonin (5-hydroxytryptamine) release and uptake in platelets from healthy persons and migrainous patients in attack-free intervals. Headache 14:26–32, 1974.

442. Dalsgaard-Nielsen T and Ulrich J: Prevalence and heredity of migraine and migrainoid headaches among 461 Danish doctors. Headache 12:168–172, 1973.

443. Dalton K: Progesterone suppositories and pessaries in the treatment of menstrual migraine. Headache 12:151–159, 1973.

444. Dalton K: Food intake prior to migraine attacks—study of 2,313 spontaneous attacks. Headache 15:188–193, 1975.

445. Dalton K: Migraine and oral contraceptives. Headache 15:247–251, 1976.

446. Damasio H and Beck D: Migraine, thrombocytopenia and serotonin metabolism. Lancet i:240–242, 1978.

447. D'Andrea G, Toldo M, Cortelazzo S, and Milone FF: Platelet activity in migraine. Headache 22:207–212, 1982.

448. Daniel EE: Pharmacology of adrenergic, cholinergic and drugs acting on other receptors in gastrointestinal muscle. In Betaccini G (ed): Medications and Drugs in Gastrointestinal Motility, Handbook of Experimental Pharmacology, Vol 59. Springer-Verlag, Berlin, 1982, pp 249–322.

449. Darling M: The use of exercise as a method of aborting migraine. Headache 31:616–618, 1991.

450. Dauphin F, Lacombe P, Sercombe R, Hamel E, and Seylez J: Hypercapnia and stimulation of the substantia innominata increase rat frontal cortical blood flow by different cholinergic mechanisms. Brain Res 553:75–83, 1991.

452. Davidsen PCB, Secher NJ, and Pedersen GT: Cyclical therapy with estradiol valerate/norgestrel at the menopause: Report of a double-blind investigation. Ugeskr Laeger 136:1805–1808, 1974.

453. Davies MJ, Moore BP, and Braimbridge MV: The floppy mitral valve. Study of incidence, pathology, and complications in surgical necropsy, and forensic material. Br Heart J 40:468–481, 1978.

454. Davies P, Bailey PJ, Goldenberg MM, and Ford-Hutchinson AW: The role of arachidonic acid oxygenation products in pain and inflammation. Annu Rev Immunol 2:335–357, 1984.

455. Davis CJ, Harding RK, Leslie RA, and Andrews PLR: The organisation of vomiting as a protective reflex. In

Davis CJ, Lake-Bakaar GV, and Grahame-Smith DG (eds): Nausea and Vomiting: Mechanisms and Treatment. Springer-Verlag, Berlin, 1986, pp 65–75.

456. Davis E and Landau J: Clinical Capillary Microscopy. Thomas, Springfield, Illinois, 1966.

457. Davis KD and Dostrovsky JO: Activation of trigeminal brain stem nociceptive neurons by dural artery stimulation. Pain 25:395–401, 1986.

458. Davis KD and Dostrovsky JO: Responses of feline trigeminal spinal tract nucleus neurons to stimulation of the middle meningeal artery and sagittal sinus. J Neurophysiol 59:648–666, 1988.

459. Davis MS: Variations in patients' compliance with doctors' advice: An empirical analysis of patterns of communication. Am J Public Health 58:274–288, 1968.

460. Davis-Jones A, Gregory MC, and Whitty CWM: Permanent sequelae in the migraine attack. In Cummings JN (ed): Background to Migraine. Springer-Verlag, New York, 1972, pp 25–27.

461. Day JW and Raskin NH: Thunderclap headache: Symptom of unruptured cerebral aneurysm. Lancet ii:1247–1248, 1986.

462. Deanovic Z, Iskric S, and Dupelj M: Fluctuation of 5-hydroxy-indole compounds in the urine of migrainous patients. Biomedicine 23:346–349, 1975.

463. De Benedittis G and De Santis A: Chronic post-traumatic headache: Clinical, psychopathological features and outcome determinants. J Neurosurg Sci 27:177–186, 1983.

464. De Benedittis G, Lorenzetti A, and Pieri A: The role of stressful life events in the onset of chronic primary headache. Pain 40:65–75, 1990.

465. Debney LM and Hedge A: Physical trigger factors in migraine—with special reference to the weather. In Amery WK and Wauquier A (eds): The Prelude to the Migraine Attack. Baillière Tindall, London, 1986, pp 8–24.

466. Debruyne J, Crevits L, and Vander Eecken H: Migraine-like headache in intraventricular tumours. Clin Neurol Neurosurg 84:51–57, 1982.

467. De Clerck F, van Nueten JM, and Reneman RS: Platelet-vessel wall interactions: Implication of 5-hydroxytryptamine. A review. Agents Actions 15:612–626, 1984.

468. De Fine Olivarius B and Jensen TS: Transient global amnesia in migraine. Headache 19:335–338, 1979.

469. De La Torre JC: Evidence for central innervation of intracerebral blood vessels: Local cerebral blood flow measurements and histofluorescence analysis by the sucrose-phosphate-glyoxylic acid (SPG) method. Neuroscience 1:455–457, 1976.

470. De La Torre JC, Surgeon JW, and Walker RH: Effect of locus coeruleus stimulation on cerebral blood flow in selected brain regions. Acta Neurol Scand 56 (Suppl 64):104–105, 1977.

471. Del Bene F, Poggioni M, Garagiola U, and Maresca V: Intramuscular treatment of migraine attacks using diclofenac sodium: A crossover clinical trial. J Int Med Res 15:44–48, 1987.

472. De Ley G, Weyne J, Demeester G, and Leusen I: Response of local blood flow in the caudate nucleus of the cat to intraventricular administration of histamine. Stroke 13:499–504, 1982.

473. Del Fiacco M, Quartu M, Floris A, and Diaz G: Substance P-like immunoreactivity in the human trigeminal ganglion. Neuroscience Lett 110:16–21, 1990.

474. Deliganis AV and Peroutka SJ: 5-Hydroxytryptamine$_{1D}$ receptor agonism predicts antimigraine efficacy. Headache 31:228–231, 1991.

475. de Lignières BD, Vincens M, Mauvais-Jarvis P, Mas JL, Touboul PJ, and Bousser MG: Prevention of menstrual migraine by percutaneous estradiol. Br Med J 293:1540, 1986.

476. Della Bella D, Carenzi A, Casacci F, Anselmi B, Baldi E, and Salmon S: Endorphins in the pathogenesis of headache. Adv Neurol 33:75–79, 1982.

477. De Marinis M, Janiri L, and Agnoli A: Headache in the use and withdrawal of opiates and other associated substances of abuse. Headache 31:159–163, 1991.

478. de Metz JE and van Zwieten PA: Differential effects of dihydroergotamine on the circulatory actions of arterial and venous dilators in the rat. J Cardiovasc Pharmacol 3:217–227, 1981.

479. den Boer MO, Villalón CM, Heiligers JPC, Humphrey PPA, and Saxena PR: Role of 5-HT$_1$-like receptors in the reduction of porcine cranial arteriovenous anastomotic shunting by sumatriptan. Br J Pharmacol 102:323–330, 1991.

480. Dennerstein L, Laby B, Burrows GD, and Hyman GJ: Headache and sex hormone therapy. Headache 18:146–153, 1978.

481. Dennerstein L, Morse C, Burrows G, Oats J, Brown J, and Smith M: Menstrual migraine: A double-blind trial of percutaneous estradiol. Gynecol Endocrinol 2:113–120, 1988.

482. Denton IC, White RP, and Robertson JT: The effects of prostaglandins E$_1$, A$_1$ and F$_{2\alpha}$ on the cerebral circulation of dogs and monkeys. J Neurosurg 36:34–42, 1972.

483. Deonna T: Paroxysmal disorders which may be migraine or may be confused with it. In Hockaday JM (ed): Migraine in Childhood. Butterworth, London, 1988, pp 75–87.

484. Deonna T and Martin D: Benign paroxysmal torticollis in infancy. Arch Dis Child 56:956–958, 1981.

485. De Silva KL, Muller PJ, and Pearce J: Acute drug-induced extrapyramidal syndromes. The Practitioner 211:316–320, 1973.

486. Desmukh SV and Meyer JS: Cyclic changes in platelet dynamics in migraine. Neurology 26:347, 1976.

487. de Trafford JC, Lafferty K, Potter CE, Roberts VC, and Cotton LT: An epidemiological survey of Raynaud's phenomenon. Eur J Vasc Surg 2:167–170, 1988.

488. Deubner DC: An epidemiologic study of migraine and headache in 10–20 year olds. Headache 17:173–180, 1977.

489. DeVoto M, Lozito A, Stafa G, D'Alessandro R, Sacquengna T, and Romeo G: Segregation analysis of migraine in 128 families. Cephalalgia 6:101–105, 1986.

490. DeWitt LD and Wechsler LR: Current concepts of cerebrovascular disease: transcranial Doppler. Stroke 19:915–921, 1988.

491. Dexter JD and Byer JA: The evaluation of 118 patients treated with low sucrose, frequent feeding diet. Headache 21:125, 1981.

492. Dexter JD, Byer JA, and Slaughter JR: The concomitant use of amitriptyline and propranolol in intractable headache. Headache 20:157, 1980.

493. Dexter JD and Riley TL: Studies in nocturnal migraine. Headache 15:51–62, 1975.

494. Dexter JD and Weitzman ED: The relationship of nocturnal headaches to sleep stage patterns. Neurology 20:513–518, 1970.

495. Dhopesh V, Maany I, and Herring C: The relationship of cocaine to headache in polysubstance abusers. Headache 31:17–19, 1991.

496. Dhuna A, Pascual-Leone A, and Belgrade M: Cocaine-related vascular headaches. J Neurol Neurosurg Psychiatry 54:803–806, 1991.

497. Diamond S: Depressive headaches. Headache 4:255–259, 1964.

498. Diamond S: Treatment of migraine with isometheptene, acetaminophen, and dichloralphenazone combination: A double-blind, crossover trial. Headache 15:282–287, 1976.

499. Diamond S: Prolonged benign exertional headache: Its clinical characteristics and response to indomethacin. Headache 22:96–98, 1982.

500. Diamond S: Ibuprofen versus aspirin and placebo in the treatment of mus-

cle contraction headache. Headache 23:206–210, 1983.

501. Diamond S and Freitag FG: Cold as an adjunctive therapy for headache. Postgrad Med 79:305–309, 1986.

502. Diamond S and Freitag FG: Do nonsteroidal anti-inflammatory agents have a role in the treatment of migraine headaches? Drugs 37:755–760, 1989.

503. Diamond S, Freitag FG, Diamond ML, and Urban G: Transnasal butorphanol in the treatment of migraine headache pain. Headache Quarterly, Current Treatment and Research 3:164–171, 1992.

504. Diamond S, Freitag FG, Gallagher RM, and Feinberg DT: Ketoprofen in the prophylaxis of migraine. Headache Quarterly, Current Treatment and Research 1:75–77, 1990.

505. Diamond S, Freitag FG, and Nursall A: The effects of weather on migraine frequency in Chicago. Headache Quarterly, Current Treatment and Research 1:136–145, 1990.

506. Diamond S, Greenberg I, Freitag FG, and Urban GJ: MRI changes in migraine. In Clifford Rose F (ed): New Advances in Headache Research: 2. Smith-Gordon, London, 1991, pp 53–61.

507. Diamond S, Kudrow L, Stevens J, and Shapiro DB: Long-term study of propranolol in the treatment of migraine. Headache 22:268–271, 1982.

508. Diamond S and Medina JL: Double-blind study of propranolol for migraine prophylaxis. Headache 16:24–27, 1976.

509. Diamond S, Medina J, Diamond-Falk J, and DeVeno T: The value of biofeedback in the treatment of chronic headache: A five-year retrospective study. Headache 19:90–96, 1979.

510. Diamond S and Montrose D: The value of biofeedback in the treatment of chronic headache: A four-year retrospective study. Headache 24:5–18, 1984.

511. Diamond S, Solomon G, Freitag F,

and Mehta N: Fenoprofen in the prophylaxis of migraine: A double-blind placebo-controlled study. Headache 27:246–249, 1987.

512. Di Carlo V: Serotoninergic innervation of extrinsic brainstem blood vessels. Neurology 31:104, 1981.

513. Di Carlo V: Perivascular serotonergic neurons: Somatodendritic contacts and axonic innervation of blood vessels. Neuroscience Lett 51:295–302, 1984.

514. Dichgans J and Diener HC: Clinical manifestations of excessive use of analgesia medication. In Diener HC and Wilkinson M (eds): Drug-Induced Headache, Springer-Verlag, Berlin, 1988, pp 8–15.

515. Dichgans J, Diener HC, Gerber WD, Verspohl EJ, Kukiolka H, and Kluck M: Analgetika-induzierter Dauerkopfschmerz. Dtsch Med Wochenschr 109:369–373, 1984.

516. Dickenson AH, Oliveras JL, and Besson JM: Role of the nucleus raphe magnus in opiate analgesia as studied by the microinjection technique in the rat. Brain Res 170:95–111, 1979.

517. Diehr P, Diehr G, Koepsell T, et al.: Cluster analysis to determine headache types. J Chron Dis 35:623–633, 1982.

518. Diehr P, Wood R, Wolcott B, Slay L, and Tomkins RK: On the relationships among headache symptoms. J Chron Dis 35:321–331, 1982.

519. Diener HC, Gerber WD, Geiselhart S, Dichgans J, and Scholz E: Short- and long-term effects of withdrawal therapy in drug-induced headache. In Diener HC and Wilkinson M (eds): Drug-Induced Headache, Springer-Verlag, Berlin, 1988, pp 133–142.

520. Diener HC, Haab J, Peters C, Ried S, Dichgans J, and Pilgrim A: Subcutaneous sumatriptan in the treatment of headache during withdrawal from drug-induced headache. Headache 31:205–209, 1991.

521. Diener HC, Peters C, Rudzio M, et al.: Ergotamine, flunarazine and sumatriptan do not change cerebral blood

flow velocity in normal subjects and migraineurs. J Neurol 238:245, 1991.

522. Dige-Petersen H, Lassen NA, Noer J, Tønnesen KH, and Olesen J: Subclinical ergotism. Lancet ii:65–66, 1977.

523. Digre K and Damassio H: Menstrual migraine: Differential diagnosis, evaluation, and treatment. Clin Obst Gynecol 30:417–430, 1987.

524. Dimitriadou V, Buzzi MG, Theoharides TC, and Moskowitz MA: Anti-inflammatory effects of dihydroergotamine and sumatriptan in blood vessels and mast cells of dura mater. Cephalalgia 11 (Suppl 11):9–10, 1991.

525. Dimitriadou V, Buzzi MG, Theoharides TC, and Moskowitz MA: Ultrastructural evidence for neurogenically mediated changes in blood vessels of the rat dura mater and tongue following antidromic trigeminal stimulation. Neuroscience 44:97–112, 1991.

526. Dimlich RVW, Keller JT, Strauss TA, and Fritts MJ: Linear arrays of homogeneous mast cells in the dura mater of the rat. J Neurocytol 20:485–503, 1991.

527. Dittrich J, Havlová M, and Nevsimalová S: Paroxysmal hemiparesis in childhood. Dev Med Child Neurol 21:800–807, 1979.

528. Donatsch P, Engel G, Richardson BP, and Stadler PA: The inhibitory effect of neuronal 5-hydroxytryptamine (5-HT) receptor antagonists on experimental pain in humans. Br J Pharmacol 81:35P, 1984.

529. Dorfman LJ, Marshall WH, and Enzmann DR: Cerebral infarction and migraine: Clinical and radiologic correlations. Neurology 29:317–322, 1979.

530. Dostrovsky JO, Davis KD, and Kawakita K: Central mechanisms of vascular headaches. Can J Physiol Pharmacol 69:652–658, 1991.

531. Dostrovsky JO, Hu JW, Sessle BJ, and Sumino R: Stimulation sites in periaqueductal gray, nucleus raphe magnus and adjacent regions effective in suppressing oral-facial reflexes. Brain Res 252:287–297, 1982.

532. Dow DJ and Whitty CWM: Electroencephalographic changes in migraine. Lancet ii:52–54, 1947.

533. Downey JA and Frewin DB: Vascular responses in the hands of patients suffering from migraine. J Neurol Neurosurg Psychiatry 35:258–263, 1972.

534. Dowson DI, Lewith GT, and Machin D: The effects of acupuncture versus placebo in the treatment of headache. Pain 21:35–42, 1985.

535. Drayer DE: Lipophilicity, hydrophilicity, and the central nervous system side effects of beta blockers. Pharmacotherapy 7:87–91, 1987.

536. Dreifuss FE, Langer DH, Moline KA, and Maxwell JE: Valproic acid hepatic fatalities. II. US experience since 1984. Neurology 39:301–207, 1989.

537. Drummond AH: Platelet-biogenic amine interactions. In Gordon JL (ed): Platelets in Biology and Pathology. Elsevier, Amsterdam, 1976, pp 203–239.

538. Drummond PD: Predisposing, precipitating and relieving factors in different categories of headache. Headache 25:16–22, 1985.

539. Drummond PD: A quantitative assessment of photophobia in migraine and tension headache. Headache 26:465–469, 1986.

540. Drummond PD: Scalp tenderness and sensitivity to pain in migraine and tension headache. Headache 27:45–50, 1987.

541. Drummond PD: Pupil diameter in migraine and tension headache. J Neurol Neurosurg Psychiatry 50:228–230, 1987.

542. Drummond PD: Autonomic disturbances in cluster headache. Brain 111:1199–1209, 1988.

543. Drummond PD: Disturbances in ocular sympathetic function and facial blood flow in unilateral migraine headache. J Neurol Neurosurg Psychiatry 53:121–125, 1990.

544. Drummond PD: Cervical sympa-

thetic deficit in unilateral migraine headache. Headache 31:669–672, 1991.

545. Drummond PD and Lance JW: Extracranial vascular changes and the source of pain in migraine headache. Ann Neurol 13:32–37, 1983.

546. Drummond PD and Lance JW: Clinical diagnosis and computer analysis of headache symptoms. J Neurol Neurosurg Psychiatry 47:128–133, 1984.

547. Drummond PD and Lance JW: Facial temperature in migraine, tension–vascular and tension headache. Cephalalgia 4:149–158, 1984.

548. Drummond PD and Lance JW: Neurovascular changes in headache patients. Clin Exp Neurol 20:93–99, 1984.

549. du Boulay GH, Ruiz JS, Clifford Rose F, Stevens JM, and Zilka KJ: CT changes associated with migraine. AJNR 4:472–473, 1983.

550. Duckro PN and Cantwell-Simmons E: A review of studies evaluating biofeedback and relaxation training in the management of pediatric headache. Headache 29:428–433, 1989.

551. Duckro PN, Tait RC, and Margolis RB: Prevalence of very severe headache in a large US metropolitan area. Cephalalgia 9:199–205, 1989.

552. Duffy GB: The warning leak in spontaneous subarachnoid hemorrhage. Med J Aust 28:514, 516, 1983.

553. Duggan AW and North RA: Electrophysiology of opioids. Pharmacol Rev 35:219–281, 1983.

554. Dukes HT and Vieth RG: Cerebral arteriography during migraine prodrome and headache. Neurology 14:636–639, 1964.

555. Dunn DW and Snyder CH: Benign paroxysmal vertigo of childhood. Am J Dis Child 130:1099–1100, 1976.

555a. Dürsteler MR: Migräne und Vestibularapparat. J Neurol 210:253–269, 1975.

556. Duthie DJR and Nimmo WS: Adverse effects of opioid analgesic drugs. Br J Anaesthesia 59:61–77, 1987.

557. Dvilansky A, Rishpon S, Nathan I, Zolotow Z, and Korczyn AD: Release of platelet 5-hydroxytryptamine by plasma taken from patients during and between migraine attacks. Pain 2:315–318, 1976.

558. Dworkin GS, Andermann F, Carpenter S, et al.: Classical migraine, intractable epilepsy amd multiple strokes: A syndrome related to mitochondrial encephalopathy. In Andermann F and Lugaresi E (eds): Migraine and Epilepsy. Butterworth, Boston, 1987, pp 203–232.

559. Eadie MJ: Ergotamine pharmacokinetics in man: An editorial. Cephalalgia 3:135–138, 1983.

560. Ebertz JM, Hirshman CA, Kettelkamp NS, Uno H, and Hanifin JM: Substance P-induced histamine release in human cutaneous mast cells. J Invest Dermatol 88:682–685, 1987.

561. Eckert H, Kiechel JR, Rosenthaler J, Schmidt R, and Schrier E: Biopharmaceutical aspects. Analytical methods, pharmacokinetics, metabolism, and bioavailability. In Berde B and Schild HO (eds): Ergot Alkaloids and Related Compounds, Handbook of Experimental Pharmacology, Vol 49. Springer-Verlag, New York, 1978, pp. 719–803.

562. Edelson RN: Menstrual migraine and other hormonal aspects of migraine. Headache 25:376–379, 1985.

563. Edes AD and Daily D: EEG studies in complex migraine. Electroencephalogr Clin Neurophysiol 23:86, 1967.

564. Editorial: Headache in multiple sclerosis. Br Med J 187:713–714, 1969.

565. Edmeads J: Management of the acute attack of migraine. Headache 13:91–95, 1973.

566. Edmeads J: Cerebral blood flow in migraine. Headache 17:148–152, 1977.

567. Edmeads J: Headaches and head pains associated with disease of the cervical spine. Med Clin North Am 62:533–544, 1978.

568. Edmeads J: The headaches of ischemic cerebrovascular disease. Headache 19:345–349, 1979.

569. Edmeads J: Complicated migraine

and headache in cerebrovascular disease. Neurol Clin 1:385–397, 1983.

570. Edmeads J: Does the neck play a role in migraine? In Blau JN (ed): Migraine. Clinical and Research Aspects. Johns Hopkins University Press, Baltimore, 1987, pp 651–656.

571. Edmeads J: Emergency management of headache. Headache 28:675–679, 1988.

572. Edmeads J: Management of migraine in the elderly. In Diamond S (ed): Migraine Headache Prevention and Management. Dekker, New York, 1990, pp 173–188.

573. Edmeads J: Controversies in complicated migraine. Headache Quarterly, Current Treatment and Research 1:45–50, 1990.

574. Edna TH and Cappelen J: Late postconcussional symptoms in traumatic head injury. An analysis of frequency and risk factors. Acta Neurochir 86:12–17, 1987.

575. Edvinsson L: Characterization of the contractile effect of neuropeptide Y in feline cerebral arteries. Acta Physiol Scand 125:33–41, 1985.

576. Edvinsson L: Beta-adrenoceptor functions and the cerebral circulation. In Clifford Rose F (ed): Advances in Headache Research, Vol 4, Libbey, London, 1987, pp 147–153.

577. Edvinsson L, Brodin E, Jansen I, and Uddman R: Neurokinin A in cerebral vessels: Characterization, localization and effects in vitro. Regulatory Peptides 20:181–197, 1988.

578. Edvinsson L, Copeland JR, Emson PC, McCulloch J, and Uddman R: Nerve fibers containing neuropeptide Y in the cerebrovascular bed: Immunocytochemistry, radioimmunoassay, and vasomotor effects. J Cereb Blood Flow Met 7:45–57, 1987.

579. Edvinsson L, Degueurce A, Duverger D, MacKenzie ET, and Scatton B: Central serotonergic nerves project to the pial vessels of the brain. Nature 306:55–57, 1983.

580. Edvinsson L and Ekman R: Distribution and dilatory effect of vasoactive intestinal polypeptide (VIP) in human cerebral arteries. Peptides 5:329–331, 1984.

581. Edvinsson L, Ekman R, Jansen I, McCulloch J, and Uddman R: Calcitonin gene-related peptide and cerebral blood vessels: Distribution and vasomotor effects. J Cereb Blood Flow Metab 7:720–728, 1987.

582. Edvinsson L, Ekman R, Jansen I, Ottosson A, and Uddman R: Peptide-containing nerve fibers in human cerebral arteries: Immunocytochemistry, radioimmunoassay, and in vitro pharmacology. Ann Neurol 21:431–437, 1987.

583. Edvinsson L, Emson P, McCulloch J, Tatemoto K, and Uddman R: Neuropeptide Y: Cerebrovascular innervation and vasomotor effects in the cat. Neuroscience Lett 43:79–84, 1983.

584. Edvinsson L, Emson P, McCulloch J, Tatemoto K, and Uddman R: Neuropeptide Y: Immunocytochemical localization to and effect upon feline pial arteries and veins in vitro and in situ. Acta Physiol Scand 122:155–163, 1984.

585. Edvinsson L, Fahrenkrug J, Hanko J, McCulloch J, and Owman C: Vasoactive intestinal polypeptide: Distribution and effects on cerebral blood flow and metabolism. In Cervós-Navarro J and Fritschka E (eds): Cerebral Microcirculation and Metabolism. Raven, New York, 1981, pp 147–155.

586. Edvinsson L, Falck B, and Owman C: Possibilities for a cholinergic action on smooth musculature and on sympathetic axons in brain vessels mediated by muscarinic and nicotinic receptors. J Pharmacol Exp Ther 200:117–126, 1977.

587. Edvinsson L and Fredholm BB: Characterization of adenosine receptors in isolated cerebral arteries of cat. Br J Pharmacol 80:631–637, 1983.

588. Edvinsson L, Lindvall K, Nielsen C, and Owman C: Are brain vessels innervated also by central (non-sympathetic) adrenergic neurons? Brain Res 63:496–499, 1973.

589. Edvinsson L and MacKenzie ET: Amine mechanisms in the cerebral circulation. Pharmacol Rev 28:275–348, 1976.

590. Edvinsson L, McCulloch J, Kingman TA, and Uddman R: On the functional role of the trigemino-cerebrovascular system in the regulation of cerebral circulation. In Owman C and Hardebo JE (eds): Neural Regulation of Brain Circulation. Elsevier, Amsterdam, 1986, pp 407–418.

591. Edvinsson L, McCulloch J, and Uddman R: Substance P: Immunohistochemical localization and effect upon cat pial arteries *in vitro* and *in situ*. J. Physiol (Lond) 318:251–258, 1981.

592. Edvinsson L, McCulloch J, and Uddman R: Feline cerebral veins and arteries: Comparison of autonomic innervation and vasomotor responses. J Physiol (Lond) 325:161–173, 1982.

593. Edvinsson L and Owman C: Sympathetic innervation and adrenergic receptors in intraparenchymal cerebral arterioles of baboon. Acta Physiol Scand 452 (Suppl):57–59, 1977.

594. Edvinsson L and Uddman R: Adrenergic, cholinergic and peptidergic nerve fibres in dura mater—involvement in headache. Cephalalgia 1:175–179, 1981.

595. Edvinsson L and Uddman R: Immunohistochemical localization and dilatatory effect of substance P on human cerebral arteries. Brain Res 232:466–471, 1982.

596. Eeg-Olofsson O, Odkvist L, Lindskog U, and Anderson B: Benign paroxysmal vertigo in childhood. Acta Otolaryngol 93:283–289, 1982.

597. Egger J, Carter CM, Wilson J, Turner MW, and Soothill JF: Is migraine food allergy? A double-blind controlled trial of oligoantigenic diet treatment. Lancet *ii*:865–869, 1983.

598. Ehde DM and Holm JE: Stress and headache: Comparisons of migraine, tension, and headache-free subjects. Headache Quarterly, Current Treatment and Research 3:54–60, 1992.

599. Ehyai A and Fenichel GM: The natural history of acute confusional migraine. Arch Neurol 35:368–369, 1978.

600. Eigler FW, Schaarschmidt K, Gross E, and Richter HJ: Anorectal ulcers as a complication of migraine therapy. J R Soc Med 79:424–426, 1986.

601. Ekbom K: Alprenolol for migraine prophylaxis. Headache 15:129–132, 1975.

602. Ekbom K: Some observations on pain in cluster headache. Headache 14:219–225, 1975.

603. Ekbom K and Lundberg PO: Clinical trial of LB-56 (d,1-4-(2-hydroxy-3-isopropylaminopropoxy)indol): An adrenergic β-receptor blocking agent in migraine prophylaxis. Headache 12:15–17, 1972.

604. Ekbom K and Zetterman M: Oxprenolol in the treatment of migraine. Acta Neurol Scand 56:181–184, 1977.

605. Elkind AH: Interval therapy of migraine: The art and science. Headache Quarterly, Current Treatment and Research 1:280–289, 1990.

606. Elkind AH, Friedman AP, Bachman A, Siegelman SS, and Sacks OW: Silent retroperitoneal fibrosis associated with methysergide therapy. JAMA 206:1041–1044, 1968.

607. Elkind AH, Friedman AP, and Grossman J: Cutaneous blood flow in vascular headaches of the migraine type. Neurology 14:24–30, 1974.

608. El-Mallakh RS: Marijuana and migraine. Headache 27:442–443, 1987.

609. El-Mallakh RS, Kranzler HR, and Kamanitz JR: The association between headaches and alcohol and drug use in substance abuse patients. Headache Quarterly, Current Treatment and Research 2:319–322, 1991.

610. Emery ES: Acute confusional state in children with migraine. Pediatrics 60:110–114, 1977.

611. Emori T, Hirata Y, Ohta K, Schichiri M, and Marumo F: Secretory mechanism of immunoreactive endothelin in cultured bovine endothelial cells.

Biochem Biophys Res Commun 160:93–100, 1989.

612. Engel D: Studies on headache produced by carbon dioxide, histamine and adrenalin. Acta Neurochir 21:269–283, 1969.

613. Engel GL: 'Psychogenic' pain and the pain-prone patient. Am J Med 26:899–918, 1959.

614. Engel GL, Webb JP, Ferris EB, Romano J, Ryder H, and Blankenhorn MA: A migraine-like syndrome complicating decompression sickness. War Med 5:304–314, 1944.

615. Epstein LH, Abel GG, Colline F, Parker L, and Cinciripini PM: The relationship between frontalis muscle reactivity and self-reports of headache pain. Behav Res Ther 16:153–160, 1978.

616. Epstein MT, Hockaday JM, and Hockaday TDR: Migraine and reproductive hormones throughout the menstrual cycle. Lancet i:543–546, 1975.

617. Evans CS, Gray S, and Kazim NO: Analysis of commercially available cheeses for the migraine inducer tyramine by thin-layer chromatography and spectrophotometry. Analyst 113:1605–1606, 1988.

618. Evans L and Spelman M: The problem of non-compliance with drug therapy. Drugs 25:63–76, 1983.

619. Evans RW: The postconcussion syndrome and the sequelae of mild head injury. Neurol Clin 10:815–847, 1992.

620. Executive Committee of the American Academy of Allergy and Immunology: Clinical ecology. J Allergy Clin Immunol 78:269–271, 1986.

621. Facchinetti F and Genazzani AR: Opioids in cerebrospinal fluid and blood of headache sufferers. In Olesen J and Edvinsson L (eds): Basic Mechanisms of Headache. Elsevier, Amsterdam, 1988, pp 262–269.

622. Facchinetti F, Nappi G, Savoldi F, and Genazzani AR: Primary headaches: Reduced circulating β-lipotropin and β-endorphin levels with impaired reactivity to acupuncture. Cephalalgia 1:195–201, 1981.

623. Fanchamps A: Why do not all beta-blockers prevent migraine? Headache 25:61–62, 1985.

624. Fanciullacci M: Iris adrenergic impairment in idiopathic headache. Headache 19:8–13, 1979.

625. Fanciullacci M, Franchi G, and Michelacci S: Indomethacin as a drug capable of provoking or breaking off headache. Res Clin Stud Headache 3:335–343, 1970.

626. Farkas V, Benninger C, and Matthis P: EEG alterations in migraine. An expression of pain hypertransmission? Adv Pain Res Ther 20:241–251, 1992.

627. Farkas V, Benninger C, Matthis P, Scheffner D, and Lindeisz F: The EEG background activity in children with migraine. Cephalalgia 7 (Suppl 6):59–64, 1987.

628. Farrell WJ, Nolan JJ, and Tessitore A: Unilateral leg edema, migraine and methysergide. JAMA 207:1909–1911, 1969.

629. Fay T: The mechanism of headache. Trans Am Neurol Assoc 62:72–77, 1936.

630. Fazekas F, Koch M, Schmidt R, et al.: The prevalence of cerebral damage varies with migraine type: A MRI study. Headache 32:287–291, 1992.

631. FDA Drug Bulletin. Use of approved drugs for unlabeled indications. 12:4–5, 1982.

632. Featherstone HJ: Low-dose propranolol therapy for aborting acute migraine. West J Med 138:416–417, 1983.

633. Featherstone HJ: Medical diagnoses and problems in individuals with recurrent idiopathic headaches. Headache 25:136–140, 1985.

634. Featherstone HJ: Migraine and muscle contraction headaches: A continuum. Headache 25:194–198, 1985.

635. Featherstone HJ: Clinical features of stroke in migraine: A review. Headache 26:128–133, 1986.

636. Fedotin MS and Hartman C: Ergotamine poisoning producing renal arterial spasm. N Engl J Med 283:518–520, 1970.

637. Feindel W, Penfield W, and Mc-Naughton F: The tentorial nerves and localization of intracranial pain in man. Neurology 10:555–563, 1960.

638. Feinmann C: Pain relief by antidepressants: Possible modes of action. Pain 23:1–8, 1985.

639. Feldman JM, Lee EM, and Castleberry CA: Catecholamine and serotonin content of foods: Effect on urinary excretion of homovanillic acid and 5-hydroxyindoleacetic acid. J Am Diet Assoc 87:1031–1035, 1987.

640. Feneley MP, Morgan JJ, McGrath MA, and Egan JD: Transient aortic arch syndrome with dysphasia due to ergotism. Stroke 14:811–814, 1983.

641. Fenichel GM: Migraine as a cause of benign paroxysmal vertigo of childhood. J Pediat 71:114–115, 1967.

642. Fenichel GM: Migraine in children. Neurol Clinics 3:77–94, 1985.

643. Feniuk W, Humphrey PPA, and Perren MJ: The selective carotid arterial vasoconstrictor action of GR 43175 in anaesthetized dogs. Br J Pharmacol 96:83–90, 1989.

644. Fentress DW, Masek BJ, Mehegan JE, and Benson H: Biofeedback and relaxation response training in the treatment of pediatric migraine. Develop Med Child Neurol 28:139–146, 1986.

645. Ferbert A, Busse D, and Thron A: Microinfarction in classic migraine? A study with magnetic resonance imaging findings. Stroke 22:1010–1014, 1991.

646. Ferrari MD, Bayliss EM, Ludlow S, and Pilgrim AJ: Subcutaneous GR43175 in the treatment of acute migraine: An international study. Cephalalgia 9 (Suppl 10):348, 1989.

647. Ferrari MD, Buruma OJS, van Laar-Ramaker M, and Dijkmans BC: A migrainous syndrome with pleocytosis. Neurology 33:813, 1983.

648. Ferrari MD, Odink J, Frölich M, Tapparelli C, and Portielje JEA: Release of platelet metenkephalin, but not serotonin, in migraine. A platelet response unique to migraine patients? J Neurol Sci 93:51–60, 1989.

649. Ferrari MD, Odink J, Tapparelli C, Van Kempen GMJ, Pennings EJM, and Bruyn GW: Serotonin metabolism in migraine. Neurology 39:1239–1242, 1989.

650. Ferreira SH and Nakamura M: Prostaglandin hyperalgesia, a cAMP/Ca^{++} dependent process. Prostaglandins 18:179–190, 1979.

651. Fields HL, Emson PC, Leigh BK, Gilbert RFT, and Iversen LL: Multiple opiate receptor sites on primary afferent fibres. Nature 284:351–353, 1980.

652. Fields HL, Heinricher MM, and Mason P: Neurotransmitters in nociceptive modulatory circuits. Annu Rev Neurosci 14:219–245, 1991.

653. Fincham RW, Perdue Z, and Dunn VD: Bilateral focal cortical atrophy and chronic ergotamine abuse. Neurology 35:720–722, 1985.

654. Finley JC, Lindström P, and Petrusz P: Immunocytochemical localization of β-endorphin–containing neurons in the rat brain. Neuroendocrinology 33:28–42, 1981.

655. Fisher CM: Headache in acute cerebrovascular disease. In Vinken PJ and Bruyn GW (eds): Handbook of Clinical Neurology, Vol 5. North-Holland, Amsterdam, 1968, pp 124–156.

656. Fisher CM: Cerebral ischemia—less familiar types. Clin Neurosurg 18:267–335, 1971.

657. Fisher CM: Late-life migraine accompaniments as a cause of unexplained transient ischemic attacks. Can J Neurol Sci 7:9–17, 1980.

658. Fisher CM: The headache and pain of spontaneous carotid dissection. Headache 22:60–65, 1982.

659. Fisher CM: Late-life migraine accompaniments—further experience. Stroke 17:1033–1042, 1986.

660. Fitterling JM, Martin JE, Gramling S, Cole P, and Milan MA: Behavioral management of exercise training in vascular headache patients: An investigation of exercise adherence

and headache activity. J Appl Behav Anal 21:9–19, 1988.

661. Fitzpatrick R and Hopkins A: Referrals to neurologists for headaches not due to structural disease. J Neurol Neurosurg Psychiatry 44:1061–1067, 1981.

662. Fitzsimons RB and Wolfenden WH: Migraine coma: Meningitic migraine with cerebral edema associated with a new form of autosomal dominant cerebellar ataxia. Brain 108:555–577, 1985.

663. Fjällbrant N and Iggo A: The effect of histamine, 5-hydroxytryptamine and acetylcholine on cutaneous afferent fibres. J Physiol (Lond) 156:578–590, 1961.

664. Fleishman JA, Segall JD, and Judge FP: Isolated transient alexia. A migrainous accompaniment. Arch Neurol 40:115–116, 1983.

665. Flodgaard H and Klenow H: Abundant amounts of diadenosine 5′,5″-P^1,P^4-tetraphosphate are present and releasable, but metabolically inactive, in human platelets. Biochem J 208:737–742, 1982.

666. Fock S and Mense S: Excitatory effects of 5-hydroxytryptamine, histamine and potassium ions on muscular group IV afferent units: A comparison with bradykinin. Brain Res 105:459–469, 1976.

667. Fog-Møller F, Bryndum B, Dalsgaard-Nielsen T, Kemp Genefke I, and Nattero G: Therapeutic effect of reserpine on migraine syndrome: Relationship to blood amine levels. Headache 15:275–278, 1976.

668. Foo Lin I, Spiga R, and Fortsch W: Insight and adherence to medication in chronic schizophrenics. J Clin Psychiatry 40:430–432, 1979.

669. Foote SL, Bloom FE, and Aston-Jones G: Nucleus locus coeruleus: New evidence of anatomical and physiological specificity. Physiol Rev 63:844–914, 1983.

670. Forbes HS, Wolff HG, and Cobb S: The cerebral circulation. X. The action of histamine. Am J Physiol 89:266–272, 1929.

671. Formisano R, Falaschi P, Cerbo R, et al.: Nimodipine in migraine: Clinical efficacy and endocrinological effects. Eur J Clin Pharmacol 41:69–71, 1991.

672. Formisano R, Zanette E, Cerbo R, et al.: Transcranial Doppler on spontaneous and induced attacks in migraine patients. Cephalalgia 9 (Suppl 10):68–69, 1989.

673. Forrester T, Harper AM, MacKenzie ET, and Thomson EM: Effect of adenosine triphosphate and some derivatives on cerebral blood flow and metabolism. J Physiol (Lond) 296:343–355, 1979.

674. Forssman B, Henriksson KG, Johannson V, Lindvall L, and Lundin HC: Propranolol for migraine prophylaxis. Headache 16:238–245, 1976.

675. Forssman B, Lindblad CJ, and Zbornikova V: Atenolol for migraine prophylaxis. Headache 23:188–190, 1983.

676. Forsythe WI: Headache: part VII—use of sedatives and tranquilizers in the treatment of headaches in adults and children. International Medicine 7:169–173, 1986.

677. Forsythe WI, Gilles D, and Sills MA: Propranolol ('Inderal') in the treatment of childhood migraine. Develop Med Child Neurol 26:737–741, 1984.

678. Forsythe WI and Redmond A: Two controlled trials of tyramine in children with migraine. Develop Med Child Neurol 16:794–799, 1974.

679. Foster RW and Ramage AG: The action of some chemical irritants on somatosensory receptors of the cat. Neuropharmacology 20:191–198, 1981.

680. Fowler PA, Lacey LF, Thomas M, Keene ON, Tanner RJN, and Baber NS: The clinical pharmacology, pharmacokinetics and metabolism of sumatriptan. Eur Neurol 31:291–294, 1991.

681. Fowler PA, Thomas M, Lacey LF, Andrew P, and Dallas FAA: Early studies with the novel 5-HT_1-like agonist

GR43175 in healthy volunteers. Cephalalgia 9 (Suppl 9):57–62, 1989.

682. Fozard JR: Serotonin, migraine and platelets. Prog Pharmacol 4:136–146, 1982.

683. Fozard JR: 5-HT$_3$ receptors and cytotoxic drug-induced vomiting. Trends Pharmacol Sci 8:44–45, 1987.

684. Fozard JR: The pharmacological basis of migraine treatment. In Blau JN (ed): Migraine. Clinical and Research Aspects. The Johns Hopkins University Press, Baltimore, 1987, pp 165–184.

685. Fozard JR: 5-HT in migraine: Evidence from 5-HT receptor antagonists for a neuronal etiology. In Sandler M and Collins GM (eds): Migraine: A Spectrum of Ideas. Oxford University Press, Oxford, 1990, pp 128–141.

686. Frank JD: Biofeedback and the placebo effect. Biofeedback Self-regulation 7:449–460, 1982.

687. Fredriksen TA, Hovdal H, and Sjaastad O: Cervicogenic headache: Clinical manifestations. Cephalalgia 7:147–160, 1987.

688. Freedman MS and Gray TA: Vascular headache: A presenting symptom of multiple sclerosis. Can J Neurol Sci 16:63–66, 1989.

689. Freitag FG and Diamond S: Nadolol and placebo comparison study in the prophylactic treatment of migraine. JAMA 84:737–741, 1984.

690. Frenken CWGM and Nuijten STM: Flunarizine, a new preventive approach to migraine: A double-blind comparison with placebo. Clin Neurol Neurosurg 86:17–20, 1984.

691. Friberg L: Cerebral blood flow changes in migraine: Methods, observations and hypotheses. J Neurol 238:S12–S17, 1991.

692. Friberg L, Kastrup J, Hansen M, and Bülow J: Cerebral effects of scalp cooling and extracerebral contribution to calculated blood flow values using the intravenous ^{133}Xe technique. Scand J Clin Lab Invest 46:375–379, 1986.

693. Friberg L, Olesen J, and Iversen HK: Regional cerebral blood flow during attacks and when free of symptoms in a large group of migraine patients. Cephalalgia 9 (Suppl 10):29–30, 1989.

694. Friberg L, Olesen J, Iversen HK, and Sperling B: Migraine pain associated with middle cerebral artery dilatation: Reversal by sumatriptan. Lancet 338:13–17, 1991.

695. Friberg L, Skyhøj Olsen T, Roland PE, and Lassen NA: Focal ischaemia caused by instability of cerebrovascular tone during attacks of hemiplegic migraine. A regional cerebral blood flow study. Brain 110:917–934, 1987.

696. Fricton JR: Myofascial pain syndrome. Adv Pain Res Ther 17:107–127, 1990.

697. Fried FE, Lamberti J, and Sneed P: Treatment of tension and migraine headaches with biofeedback techniques. Missouri Med 74:253–255, 1977.

698. Friedman AP: Migraine headaches. JAMA 222:1399–1402, 1972.

699. Friedman AP: Migraine: An overview. In Pearce J (ed): Modern Topics in Migraine. Heinemann, London, 1975, pp 159–167.

700. Friedman AP: Characteristics of tension headache: A profile of 1420 cases. Psychosomatics 20:451–461, 1979.

701. Friedman AP: Overview of migraine. Adv Neurol 33:1–17, 1982.

702. Friedman AP and Brenner C: Posttraumatic and histamine headache. Arch Neurol Psychiatry 52:126–130, 1944.

703. Friedman AP, Harter DH, and Merritt HH: Ophthalmoplegic migraine. Arch Neurol 7:320–327, 1962.

704. Friedman AP, von Storch TJC, and Merritt HH: Migraine and tension headaches. A clinical study of 2000 cases. Neurology 4:773–788, 1954.

705. Friedman AP and Wood EH: Thermography in vascular headache. In

Uematsu S (ed): Medical Thermography, Theory and Clinical Applications. Brentwood, Los Angeles, 1976, pp 80–84.

706. Friedman H and Traub HA: Brief psychological training procedures in migraine treatment. Am J Clin Hypnosis 26:187–200, 1984.

707. Friedman MD and Wilson EJ: Migraine: Its treatment with dihydroergotamine. Ohio State Med J 43:934–938, 1947.

708. Fries JF, Williams CA, Bloch DA, and Michel BA: Nonsteroidal anti-inflammatory drug-associated gastropathy: Incidence and risk factor models. Am J Med 91:213–222, 1991.

709. Frishman WH: Beta-adrenergic blocker withdrawal. Am J Cardiol 59:26F–32F, 1987.

710. Froelich WA, Carter CC, O'Leary JL, and Rosenbaum HE: Headache in childhood. Electroencephalographic evaluation of 500 cases. Neurology 10:639–42, 1960.

711. Fromm-Reichmann F: Contribution to the psychogenesis of migraine. Psychoanal Rev 24:26–33, 1937.

712. Fuchs M and Blumenthal LS: Use of ergot preparations in migraine. JAMA 143:1462–1464, 1950.

713. Fukushima T and Kerr FWL: Organization of trigeminothalamic tracts and other thalamic afferent systems of the brainstem in the rat: Presence of gelatinosa neurons with thalamic connections. J Comp Neurol 183:169–184, 1979.

714. Fuller GN and Guiloff RJ: Migrainous olfactory hallucinations. J Neurol Neurosurg Psychiatry 50:1688–1690, 1987.

715. Fuller RW, Snoddy HD, and Hemrick SK: Effects of fenfluramine and norfenfluramine on brain serotonin metabolism in rats. Proc Soc Exp Biol Med 157:202–205, 1978.

716. Furchgott RF and Vanhoutte PM: Endothelium-derived relaxing and contracting factors. FASEB J 3:2007–2018, 1989.

717. Furmanski AR: Dynamic concepts of migraine. A character study of one hundred patients. Arch Neurol Psychiatry 67:23–31, 1952.

718. Gale EN: Psychological characteristics of long-term female temporomandibular joint pain patients. J Dent Res 57:481–483, 1978.

719. Gale EN and Gross A: An evaluation of temporomandibular joint sounds. J Am Dent Assoc 111:62–63, 1985.

720. Galer BS, Lipton RB, Solomon S, Newman LC, and Spierings ELH: Myocardial ischemia related to ergot alkaloids: A case report and literature review. Headache 31:446–450, 1991.

721. Gallagher RM: Emergency treatment of intractable migraine. Headache 26:74–75, 1986.

722. Gamberini G, D'Alessandro R, Labriola E, et al.: Further evidence on the association of mitral valve prolapse and migraine. Headache 24:39–40, 1984.

723. Gammie KM and Waters WE: Headache and migraine in a biscuit factory. In Waters WE (ed): The Epidemiology of Migraine. Boehringer Ingelheim, Bracknell-Berkshire. 1974, pp 44–48.

724. Gamsa A: Is emotional disturbance a precipitator or a consequence of chronic pain? Pain 42:183–195, 1990.

725. Gamse R, Holzer P, and Lembeck F: Indirect evidence for presynaptic location of opiate receptors on chemosensitive primary sensory neurons. Naunyn-Schmiedebergs Arch Pharmacol 308:281–285, 1979.

726. Gamse R, Leeman SE, Holzer P, and Lembeck F: Differential effects of capsaicin on the content of somatostatin, substance P, and neurotensin in the nervous system of the rat. Naunyn-Schmiedebergs Arch Pharmacol 317:140–148, 1981.

727. Garattini S, Buczko W, Jori A, and Samanin R: The mechanism of action of fenfluramine. Postgrad Med J 51 (Suppl 1):27–35, 1975.

728. Garcia Leme J: Bradykinin system. In Vane JR and Ferreira SH (eds): Inflammation, Handbook of Experimental Pharmacology, Vol 50, Part I.

Springer-Verlag, Berlin, 1978, pp 464–522.

729. Gardner JH, Hornstein S, and Van den Noort S: The clinical characteristics of headache during impending cerebral infarction in women taking oral contraceptives. Headache 8:108–111, 1968.

730. Gardner-Medwin AR: Possible roles of vertebrate neuroglia in potassium dynamics, spreading depression and migraine. J Exp Biol 95:111–127, 1981.

731. Gardner-Medwin AR, Tepley N, Barkley GL, et al.: Magnetic fields associated with spreading depression in anaesthetized rabbits. Brain Res 540:153–158, 1991.

732. Garnic JD and Schellinger D: Arterial spasm as a finding intimately associated with the onset of vascular headache. A case report. Neuroradiology 24:273–276, 1983.

733. Garvey MJ, Tollefson GD, and Schaffer CB: Migraine headaches and depression. Am J Psychiatry 141:986–988, 1984.

734. Gascon G and Barlow C: Juvenile migraine presenting as an acute confusional state. Pediatrics 45:628–635, 1970.

735. Gastaut H, Navarranne P, and Simon y Canton L: EEG characteristics of migrainous cerebral attacks of a deficitory type (hemiplegic migraine). Electroencephalogr Clin Neurophysiol 23:381, 1967.

736. Gastaut H and Zifkin BG: Benign epilepsy of childhood with occipital spike and wave complexes. In Andermann F and Lugaresi E (eds): Migraine and Epilepsy, Butterworth, Boston, 1987, pp 47–82.

737. Gastaut JL, Yermenos E, Bonnefoy M, and Cros D: Familial hemiplegic migraine: EEG and CT scan study of two cases. Ann Neurol 10:392–395, 1981.

738. Gauthier JG, Bois R, Allaire D, and Drolet M: Evaluation of skin temperature biofeedback training at two different sites for migraine. J Behav Med 4:407–419, 1981.

739. Gauthier JG, Fournier AL, and Roberge C: The differential effects of biofeedback in the treatment of menstrual and nonmenstrual migraine. Headache 31:82–90, 1991.

740. Gauthier JG, Fradet C, and Roberge C: The differential effects of biofeedback in the treatment of classical and common migraine. Headache 28:39–46, 1988.

741. Gawel MJ, Burkitt M, and Clifford Rose F: The platelet release reaction during migraine attacks. Headache 19:323–327, 1979.

742. Gawel MJ, Connolly JF, and Clifford Rose F: Migraine patients exhibit abnormalities in the visual evoked potential. Headache 23:49–52, 1983.

743. Gawel MJ, Kreeft J, Nelson RF, Simard D, and Arnott WS: Comparison of the efficacy and safety of flunarazine to propranolol in the prophylaxis of migraine. Can J Neurol Sci 19:340–345, 1992.

744. Gazzaniga PP, Ferroni P, Lenti L, et al.: Identification of blood leukotrienes in classical migraine. Headache 27:211–215, 1987.

745. Gebhart GF: Modulatory effects of descending systems on spinal dorsal horn neurons. In Yaksh TL (ed): Spinal Afferent Processing. Academic, New York, 1986, pp 391–416.

746. Gelford GJ and Cromwell DK: Methysergide, retroperitoneal fibrosis and rectosigmoid stricture. Am J Roentgen 104:566–570, 1968.

747. Gelford GJ, Wilets AJM, Nelson D, and Kroil L: Retroperitoneal fibrosis and methysergide: Report of three cases. Radiology 88:976–980, 1967.

748. Gelmers HJ: Common migraine attacks proceeded by focal hyperemia and parietal oligemia in the rCBF pattern. Cephalalgia 2:29–32, 1982.

749. Gelmers HJ: Nimodipine, a new calcium antagonist, in the prophylactic treatment of migraine. Headache 23:106–109, 1983.

750. Genazzani AR, Nappi G, Facchinetti F, et al.: Progressive impairment of CSF β-EP levels in migraine sufferers. Pain 18:127–133, 1984.

751. Geppetti P, Maggi CA, Perretti F, Frilli S, and Manzini S: Simulta-

neous release by bradykinin of substance P- and calcitonin gene-related peptide immunoreactivities from capsaicin-sensitive structures in guinea-pig heart. Br J Pharmacol 94:288–290, 1988.

752. Gerard G and Weisberg LA: MRI periventricular lesions in adults. Neurology 36:998–1001, 1986.

753. Gerber WD, Miltner W, and Niederberger U: The role of behavioral and social factors in the development of drug-induced headache. In Diener HC and Wilkinson M (eds): Drug-Induced Headache. Springer-Verlag, Berlin, 1988, pp 65–74.

754. Ghose K: Migraine, antimigraine drugs and tyramine pressor test. In Amery WK, Van Nueten JM, and Wauquier A (eds): The Pharmacological Basis of Migraine Therapy. Pitman, London, 1984, pp 213–229.

755. Ghose K and Carroll JD: Mechanism of tyramine-induced migraine: Similarity with dopamine and interactions with disulfiram and propranolol in migraine patients. Neuropsychobiol 12:122–126, 1984.

756. Ghose K, Coppen A, and Carroll D: Intravenous tyramine response in migraine before and during treatment with indoramin. Br Med J i:1191–1193, 1977.

757. Giacovazzo M, Martelletti P, and Valducci G: Computerized telethermographic assessment in migraine, with particular reference to the prodromal phase. Cephalalgia 6:219–222, 1986.

758. Giardina EGV, Cooper TB, Suckow R, and Saroff AL: Cardiovascular effects of doxepin in cardiac patients with ventricular arrhythmias. Clin Pharmacol Ther 42:20–27, 1987.

759. Gibb CM, Davies PTG, Glover V, Steiner TJ, Clifford Rose F, and Sandler M: Chocolate is a migraine-provoking agent. Cephalalgia 11:93–95, 1991.

760. Gibbins I, Brayden JE, and Bevan JA: Perivascular nerves with immunoreactivity to vasoactive intestinal polypeptide in cephalic arteries of the cat: Distribution, possible origins and functional implications. Neuroscience 13:1327–1346, 1984.

761. Gibbs FA and Gibbs EL: Atlas of Electroencephalography. Methodology and Controls. Addison-Wesley, Cambridge, 1950.

762. Giel R, de Vlieger M, and van Vliet AGM: Headache and the EEG. Electroencephalogr Clin Neurophysiol 2:492–495, 1966.

763. Gilbert GJ: An occurrence of complicated migraine during propranolol therapy. Headache 22:81–83, 1982.

764. Gilchrist JM and Coleman RA: Ornithine transcarbamylase deficiency: Adult onset of severe symptoms. Ann Intern Med 106:556–558, 1987.

765. Giuseffi V, Wall M, Siegel PZ, and Rojas PB: Symptoms and disease associations in idiopathic intracranial hypertension (pseudotumor cerebri): A case control study. Neurology 41:239–244, 1991.

766. Glaros AG: Incidence of diurnal and nocturnal bruxism. J Prosthet Dent 45:545–549, 1981.

767. Glassman AH and Bigger JT: Cardiovascular effects of therapeutic doses of tricyclic antidepressants. A review. Arch Gen Psychiatry 38:815–820, 1981.

768. Glassman AH, Bigger JT, Giardina EV, Kantor SJ, Perel JM, and Davies M: Clinical characteristics of imipramine-induced orthostatic hypotension. Lancet i:468–472, 1979.

769. Glaum SR, Proudfit HK, and Anderson EG: Reversal of the antinociceptive effects of intrathecally administered serotonin in the rat by a selective 5-HT$_3$ receptor antagonist. Neurosci Lett 95:313–317, 1988.

770. Glista GG, Mellinger JF, and Rooke ED: Familial hemiplegic migraine. Mayo Clin Proc 50:307–311, 1975.

771. Gloor P: Migraine and regional cerebral blood flow. Trends Neurosci 9:21, 1986.

772. Glover V, Littlewood J, Sandler M, Peatfield R, Petty R, and Clifford Rose F: Biochemical predisposition

to dietary migraine: The role of phenolsulphotransferase. Headache 23:53–58, 1983.

773. Glover V, Littlewood J, Sandler M, Peatfield R, Petty R, and Clifford Rose F: Dietary migraine: Looking beyond tyramine. In Clifford Rose F (ed): Progress in Migraine Research. Pitman, London, 1984, pp 113–119.

774. Glover V, Peatfield RC, Zammit-Pace R, et al.: Platelet monoamine oxidase activity and headache. J Neurol Neurosurg Psychiatry 44:786–790, 1981.

775. Glover V and Sandler M: The biochemical basis of migraine predisposition. In Sandler M and Collins GM (eds): Migraine: A Spectrum of Ideas. Oxford University Press, Oxford, 1990, pp 228–241.

776. Goadsby PJ and Duckworth JW: Low frequency stimulation of the locus coeruleus reduces regional cerebral blood flow in the spinalized cat. Brain Res 476:71–77, 1989.

777. Goadsby PJ, Edvinsson L, and Ekman R: Release of vasoactive peptides in the extracerebral circulation of humans and the cat during activation of the trigeminovascular system. Ann Neurol 23:193–196, 1988.

778. Goadsby PJ, Edvinsson L, and Ekman R: Vasoactive peptide release in the extracerebral circulation of humans during migraine headache. Ann Neurol 28:183–187, 1990.

779. Goadsby PJ and Gundlach AL: Localization of ^{3}H-dihydroergotamine-binding sites in the cat central nervous system: Relevance to migraine. Ann Neurol 29:91–94, 1991.

780. Goadsby PJ, Lambert GA, and Lance JW: Differential effects on the internal and external carotid circulation of the monkey evoked by locus coeruleus stimulation. Brain Res 249:247–254, 1982.

781. Goadsby PJ, Lambert GA, and Lance JW: Effects of locus coeruleus stimulation on carotid vascular resistance in the cat. Brain Res 278:175–183, 1983.

782. Goadsby PJ, Lambert GA, and Lance JW: The peripheral pathway for extracranial vasodilatation in the cat. J Auton Nerv Syst 10:145–155, 1984.

783. Goadsby PJ, Lambert GA, and Lance JW: The mechanism of cerebrovascular vasoconstriction in response to locus coeruleus stimulation. Brain Res 326:213–217, 1985.

784. Goadsby PJ and Lance JW: Brain stem effects on intra- and extracerebral circulations. Relation to migraine and cluster headache. In Olesen J and Edvinsson L (eds): Basic Mechanisms of Headache. Elsevier, Amsterdam, 1988, pp 413–427.

785. Goadsby PJ, Piper RD, Lambert GA, and Lance JW: The effect of stimulation of the nucleus raphe dorsalis (DRN) on carotid blood flow. I. The monkey. Am J Physiol 248:R257–R267, 1985.

786. Goadsby PJ, Piper RD, Lambert GA, and Lance JW: The effect of stimulation of the nucleus raphe dorsalis (DRN) on carotid blood flow. II. The cat. Am J Physiol 248:R263–R269, 1985.

787. Goadsby PJ and Zagami AS: Stimulation of the superior sagittal sinus increases metabolic activity and blood flow in certain regions of the brain stem and upper cervical spinal cord of the cat. Brain 114:1001–1011, 1991.

788. Goadsby PJ, Zagami AS, Donnan GA, et al.: Oral sumatriptan in acute migraine. Lancet 338:782–783, 1991.

789. Goadsby PJ, Zagami AS, and Lambert GA: Neural processing of craniovascular pain: A synthesis of the central structures involved in migraine. Headache 31:365–371, 1991.

790. Gold MS, Potash C, Sweeney DR, and Kleber WD: Opiate withdrawal using clonidine. JAMA 243:343–346, 1980.

791. Golden GS and French JH: Basilar artery migraine in young children. Pediatrics 56:722–726, 1975.

792. Goldensohn ES: Paroxysmal and other features of the electroenceph-alogram in migraine. Res Clin Stud Headache 4:118–128, 1976.

793. Goldfischer JD: Acute myocardial infarction secondary to ergot therapy. Report of a case and review of the literature. N Engl J Med 262:860–863, 1960.

794. Goldhammer L: Spectrum of cervicocranial junction syndromes involving occipital neuralgias. Occipital trigeminal syndrome. Headache Quarterly, Current Treatment and Research 1:230–238, 1990.

795. Goldstein AS, Kaizer S, and Warren R: Psychotropic effects of caffeine in man. II. Alertness, psychomotor coordination, and mood. J Pharmacol Exp Ther 150:146–151, 1965.

796. Goldstein J: Headache in AIDS. In Clifford Rose F (ed): New Advances in Headache Research. Smith-Gordon, London, 1989, pp 31–38.

797. Goldstein J: Headache and acquired immunodeficiency syndrome. Neurol Clin 8:947–960, 1990.

798. Goldstein J: Posttraumatic headache and the postconcussion syndrome. Med Clin North Am 75:641–651, 1991.

799. Goldstein M and Chen TC: The epidemiology of disabling headache. Adv Neurol 33:377–390, 1982.

800. Goldzieher JW, Moses LE, Averkin E, Scheel C, and Taber BZ: A placebo-controlled double-blind crossover investigation of the side effects attributed to oral contraceptives. Fertil Steril 22:609–623, 1971.

801. Golla FL and Winter AL: Analysis of cerebral responses to flicker in patients complaining of episodic headache. Electroencephalogr Clin Neurophysiol 11:539–549, 1959.

802. Gomersall JD and Stuart A: Amitriptyline in migraine prophylaxis. J Neurol Neurosurg Psychiatry 36:684–690, 1973.

803. Gomersall JD and Stuart A: Variations in migraine attacks with changes in weather conditions. Int J Biometeorol 17:285–299, 1973.

804. Gomi S, Gotoh F, Komatsumoto S, Ishikawa Y, Araki N, and Hamada J: Sweating function and retinal vasomotor reactivity in migraine. Cephalalgia 9:179–185, 1989.

805. Goodell H, Lewontin R, and Wolff H: Familial occurrence of migraine headache: A study of heredity. Arch Neurol Psychiatry 72:325–334, 1954.

806. Goodman BW: Temporal arteritis. Am J Med 67:839–852, 1979.

807. Gorelick PB, Hier DB, Caplan LR, and Langenberg P: Headache in acute cerebrovascular disease. Neurology 36:1445–1450, 1986.

808. Gotoh F, Komatsumoto S, Araki N, and Gomi S: Noradrenergic nervous activity in migraine. Arch Neurol 41:951–955, 1984.

809. Gowers WR: Subjective Sensations of Sight and Sound. Abiotrophy and Other Lectures. Churchill, London, 1907.

810. Graffenreid BV, Hill RC, and Nuesch E: Headache as a model for assessing mild analgesic drugs. J Clin Pharmacol 20:131–144, 1980.

811. Graff-Radford SB: Oromandibular disorders and headache: A critical appraisal. Neurol Clin 8:947–960, 1990.

812. Graff-Radford SB, Jaeger B, and Reeves JL: Myofascial pain may present clinically as occipital neuralgia. Neurosurgery 19:610–613, 1986.

813. Grafstein B: Mechanism of spreading cortical depression. J Neurophysiol 19:154–171, 1956.

814. Graham AN, Johnson ES, Persand NP, Turner P, and Wilkinson MG: Ergotamine toxicity and serum concentrations of ergotamine in migraine patients. Hum Toxicol 3:193–199, 1984.

815. Graham JR: Methysergide for prevention of headache: Experience in five hundred patients over three years. N Engl J Med 270:67–72, 1964.

816. Graham JR: Cardiac and pulmonary fibrosis during methysergide ther-

apy for headache. Am J Med Sci 254:23–34, 1967.

817. Graham JR: Migraine, clinical aspects. In Vinken PJ and Bruyn GW (eds): Handbook of Clinical Neurology, Vol 5. North-Holland, Amsterdam, 1968, pp 45–58.

818. Graham JR: Cluster headache. Headache 11:175–185, 1972.

819. Graham JR: Some clinical and theoretical aspects of cluster headache. In Saxena PR (ed): Migraine and Related Headaches. Erasmus Universiteit, Rotterdam, 1975, pp 27–40.

820. Graham JR, Rogado AZ, Rahman M, and Gramer IV: Some physiological and psychological characteristics of patients with cluster headache. In Cochrane AL (ed): Background to Migraine. Heinemann, London, 1970, pp 38–51.

821. Graham JR, Suby HI, Le Compte PM, and Sadowsky NL: Fibrotic disorders associated with methysergide therapy for headache. N Engl J Med 274:359–369, 1966.

822. Graham JR and Wolff HG: Mechanism of migraine headache and action of ergotamine tartrate. Arch Neurol Psychiatry 39:737–763, 1938.

823. Granella F, Farina S, Malferrari G, and Manzoni GC: Drug abuse in chronic headache: A clinico-epidemiologic study. Cephalalgia 7:15–19, 1987.

824. Grant ECG: Food allergies and migraine. Lancet i:966–968, 1979.

825. Grant ECG, Albuquerque M, Steiner TJ, and Clifford Rose F: Oral contraceptives, smoking, and ergotamine in migraine. In Greene R (ed): Current Concepts in Migraine Research. Raven, New York, 1978, pp 97–100.

826. Grässler W and Olthoff KH: Migräne und hormonelle Antikonzeptiva. Z Ärztl Fortbild (Jena) 78:229–232, 1984.

827. Gray LA: The use of progesterone in nervous tension states. South Med J 34:1004–1006, 1941.

828. Gray PA and Burtness HI: Hypoglycemic headache. Endocrinology 19:549–560, 1935.

829. Greenberg DA: Migraine. In Klawans HL, Goetz CG, and Tanner CM (eds): Textbook of Clinical Neuropharmacology and Therapeutics, 2nd ed. Raven, New York, 1992, pp 373–387.

830. Greenberg RN: Overview of patient compliance with medication dosing: A literature review. Clin Ther 6:592–599, 1984.

831. Greene R: Menstrual headache. Res Clin Stud Headache 1:62–73, 1967.

832. Griesbacher T and Lembeck F: Effect of bradykinin antagonists on bradykinin-induced plasma extravasation, venoconstriction, prostaglandin E_2 release, nociceptor stimulation, and contraction of the iris sphincter muscle in the rabbit. Br J Pharmacol 92:333–340, 1987.

833. Griffin MR, Ray WA, and Schaffner W: Nonsteroidal anti-inflammatory drug use and death from peptic ulcer in elderly persons. Ann Intern Med 109:359–363, 1988.

834. Griffith JF and Dodge PR: Transient blindness following head injury in children. N Engl J Med 278:648–651, 1968.

835. Griffith RW, Grauwiler J, Hodel CH, Leist KH, and Matter B: Toxicologic considerations. In Berde B and Schild HO (eds): Ergot Alkaloids and Related Compounds, Handbook of Experimental Pharmacology, Vol 49. Springer-Verlag, New York, 1978, pp. 805–851.

836. Griffiths RR and Woodson PP: Caffeine physical dependence: A review of human and laboratory animal studies. Psychopharmacology 94:437–451, 1988.

837. Grindal AB, Cohen RJ, Saul RF, and Taylor JR: Cerebral infarction in young adults. Stroke 9:39–42, 1978.

838. Gross PM, Harper AM, and Teasdale GM: Cerebral circulation and histamine: 2. Responses of pial veins and arterioles to receptor agonists. J

Cereb Blood Flow Metab 1:219–225, 1981.

839. Grosskreutz SR and Osborn RE: Computed tomography of the brain in the evaluation of the headache patient. Military Med 156:137–140, 1991.

840. Grotemeyer KH, Scharafinski HW, Husstedt I, and Schlake HP: Acetylsalicylic acid vs. metoprolol in migraine prophylaxis. A double-blind cross-over study. Headache 30:639–641, 1990.

841. Grotemeyer KH, Schlake HP, and Husstedt IW: Migräneprophylaxe mit Metoprolol und Flunarazine. Eine Doppelblind-cross-over-Studie. Nervenarzt 52:549–552, 1988.

842. Grotemeyer KH, Viand R, and Beykirch K: Thrombozytenfunktion bei vasomotorischen Kopfschmerzen und Migränekopfschmerzen. Dtsch Med Wochenschr 108:775–778, 1983.

843. Grzelewska-Rzymowska I, Bogucki A, Szmidt M, Kowalski ML, Prusinski A, and Rozniecki J: Migraine in aspirin-sensitive asthmatics. Allergol Immunopathol 13:13–16, 1985.

844. Guest IA and Woolf AL: Fatal infarction of the brain. Br Med J i:225–226, 1964.

845. Guiloff RJ and Fruns M: Limb pain in migraine and cluster headache. J Neurol Neurosurg Psychiatry 51:1022–1031, 1988.

846. Guiloff RJ and Fruns M: Migrainous limb pain. Headache 30:138–141, 1990.

847. Gulbenkian S, Merighi A, Wharton J, Varndell IM, and Polak JM: Ultrastructural evidence for the coexistence of calcitonin gene-related peptide and substance P in secretory vesicles of peripheral nerves in the guinea pig. J Neurocytol 15:535–542, 1986.

848. Gulliksen G and Enevoldsen E: Prolonged changes in rCBF following attacks of migraine accompagnée. Acta Neurol Scand 69 (Suppl 98):270–271, 1984.

849. Guralnick W, Kaban LB, and Merrill RG: Temporomandibular joint afflictions. N Engl J Med 299:123–129, 1978.

850. Guthkelch AN: Benign post-traumatic encephalopathy in young people and its relation to migraine. Neurosurgery 1:101–106, 1977.

851. Gwyn DG, Leslie RA, and Hopkins DA: Gastric afferents to the nucleus of the solitary tract in the cat. Neuroscience Lett 14:13–17, 1979.

852. Haas DC: Arteriovenous malformations and migraine: Case reports and an analysis of the relationship. Headache 31:509–513, 1991.

853. Haas DC and Lourie H: Trauma-triggered migraine: An explanation for common neurological attacks after mild head trauma. J Neurosurg 68:181–188, 1988.

854. Haber JD, Kuczmierczyk AR, and Adams HE: Tension headaches: Muscle overactivity or psychogenic pain. Headache 25:23–29, 1985.

855. Hachinski V, Norris JW, Edmeads J, and Cooper PW: Ergotamine and cerebral blood flow. Stroke 9:594–596, 1978.

856. Hachinski VC, Olesen J, Norris JW, Larsen B, Enevoldsen E, and Lassen NA: Cerebral hemodynamics in migraine. Can J Neurol Sci 4:245–249, 1977.

857. Hachinski VC, Porchawka J, and Steele JC: Visual symptoms in the migraine syndrome. Neurology 23:570–579, 1973.

858. Hagberg H, Andersson P, Lacarewicz J, Jacobson I, Butcher S, and Sandberg M: Extracellular adenosine, inosine, hypoxanthine and xanthine in relation to tissue nucleotides and purines in rat striatum during transient ischemia. J Neurochem 49:227–231, 1987.

859. Hage P: Exercise may reduce frequency of migraine. The Physician and Sports Medicine 9:24–25, 1981.

860. Hagen I, Nesheim BI, and Tuntland T: No effect of vitamin B-6 against premenstrual tension. A controlled clinical study. Acta Obstet Gynecol Scand 64:667–670, 1986.

861. Haimart M, Pradalier A, Launay JM, Dreux C, and Dry J: Whole blood and plasma histamine in common migraine. Cephalalgia 7:39–42, 1987.

862. Hakkarainen H and Allonen H: Ergotamine vs. metoclopramide vs. their combination in acute migraine attacks. Headache 22:10–12, 1982.

863. Hakkarainen H, Vapaatalo H, Gothoni G, and Parantainen J: Tolfenamic acid is as effective as ergotamine during migraine attacks. Lancet ii:326–328, 1979.

864. Hamik A and Peroutka SJ: 1-(m-Chlorophenyl)piperazine (mCPP) interactions with neurotransmitter receptors in the human brain. Biol Psychiatry 25:569–575, 1989.

865. Hamilton CR, Shelley WM, and Tumulty PA: Giant cell arteritis: Including temporal arteritis and polymyalgia rheumatica. Medicine 50:1–27, 1971.

866. Hamilton RB and Norgren R: Central projections of gustatory nerves in the rat. J Comp Neurol 222:560–577, 1984.

867. Hammarström S: Leukotrienes. Annu Rev Biochem 52:355–377, 1983.

868. Hammer B, Tarnecki R, Vyklicky L, and Wiesendanger M: Corticofugal control of presynaptic inhibition in the spinal trigeminal complex of the cat. Brain Res 2:216–218, 1966.

869. Hammond J: The late sequelae of recurrent vomiting of childhood. Develop Med Child Neurol 16:15–22, 1974.

870. Hammond SR and Danta G: Occipital neuralgia. Clin Exp Neurol 15:258–270, 1978.

871. Hanakoglu A, Somekh E, and Fried D: Benign paroxysmal torticollis in infancy. Clin Pediatr (Phila) 23:272–274, 1984.

872. Hanaoka K, Ohtani M, Toyooka H, et al.: The relative contribution of direct and supraspinal descending effects upon spinal mechanisms of morphine analgesia. J Pharmacol Exp Ther 207:476–484, 1978.

873. Handwerker HO, Reeh PW, and Steen KH: Effects of 5-HT on nociceptors. In Besson JM (ed): Serotonin and Pain. Elsevier, Amsterdam, 1990, pp 1–15.

874. Hanin G, Bousser MG, Olesen J, Vargaftig BB, Jensen K, and Jacobson B: Platelet aggregation study in migraine patients between and during attacks. Cephalalgia 3 (Suppl 3):345–347, 1985.

875. Hanington E: Migraine: A blood disorder? Lancet ii:501–503, 1978.

876. Hanington E: Diet and migraine. J Human Nutrition 34:175–180, 1980.

877. Hanington E: Platelet behaviour in migraine. Panminerva Med 24:63–66, 1982.

878. Hanington E: Migraine: The platelet hypothesis after 10 years. Biomed Pharmacother 43:719–726, 1989.

879. Hanington E and Harper AM: The role of tyramine in the aetiology of migraine, and related studies on the cerebral and extracerebral circulations. Headache 8:84–97, 1968.

880. Hanington E, Jones RJ, Amess JAL, and Wachowicz B: Migraine: A platelet disorder. Lancet ii:720–723, 1981.

881. Hanko J, Hardebo JE, Kåhrstrom J, Owman C, and Sundler F: Calcitonin gene-related peptide is present in mammalian cerebrovascular nerve fibres and dilates pial and peripheral arteries. Neuroscience Lett 57:91–95, 1985.

882. Hanko J, Hardebo JE, Kåhrstrom J, Owman C, and Sundler F: Existence and coexistence of calcitonin gene-related peptide (CGRP) and substance P in cerebrovascular nerves and trigeminal ganglion cells. Acta Physiol Scand 127 (Suppl 552):29–32, 1986.

883. Hannah P, Glover V, and Sandler M: Tyramine in wine and beer. Lancet i:879, 1988.

884. Hannah P, Jarman J, Glover V, Sandler M, Davies PTG, and Clifford Rose F: Kinetics of platelet 5-hydroxytryptamine uptake in head-

ache patients. Cephalalgia 11:141–145, 1991.

885. Hansen AJ: Effects of anoxia on ion distribution in the brain. Physiol Rev 65:101–148, 1985.

886. Hansen AJ, Quistorff B, and Gjedde A: Relationship between local changes in cortical blood flow and extracellular K^+ during spreading depression. Acta Physiol Scand 109:1–6, 1980.

887. Hansen HJ and Drewes VM: The nitroglycerine ointment test—a double-blind examination. Dan Med Bull 17:226–229, 1970.

888. Hansen SL, Borelli-Møller L, Strange P, Nielsen BM, and Olesen J: Ophthalmoplegic migraine: Diagnostic criteria, incidence of hospitalization and possible etiology. Acta Neurol Scand 81:54–60, 1990.

889. Hara H, Hamill GS, and Jacobowitz DM: Origin of cholinergic nerves to the rat major cerebral arteries: Coexistence with vasoactive intestinal polypeptide. Brain Res Bull 14:179–188, 1985.

890. Hara H, Jansen I, Ekman R, et al.: Acetylcholine and vasoactive intestinal peptide in cerebral blood vessels: Effect of extirpation of the sphenopalatine ganglion. J Cereb Blood Flow Metab 9:204–211, 1989.

891. Hara H and Weir B: Pathway of acetylcholinesterase containing nerves to the major cerebral arteries in rats. J Comp Neurol 250:245–252, 1986.

892. Hardebo JE, Arbab M, Suzuki N, and Svendgaard NA: Pathways of parasympathetic and sensory cerebrovascular nerves in monkeys. Stroke 22:331–342, 1991.

893. Hardebo JE and Edvinsson L: Adenine compounds: Cerebrovascular effects in vitro with reference to their possible involvement in migraine. Stroke 10:58–62, 1979.

894. Hardebo JE and Suzuki N: Evidence for neurogenic inflammation upon activation of trigeminal fibers to the internal carotid artery and dural vessels, but not to pial arteries and their cortical branches. In Clifford Rose F (ed): New Advances in Headache Research: 2. Smith-Gordon, London, 1991, pp 173–176.

895. Harden RN, Carter TD, Gilman CS, Gross AJ, and Peters JR: Ketorolac in acute headache management. Headache 31:463–464, 1991.

896. Harik SI, Sharma VK, Wetherbee JR, Warren RH, and Banerjee SP: Adrenergic receptors of cerebral microvessels. Eur J Pharmacol 61:207–208, 1980.

897. Harper AM, Deshmukh VD, Rowan JO, and Jennett WB: The influence of sympathetic nervous activity on cerebral blood flow. Arch Neurol 27:1–6, 1972.

898. Harper AM and MacKenzie ET: Cerebral circulatory and metabolic effects of 5-hydroxytryptamine in anaesthetized baboons. J Physiol (Lond) 271:721–733, 1977.

899. Harrigan JA, Kues JR, Ricks DF, and Smith R: Moods that predict coming migraine headaches. Pain 20:385–396, 1984.

900. Harrison MJG and Bevan AT: Early symptoms of temporal arteritis. Lancet ii:638–640, 1967.

901. Harrison MJG, Emmons PR, and Mitchell JRA: The variability of human platelet aggregation. J Atheroscler Res 7:197, 1967.

902. Harrison TE: Ergotaminism. JACEP 7:162–169, 1978.

903. Harrison WM, McGrath PJ, Stewart PJ, and Quitkin F: MAOIs and hypertensive crises. The role of OTC drugs. J Clin Psychiatry 50:64–65, 1989.

904. Hart RG and Miller VT: Cerebral infarction in young adults: A practical approach. Stroke 14:110–114, 1983.

905. Hartman BK: Immunofluorescence of dopamine-hydroxylase. Application of improved methodology to the localization of the peripheral and central noradrenergic nervous system. J Histochem Cytochem 21:312–332, 1973.

906. Hartman BK, Zide D, and Udenfriend S: The use of dopamine-hydroxylase as a marker for the central noradren-

ergic nervous system in the rat brain. Proc Natl Acad Sci USA 69:2722–2726, 1972.

907. Hartman MM: Parenteral use of dihydroergotamine in migraine. Ann Allergy 3:440–442, 1945.

908. Harto-Truax N, Stern WC, Miller LL, Sato TL, and Cato AE: Effects of bupropion on body weight. J Clin Psychiat 44:183–186, 1983.

909. Harvald B and Hauge M: A catamnestic investigation of Danish twins. Dan Med Bull 3:150–158, 1956.

910. Hass DC and Lourie H: Trauma-triggered migraine: An explanation for common neurological attacks after mild head trauma. J Neurosurg 68:181–188, 1988.

911. Hauge T: Catheter vertebral angiography. Acta Radiol 42(Suppl 109):1–23, 1954.

912. Havanka-Kanniainen H: Cardiovascular reflex responses during migraine attack. Headache 26:442–446, 1986.

913. Havanka-Kanniainen H: Treatment of acute migraine attack: Ibuprofen and placebo compared. Headache 29:507–509, 1989.

914. Havanka-Kanniainen H, Hokkanen E, and Myllyla VV: Efficacy of nimodipine in the prophylaxis of migraine. Cephalalgia 5:39–43, 1985.

915. Havanka-Kanniainen H, Hokkanen E, and Myllyla VV: Efficacy of nimodipine in comparison with pizotifen in the prophylaxis of migraine. Cephalalgia 7:7–13, 1987.

916. Havanka-Kanniainen H, Tolonen U, and Myllyla VV: Cardiovascular reflexes in young migraine patients. Headache 26:420–424, 1986.

917. Headache Classification Committee of the International Headache Society: Classification and diagnostic criteria for headache disorders, cranial neuralgias and facial pain. Cephalalgia 8 (Suppl 7):1–96, 1988.

918. Healey LA and Wilske KR: Manifestations of giant cell arteritis. Med Clin North Am 61:261–270, 1977.

919. Heathfield KWG, Stone P, and Crowder D: Pizotifen in the treatment of migraine. Practitioner 218:428–430, 1977.

920. Heatley RV, Denburg JA, Bayer N, and Bienenstock J: Increased plasma histamine levels in migraine patients. Clin Allergy 12:145–149, 1982.

921. Hedges TR: An ophthalmologist's view of headache. Headache 19:151–155, 1979.

922. Heistad DD and Kontos HA: Cerebral circulation. In Shepherd JT and Abboud FM (eds): Handbook of Physiology, The Cardiovascular System, Peripheral Circulation and Organ Blood Flow, Vol 3. American Physiological Society, Bethesda, 1983, pp 137–182.

923. Heistad DD and Marcus ML: Evidence that neural mechanisms do not have important effects on cerebral blood flow. Circ Res 42:295–302, 1978.

924. Heistad DD, Marcus ML, and Gross PM: Effects of sympathetic nerves on cerebral vessels in dog, cat and monkey. Am J Physiol 235:H544–H552, 1978.

925. Heistad DD, Marcus ML, Said SI, and Gross PM: Effect of acetylcholine and vasoactive intestinal peptide on cerebral blood flow. Am J Physiol 239:H73–H80, 1980.

926. Helkimo M: Studies on function and dysfunction of the masticatory system. Acta Odont Scand 37:255–267, 1974.

927. Henderson KM and Tsang BK: Danazol suppresses luteal function in vitro and in vivo. Fertil Steril 33:550–556, 1980.

928. Henderson WR and Raskin NH: "Hot-dog" headache: Individual susceptibility to nitrite. Lancet ii:1162–1163, 1972.

929. Henrich JB: The association between migraine and cerebral vascular events: An analytical review. J Chron Dis 40:329–335, 1987.

930. Henrich JB and Horwitz RI: A controlled study of ischemic stroke risk in migraine patients. J Clin Epidemiol 42:773–780, 1989.

931. Henrich JB, Sandercock PAG, Warlow CP, and Jones LN: Stroke and migraine in the Oxfordshire Community stroke project. J Neurol 233:257–262, 1986.

932. Henry LG, Blackwood JS, Conley JE, and Bernhard VM: Ergotism. Arch Surg 110:929–932, 1975.

933. Henry P, Baille HM, Dartigues JF, and Jogeix M: Headaches and acupuncture. In Pfaffenrath V, Lundberg PO, and Sjaastads O (eds): Updating in Headache. Springer-Verlag, Berlin, 1985, pp 208–216.

934. Henry PY, Larre P, Aupy M, Lafforgue JL, and Orgogozo JM: Reversible cerebral arteriopathy associated with the administration of ergot derivatives. Cephalalgia 4:171–178, 1984.

935. Henryk-Gutt R and Rees WL: Psychological aspects of migraine. J Psychosom Res. 17:141–153, 1973.

936. Herberg LJ: The hypothalamus and aminergic pathways. In Pearce J (ed): Modern Topics in Migraine. Heinemann, London, 1975, pp 85–95.

937. Hering R, Couturier EGM, Steiner TJ, Asherson RA, and Clifford Rose F: Anticardiolipin antibodies in migraine. Cephalalgia 11:19–21, 1991.

938. Hering R and Kuritzky A: Sodium valproate in the prophylactic treatment of migraine: A double-blind study versus placebo. Cephalalgia 12:81–84, 1992.

939. Hering R and Steiner TJ: Abrupt outpatient withdrawal of medication in analgesic-abusing migraineurs. Lancet 337:1442–1443, 1991.

940. Herold S, Gibbs JM, Jones AKP, Brooks DJ, Frackowiak RSJ, and Legg NJ: Oxygen metabolism in migraine. J Cereb Blood Flow Metab 5(Suppl 1):S445–S446, 1985.

941. Herrmann WM, Horowski R, Dannehl K, Kramer U, and Lurati K: Clinical effectiveness of lisuride hydrogen maleate: A double-blind trial versus methysergide. Headache 17:54–60, 1977.

942. Heyck H: Der Kopfschmerz. Georg Thieme Verlag, Stuttgart, 1958.

943. Heyck H: Pathogenesis of migraine. Res Clin Stud Headache 2:1–28, 1969.

944. Heyck H: Varieties of hemiplegic migraine. Headache 12:135–142, 1973.

945. Heyck H: Headache and Facial Pain. Georg Thieme Verlag, Stuttgart, 1981.

946. Hilke H, Kanto J, and Kleimola T: Intramuscular absorption of dihydroergotamine in man. Int J Clin Pharmacol 16:277–278, 1978.

947. Hilton BP: Effects of reserpine and chlorpromazine on 5-hydroxytryptamine uptake of platelets from migrainous and control subjects. J Neurol Neurosurg Psychiatry 37:711–714, 1974.

948. Hilton BP and Cumings JN: An assessment of platelet aggregation induced by 5-hydroxytryptamine. J Clin Pathol 24:250–258, 1971.

949. Hilton BP and Cumings JN: 5-hydroxytryptamine levels and platelet aggregation responses in subjects with acute migraine headache. J Neurol Neurosurg Psychiatry 35:505–509, 1972.

950. Hindfelt B and Nilsson O: Brain infarction in young adults with particular reference to pathogenesis. Acta Neurol Scand 55:145–157, 1977.

951. Hiner BC, Roth HL, and Peroutka SJ: Antimigraine drug interactions with 5-hydroxytryptamine$_{1A}$ receptors. Ann Neurol 19:511–513, 1986.

952. Hinge HH, Jensen TS, Kjaer M, Marquardsen J, and De Fine Olivarius B: The prognosis of transient global amnesia. Results of a multicenter study. Arch Neurol 43:673–676, 1986.

953. Hirayama K and Ito N: Clinical aspects of migraine in Japan. In Clifford Rose F (ed): Advances in Migraine Research and Therapy. Raven, New York, 1982, pp 13–23.

954. Ho AKS, Loh HH, Craves F, Hitzemann RJ, and Gershon S: The effect of prolonged lithium treatment on

the synthesis rate and turnover of monoamines in brain regions of rats. Eur J Pharmacol 10:72–78, 1970.

955. Hockaday JM: Basilar migraine in childhood. Develop Med Child Neurol 21:455–463, 1979.

956. Hockaday JM: Definitions, clinical features, and diagnosis of childhood migraine. In Hockaday JM (ed): Migraine in Childhood. Butterworth, London, 1988, pp 5–24.

957. Hockaday JM: Is there a place for the "abdominal migraine" as a separate entity in the IHS classification? Yes! Cephalalgia 12:346–348, 1992.

958. Hockaday JM and Debney LM: The EEG in migraine. In Olesen J and Edvinsson L (eds): Basic Mechanisms of Headache, Elsevier, Amsterdam, 1988, pp 365–376.

959. Hockaday JM and Whitty CWM: Factors determining the electroencephalogram in migraine: A study of 560 patients, according to the clinical type of migraine. Brain 92:769–788, 1969.

960. Hockaday JM, Williamson DH, and Whitty CMW: Blood-glucose levels and fatty-acid metabolism in migraine related to fasting. Lancet i:1153–1156, 1971.

961. Hodges JR and Warlow CP: The aetiology of transient global amnesia. A case control study of 114 cases with prospective follow-up. Brain 113:639–657, 1990.

962. Hoffert MJ, Scholz MJ, and Kanter R: A double-blind controlled study of nifedipine as an abortive treatment in acute attacks of migraine with aura. Cephalalgia 12:323–324, 1992.

963. Hogan MJ, Brunet DG, Ford PM, and Lillicrap D: Lupus anticoagulant, antiphospholipid antibodies and migraine. Can J Neurol Sci 15:420–425, 1988.

964. Hokkanen E, Waltino O, and Kallanranta T: Toxic effects of ergotamine used for migraine. Headache 18:95–98, 1978.

965. Holdorff B, Sinn M, and Roth G: Propranolol in der Migräneprophylaxie. Eine Doppelblind-studie. Medizinische Klinik 72:1115–1118, 1977.

966. Hollenberg NK: Serotonin and vascular responses. Annu Rev Pharmacol Toxicol 28:41–59, 1988.

967. Hollnagel H and Nørrelund N: Headache among 40 year-olds in Glostrup. Ugeskr Laeger 142:3071–3077, 1980.

968. Holmes DS and Burish TG: Effectiveness of biofeedback for treating migraine and tension headaches: A review of the evidence. J Psychosom Res 27:515–532, 1983.

969. Holmes GP, Kaplan JE, Gantz NM, et al.: Chronic fatigue syndrome: A working case definition. Ann Intern Med 108:387–389, 1988.

970. Holmsen H, Day HJ, and Setkowsky CA: Behaviour of adenine nucleotides during the platelet release reaction induced by adenosine diphosphate and adrenaline. Biochem J 129:67–82, 1972.

971. Holroyd KA and Penzien DB: Client variables and the behavioral treatment of recurrent tension headache: A meta-analytic review. J Behav Med 9:515–536, 1986.

972. Holroyd KA and Penzien DB: Pharmacological versus non-pharmacological prophylaxis of recurrent migraine headache: A meta-analytic review of clinical trials. Pain 42:1–13, 1990.

973. Holroyd KA, Penzien DB, and Cordingley GE: Propranolol in the management of recurrent migraine: A meta-analytic review. Headache 31:333–340, 1991.

974. Holstege G and Kuypers HGM: The anatomy of brain stem pathways to the spinal cord in cat. A labeled amino acid tracing study. Prog Brain Res 57:145–175, 1982.

975. Holzer P: Local effector functions of capsaicin-sensitive sensory nerve endings: Involvement of tachykinins, calcitonin gene-related peptide and other neuropeptides. Neuroscience 24:739–768, 1988.

976. Holzner F, Wessely P, Zeiler K, and Ehrmann L: Cerebral angiography

in complicated migraine—reactions, incidents. Klin Wochenschr 63:116–122, 1985.

977. Honig PJ and Charney EP: Children with brain tumor headaches. Distinguishing features. Am J Dis Child 136:121–124, 1982.

978. Hood JD and Kayan A: Neuro-otology and migraine. In Blau JN (ed): Migraine. Clinical and Research Aspects. Johns Hopkins University Press, Baltimore, 1987, pp 597–624.

979. Hooker WD and Raskin NH: Neuropsychologic alterations in classic and common migraine. Arch Neurol 43:709–712, 1986.

980. Hornabrook RW: Migrainous neuralgia. NZ Med J 63:774–779, 1964.

981. Horthe CE, Wainscott G, Neylan C, and Wilkinson MIP: Progesterone, estradiol and aldosterone levels in plasma during the menstrual cycle of women suffering from migraine. J Endocrinol 65:24–29, 1975.

982. Horton BT: Complications of temporal arteritis. Br Med J i:105–106, 1966.

983. Horton BT and Peters GA: Clinical manifestations of excessive use of ergotamine preparations and management of withdrawal effect: Report of 52 cases. Headache 2:214–227, 1963.

984. Horton BT, Ryan R, and Reynolds JL: Clinical observations on the use of E.C. 110, a new agent for the treatment of headache. Mayo Clin Proc 23:105–108, 1948.

985. Horton EW: Hypotheses on physiological roles of prostaglandins. Physiol Rev 49:122–161, 1969.

986. Hosking GP, Cavanagh NP, and Wilson J: Alternating hemiplegia: Complicated migraine of infancy. Arch Dis Child 53:656–659, 1978.

987. Hoskins PJ and Hansk GW: Opioid agonist–antagonist drugs in acute and chronic pain states. Drugs 41:326–344, 1991.

988. Hosobuchi Y, Rossier J, Bloom FE, and Guillemin R: Stimulation of human periaqueductal gray for pain relief increases immunoreactive β-endorphin in ventricular fluid. Science 203:279–281, 1979.

989. Houston DS, Shepherd JT, and Vanhoutte PM: Adenine nucleotides, serotonin, and endothelium-dependent relaxations to platelets. Am J Physiol 248:H389–H395, 1985.

990. Hsu LKG, Crisp AH, Kalucy RS, et al.: Nocturnal plasma levels of catecholamines, tryptophan, glucose and free fatty acids and the sleeping encephalographs of subjects experiencing early morning migraine. In Greene R (ed): Current Concepts in Migraine Research. Raven, New York, 1978, pp 121–130.

991. Hua XY, Saria A, Gamse R, Theodorsson-Norheim E, Brodin E, and Lundberg JM: Capsaicin induced release of multiple tachykinins (substance P, neurokinin A and eledoisin-like material) from guinea-pig spinal cord and ureter. Neuroscience 19:313–319, 1986.

992. Hudgson P and Hart JA: Acute ergotism: Report of a case and review of the literature. Med J Aust 2:589–591, 1964.

993. Hughes EC, Gott PS, Weinstein RC, and Binggeli R: Migraine: A diagnostic test for etiology of food sensitivity by a nutritionally supported fast and confirmed by long-term report. Ann Allergy 55:28–32, 1985.

994. Hughes HE and Goldstein DA: Birth defects following maternal exposure to ergotamine, beta blockers, and caffeine. J Med Genetics 25:396–399, 1988.

995. Hughes JB: Metoclopramide in migraine. Med J Aust 2:580, 1977.

996. Hughes JR: EEG in headache. Headache 11:161–170, 1972.

997. Hughes RC and Foster JB: BC 105 in the prophylaxis of migraine. Curr Ther Res 13:63–68, 1971.

998. Humphrey PPA: 5-Hydroxytryptamine and the pathophysiology of migraine. J Neurol 238 (Suppl 1):S38–S44, 1991.

999. Humphrey PPA, Connor HE, Stubbs CM, and Feniuk W: Effect of sumatriptan on pial vessel diameter *in vivo*. In Olesen J (ed): Migraine and

Other Headaches: The Vascular Mechanisms. Raven, New York, 1991, pp 335–338.

1000. Humphrey PPA, Feniuk W, Perren MJ, Connor HE, and Oxford AW: The pharmacology of the novel 5-HT$_1$-like receptor agonist, GR43175. Cephalalgia 9 (Suppl 9):23–33, 1989.

1001. Humphrey PPA, Feniuk W, Perren MJ, Beresford IJM, Skingle M, and Whalley ET: Serotonin and migraine. Ann NY Acad Sci 600:587–600, 1990.

1002. Hungerford GD, du Boulay GH, and Zilkha KJ: Computerized axial tomography in patients with severe migraine: A preliminary report. J Neurol Neurosurg Psychiatry 39:990–994, 1976.

1003. Hunt SP, Nagy JI, and Ninkovic M: Peptides and the organization of the dorsal horn. In Sjölund BH and Björklund A (eds): Brain Stem Control of Spinal Mechanisms. Elsevier, Amsterdam, 1982, pp 159–178.

1004. Hunter CR and Mayfield FH: Role of the upper cervical roots in the production of pain in the head. Am J Surg 78:743–751, 1949.

1005. Hupp SL, Kline LB, and Corbett JJ: Visual disturbances of migraine. Surv Ophthalmol 33:221–236, 1989.

1006. Hurst WJ, Martin RA, and Zoumas BL: Biogenic amines in chocolate—a review. Nutr Reports Int 26:1081–1086, 1982.

1007. Hurst WJ and Toomey PB: High performance liquid chromatographic determination of four biogenic amines in chocolate. Analyst 106:394–402, 1981.

1008. Ibraheem JJ, Paalzow L, and Tfelt-Hansen P: Low bioavailability of ergotamine tartrate after oral and rectal administration in migraine sufferers. Br J Clin Pharmacol 16:695–699, 1983.

1009. Igarashi H, Sakai F, Kan S, Okada J, and Tazaki Y: Magnetic resonance imaging in patients with migraine. Cephalalgia 11:69–74, 1991.

1010. Ignarro LJ: Biosynthesis and metabolism of endothelium-derived nitric oxide. Annu Rev Pharmacol Toxicol 30:535–560, 1990.

1011. Inoue A, Yanagisawa M, Kimura S, et al.: The human endothelin family: Three structurally and pharmacologically distinct isopeptides predicted by three separate genes. Proc Natl Acad Sci USA 86:2863–2867, 1989.

1012. Iñiguez C, Pascual C, Pardo A, Martinez-Castrillo JC, and Alvarez-Cermeño JC: Antiphospholipid antibodies in migraine. Headache 31:666–668, 1991.

1013. Isenberg DA, Meyrick-Thomas D, Snaith ML, McKeran RO, and Royston JP: A study of migraine in systemic lupus erythematosus. Ann Rheum Dis 41:30–32, 1982.

1014. Iserson KV: Parenteral chlorpromazine treatment of migraine. Ann Emerg Med 12:756–758, 1983.

1015. Isler H: Migraine treatment as a cause of chronic migraine. In Clifford Rose F (ed): Advances in Migraine Research and Therapy. Raven, New York, 1982, pp 159–163.

1016. Isler H: Frequency and time course of premonitory phenomena. In Amery WK and Wauquier A (eds): The Prelude to the Migraine Attack. Bailliere Tindall, London, 1986, pp 44–53.

1017. Jackowski A, Crockard A, and Burnstock G: 5-Hydroxytryptamine demonstrated immunohistochemically in rat cerebrovascular nerves largely represents 5-hydroxytryptamine uptake into sympathetic nerve fibres. Neuroscience 29:453–462, 1989.

1018. Jackson CD and Fishbein L: A toxicological review of beta-adrenergic blockers. Fundamental Appl Toxicol 6:395–422, 1986.

1019. Jacobs BL, Wilkinson LO, and Fornal CA: The role of brain serotonin. A neurophysiologic perspective. Neuropsychopharmacology 3:473–479, 1990.

1020. Jacobson E: Progressive Relaxation. University of Chicago Press, Chicago, 1929.

1021. Jacobson SA: The Post-Traumatic Syndrome Following Head Injury. Thomas, Springfield, 1963.

1022. Jacome DE and Leborgne JL: MRI studies in basilar artery migraine. Headache 30:88–90, 1990.

1023. Jacquin MF, Semba K, Rhoades RW, and Egger MD: Trigeminal primary afferents project bilaterally to dorsal horn and ipsilaterally to cerebellum, reticular formation, and cuneate, solitary, supratrigeminal and vagal nuclei. Brain Res 246:285–291, 1982.

1024. Jaeger B: Are "cervicogenic" headaches due to myofascial pain and cervical spine dysfunction? Cephalalgia 9:157–164, 1989.

1025. Jain S and Ahuja GK: Unusual transient high and low density CT lesion in migraine: A case report. Headache 26:19–21, 1986.

1026. James IM, Millar RA, and Purves MJ: Observations on the extrinsic neural control of cerebral blood flow in the baboon. Circ Res 25:77–93, 1969.

1027. Jansen K, Edvinsson L, Mortensen A, and Olesen J: Sumatriptan is a potent vasoconstrictor of human dural arteries via a 5-HT$_1$-like receptor. Cephalalgia 12:202–205, 1992.

1028. Janzen R, Tanzer A, Zsochke S, and Diekmann H: Post-angiographische Spätreaktionen der Hirngefässe bei Migräne-Kranken. Beitrag zum Pathomechanisms des Migräne-Anfalles. Z Neurol 201:24–42, 1972.

1029. Jefferson JW and Greist JH: Adverse reactions—neurological tremor. In Jefferson JW and Greist JH (eds): Primer of Lithium Therapy. William &Wilkins, Baltimore, 1977, pp 139–150.

1030. Jenner P, Clow A, Reavill C, Theodorou A, and Marsden CD: A behavioral and biochemical comparison of dopamine receptor blockade produced by haloperidol with that produced by substituted benzamide drugs. Life Sci 23:545–549, 1978.

1031. Jensen K: Subcutaneous blood flow in the temporal region of migraine patients. Acta Neurol Scand 75:310–318, 1987.

1032. Jensen K and Olesen J: Temporal muscle blood flow in common migraine. Acta Neurol Scand 72:561–570, 1985.

1033. Jensen K, Tfelt-Hansen P, Lauritzen M, and Olesen J: Clinical trial of nimodipine for single attacks of classic migraine. Cephalalgia 5:125–131, 1985.

1034. Jensen K, Tfelt-Hansen P, Lauritzen M, and Olesen J: Classic migraine. A prospective recording of symptoms. Acta Neurol Scand 73:359–362, 1986.

1035. Jensen TS and Gebhart GF: General anatomy of antinociceptive systems. In Olesen J and Edvinsson L (eds): Basic Mechanisms of Headache. Elsevier, Amsterdam, 1988, pp 189–200.

1036. Jensen TS and Smith DF: Stimulation of spinal dopaminergic receptors: Differential effects on tail reflexes in rats. Neuropharmacology 22:477–483, 1983.

1038. Jensen TS, Voldby B, De Fine Olivarius BF, and Jensen FT: Cerebral hemodynamics in familial hemiplegic migraine. Cephalalgia 1:121–125, 1981.

1039. Jensen TS and Yaksh TL: Effects of an intrathecal dopamine agonist, apomorphine on thermal and chemical evoked noxious responses in rats. Brain Res 296:285–293, 1984.

1040. Jerzmanowski A and Klimek A: Immunoglobulins and complement in migraine. Cephalalgia 3:119–123, 1983.

1041. Jessup BA: Relaxation and biofeedback. In Wall PD and Melzack PR (eds): Textbook of Pain, 2nd ed. Churchill Livingstone, New York, 1989, pp 989–1000.

1042. Jessup BA, Neufeld RWJ, and Merskey H: Biofeedback therapy for headache and other pain: An evaluative review. Pain 7:225–270, 1979.

1043. Jick H, Holmes LB, Hunter JR, Madsen S, and Steragachis A: First-trimester drug use and congenital disorders. JAMA 246:343–346, 1981.

1044. Johansson O, Hökfelt T, Pernow B, et al.: Immunohistochemical support for three putative transmitters in one neuron: Coexistence of 5-hydroxytryptamine, substance P- and thyrotropin releasing hormone-like immunoreactivity in medullary neurons projecting to the spinal cord. Neuroscience 6:1857–1881, 1981.

1045. Johansson V, Nilsson LR, Widelius T, Jäverfalk T, Hellman P, and Åkesson JA: Atenolol in migraine prophylaxis: A double-blind crossover multicenter study. Headache 27:372–374, 1987.

1046. John ER: The role of quantitative EEG topographic mapping or "neurometrics" in the diagnosis of psychiatric and neurological disorders: The pros. Electroencephalogr Clin Neurophysiol 73:2–4, 1989.

1047. Johnson ES: A basis for migraine therapy—the autonomic theory reappraised. Postgrad Med J 54:231–243, 1978.

1048. Johnson ES, Ratcliffe DM, and Wilkinson M: Naproxen sodium in the treatment of migraine. Cephalalgia 5:5–10, 1985.

1049. Johnson RH, Hornabrook RW, and Lambie DG: Comparison of mefenamic acid and propranolol with placebo in migraine prophylaxis. Acta Neurol Scand 76:490–492, 1986.

1050. Johnston BM and Saxena PR: The effect of ergotamine on tissue blood flow and the arteriovenous shunting of radioactive microspheres in the head. Br J Pharmacol 63:541–549, 1978.

1051. Johnston I and Paterson A: Benign intracranial hypertension. II. CSF pressure and circulation. Brain 97:301–312, 1974.

1052. Jones EG: The Thalamus. Plenum, New York, 1985.

1053. Jones J, Sklar D, Dougherty J, and White W: Randomized double-blind trial of intravenous prochlorperazine for the treatment of acute headaches. JAMA 261:1174–1176, 1989.

1054. Jones RJ, Forsythe AM, and Amess JAL: Platelet aggregation in migraine patients during the head-

ache-free interval. Adv Neurol 33:275–288, 1982.

1055. Jones SL and Gebhart GF: Characterization of coeruleospinal inhibition of the nociceptive tail-flick reflex in the rat: Mediation by spinal α_2-adrenoceptors. Brain Res 364:315–330, 1986.

1056. Jones SL and Gebhart GF: Quantitative characterization of coeruleospinal inhibition of nociceptive transmission in the rat. J Neurophysiol 56:1397–1410, 1986.

1057. Jonkman EJ and Lelieveld MHJ: EEG computer analysis in patients with migraine. Electroencephalogr Clin Neurophysiol 52:652–655, 1981.

1058. Jonsdottir M, Meyer JS, and Rogers RL: Efficacy, side effects and tolerance compared during headache treatment with three different calcium blockers. Headache 27:364–369, 1987.

1059. Joseph R, Cooke GE, Steiner TJ, and Clifford Rose F: Intracranial space-occupying lesions in patients attending a migraine clinic. Practitioner 229:477–481, 1985.

1060. Joseph R and Welch KMA: The platelet and migraine: A nonspecific association. Headache 27:375–380, 1987.

1061. Joseph R, Welch KMA, Grunfeld S, Oster SB, and D'Andrea G: Cytosolic ionized calcium homeostasis in platelets: An abnormal sensitivity to PAF-activation in migraine. Headache 28:396–402, 1988.

1062. Jost WH, Raulf H, and Müller-Lobeck H: Anorectal ergotism. Induced by migraine therapy. Acta Neurol Scand 84:73–74, 1991.

1063. Juan H: Mechanism of action of bradykinin-induced release of prostaglandin E. Naunyn Schmiedebergs Arch Pharmacol 300:77–85, 1977.

1064. Juan H and Lembeck F: Release of prostaglandins from the isolated perfused rabbit ear by bradykinin and acetylcholine. Agents Actions 6:642–645, 1976.

1065. Juan H and Sametz W: Histamine-induced release of arachidonic acid and of prostaglandins in the peripheral vascular bed: Mode of action. Naunyn Schmiedebergs Arch Pharmacol 314:183–190, 1980.

1066. Juan H, Sametz W, Petronijevic S, and Lembeck F: Prostaglandin release and nociceptor stimulation by peptides. Naunyn Schmiedebergs Arch Pharmacol 326:64–68, 1984.

1067. Juel-Nielsen N: Individual and environment. A psychiatric–psychological investigation of monozygotic twins reared apart. Acta Psychiatrica Scand 40 (Suppl 183):1–292, 1965.

1068. Juge O and Gauthier G: Mesures de débit sanguin cérébral régional (DSR) par inhalation de Xénon 133: applications cliniques. Bull Schweiz Akad Med Wiss 36:101–115, 1980.

1069. Jurna I and Brune K: Central effect of the non-steroid anti-inflammatory agents, indomethacin, ibuprofen, and diclofenac determined in C-fibre-evoked activity on single neurons of the rat thalamus. Pain 41:71–80, 1990.

1070. Kafka MS, Tallman JF, Smith CC and Costa JL: Alpha-adrenergic receptors on human platelets. Life Sci 21:1429–1438, 1977.

1071. Kahan A, Weber S, Amor B, Guerin F, and Degeorges M: Nifedipine in the treatment of migraine in patients with Raynaud's phenomenon. N Engl J Med 308:1102–1103, 1983.

1072. Kalendovsky Z and Austin JH: Complicated migraine: Its association with increased platelet aggregability and abnormal coagulation factors. Headache 15:18–35, 1975.

1073. Kallanranta T, Hakkarainen H, Hokkanen E, and Tuovinen T: Clonidine in migraine prophylaxis. Headache 17:169–172, 1977.

1074. Kallos P and Kallos-Deffner L: Allergy and migraine. Int Arch Allergy Appl Immunol 7:367–372, 1955.

1075. Kamakura S, Kamo J, and Tsurufuji S: Role of bradykinin in the vascular permeability response induced by carrageenan in rats. Br J Pharmacol 93:739–746, 1988.

1076. Kangasniemi P, Andersen AR, Andersson PG, et al.: Classic migraine: Effective prophylaxis with metoprolol. Cephalalgia 7:231–238, 1987.

1077. Kangasniemi P and Hedman C: Metoprolol and propranolol in the prophylactic treatment of classical and common migraine: A double-blind study. Cephalalgia 4:91–96, 1984.

1078. Kangasniemi P, Sonninen V, and Rinne UK: Excretion of free and conjugated 5-HIAA and VMA in urine and concentration of 5-HIAA and HVA in CSF during migraine attacks and free intervals. Headache 12:62–65, 1972.

1079. Kanto J: Clinical pharmacokinetics of ergotamine, dihydroergotamine, ergotoxine, bromocriptine, methysergide and lergotrile. Int J Clin Pharmacol 21:135–142, 1983.

1080. Kaplan AP: Hageman factor-dependent pathways: Mechanisms of initiation and bradykinin formation. Fed Proc 42:3123–3127, 1983.

1081. Kaplan KL and Owen J: Plasma level of beta-thromboglobulin and platelet factor 4 as indices of platelet activation in vivo. Blood 57:199–202, 1981.

1082. Karachalios GN, Fotiadou A, Chrisikos N, Karabetsos A, and Kehagioglou K: Treatment of acute migraine attack with diclofenac sodium: A double-blind study. Headache 32:98–100, 1992.

1083. Kåss B and Nestvold K: Propranolol (Inderal) and clonidine (Catapressen) in the prophylactic treatment of migraine: A comparative trial. Acta Neurol Scand 61:351–356, 1980.

1084. Katayama Y, Ueno Y, Tsukiyama T, and Tsubokawa T: Long-lasting suppression of firing of cortical neurons and decrease in cortical blood flow following train pulse stimulation of the locus coeruleus in the cat. Brain Res 216:173–179, 1981.

1085. Katz RI, Chase TN, and Kopin IJ: Evoked release of norepinephrine and serotonin from brain slices: Inhibition by lithium. Science 162:466–467, 1968.

1086. Kaul SN, Du Boulay GH, Kendall BE, and Ross-Russell RW: Relationship between visual field defect and arterial occlusion in the posterior cerebral circulation. J Neurol Neurosurg Psychiatry 37:1022–1030, 1974.

1087. Kayan A and Hood JD: Neuro-otological manifestations of migraine. Brain 107:1123–1142, 1984.

1088. Keele CA and Armstrong D: Substances Producing Pain and Itch. Arnold, London, 1964.

1089. Keinanen-Kiukaanniemi S, Kaapa P, Saukkonen AL, Viinikka L, and Ylikorkala O: Decreased thromboxane production in migraine patients during headache-free period. Headache 24:339–341, 1984.

1090. Keller JT, Beduk A, and Saunders MC: Origin of fibers innervating the basilar artery of the cat. Neuroscience Lett 58:263–268, 1985.

1091. Keller JT, Dimlich RVW, Zuccarello M, Lanker L, Strauss TA, and Fritts MJ: Influence of the sympathetic nervous system as well as trigeminal sensory fibres on rat dural mast cells. Cephalalgia 11:215–221, 1991.

1092. Keller JT, Saunders MC, Beduk A, and Jollis JG: Innervation of the posterior fossa dura of the cat. Brain Res Bull 14:97–102, 1985.

1093. Kellgren JH: Observation on referred pain arising from muscle. Clin Sci 3:175–190, 1938.

1094. Kellgren JH: On the distribution of pain arising from deep somatic structures with charts of segmental pain areas. Clin Sci 4:35–46, 1939.

1095. Kelly R: Colloid cysts of the third ventricle. Brain 74:23–65, 1951.

1096. Kelly RE: Methysergide and coronary thrombosis. Practitioner 195:565–566, 1965.

1097. Kendall B: Neuro-radiological investigations. In Warlow C and Morris PJ (eds): Transient Ischemic Attacks. Dekker, New York, 1982, pp 154–172.

1098. Kennard C, Gawel M, Rudolf N deM, and Clifford Rose F: Visual evoked potentials in migraine subjects. Res Clin Stud Headache 6:73–80, 1978.

1099. Kennedy C, Delbro D, and Burnstock G: P_2-purinoreceptors mediate both vasodilatation via the endothelium and vasoconstriction of the isolated rat femoral artery. Eur J Pharmacol 107:161–168, 1985.

1100. Kerber CW and Newton TH: The macro- and microvasculature of the dura mater. Neuroradiology 6:175–179, 1973.

1101. Kerr FWL: A mechanism to account for frontal headache in cases of posterior fossa tumors. J Neurosurg 18:605–609, 1961.

1102. Kewman D and Roberts AH: Skin temperature biofeedback and migraine headaches: A double-blind study. Biofeedback Self Regul 5:327–345, 1980.

1103. Khachaturian H, Lewis ME, Schäfer MKH, and Watson SJ: Anatomy of the CNS opioid systems. Trends Neurosci 8:111–119, 1985.

1104. Khachaturian H, Lewis ME, and Watson SJ: Immunocytochemical studies with antisera against Leu-enkephalin and an enkephalin precursor fragment (BAM-22P) in the rat brain. Life Sci 31:1879–1882, 1982.

1105. Khachaturian H, Watson SJ, Lewis ME, Coy D, Goldstein A, and Akil H: Dynorphin immunocytochemistry in the rat central nervous system. Peptides 3:941–954, 1982.

1106. Kilbinger H and Weinrauch TR: Drugs increasing gastrointestinal motility. Pharmacol 25:61–72, 1982.

1107. Kim CK: The effect of acupuncture on migraine headache. Am J Chin Med 2:407–411, 1974.

1108. Kim M and Blanchard EB: Two studies of the non-pharmacological treatment of menstrually related migraine headaches. Headache 32:197–202, 1992.

1109. Kimball RW, Friedman A, and Vallejo E: Effects of serotonin in migraine patients. Neurology 10:107–111, 1960.

1110. Kimmel DL: Innervation of spinal dura mater and dura mater of the posterior cranial fossa. Neurology 11:800–809, 1961.

1111. Kimmel DL: The nerves of the cranial dura mater and their significance in dural headache and referred pain. Chicago Med School Quarterly 22:16–26, 1961.

1112. Kinast M, Lueders H, Rothner AD, and Erenberg G: Benign focal epileptiform discharges in childhood migraine. Neurology 32:1309–1311, 1982.

1113. King RB and Saba MI: Forewarnings of major subarachnoid hemorrhage due to congenital berry aneurysm. NY State J Med 74:638–639, 1974.

1114. Klapper JA: The efficacy of migraine prophylaxis. Headache Quarterly, Current Treatment and Research 2:278–284, 1991.

1115. Klee A: A Clinical Study of Migraine with Particular Reference to the Most Severe Cases. Munksgaard, Copenhagen, 1968.

1116. Klee A: Perceptual disorders in migraine. In Pearce J (ed): Modern Topics in Migraine. Heinemann, London, 1975, pp 45–51.

1117. Klee A and Willanger R: Disturbances of visual perception in migraine. Acta Neurol Scand 42:400–414, 1966.

1118. Klein LS, Simpson RJ, Stern R, Hayward JC, and Foster JR: Myocardial infarction following administration of sublingual ergotamine. Chest 82:375–376, 1982.

1119. Kline LB and Kelly CL: Ocular migraine in a patient with cluster headaches. Headache 20:253–257, 1980.

1120. Kloster R, Nestvold K, and Vilming ST: A double-blind study of ibuprofen versus placebo in the treatment of acute migraine attacks. Cephalalgia 12:169–171, 1992.

1121. Klysner R, Geisler A, Hansen KW, Skov PS, and Norn S: Histamine H_2 receptor-mediated cyclic AMP formation in human platelets. Acta Pharmacol Toxicol 47:1–4, 1980.

1122. Knapp S and Mandell AJ: Short- and long-term lithium administration: Effects on the brain serotonergic biosynthetic systems. Science 180:645–647, 1973.

1123. Knapp TW and Florin I: The treatment of migraine headache by training in vasoconstriction of the temporal artery and a cognitive stress-coping training. Behav Anal Modif 4:267–274, 1981.

1124. Kobari M, Meyer JS, and Ichijo M: Cerebral hemodynamic changes during migraine and cluster headaches—pharmacological implications. Headache Quarterly, Current Treatment and Research 1:23–37, 1990.

1125. Kobari M, Meyer JS, Ichijo M, Imai A, and Oravez WT: Hyperperfusion of cerebral cortex, thalamus and basal ganglia during spontaneously occurring migraine headaches. Headache 29:282–289, 1989.

1126. Kobari M, Meyer JS, Ichijo M, and Kawamura J: Cortical and subcortical hyperperfusion during migraine and cluster headache measured by Xe CT-CBF. Neuroradiology 32:4–11, 1990.

1127. Koehler SM and Glaros A: The effect of aspartame on migraine headache. Headache 28:10–13, 1988.

1128. Koella WP: CNS-related (side-) effects of β-blockers with special reference to mechanisms of action. Eur J Clin Pharmacol 28(Suppl):55–63, 1985.

1129. Kohlenberg RJ: Tyramine sensitivity in dietary migraine: A critical review. Headache 22:30–34, 1982.

1130. Köhler T and Haimerl C: Daily stress as a trigger of migraine attacks: Results of thirteen single-subject studies. J Consult Clin Psychol 58:870–872, 1990.

1131. Kontos HA, Wei EP, Raper AJ, et al.: Role of tissue hypoxia in local regulation of cerebral microcirculation. Am J Physiol 234:H582–H591, 1978.

1132. Kopera H and Pinder R: Psychomimetic and psychotherapeutic drugs. In Kuemmerle HP and Brendel K (eds): Clinical Pharmacology of Pregnancy. Thieme-Stratton, New York, 1984, pp 345–351.

1133. Kosterlitz HW and Paterson SJ: Types of opioid receptors: Relation to antinociception. Philos Trans R Soc Lond 308B:291–297, 1985.

1134. Kozubski W and Stanczyk L: The influence of plasma free fatty acids and cholesterol on the aggregation of blood platelets in migraine patients. Headache 25:199–203, 1985.

1135. Krabbe AA: Cluster headache: A review. Acta Neurol Scand 74:1–9, 1986.

1136. Krabbe AA and Olesen J: Headache provocation by continuous intravenous infusion of histamine. Clinical results and receptor mechanisms. Pain 8:253–259, 1980.

1137. Krabbe AA and Olesen J: Effect of histamine on regional cerebral blood flow in man. Cephalalgia 2:15–18, 1982.

1138. Krägeloh I and Aicardi J: Alternating hemiplegia in infants: Report of five cases. Develop Med Child Neurol 22:784–791, 1980.

1139. Kraig RP and Nicholson C: Extracellular ionic variations during spreading depression. Neuroscience 3:1045–1059, 1978.

1140. Kreel L: The use of metoclopramide in radiology. Postgrad Med J 49:42–45, 1973.

1141. Kremenitzer M and Golden GS: Hemiplegic migraine: Cerebrospinal fluid abnormalities. J Pediatr 85:139, 1974.

1142. Kropp P and Gerber WD: Contingent negative variation—findings and perspectives in migraine. Cephalalgia 13:33–36, 1993.

1143. Kruglak KL, Nathan I, Korczyn AD, Zolotov Z, Bergner V, and Dvilansky A: Platelet aggregability, disaggregability and serotonin uptake in migraine. Cephalalgia 4:221–225, 1984.

1144. Kudrow L: The relationship of headache frequency to hormone use in migraine. Headache 15:36–40, 1975.

1145. Kudrow L: Cluster Headache. Mechanisms and Management. Oxford University Press, Oxford, 1980.

1146. Kudrow L: Paradoxical effects of frequent analgesic use. Adv Neurol 33:335–341, 1982.

1147. Kugler J and Laub M: Headache determination by meteorotropic influences. Res Clin Stud Headache 6:117–122, 1977.

1148. Kuhn MJ and Shekar PC: A comparative study of magnetic resonance imaging and computed tomography in the evaluation of migraine. Comput Med Imag Graphics 14:149–152, 1990.

1149. Kumazawa T and Mizumura K: Effects of synthetic substance P on unit discharges of testicular nociceptors of dogs. Brain Res 170:553–557, 1979.

1150. Kunkel RS: Acephalgic migraine. Headache 26:198–201, 1986.

1151. Kunkel R: Headache. In Rakel RE (ed): Conn's Current Therapy. WB Saunders, Philadelphia, 1988, pp 772–781.

1152. Kunkle EC and Anderson WB: Significance of minor eye signs in headache of migraine type. Arch Ophthal 65:504–507, 1961.

1153. Kuritzky A, Ziegler DK, and Hassanein R: Vertigo, motion sickness and migraine. Headache 21:227–231, 1981.

1154. Kuritzky A, Ziegler DK, Hassanein R, Sood P, and Hirwitz A: Relation between plasma concentration of propranolol, beta blocking and migraine. In Clifford Rose F (ed): Migraine Clinical and Research Advances Symposium. Karger, Basel, 1985, pp 250–255.

1155. Kuschinsky W and Wahl M: Alpha receptor stimulation by endogenous and exogenous norepinephrine and blockade by phentolamine in pial arteries of cats. Circ Res 37:168–174, 1975.

1156. Labbe EL and Williamson DA: Treatment of childhood migraine using autogenic feedback training. J Consult Clin Psychol 52:968–976, 1984.

1157. Lacombe P, Sercombe R, Verrecchia C, Philipson V, MacKenzie ET, and Seylaz J: Cortical blood flow increases induced by stimulation of the substantia innominata in the unanesthetized rat. Brain Res 491:1–14, 1989.

1158. Lacroix JM, Clarke MA, Bock JC, Doxey N, Wood A, and Lavis S: Biofeedback and relaxation in the treatment of migraine headaches: Comparative effectiveness and physiological correlates. J Neurol Neurosurg Psychiatry 46:525–532, 1983.

1159. Lagier G, Castot A, Riboulet G, and Boesh C: Un cas d'ergotisme mineur semblant en rapport avec une potentialisation de l'ergotamine par l'éthylsuccinate d'érythromycine. Therapie 34:515–521, 1979.

1160. Lagrèze HL, Dettmers C, and Hartmann A: Abnormalities of interictal cerebral perfusion in classic but not common migraine. Stroke 19:1108–1111, 1988.

1161. Lake A, Rainey J, and Papsdorf JD: Biofeedback and rational-emotive therapy in the management of migraine headache. J Appl Behav Anal 12:127–140, 1979.

1162. Lambert GA: Central trigeminal craniovascular pathways. Cephalalgia 9(Suppl 10):12–13, 1989.

1163. Lambert GA, Bogduk N, Goadsby PJ, Duckworth JW, and Lance JW: Decreased carotid arterial resistance in cats in response to trigeminal stimulation. J Neurosurg 61:307–315, 1984.

1164. Lambert GA, Lowy AJ, Boers PM, Angus-Leppan H, and Zagami AS: The spinal cord processing of input from the superior sagittal sinus: Pathway and modulation by ergot alkaloids. Brain Res 597:321–330, 1992.

1165. Lambert GA, Zagami AS, Bogduk N, and Lance JW: Cervical spinal cord neurons receiving sensory input from the cranial vasculature. Cephalalgia 11:75–85, 1991.

1166. LaMotte RH: Psychophysical and neurophysiological studies of chemically induced cutaneous pain and itch. The case of the missing nociceptor. Prog Brain Res 74:331–335, 1988.

1167. Lance JW: Mechanisms and Management of Headache, 4th ed. Butterworth, London, 1982.

1168. Lance JW: Migraine and cluster headache. In Johnson RT (ed): Current Therapy in Neurologic Disease. CV Mosby, St Louis, 1985, pp 85–91.

1169. Lance JW: Fifty years of migraine research. Aust NZ J Med 18:311–317, 1988.

1170. Lance JW: The controlled application of cold and heat by a new device (Migra-lief apparatus) in the treatment of headache. Headache 28:458–461, 1988.

1171. Lance JW: Headache: Classification, mechanism and principles of therapy, with particular reference to migraine. Recenti Progressi in Medicina 80:673–680, 1989.

1172. Lance JW and Anthony M: Some clinical aspects of migraine. A prospective study of 500 patients. Arch Neurol 15:356–361, 1966.

1173. Lance JW and Anthony M: Migrainous neuralgia or cluster headache? J Neurol Sci 13:401–414, 1971.

1174. Lance JW and Anthony M: Thermographic studies in vascular headache. Med J Aust 58:240–243, 1971.

1175. Lance JW, Anthony M, and Hinterberger H: The control of cranial arteries by humoral mechanisms and its relation to the migraine syndrome. Headache 7:93–102, 1967.

1176. Lance JW, Anthony M, and Somerville B: Comparative trial of serotonin antagonists in the management of migraine. Br Med J 2:327–330, 1970.

1177. Lance JW, Anthony M, and Somerville B: Thermographic, hormonal and clinical studies in migraine. Headache 9:93–104, 1970.

1178. Lance JW and Curran DA: Treatment of chronic tension headache. Lancet i:1236–1239, 1964.

1179. Lance JW, Curran DA, and Anthony M: Investigations into the mechanism and treatment of chronic headache. Med J Aust 2:909–914, 1965.

1180. Lance JW, Lamberg GA, Goadsby PJ, and Duckworth JW: Brainstem influences on the cephalic circulation: Experimental data from cat and monkey of relevance to the mechanism of migraine. Headache 23:258–265, 1983.

1181. Lance JW, Spira PJ, Mylecharane EJ, Lord GDA, and Duckworth JW: Evaluation of drugs applicable to treatment of migraine in the cranial circulation of the monkey. Res Clin Stud Headache 6:13–18, 1978.

1182. Lane PH and Ross R: Intravenous chlorpromazine: Preliminary results in acute migraine. Headache 25:302–304, 1985.

1183. Lane PL, McLellan BA, and Baggoley CJ: Comparative efficacy of chlorpromazine and meperidine with dimenhydrinate in migraine headache. Ann Emerg Med 18:360–365, 1989.

1184. Langemark M and Olesen J: Drug abuse in migraine patients. Pain 19:81–86, 1984.

1185. Langemark M and Olesen J: Pericranial tenderness in tension headache. A blind, controlled study. Cephalalgia 7:249–255, 1987.

1186. Lansky MR and Selzer J: Priapism associated with trazodone therapy: Case report. J Clin Psychiatry 45:232–233, 1984.

1187. Lapkin ML, French JH, and Golden GS: The electroencephalogram in childhood basilar artery migraine. Neurology 27:580–583, 1977.

1188. Lapkin ML and Golden GS: Basilar artery migraine: A review of 30 cases. Am J Dis Child 132:276–281, 1978.

1189. Largen JW, Mathew RJ, Dobbins K, and Claghorn JL: Specific and nonspecific effects of skin temperature control in migraine management. Headache 21:36–44, 1981.

1190. Larson EB, Omenn GS, and Lewis H: Diagnostic evaluation of headache. Impact of computerized tomography and cost-effectiveness. JAMA 243:359–362, 1980.

1191. Larson-Cohn U and Lundberg PO: Headache and treatment with oral contraceptives. Acta Neurol Scand 46:267–278, 1970.

1192. Larsson LI, Edvinsson L, Fahrenkrug J, et al.: Immunohistochemical localization of a vasodilatory peptide (VIP) in cerebrovascular nerves. Brain Res 113:400–404, 1976.

1193. Lasater GM: Primary intracranial hypotension. Headache 10:63–66, 1970.

1194. Lashley KS: Patterns of cerebral integration indicated by the scotomas of migraine. Arch Neurol Psychiatry 46:331–339, 1941.

1195. Laska EM, Sunshine A, Mueller F, Elvers WB, Siegel C, and Rubin A: Caffeine as an analgesic adjuvant. JAMA 251:1711–1718, 1984.

1196. Launay JM and Pradalier A: Common migraine attack: Platelet modifications are mainly due to plasma factor(s). Headache 25:262–267, 1985.

1197. Launay JM, Pradalier A, Dreux C, and Dry J: Platelet serotonin uptake and migraine. Cephalalgia 2:57–59, 1982.

1198. Laurence KM: Genetics of migraine. In Blau JN (ed): Migraine. Clinical and Research Aspects. Johns Hopkins University Press, Baltimore, 1987, pp 479–484.

1199. Lauritzen M: Long-lasting reduction of cortical blood flow of the brain after spreading depression with preserved autoregulation and impaired CO_2 response. J Cereb Blood Flow Metab 4:546–554, 1984.

1200. Lauritzen M: Cerebral blood flow in migraine and cortical spreading depression. Acta Neurol Scand 76(Suppl 113):1–40, 1987.

1201. Lauritzen M: Cortical spreading depression as a putative migraine mechanism. Trends Neurosci 10:8–12, 1987.

1202. Lauritzen M, Joergensen MB, Diemer NH, Gjedde A, and Hansen AJ: Persistent oligemia of rat cerebral cortex in the wake of spreading depression. Ann Neurol 12:469–474, 1982.

1203. Lauritzen M and Olesen J: Regional cerebral blood flow during migraine attacks by Xenon-133 inhalation and emission tomography. Brain 107:447–461, 1984.

1204. Lauritzen M, Skyhøj Olsen T, Lassen NA, and Paulson OB: Changes of regional cerebral blood flow during the course of classical migraine attacks. Ann Neurol 13:633–641, 1983.

1205. Lauritzen M, Skyhøj Olsen T, Lassen NA, and Paulson OB: Regulation of regional cerebral blood flow during and between migraine attacks. Ann Neurol 14:569–572, 1983.

1206. Lauritzen M, Trojaborg W, and Olesen J: The EEG in common and classic migraine attacks. In Clifford Rose F (ed): Advances in Migraine Research and Therapy. Raven, New York, 1982, pp 79–84.

1207. Leahey WJ, Neill JD, Varma MPS, and Shanks RG: Comparison of the efficacy and pharmacokinetics of conventional propranolol and a long acting preparation of propranolol. Br J Clin Pharmacol 9:33–40, 1980.

1208. Leão AAP: Spreading depression of activity in the cerebral cortex. J Neurophysiol 7:359–390, 1944.

1209. Leão AAP: Further observations on the spreading depression of activity in the cerebral cortex. J Neurophysiol 10:409–414, 1947.

1210. Leão AAP and Morison RS: Propagation of spreading cortical depression. J Neurophysiol 8:33–45, 1945.

1211. LeBars D, Dickenson AH, and Besson JM: Microinjection of morphine within nucleus raphe magnus and dorsal horn neuron activities related to nociception in the rat. Brain Res 189:467–481, 1980.

1212. Lebensohn JE: The nature of photophobia. Arch Ophthalmol 12:380–390, 1934.

1213. Leblanc R: The minor leak preceding subarachnoid hemorrhage. J Neurosurg 66:35–39, 1987.

1214. Lechner H, Ott E, Fazekas F, and Pilger E: Evidence of enhanced platelet aggregation and platelet sensitivity in migraine patients. Cephalalgia 5(Suppl 2):89–91, 1985.

1215. Lee CH and Lance JW: Migraine stupor. Headache 17:32–38, 1977.

1216. Lee Y, Kawai Y, Shiosaka S, et al.: Coexistence of calcitonin gene related peptide and substance P-like peptide in single cells of the trigeminal ganglion of the rat: Immunohistochemical analysis. Brain Res 330:194–196, 1985.

1217. Lees F and Watkins SM: Loss of consciousness in migraine. Lancet ii:647–650, 1963.

1218. Lehtonin JB: Visual evoked cortical potentials for single flashes and flickering light in migraine. Headache 14:1–12, 1974.

1219. Lehtonin J, Hyyppä MT, Kaihola HL, Kangasiemi P, and Lang AH: Visual evoked potentials in menstrual migraine. Headache 19:63–70, 1979.

1220. Lembeck F and Donnerer J: Opioid control of the function of primary afferent substance P fibers. Eur J Pharmacol 114:241–246, 1985.

1221. Lembeck F, Donnerer J, and Barthó L: Inhibition of neurogenic vasodilation and plasma extravasation by substance P antagonists, somatostatin and [D-met^2, pro^5]enkephalinamide. Eur J Pharmacol 85:171–176, 1982.

1222. Lembeck F, Popper H, and Juan H: Release of prostaglandins by bradykinin as an intrinsic mechanism of its algesic effect. Naunyn Schmiedebergs Arch Pharmacol 294:69–73, 1976.

1223. Lenarduzzi P, Delmotte P, Bigilimana I, and Schoenen J: Pirprofen in migraine attacks during the weaning period in drug abuse headache, an open study. New Trends Clin Neuropharm 2:42–43, 1988.

1224. Lennox WG: Ergonovine versus ergotamine as a terminator of migraine headaches. Am J Med Sci 195:458–468, 1938.

1225. Lennox WG: Epilepsy and Related Disorders. Little, Brown, Boston, 1960.

1226. Lennox WG and von Storch TJC: Experience with ergotamine tartrate in 120 patients with migraine. JAMA 105:169–171, 1935.

1227. Leonards JR: The influence of solubility on the rate of gastrointestinal asborption of aspirin. Clin Pharmacol Ther 4:476–479, 1963.

1228. Leonards JR and Levy G: Reduction or prevention of aspirin-induced occult gastrointestinal blood. Clin Pharmacol Ther 10:571–575, 1969.

1229. Leon-Sotomayor LA: Cardiac migraine—report of twelve cases. Angiology 25:161–171, 1974.

1230. Levine J and Swanson PD: Nonatherosclerotic causes of stroke. Ann Int Med 70:807–816, 1969.

1231. Levine JD, Lau W, Kwait G, and Goetzl EJ: Leukotriene B$_4$ produces hyperalgesia that is dependent on polymorphonuclear leukocytes. Science 225:743–745, 1984.

1232. Levine SR, Deegan MJ, Futrell N, and Welch KMA: Cerebrovascular and neurologic disease associated with antiphospholipid antibodies: 48 cases. Neurology 40:1181–1189, 1990.

1233. Levine SR, Joseph R, D'Andrea G, and Welch KMA: Migraine and the lupus anticoagulant. Case reports and review of the literature. Cephalalgia 7:93–99, 1987.

1234. Levine SR, Welch KMA, Ewing JR, Joseph R, and D'Andrea G: Cerebral blood flow asymmetries in headache-free migraineurs. Stroke 18:1164–1165, 1987.

1235. Leviton A, Malvea B, and Graham JR: Vascular diseases, mortality and migraine in the parents of migraine patients. Neurology 24:669–672, 1974.

1236. Levor RM, Cohen MJ, Naliboff BD, McArthur D, and Heuser G: Psychosocial precusors and correlates of migraine headache. J Consult Clin Psychol 54:347–353, 1986.

1237. Levy L: An epidemiological study of headache in an urban population in Zimbabwe. Headache 23:2–9, 1983.

1238. Ley P: Memory for medical information. Br J Social Clin Psychol 18:245–255, 1979.

1239. Leysen JE, Geerts R, Gommeren W, Verwimp M, and Van Gompel P: Regional distribution of serotonin-2 receptor sites in the brain and the effects of neuronal lesions. Arch Int Pharmacodyn 256:301–305, 1982.

1240. Leysen JE and Gommeren W: In vitro receptor binding profile of drugs used in migraine. In Amery WK, Van Neuten JM, and Wauquier A (eds): The Pharmacological Basis of Migraine Therapy. Pitman, London, 1984, pp 255–266.

1241. Lichten EM, Bennett RS, Whitty AJ, and Daoud Y: Efficacy of danazol in the control of hormonal migraine. J Reproduct Med 36:419–424, 1991.

1242. Lieberman AN, Jonas S, Hass WK, et al.: Bilateral cervical carotid and intracranial vasospasm causing cerebral ischemia in a migrainous patient: A case of 'diplegic migraine.' Headache 24:245–248, 1984.

1243. Lindegaard KF, Ovrelid L, and Sjaastaad O: Naproxen in the prevention of migraine attacks. A double-blind placebo-controlled cross-over study. Headache 20:96–98, 1980.

1244. Lindvall O, Björklund A, and Skagerberg G: Dopamine-containing neurons in the spinal cord: Anatomy and some functional aspects. Ann Neurol 14:255–260, 1983.

1245. Linet MS, Celentano DD, and Stewart WF: Headache characteristics associated with physician consultation: A population-based survey. Am J Prev Med 7:40–46, 1991.

1246. Linet MS and Stewart WF: Migraine headache: Epidemiologic perspectives. Epidemiol Rev 6:107–139, 1984.

1247. Linet MS and Stewart WF: The epidemiology of migraine headache. In Blau JN (ed): Migraine. Clinical and Research Aspects. Johns Hopkins University Press, Baltimore, 1987, pp 451–477.

1248. Linet MS, Stewart WF, Celentano DD, Ziegler D, and Sprecher M: An epidemiologic study of headache among adolescents and young adults. JAMA 261:2211–2216, 1989.

1249. Lingjaerde O: Platelet uptake and storage of serotonin. In Essman WB (ed): Serotonin in Health and Disease. Spectrum, New York, 1977, pp 139–199.

1250. Lingjaerde O and Monstad P: The uptake, storage, and efflux of serotonin in platelets from migraine patients. Cephalalgia 6:135–139, 1986.

1251. Lippman CW: Certain hallucinations peculiar to migraine. J Nerv Ment Dis 116:346–351, 1952.

1252. Lippman CW: Characteristic headache resulting from prolonged use of ergot derivatives. J Nerv Ment Dis 121:270–273, 1955.

1253. Lipson EH and Robertson WC: Paroxysmal torticollis in infancy: Familial occurrence. Am J Dis Child 132:422–423, 1978.

1254. Lipton RB, Choy-Kwong M, and Solomon S: Headaches in hospitalized cocaine users. Headache 29:224–227, 1989.

1255. Lipton RB, Newman LC, Cohen JS, and Solomon S: Aspartame as a dietary trigger of headache. Headache 29:90–92, 1989.

1256. Lipton RB, Stewart WF, Celentano DD, and Reed ML: Undiagnosed migraine headaches. A comparison of symptom-based and reported physician diagnosis. Arch Intern Med 152:1273–1278, 1992.

1257. Litman GI and Friedman HM: Migraine and the mitral valve prolapse syndrome. Am Heart J 96:610–614, 1978.

1258. Little JR and MacCarty CS: Colloid cysts of the third ventricle. J Neurosurg 40:230–235, 1974.

1259. Littlewood J, Gibb C, and Glover V: Red wine as migraine trigger. In Clifford Rose F (ed): Advances in Headache Research, Vol 4. Libbey, London, 1987, pp 123–127.

1260. Littlewood JT, Gibb C, Glover V, Sandler M, Davies PTG, and Clifford Rose F: Red wine as a cause of migraine. Lancet i:558–559, 1988.

1261. Littlewood J, Glover V, Sandler M, Petty R, Peatfield R, and Clifford Rose F: Platelet phenolsulphotransferase deficiency in dietary migraine. Lancet i:983–986, 1982.

1262. Liu-Chen LY, Gillespie SA, Norregaard TV, and Moskowitz MA: Co-lo-

calization of retrogradely transported wheat germ agglutinin and putative neurotransmitter substance P within trigeminal ganglion cells projecting to cat middle cerebral artery. J Comp Neurol 225:187–192, 1984.

1263. Liu-Chen LY, Mayberg MR, and Moskowitz MA: Immunohistochemical evidence for a substance P-containing trigeminovascular pathway to pial arteries in cats. Brain Res 268:162–166, 1983.

1264. Lloyd AR, Wakefield D, Boughton CR, and Dwyer JM: Immunological abnormalities in the chronic fatigue syndrome. Med J Aust 151:122–124, 1989.

1265. Logan W and Sherman DG: Transient global amnesia. Stroke 14:1005–1007, 1983.

1266. Logar C, Grabmair W, and Lechner H: Das EEG bei Migrane. EEG EMG Z Elektoenzephalogr Elelektromyogr Verwandte Geb 17:153–156, 1986.

1267. Loh L, Nathan PW, Schott GD, and Zilkha KJ: Acupuncture versus medical treatment for migraine and muscle tension headaches. J Neurol Neurosurg Psychiatry 47:333–337, 1984.

1268. Loisy C, Arnaud JL, and Amelot A: Contribution to the study of histamine metabolism in migrainous subjects. Res Clin Stud Headache 3:252–259, 1970.

1269. Lord GDA and Duckworth JW: Immunoglobulin and complement studies in migraine. Headache 17:163–168, 1977.

1270. Lord GDA and Duckworth JW: Complement and immune complex studies in migraine. Headache 18:255–260, 1978.

1271. Lord GDA, Duckworth JW, and Charlesworth JA: Complement activation in migraine. Lancet i:781–782, 1977.

1272. Louis P: A double-blind placebo-controlled prophylactic study of flunarizine (Sibelium) in migraine. Headache 21:235–239, 1981.

1273. Lous I and Olesen J: Evaluation of pericranial tenderness and oral function in patients with common migraine, muscle contraction headache and 'combination headache.' Pain 12:385–393, 1982.

1274. Love PE and Santoro SA: Antiphospholipid antibodies: Anticardiolipin and the lupus anticoagulant in systemic lupus erythematosus (SLE) and in non-SLE disorders. Prevalence and clinical significance. Ann Intern Med 112:682–698, 1990.

1275. Lovshin LL: Vascular neck pain—a common syndrome seldom recognized. Cleveland Clinical Quarterly 27:5–13, 1960.

1276. Lowe DA, Matthews EK, and Richardson PB: The calcium antagonistic effects of cyproheptadine on contraction, membrane electrical events and calcium influx in the guinea-pig taenia coli. Br J Pharmacol 74:651–663, 1981.

1277. Lowe RF: Aetiology of the anatomical basis for primary angle closure glaucoma. Br J Ophthalmol 54:161–169, 1970.

1278. Lowenstein DH, Massa SM, Rowbotham MC, Collins SD, McKinney HE, and Simon RP: Acute neurologic and psychiatric complications associated with cocaine abuse. Am J Med 83:841–846, 1987.

1279. Lucas RN: Migraine in twins. J Psychosom Res 21:147–156, 1977.

1280. Lucas RN and Falkowski W: Ergotamine and methysergide abuse in patients with migraine. Br J Psychiatry 122:199–203, 1973.

1281. Lucas RV and Edwards JE: The floppy mitral valve. Curr Probl Cardiol 7:1–48, 1982.

1282. Ludin HP: Flunarazine and propranolol in the treatment of migraine. Headache 29:218–223, 1989.

1283. Ludvigsson J: Propranolol used in prophylaxis of migraine in children. Acta Neurol Scand 50:109–115, 1974.

1284. Lundberg JM, Hökfelt T, Schultzberg M, Uvnäs-Wallenstein K, Köhler C, and Said SI: Occurrence of vasoactive intestinal polypeptide (VIP)-like immunoreactivity in certain cholinergic neurons of the cat: Evidence from combined immunohistochemistry and acetylcholinesterase staining. Neuroscience 4:1539–1559, 1979.

1285. Lundberg PO: Migraine prophylaxis with progestogens. Acta Endocrinol 40 (Suppl 68):1–22, 1962.

1286. Lundberg PO: Abdominal migraine—diagnosis and therapy. Headache 15:122–125, 1975.

1287. Lüscher TF and Vanhoutte PM: The Endothelium: Modulator of Cardiovascular Function. CRC, Boca Raton, 1990.

1288. MacLean C, Appenzeller O, Cordaro JT, and Rhodes J: Flash evoked potentials in migraine. Headache 14:193–198, 1975.

1289. Maertens de Noordhout A, Timsit-Berthier M, Timsit M, and Schoenen J: Contingent negative variation in headache. Ann Neurol 19:78–80, 1986.

1290. Magos AL, Brincat M, and Studd JW: Treatment of the premenstrual syndrome by subcutaneous estradiol implants and cyclical norethisterone: Placebo controlled study. Br Med J 292:1629–1633, 1986.

1291. Magos AL, Zikha KJ, and Studd JW: Treatment of menstrual migraine by estradiol implants. J Neurol Neurosurg Psychiatry 46:1044–1046, 1983.

1292. Malmgren R, Olsson P, Tornling G, and Unge G: Acetylsalicyclic asthma and migraine—a defect in serotonin (5-HT) uptake in platelets. Thromb Res 13:1137–1139, 1978.

1293. Manotti C, Quintavalla R, and Manzoni GC: Platelet activation in migraine. Thromb Haemost 50:758, 1983.

1294. Mansfield LE: Food allergy and headache. Whom to evaluate and how to treat. Postgrad Med 83:46–51, 1988.

1295. Mansfield LE, Vaughan TR, Waller SF, Haverly RW, and Ting S: Food allergy and adult migraine: Double-blind and mediator confirmation of an allergic etiology. Ann Allergy 55:126–129, 1985.

1296. Manzoni GC, Farina S, Granella F, Alfieri M, and Bisi M: Classic and common migraine: Suggestive clinical evidence of two separate entities. Funct Neurol 1:112–122, 1986.

1297. Manzoni GC, Farina S, Lanfranchi M, and Solari A: Classic migraine—clinical findings in 164 patients. Eur Neurol 24:163–169, 1985.

1298. Manzoni GC, Terzano MG, Bono G, Micieli G, Martucci N, and Nappi G: Cluster headache—clinical findings in 180 patients. Cephalalgia 3:21–30, 1983.

1299. Maratos J and Wilkinson M: Migraine in children: A medical and psychiatric study. Cephalalgia 2:179–187, 1982.

1300. Marcus DA and Soso MJ: Migraine and stripe-induced visual discomfort. Arch Neurol 46:1129–1132, 1989.

1301. Marcussen RM and Wolff HG: Studies on headache: (1) Effects of carbon dioxide–oxygen mixtures given during preheadache phase of the migraine attack; (2) further analysis of the pain mechanisms in headache. Arch Neurol Psychiatry 63:42–51, 1950.

1302. Markley HG, Cheronis J, and Piepho RW: Verapamil in prophylactic therapy of migraine. Neurology 34:973–976, 1984.

1303. Markowitz S, Saito K, and Moskowitz MA: Neurogenically mediated leakage of plasma protein occurs from blood vessels in dura mater but not brain. J Neurosci 7:4129–4136, 1987.

1304. Markowitz S, Saito K, and Moskowitz MA: Neurogenically mediated plasma extravasation in dura mater: Effect of ergot alkaloids. A possible mechanism of action in vascular headaches. J Neurosci 8:83–91, 1988.

1305. Markus HS: A prospective follow up of thunderclap headache mimicking subarachnoid hemorrhage. J Neurol Neurosurg Psychiatry 54:1117–1118, 1991.

1306. Markus HS and Hopkinson N: Migraine and headache in systemic lupus erythematosus and their relationship with antibodies against phospholipids. J Neurol 239:39–42, 1992.

1307. Markush RE, Karp HR, Heyman A, and O'Fallon WM: Epidemiologic study of migraine symptoms in young women. Neurology 25:430–435, 1975.

1308. Marshall J: The cause and prognosis of strokes in people under 50 years. J Neurol 53:473–478, 1982.

1309. Marshall WH: Spreading cortical depression of Leão. Physiol Rev 39:239–279, 1959.

1310. Marsters JB, Mortimer MJ, and Hay KM: Glucose and diet in the fasting migraineur. Headache 26:243–247, 1986.

1311. Martin EA: Headache during sexual intercourse (coital cephalalgia). A report of six cases. Irish J Med Sci 148:342–345, 1974.

1312. Martin PR and Mathews AM: Tension headaches: Psychophysiological investigation and treatment. J Psychosomatic Res 22:389–399, 1978.

1313. Marzillier JS: Cognitive therapy and behavioral practice. Behav Res Ther 18:249–258, 1980.

1314. Masel BE, Chesson AL, Peters BH, Levin HS, and Alperin JB: Platelet antagonists in migraine prophylaxis. A clinical trial using aspirin and dipyridamole. Headache 20:13–18, 1980.

1315. Masi AT and Dugdale M: Cerebrovascular diseases associated with the use of oral contraceptives. A review of the English-language literature. Ann Intern Med 72:111–121, 1970.

1316. Masland WS, Friedman AP, and Buchsbaum HW: Computerized axial tomography of migraine. Res Clin Stud Headache 6:136–140, 1978.

1317. Mason P and Fields HL: Axonal trajectories and terminations of on- and off-cells in the cat lower brainstem. J Comp Neurol 288:185–207, 1989.

1318. Massey EW: Migraine during pregnancy. Obstet Gynecol Surv 32:693–696, 1977.

1319. Massey EW: Effort headache in runners. Headache 22:99–100, 1982.

1320. Massiou H, Seerurier D, Lasserre O, and Bousser MG: Effectiveness of oral diclofenac in the acute treatment of common migraine attacks: A double-blind study versus placebo. Cephalalgia 11:59–63, 1991.

1321. Masuzawa T, Shinoda S, Furuse M, Nakahara N, Abe F, and Sato F: Cerebral angiographic changes on serial examination of a patient with migraine. Neuroradiology 24:277–281, 1983.

1322. Mathew NT: Computerized axial tomography in migraine. In Greene R (ed): Current Concepts in Migraine Research. Raven, New York, 1978, pp 63–71.

1323. Mathew NT: Prophylaxis of migraine and mixed headache: A randomized controlled study. Headache 21:105–109, 1981.

1324. Mathew NT: Indomethacin responsive headache variant. Spectrum of a new headache syndrome. Headache 21:147–150, 1981.

1325. Mathew NT: Management of ergotamine withdrawal. In Diener HC and Wilkinson M (eds): Drug-Induced Headache. Springer-Verlag, Berlin, 1988, pp 150–156.

1326. Mathew NT: Chronic daily headache: Clinical features and natural history. In Nappi G, Bono G, Sandrini G, Martignoni E, and Micieli G (eds): Headache and Depression: Serotonin Pathways as a Common Clue. Raven, New York, 1991, pp 49–58.

1327. Mathew NT: The abortive treatment of migraine. In Gallagher RM (ed): Drug Therapy for Headache. Dekker, New York, 1991, pp 95–113.

1328. Mathew NT and Ali S: Valproate in the treatment of persistent chronic daily headache. An open label study. Headache 31:71–74, 1991.

1329. Mathew NT and Alvarez L: The usefulness of thermography in headache. In Clifford Rose F (ed): Progress in Migraine Research, Vol 2. Pittman, London, 1984, pp 232–245.

1330. Mathew NT, Dexter J, Couch J, et al.: Dose ranging efficacy and safety of subcutaneous sumatriptan in the acute treatment of migraine. Arch Neurol 49:1271–1276, 1992.

1331. Mathew NT, Hrastnik F, and Meyer JS: Regional cerebral blood flow in the diagnosis of vascular headache. Headache 15:252–260, 1975.

1332. Mathew NT, Kurman R, and Perez F: Drug-induced refractory headache: Clinical features and management. Headache 30:634–638, 1990.

1333. Mathew NT, Meyer JS, Welch KMA, and Neblett CR: Abnormal CT scans in migraine. Headache 16:272–279, 1977.

1334. Mathew NT, Reuveni U, and Perez F: Transformed or evolutive migraine. Headache 27:102–106, 1987.

1335. Mathew NT, Stubits E, and Nigam MP: Transformation of episodic migraine into daily headache: Analysis of factors. Headache 22:66–68, 1982.

1336. Mathew RJ, Weinman ML, and Largen JW: Sympathetic–adrenomedullary activation and migraine. Headache 22:13–19, 1982.

1337. Mathew RJ and Wilson WH: Regional cerebral blood flow changes associated with ethanol intoxication. Stroke 17:1156–1159, 1986.

1338. Matsuyama T, Wanaka A, Yoneda S, et al.: Two distinct calcitonin gene-related peptide-containing peripheral nervous systems: Distribution and quantitative differences between the iris and cerebral artery with special reference to substance P. Brain Res 373:205–212, 1986.

1339. Matthews WB: Footballer's migraine. Br Med J ii:326–327, 1972.

1340. Matthysse S: Antipsychotic drug actions: A clue to the neuropathology of schizophrenia. Fed Proc 32:200–205, 1973.

1341. Mayberg MR, Langer RS, Zervas NT, and Moskowitz MA: Perivascular meningeal projections from cat trigeminal ganglia: Possible pathway for vascular headaches in man. Science 213:228–230, 1981.

1342. Mayberg MR, Zervas NT, and Moskowitz MA: Trigeminal projections to supratentorial pial and dural blood vessels in cats demonstrated by horseradish peroxidase histochemistry. J Comp Neurol 223:46–56, 1984.

1343. McArthur DL and Cohen J: Measures of forehead and finger temperature, frontalis EMG, heart rate and finger pulse amplitude during and between migraine headaches. Headache 20:134–136, 1980.

1344. McArthur JC, Marek K, Pestronk A, McArthur J, and Peroutka SJ: Nifedipine in the prophylaxis of classic migraine: A cross-over, double-masked, placebo-controlled study of headache frequency and side effects. Neurology 39:284–286, 1989.

1345. McArthur MB: Neurologic manifestations of AIDS. Medicine 66:407–437, 1987.

1346. McBean DE, Sharkey J, Ritchie IM, and Kelly PAT: Evidence for a possible role of serotonergic systems in the control of cerebral blood flow. Brain Res 537:307–310, 1990.

1347. McCabe BJ: Dietary tyramine and other pressor amines in MAOI regimens: A review. J Am Diet Assoc 86:1059–1064, 1986.

1348. McCarthy BG and Peroutka SJ: Comparative neuropharmacology of dihydroergotamine and sumatriptan (GR 43175). Headache 29:420–422, 1989.

1349. McCulloch J and Edvinsson L: Calcitonin gene-related peptide and the trigeminal innervation of the cerebral circulation. In Edvinsson L and McCulloch J (eds): Peptidergic Mechanisms in the Cerebral Circulation. VPH Verlagsgesellschaft, Weinheim, 1987, pp 132–151.

1350. McCulloch J, Uddman R, Kingman TA, and Edvinsson L: Calcitonin gene-related peptide: Functional role in cerebrovascular regulation. Proc Natl Acad Sci USA 83:5731–5735, 1986.

1351. McEwen JI, O'Connor HM, and Dinsdale HB: Treatment of migraine with intramuscular chlorpromazine. Ann Emerg Med 16:758–763, 1987.

1352. McMahon MS, Norregaard TV, Beyerl BD, Borges LF, and Moskowitz MA: Trigeminal afferents to cerebral arteries are not divergent axon collaterals. Neurosci Lett 60:63–68, 1985.

1353. McNaughton FL: The innervation of the intracranial blood vessels and dural sinuses. Res Publ Assoc Nerv Ment Dis 18:178–200, 1938.

1354. McNeil G, Shaw P, and Dock D: Substitution of atenolol for propranolol in a case of propranolol related depression. Am J Psychiatry 139:1187–1188, 1982.

1355. Meade TW, Greenberg G, and Thompson SG: Progestogens and cardiovascular reactions associated with oral contraceptives and a comparison of the safety of 50- and 30-microgram estrogen preparations. Br Med J 280:1157–1161, 1980.

1356. Medina JL and Diamond S: Migraine and atopy. Headache 16:271–274, 1976.

1357. Medina JL and Diamond S: The role of diet in migraine. Headache 18:31–34, 1978.

1358. Medina JL and Diamond S: Cyclical migraine. Arch Neurol 38:343–344, 1981.

1359. Medina JL, Diamond S, and Franklin MA: Biofeedback therapy for migraine. Headache 16:115–118, 1976.

1360. Medina JL, Diamond S, and Rubino F: Headache in patients with transient ischemic attacks. Headache 15:194–197, 1975.

1361. Meier J and Schreier E: Human plasma levels of some anti-migraine drugs. Headache 15:96–104, 1976.

1362. Meltzer HY and Lowy MT: The serotonin hypothesis of depression. In Meltzer HY (ed): Psychopharmacology: The Third Generation of Progress. Raven, New York, 1987, pp 513–526.

1363. Melzack R and Casey KL: Sensory, motivational, and central control determinants of pain. A new conceptual model. In Kenshalo D (ed): The Skin Senses. Thomas, Springfield, 1968, pp 423–439.

1364. Mendenopoulos G, Manafi T, Logothetis I, and Bostantjopoulou S: Flunarizine in the prevention of classical migraine: A placebo-controlled evaluation. Cephalalgia 5:31–37, 1985.

1365. Mense S and Schmidt RF: Activation of group IV afferent units from muscle by algesic agents. Brain Res 72:305–310, 1974.

1366. Merhoff GC and Porter JM: Ergot intoxication: Historical review and description of unusual clinical manifestations. Ann Surg 180:773–779, 1974.

1367. Merikangas KR: Genetic epidemiology of migraine. In Sandler M and Collins GM (eds): Migraine: A Spectrum of Ideas. Oxford University Press, Oxford, 1990, pp 40–48.

1368. Merikangas KR and Angst J: Depression and migraine. In Sandler M and Collins GM (eds): Migraine: A Spectrum of Ideas. Oxford University Press, Oxford, 1990, pp 248–258.

1369. Merikangas KR, Angst J, and Isler H: Migraine and psychopathology. Results of the Zurich cohort study of young adults. Arch Gen Psychiatry 47:849–853, 1990.

1370. Merikangas KR, Risch NJ, Merikangas JR, Weissman MM, and Kidd KK: Migraine and depression: Association and familial transmission. J Psychiatry Res 22:119–129, 1988.

1371. Merrett J, Peatfield RC, Clifford Rose F, and Merrett JG: Food related antibodies in headache patients. J Neurol Neurosurg Psychiatry 46:738–742, 1983.

1372. Messinger HB, Spierings ELH, and Vincent AJP: Overlap of migraine and tension-type headache in the International Headache Society classification. Cephalalgia 11:233–237, 1991.

1373. Meyboom RHB, Ferrari MD, and Dieleman BP: Parkinsonism, tardive dyskinesia, akathisia, and depression induced by flunarizine. Lancet ii:292, 1986.

1374. Meyer JS, Dowell R, Mathew N, and Hardenberg J: Clinical and hemodynamic effects during treatment of vascular headaches with verapamil. Headache 24:313–321, 1984.

1375. Meyer JS and Hardenberg J: Clinical effectiveness of calcium entry blockers in prophylactic treatment of migraine and cluster headaches. Headache 23:266–277, 1983.

1376. Meyer JS, Kawamura J, and Terayama Y: CT-CBF and ^{133}Xe CBF studies in migraine without aura. In Olesen J (ed): Migraine and Other Headaches: The Vascular Mechanisms. Raven, New York, 1991, pp 227–234.

1377. Meyer JS, Nance M, Walker M, Zetusky WJ, and Dowell RE: Migraine and cluster headache treatment with calcium antagonists supports a vascular pathogenesis. Headache 25:358–367, 1985.

1378. Meyer JS, Zetusky W, Jónsdóttir M, and Mortel K: Cephalic hyperemia during migraine headaches. A prospective study. Headache 26:388–397, 1986.

1379. Michael MI and Williams JM: Migraine in children. J Pediatr 41:18–24, 1952.

1380. Michultka DM, Blanchard EB, Appelbaum KA, Jaccard J, and Dentinger MP: The refractory headache patient: II. High medication consumption (analgesic rebound) headache. Behav Res Ther 27:411–420, 1989.

1381. Micieli G, Tassorelli C, Magri M, Sandrini G, Cavallini A, and Nappi G: Vegetative imbalance in migraine. A dynamic TV pupillometric evaluation. Funct Neurol 4:105–111, 1989.

1382. Middlemiss DN: Blockade of the central 5-HT autoreceptor by β-adrenoceptor antagonists. Eur J Pharmacol 120:51–56, 1986.

1383. Middlemiss DN, Buxton DA, and Greenwood DT: Beta-adrenoceptor antagonists in psychiatry and neurology. Pharmacol Ther 12:419–437, 1981.

1384. Migraine-Nimodipine European Study Group (MINES): European multicenter trial in the prophylaxis of common migraine (migraine without aura). Headache 29:633–638, 1989.

1385. Migraine-Nimodipine European Study Group (MINES): European multicenter trial in the prophylaxis of classic migraine (migraine with aura). Headache 29:639–642, 1989.

1386. Mikkelsen BM and Falk JV: Prophylactic treatment of migraine with tolfenamic acid. A comparative double-blind crossover study between tolfenamic acid and placebo. Acta Neurol Scand 66:105–111, 1982.

1387. Millan MH, Millan MJ, and Herz A: Midbrain stimulation-induced antinociception in the rat: Characterization of role of β-endorphin. Adv Pain Res Ther 9:493–498, 1985.

1388. Miller AD and Wilson VJ: 'Vomiting center' reanalyzed: An electrical stimulation study. Brain Res 270:154–158, 1983.

1389. Miller D, Waters DD, Warnica W, Szlachcic J, Kreeft J, and Théroux P: Is variant angina the coronary manifestation of a generalized vasospastic disorder? N Engl J Med 304:763–771, 1981.

1390. Millichap J: Recurrent headache in 100 children. EEG changes and response to phenytoin. Child's Brain 4:95–105, 1978.

1391. Mills DCB and Smith JB: The influence on platelet aggregation of drugs that affect the accumulation of adenosine 3′:5′-cyclic monophosphate in platelets. Biochem J 121:185–196, 1971.

1392. Milne G: Hypnotherapy with migraine. Aust J Clin Exp Hypnosis 11:23–32, 1983.

1393. Milner PM: Note on a possible correspondence between the scotomas of migraine and spreading depression of Leão. Electroencephalogr Clin Neurophysiol 10:705, 1958.

1394. Minervini MG, Balducci M, and Puca F: Diclofenac sodium in the treatment of migraine attack. In Clifford Rose F (ed): New Advances in Headache Research: 2. Smith-Gordon, London, 1991, pp 303–306.

1395. Mira M, McNeil D, Fraser IS, Vizzard J, and Abraham S: Mefenamic acid in the treatment of premenstrual syndrome. Obstet Gynecol 68:395–398, 1986.

1396. Mitchell KR and White RG: Behavioral self-management: An application to the problem of migraine headaches. Behavior Therapy 24:241–248, 1982.

1397. Mizumura K, Sato J, and Kumazawa T: Effects of prostaglandins and other putative chemical intermediaries on the activity of the canine testicular polymodal receptors studied in vitro. Pfluegers Arch 408:565–572, 1987.

1398. Mochi M, Sangiorgi S, and Cortelli P: Migraine with aura: A threshold character with mitochondrial enzyme deficiency. Neurology 41(Suppl 1):369, 1991.

1399. Moffett AM, Swash M, and Scott DF: Effect of tyramine in migraine: A double-blind study. J Neurol Neurosurg Psychiatry 35:496–499, 1972.

1400. Moffett AM, Swash M, and Scott DF: Effect of chocolate in migraine: A double-blind study. J Neurol Neurosurg Psychiatry 37:445–448, 1974.

1401. Mohr JP: Neurological manifestations and factors related to therapeutic decisions. In Wilson CB and Stein BM (eds): Intracranial Arteriovenous Malformations. Williams & Wilkins, Baltimore, 1984, pp 1–11.

1402. Mokha SS, McMillan JA, and Iggo A: Descending control of spinal nociceptive transmission. Actions produced on spinal multireceptive neurons from the nuclei locus coeruleus (LC) and raphe magnus (NRM). Exp Brain Res 58:213–226, 1985.

1403. Molaie M, Olson CM, and Koch J: The effect of intravenous verapamil on acute migraine headache. Headache 27:51–53, 1987.

1404. Moncada S, Ferreira SH, and Vane JR: Pain and inflammatory mediators. In Vane JR and Ferreira SH (eds): Inflammation, Handbook of Experimental Pharmacology, Vol 50, Part I. Springer-Verlag, Berlin, 1978, pp 588–616.

1405. Mondrup K and Moller CE: Prophylactic treatment of migraine with clonidine: A controlled clinical trial. Acta Neurol Scand 56:405–412, 1977.

1406. Monro J: Food allergy and migraine. Clin Immunol Allergy 2:137–163, 1982.

1407. Monro J, Brostoff J, Carini C, and Zilkha K: Food allergy in migraine: Study of dietary exclusion and RAST. Lancet *ii*:1–4, 1980.

1408. Monstad P and Lingjaerde O: Platelet serotonin uptake and efflux in migraine. Acta Neurol Scand 69:273–274, 1984.

1409. Montagna P, Cortelli P, Monari L, et al.: Brain and muscle energy metabolism in migraine studied by ^{31}P magnetic resonance spectroscopy (^{31}P-MRS). Neurology 41(Suppl 1):369, 1991.

1410. Montagna P, Gallassi R, Medori R, et al.: MELAS syndrome: Characteristic migrainous and epileptic features and maternal transmission. Neurology 38:751–754, 1988.

1411. Montalban J, Cervera R, Font J, et al.: Lack of association between anticardiolipin antibodies and migraine in systemic lupus erythematosus. Neurology 42:681–682, 1992.

1412. Moore KL: Valproate in the treatment of refractory recurrent headaches: A retrospective analysis of 207 patients. Headache Quarterly, Current Treatment and Research 3:323–325, 1992.

1413. Moore KL: Documentation and risk management for the headache specialist: Potential pitfalls of practice parameters. Headache Quarterly, Current Treatment and Research 4:68–83, 1993.

1414. Moore RY and Bloom FE: Central catecholamine neuron systems: Anatomy and physiology of the norepinephrine and epinephrine systems. Annu Rev Neurosci 2:113–168, 1979.

1415. Moore TL, Ryan RE, Pohl DA, Roodman ST, and Ryan RE: Immunoglobulin, complement, and immune complex levels during a migraine attack. Headache 20:9–12, 1980.

1416. Moreland TJ, Storli OV, and Mogstad TE: Doxepin in the prophylactic treatment of mixed vascular and tension headache. Headache 19:382–383, 1979.

1417. Moretti G, Manzoni GC, Caffarra P, and Parma M: "Benign recurrent vertigo" and its connection with migraine. Headache 20:344–346, 1980.

1418. Morrison DP: Occupational stress in migraine—is weekend headache a myth or reality? Cephalalgia 10:189–193, 1990.

1419. Moser M, Wish H, and Friedman AP: Headache and hypertension. JAMA 180:301–306, 1962.

1420. Moskowitz MA: The neurobiology of vascular head pain. Ann Neurol 16:157–168, 1984.

1421. Moskowitz MA: Basic mechanisms of headache. Neurol Clin 8:801–815, 1990.

1422. Moskowitz MA: The visceral organ brain: Implications for the pathophysiology of vascular headache. Neurology 41:182–186, 1991.

1423. Moskowitz MA: Neurogenic versus vascular mechanisms of sumatriptan and ergot alkaloids in migraine. Trends Pharmacol Sci 13:307–311, 1992.

1424. Moskowitz MA, Brody M, and Liu-Chen LY: In vitro release of immunoreactive substance P from putative afferent nerve endings in bovine pia arachnoid. Neuroscience 9:809–814, 1983.

1425. Moskowitz MA and Buzzi MG: Neuroeffector functions of sensory fibers: Implications for headache mechanisms and drug actions. J Neurol 238(Suppl 1):S18–S22, 1991.

1426. Moskowitz MA, Buzzi MG, Sakas DE, and Linnik MD: Pain mechanisms underlying vascular headaches. Rev Neurol 145:181–193, 1989.

1427. Moskowitz MA, Henrickson BM, Markowitz S, and Saito K: Intra- and extracraniovascular nociceptive mechanisms and the pathogenesis of head pain. In Olesen J and Edvinsson L (eds): Basic Mechanisms of Headache. Elsevier, Amsterdam, 1988, pp 429–437.

1428. Moskowitz MA, Sakas D, Wei EP, et al.: Postocclusive hyperemia is markedly attenuated by chronic trigeminal ganglionectomy. Am J Physiol 257:H1736–H1739, 1989.

1429. Moskowitz MA, Wei EP, Saito K, and Kontos HA: Trigeminalectomy modifies pial arteriolar responses to hypertension or norepinephrine. Am J Physiol 255:H1–H6, 1988.

1430. Mosnaim AD, Huprikar S, Wolf ME, and Diamond S: Platelet monoamine oxidase activity in female migraine patients. Headache 30:488–490, 1990.

1431. Moss G and Waters WE: Headache and migraine in a girls' grammar school. In Waters WE (ed): The Epidemiology of Migraine. Boehringer Ingelheim, Bracknell-Berkshire, 1974, pp 49–58.

1432. Moss RA, Garret J, and Chiodo JF: Temporomandibular joint dysfunction syndromes: Parameters, etiology, and treatment. Psychol Bull 92:331–346, 1982.

1433. Moyer S: Pharmacokinetics of naproxen sodium. Cephalalgia 6 (Suppl 4):77–80, 1986.

1434. Mück-Seler D, Deanovic Z, and Dupelj M: Platelet serotonin (5-HT) and 5-HT releasing factor in plasma of migrainous patients. Headache 19:14–17, 1979.

1435. Mück-Seler D, Deanovic Z, and Dupelj M: Serotonin-releasing factors in migrainous patients. Adv Neurol 33:257–264, 1982.

1436. Mueller SM, Heistad DD, and Marcus ML: Effect of sympathetic nerves on cerebral vessels during seizures. Am J Physiol 237:H178–H184, 1979.

1437. Mullinex JM, Norton BJ, Hack S, and Fishman MA: Skin temperature biofeedback and migraine. Headache 17:242–244, 1978.

1438. Muramatsu I, Fujiwara M, Miura A, and Sakakibara Y: Possible involvement of adenine nucleotides in sympathetic neuroeffector mechanisms of dog basilar artery. J Pharmacol Exp Ther 216:401–409, 1981.

1439. Muramatsu I, Fujiwara M, Miura A, and Shibata S: Reactivity of isolated canine cerebral arteries to adenine nucleotides and adenosine. Pharmacology 21:198–205, 1980.

1440. Murialdo G, Martignoni E, De Maria A, et al.: Changes in the dopaminergic control of prolactin secretion and in ovarian steroids in migraine. Cephalalgia 6:43–49, 1986.

1441. Mylecharane EJ: 5-HT$_2$ receptor antagonists and migraine therapy. J Neurol 238:S45–S52, 1991.

1442. Nachman RL and Weksler B: The platelet as an inflammatory cell. Ann NY Acad Sci 201:131–137, 1972.

1443. Nadelmann JW, Stevens J, and Saper JR: Propranolol in the prophylaxis of migraine. Headache 26:175–182, 1986.

1444. Nagel-Leiby S, Welch KMA, Grunfeld S, and D'Andrea G: Ovarian steroid levels in migraine with and without aura. Cephalalgia 10:147–152, 1990.

1445. Nahorski SR and Wilcocks AL: Interactions of β-adrenoceptor antagonists with 5-hydroxytryptamine receptor subtypes in rat cerebral cortex. Br J Pharmacol 78:107P, 1983.

1446. Nanda RN, Johnson RH, Gray J, Keogh HJ, and Melville ID: A double blind trial of acebutolol for migraine prophylaxis. Headache 18:20–22, 1978.

1447. Nappi G, Facchinetti F, Legnante G, et al.: Impairment of the central and peripheral opioid systems in headache. In Clifford Rose F (ed): Progress in Migraine Research, Vol 2. Pitman, London, 1984, pp 162–166.

1448. Nappi G, Facchinetti F, Martignoni E, et al.: Plasma and CSF endorphin levels in primary and symptomatic headaches. Headache 25:141–144, 1985.

1449. Nathanson JA and Glaser GH: Identification of beta-adrenergic-sensitive adenylate cyclase in intracranial blood vessels. Nature 278:567–569, 1979.

1450. Nattero G: Menstrual headache. Adv Neurol 33:215–226, 1982.

1451. Nattero G, Bisbocci D, and Ceresa F: Sex hormones, prolactin levels, osmolarity and electrolyte patterns in menstrual migraine—relationship with fluid retention. Headache 19:25–30, 1979.

1452. Needleman P, Turk J, Jakschik BA, Morrison AR, and Lefkowith JB: Arachidonic acid metabolism. Annu Rev Biochem 55:69–102, 1986.

1453. Nestvold K: Naproxen and naproxen sodium in acute migraine attacks. Cephalalgia 6(Suppl 4):81–84, 1986.

1454. Nestvold K, Kloster R, Partinen M, and Sulkava R: Treatment of acute migraine attack: Naproxen and placebo compared. Cephalalgia 5:115–119, 1985.

1455. Nichols FT, Mawad M, Mohr JP, Stein B, Hilal S, and Michelsen WJ: Focal headache during balloon inflation in the internal carotid and middle cerebral arteries. Stroke 21:555–559, 1990.

1456. Nicol AR: Psychogenic abdominal pain in childhood. Br J Hosp Med 27:351–353, 1982.

1457. Nieman EA and Hurwitz LJ: Ocular sympathetic palsy in periodic migrainous neuralgia. J Neurol Neurosurg Psychiatry 24:369–373, 1961.

1458. Nieper HA: The clinical applications of lithium orotate. A two year study. Aggressiologie 14:407–411, 1973.

1459. Nies AS and Shand DG: Clinical pharmacology of propranolol. Circulation 52:6–15, 1975.

1460. Nikiforow R: Headache in a random sample of 200 persons: A clinical study of a population in northern Finland. Cephalalgia 1:99–107, 1981.

1461. Nikiforow R and Hokkanen E: An epidemiological study of headache in an urban and a rural population in northern Finland. Headache 18:137–145, 1978.

1462. Nimmerfall F and Rosenthaler J: Ergot alkaloids: Hepatic distribution and estimation of absorption by measurement of total radioactivity in bile and urine. J Pharmacokin Biopharmac 4:57–62, 1976.

1463. Nitta M and Symon L: Colloid cysts of the third ventricle. A review of 36 cases. Acta Neurochir 76:99–104, 1985.

1464. Nolan L and O'Malley K: Prescribing for the elderly. Part I. Sensitivity of the elderly to adverse drug reactions. J Am Geriatr Soc 36:142–149, 1988.

1465. Noronha MJ: Double-blind randomized crossover trial of timolol in migraine prophylaxis in children. Cephalalgia 5(Suppl 3):174–175, 1985.

1466. Norregaard TV and Moskowitz MA: Substance P and the sensory innervation of intracranial and extracranial feline cephalic arteries. Brain 108:517–533, 1985.

1467. Norris JW, Hachinski VC, and Cooper PW: Changes in cerebral blood flow during a migraine attack. Br Med J iii:676–677, 1975.

1468. Northfield DWC: Some observations on headache. Brain 61:133–162, 1938.

1469. Nybäck HV, Walters JR, Aghajanian GK, and Roth RH: Tricyclic antidepressants: Effects on the firing rate of brain noradrenergic neurones. Eur J Pharmacol 32:302–312, 1975.

1470. Nyrke T and Lang AH: Spectral analysis of visual potentials evoked by sine wave modulated light in migraine. Electroencephalogr Clin Neurophysiol 53:436–442, 1982.

1471. O'Brien MD: Cerebral-cortex-perfusion rates in migraine. Lancet i:1036, 1967.

1472. O'Brien MD: Cerebral blood changes in migraine. Headache 10:139–143, 1971.

1473. Ochs S: The nature of spreading depression in neural networks. Int Rev Neurobiol 4:1–69, 1962.

1474. O'Connor PJ: Acephalgic migraine. Ophthalmology 88:999–1003, 1981.

1475. O'Connor PJ and Tredici TJ: Acephalgic migraine, 15 years experience. Ophthalmology 88:999–1002, 1982.

1476. O'Connor RP and van der Kooy D: Pattern of intracranial and extracranial projections of trigeminal ganglion cells. J Neurosci 6:2200–2207, 1986.

1477. O'Connor RP and van der Kooy D: Enrichment of a vasoactive neuropeptide (calcitonin gene related peptide) in the trigeminal sensory projections to the intracranial arteries. J Neurosci 8:2468–2476, 1988.

1478. O'Dea JPK and Davis EH: Tamoxifen in the treatment of menstrual migraine. Neurology 40:1470–1471, 1990.

1479. O'Grady J, Warrington S, Moti MJ, et al.: Effects of intravenous infusion of prostacyclin (PGI₂) in man. Prostaglandins 19:319–332, 1980.

1480. Ogunyemi AO: Prevalence of headache among Nigerian university students. Headache 24:127–130, 1984.

1481. O'Hare JA, Feely MJ, and Callaghan N: Clinical aspects of familial hemiplegic migraine in two families. Irish Med J 74:291–295, 1981.

1482. Okada YC, Lauritzen M, and Nicholson C: Magnetic field associated with spreading depression: A model for the detection of migraine. Brain Res 442:185–190, 1988.

1483. Okawara SH: Warning signs prior to rupture of an intracranial aneurysm. J Neurosurg 38:575–580, 1973.

1484. O'Keefe ST, Tsapatsaris NP, and Beetham WP: Increased prevalence of migraine and chest pain in patients with primary Raynaud disease. Ann Intern Med 116:985–989, 1992.

1485. Okogbo ME: Migraine in Nigerian children—a study of 51 patients. Headache 31:673–676, 1991.

1486. Oldendorf WH: Brain uptake of radiolabeled amino acids, amines, and hexoses after arterial injection. Am J Physiol 221:1629–1639, 1971.

1487. Olerud B, Gustavsson C, and Furberg B: Nadolol and propranolol in migraine management. Headache 26:490–493, 1986.

1488. Olesen J: Effect of intracarotid prostaglandin E₁ on the regional cerebral blood flow in man. Stroke 7:566–569, 1976.

1489. Olesen J: Some clinical features of the acute migraine attack. An analysis of 750 patients. Headache 18:268–271, 1978.

1490. Olesen J: Effect of serotonin on regional cerebral blood flow (rCBF) in man. Cephalalgia 1:7–10, 1981.

1491. Olesen J: Beta-adrenergic effects on cerebral circulation. Cephalalgia 6 (Suppl 5):41–46, 1986.

1492. Olesen J: Pathophysiological implications of migraine aura symptomatology. In Olesen J and Edvinsson L (eds): Basic Mechanisms of Headache. Elsevier, Amsterdam, 1988, pp 353–363.

1493. Olesen J: A review of current drugs for migraine. J Neurol 238:S23–S27, 1991.

1494. Olesen J, Aebelholt A, and Veilis B: The Copenhagen acute headache clinic: Organization, patient material and treatment of results. Headache 19:223–227, 1979.

1495. Olesen J, Friberg L, Skyhøj Olsen T, et al.: Timing and topography of cerebral blood flow, aura, and headache during migraine attacks. Ann Neurol 28:791–798, 1990.

1496. Olesen J, Larsen B, and Lauritzen M: Focal hyperemia followed by spreading oligemia and impaired activation of rCBF in classic migraine. Ann Neurol 9:344–352, 1981.

1497. Olgart L: Excitation of intradental sensory units by pharmacological agents. Acta Physiol Scand 92:48–55, 1974.

1498. Olivecrona H: Notes on the surgical treatment of migraine. Acta Med Scand 196:229–238, 1947.

1499. Oliveras JL, Redjemi F, Guilbaud G, and Besson JM: Analgesia induced by electrical stimulation of the inferior centralis nucleus of the raphe in the cat. Pain 1:139–145, 1975.

1500. Olness K, MacDonald JT, and Uden DL: Comparison of self-hypnosis and propranolol in the treatment of juvenile classic migraine. Pediatrics 79:93–97, 1987.

1501. Olsson JE: Neurotologic findings in basilar migraine. Laryngoscope 101(Suppl 52):1–41, 1991.

1502. Olsson JE, Behring HC, Forssmann B, et al.: Metoprolol and propranolol in migraine prophylaxis: A double-blind multicentre study. Acta Neurol Scand 70:160–168, 1984.

1503. Olszewski J: On the anatomical and functional organization of the spinal trigeminal nucleus. J Comp Neurol 92:401–413, 1950.

1504. O'Neill BP and Mann JD: Aspirin prophylaxis in migraine. Lancet *ii*:1179–1181, 1978.

1505. Onghena P and Van Houdenhove B: Antidepressant-induced analgesia in chronic non-malignant pain: A meta-analysis of 39 placebo-controlled studies. Pain 49:205–219, 1992.

1506. Oral Sumatriptan and Aspirin plus Metoclopramide Comparative Study Group: A study to compare oral sumatriptan with oral aspirin plus metoclopramide in the acute treatment of migraine. Eur Neurol 32:177–184, 1992.

1507. Orlando RC, Moyer P, and Barnett TB: Methysergide therapy and constrictive pericarditis. Ann Intern Med 88:213–214, 1978.

1508. Orne MT: Assessment of biofeedback therapy: Specific versus non-specific effects. In Orne MT, Weiss T, Callaway E, and Stroebel CF (eds): American Psychiatric Association Task Force Report on Biofeedback. American Psychiatric Association, Washington DC, 1980, pp 12–32.

1509. Orton DA and Richardson RJ: Ergotamine absorption and toxicity. Postgrad Med J 58:6–11, 1982.

1510. Osborn RE, Alder DC, and Mitchell CS: MR imaging of the brain in patients with migraine headaches. AJNR 12:521–524, 1991.

1511. Osterman PO, Lövstrand KG, Lundberg PO, Lundquist S, and Muhr C: Weekly headache periodicity and the effect of weather changes on headache. Int J Biometeorol 25:39–45, 1981.

1512. Ostfeld AM, Reis DJ, Goodell H, and Wolff HG: Headache and hydration. The significance of two varieties of fluid accumulation in patients with vascular headache of the migraine type. Arch Intern Med 96:142–152, 1955.

1513. Ostfeld AM and Wolff HG: Identification, mechanisms and management of the migraine syndrome. Med Clin North Am 42:1497–1509, 1958.

1514. O'Sullivan ME: Termination of one thousand attacks of migraine with ergotamine tartrate. JAMA 107:1208–1212, 1936.

1515. Osuntokun BO, Bademosi O, and Osuntokun O: Migraine in Nigeria. In Clifford Rose F (ed): Advances in Migraine Research and Therapy. Raven Press, New York, 1982, pp 25–38.

1516. Owman C, Hanko J, Hardebo JE, and Kahrstrom J: Neuropeptides and classical autonomic transmitters in the cardiovascular system: Existence, coexistence, action, interaction. In Owman C and Hardebo JE (eds): Neural Regulation of Brain Circulation. Elsevier, Amsterdam, 1986, pp 299–331.

1517. Packard RC: What does the headache patient want? Headache 19:370–374, 1979.

1518. Pajewski M, Modai D, Wisgarten J, Freund E, Manor A, and Starinski R: Iatrogenic arterial aneurysm associated with ergotamine therapy. Lancet ii:934–935, 1981.

1519. Pakovits M and Jacobowitz DM: Topographic atlas of catecholamine and acetylcholinesterase-containing neurons in the rat brain. II. Hindbrain (mesencephalon, rhombencephalon). J Comp Neurol 157:29–42, 1974.

1520. Panayiotopoulos CP: Basilar migraine? Seizures and severe epileptic EEG abnormalities. Neurology 30:1122–1125, 1980.

1521. Panayiotopoulos CP: Benign childhood epilepsy with occipital paroxysms: A 15-year prospective study. Ann Neurol 26:51–56, 1989.

1522. Papatheophilou R, Jeavons PM, and Disney ME: Recurrent abdominal pain: A clinical and electroencephalographic study. Develop Med Child Neurol 14:31–44, 1972.

1523. Parain D and Samson-Dollfus D: Electroencephalograms in basilar artery migraine. Electroencephalogr Clin Neurophysiol 58:392–399, 1984.

1524. Parker W: Migraine and the vestibular system in adults. Am J Otology 12:25–34, 1991.

1525. Parrino L, Pietrini V, Spaggiari MC, and Terzano MG: Acute confusional migraine attacks resolved by sleep: Lack of significant abnormalities in post-ictal polysomnograms. Cephalalgia 6:95–100, 1986.

1526. Parsonage M: Electroencephalographic studies in migraine. In Pierce J (ed): Modern Topics in Migraine. Heinemann, London. 1975, pp 72–84.

1527. Parsons AA: 5-HT receptors in human and animal cerebrovasculature. Trends Pharmacol Sci 12:310–315, 1991.

1528. Parsons AA and Whalley ET: Characterization of the 5-hydroxytryptamine receptor which mediates contraction of the human isolated basilar artery. Cephalalgia 9(Suppl 9):47–51, 1989.

1529. Parsons AA, Whalley ET, Feniuk W, Connor HE, and Humphrey PPA: 5-HT$_1$-like receptors mediate 5-hydroxytryptamine-induced contraction of human isolated basilar artery. Br J Pharmacol 96:434–440, 1989.

1530. Pascual J, Polo JM, and Berciano J: The dose of propranolol for migraine prophylaxis. Efficacy of low doses. Cephalalgia 9:287–291, 1989.

1531. Passchier J, Van Der Helm-Hylkema H, and Orlebeke JF: Psychophysiological characteristics of migraine and tension headache patients. Differential effects of sex and pain state. Headache 24:131–139, 1984.

1532. Paterson JH and McKissock W: A clinical survey of intracranial angiomas with special reference to their mode of progression and surgical treatment: A report of 110 cases. Brain 79:233–266, 1956.

1533. Patterson RH, Goodell H, and Dunning HS: Complications of carotid arteriography. Arch Neurol 10:513–520, 1964.

1534. Paulsen GW and Klawans HL: Benign orgasmic cephalgia. Headache 13:181–187, 1974.

1535. Paulson GW, Zipf RE, and Beekman JF: Pheochromocytoma causing exercise-related headache and pulmonary edema. Ann Neurol 5:96–99, 1979.

1536. Pavy-Le Traon A, Cesari JB, Fabre N, Morales MP, Geraud G, and Bes A: Contribution of transcranial Doppler to the study of cerebral circulation in the migraineur. In Clifford Rose F (ed): Advances in Migraine Research. Smith-Gordon, London, 1989, pp 157–161.

1537. Payne TJ, Stetson B, Stevens VM, Johnson CA, Penzien DB, and Van Dorsten B: The impact of cigarette smoking on headache activity in headache patients. Headache 31:329–332, 1991.

1538. Pearce I, Frank GJ, and Pearce JMS: Ibuprofen compared with paracetamol in migraine. Practitioner 227:465–467, 1983.

1539. Pearce J: The ophthalmological complications of migraine. J Neurol Sci 6:73–81, 1968.

1540. Pearce J: Some etiological factors in migraine. In Cummings JN (ed): Background to Migraine. Heinneman, London 1971, pp 1–7.

1541. Pearce J: Insulin induced hypoglycemia in migraine. J Neurol Neurosurg Psychiatry 34:154–156, 1971.

1542. Pearce J: Complicated migraine. In Pearce J (ed): Modern Topics in Migraine. Heinemann, London, 1975, pp 30–44.

1543. Pearce J: Hazards of ergotamine tartrate. Br Med J i:834–835, 1976.

1544. Pearce JM and Foster JB: An investigation of complicated migraine. Neurology 15:333–340, 1965.

1545. Pearce JMS: Whiplash injury: Fact or fiction? Headache Quarterly, Current Treatment and Research 3:45–49, 1992.

1546. Peatfield R and Clifford Rose F: Exacerbation of migraine by treatment with lithium. Headache 21:140–142, 1981.

1547. Peatfield RC, Fozard JR, and Clifford Rose F: Drug treatment of migraine. In Clifford Rose F (ed): Handbook of Clinical Neurology, Vol 4. Elsevier, Amsterdam, 1986, pp 173–216.

1548. Peatfield RC, Gawel MJ, and Clifford Rose F: Asymmetry of the aura and pain in migraine. J Neurol Neurosurg Psychiatry 44:846–848, 1981.

1549. Peatfield RC, Gawel MJ, and Clifford Rose F: The effect of infused prostacyclin in migraine and cluster headache. Headache 21:190–195, 1981.

1550. Peatfield RC, Glover V, Littlewood JT, Sandler M, and Clifford Rose F: The prevalence of diet-induced migraine. Cephalalgia 4:179–183, 1984.

1551. Peatfield RC, Petty RG, and Clifford Rose F: Double blind comparison of mefenamic acid and acetaminophen (paracetamol) in migraine. Cephalalgia 3:129–134, 1983.

1552. Peck DF and Attfield ME: Migraine symptoms on the Waters headache questionnaire: A statistical analysis. J Psychosom Res 25:281–288, 1981.

1553. Pedersen E and Møller CE: Methysergide in migraine prophylaxis. Clin Pharmacol Ther 7:520–526, 1966.

1554. Pelofsky S, Jacobson ED, and Fisher RG: Effects of prostaglandin E_1 on experimental cerebral vasospasm. J Neurosurg 36:634–639, 1972.

1555. Penfield W: Intracerebral vascular nerves. Arch Neurol Psychiatry 27:30–44, 1932.

1556. Penfield W and McNaughton FL: Dural headache and innervation of the dura mater. Arch Neurol Psychiatry 44:43–75, 1940.

1557. Pepin EP: Cerebral metastases presenting as migraine with aura. Lancet 336:127–128, 1990.

1558. Pepin EP: Symptomatic headache of recent onset posing as migraine with aura. Headache Quarterly, Current Treatment and Research 2:23–27, 1991.

1559. Peppercorn MA, Herzog AG, Dichter MA, and Mayman CI: Abdominal epilepsy. JAMA 240:2450–2451, 1978.

1560. Pereira Monteiro JM, Leite Carneiro A, Bastos Lima AF, and Castro Lopes JRC: Migraine and cerebral infarction: Three case studies. Headache 25:429–433, 1985.

1561. Perkin GD: Ischaemic lateral popliteal nerve palsy due to ergot intoxication. J Neurol Neurosurg Psychiatry 37:1389–1391, 1974.

1562. Perl ER: Pain and nociception. In Brookhart JM and Mountcastle VB (eds): Handbook of Physiology, Section 1, The Nervous System, Vol III, Sensory Processes, Part II. American Physiological Society, Bethesda, 1984, pp 915–975.

1563. Pernow J: Co-release and functional interactions of neuropeptide Y and noradrenaline in peripheral sympathetic vascular control. Acta Physiol Scand 133(Suppl 568):1–56, 1988.

1564. Peroutka SJ: The pharmacology of calcium channel antagonists: A novel class of anti-migraine drugs? Headache 23:278–283, 1983.

1565. Peroutka SJ: 5-Hydroxytryptamine receptor subtypes. Annu Rev Neurosci 11:45–60, 1988.

1566. Peroutka SJ: Developments in 5-hydroxytryptamine receptor pharmacology in migraine. Neurol Clin 8:829–837, 1990.

1567. Peroutka SJ and Allen GS: The calcium antagonist properties of cyproheptadine: Implications for antimigraine action. Neurology 34:304–309, 1984.

1568. Peroutka SJ, Banghart SB, and Allen GS: Relative potency and selectivity of calcium antagonists used in the treatment of migraine. Headache 24:55–58, 1984.

1569. Peroutka SJ, Banghart SB, and Allen GS: Calcium channel antagonism by pizotifen. J Neurol Neurosurg Psychiatry 48:381–383, 1985.

1570. Peroutka SJ and McCarthy BG: Sumatriptan (GR 43175) interacts selectively with 5-HT$_{1B}$ and 5-HT$_{1D}$ binding sites. Eur J Pharmacol 163:133–136, 1989.

1571. Peroutka SJ and Snyder SH: Long-term antidepressant treatment decreases spiroperidol-labeled serotonin receptor binding. Science 210:88–90, 1980.

1572. Peroutka SJ and Snyder SH: Antiemetics: Neurotransmitter receptor binding predicts therapeutic action. Lancet *ii*:658–659, 1982.

1573. Perren MJ, Feniuk W, and Humphrey PPA: The selective closure of feline carotid arteriovenous anastomoses (AVAs) by GR43175. Cephalalgia 9 (Suppl 9):41–46, 1989.

1574. Perrin VL: Clinical pharmacokinetics of ergotamine in migraine and cluster headache. Clin Pharmacokinet 10:334–352, 1985.

1575. Perry HT: The symptomatology of temporomandibular joint disturbance. J Prosthet Dentistry 19:288–298, 1968.

1576. Peters BH, Fraim CJ, and Masel BE: Comparison of 650 mg aspirin and 1000 mg acetaminophen with each other, and with placebo in moderately severe headache. Am J Med 76:36–42, 1983.

1577. Peters GA and Horton BT: Headache: With special reference to the excessive use of ergotamine preparations and withdrawal effects. Mayo Clin Proc 26:153–161, 1951.

1578. Peterson DL: Headache. Part IX: Nonsteroidal anti-inflammatory drugs for the treatment of headache. Intern Med Spec 7:69–77, 1986.

1579. Peto R, Gray R, Collins R, Wheatley K, Hennekens C, and Tamrozik K: Randomised trial of prophylactic daily aspirin in British male doctors. Br Med J 296:313–316, 1988.

1580. Pfaffenrath V, Dandekar R, and Pöllmann W: Cervicogenic headache—the clinical picture, radiologic findings and hypotheses on its pathophysiology. Headache 27:495–499, 1987.

1581. Pfaffenrath V, Oestreich W, and Haase W: Flunarazine (10 and 20 mg) i.v. versus placebo in the treatment of acute migraine attacks: A multi-centre double-blind study. Cephalalgia 10:77–81, 1990.

1582. Philips C: Headache in general practice. Headache 16:322–329, 1976.

1583. Philips C: The modification of tension headache pain using EMG biofeedback. Behav Res Ther 15:119–129, 1977.

1584. Philips HC: Avoidance behavior and its role in sustaining chronic pain. Behav Res Ther 25:273–279, 1987.

1585. Philips HC and Hunter M: Pain behavior in headache sufferers. Behav Anal Modif 4:257–266, 1981.

1586. Philips HC and Hunter M: Headache in a psychiatric population. J Nerv Ment Dis 170:34–40, 1982.

1587. Philips HC and Jahanshahi M: The effects of persistent pain: The chronic headache sufferer. Pain 21:163–176, 1985.

1588. Pickard JD, MacDonell LA, MacKenzie ET, and Harper AM: Prostaglandin-induced effects in the primate cerebral circulation. Eur J Pharmacol 43:343–351, 1977.

1589. Pickard JD, Tamura A, Stewart M, McGeorge A, and Firth W: Prostacyclin, indomethacin and the cerebral circulation. Brain Res 197:425–431, 1980.

1590. Pietrini V, Terzano MG, D'Andrea G, Parrino L, Canzani AR, and Ferro-Milino F: Acute confusional migraine: Clinical and electroencephalographic aspects. Cephalalgia 7:29–37, 1987.

1591. Pikoff H: Is the muscular model of headache still viable? A review of conflicting data. Headache 24:186–198, 1984.

1592. Pinard E, Purves MJ, Seylaz J, and Vasquez JV: The cholinergic pathway to cerebral blood vessels. II. Physiological studies. Pfluegers Arch 379:165–172, 1979.

1593. Piotrowski W and Foreman JC: Some effects of calcitonin gene-related peptide in human skin and on histamine release. Br J Derm 114:37–46, 1986.

1594. Piper PJ: Pharmacology of leukotrienes. Br Med Bull 39:255–259, 1983.

1595. Pitt B: Maternity blues. Br J Psychiatry 122:431–433, 1973.

1596. Pletscher A and Affolter H: The 5-hydroxytryptamine receptor of blood platelets. J Neural Transm 57:233–242, 1983.

1597. Poggioni M, Bonazzi A, Del Bene E, and Sicuteri F: Focus on latent nociceptive dysfunction in humans. Adv Pain Res Ther 20:269–280, 1992.

1598. Pointinen PJ and Salmela TM: Acupuncture treatment of migraine. In Sicuteri F (ed): Headache: New Vistas. Biomedical Press, Florence, 1977, pp 251–257.

1599. Polich J, Ehlers CL, and Dalessio DJ: Pattern-shift visual evoked responses and EEG in migraine. Headache 26:451–456, 1986.

1600. Pollack MH, Rosenbaum JF, and Cassem NH: Propranolol and depression revisited, three cases and a review. J Nerv Ment Dis 173:118–119, 1985.

1601. Portenoy RK, Abissi CJ, Lipton RB, et al.: Headache in cerebrovascular disease. Stroke 15:1009–1012, 1984.

1602. Porter J, Hunter J, and Danielson D: Oral contraceptives and nonfatal vascular disease: Recent experience. Obstet Gynecol 59:299–302, 1982.

1603. Porter J, Jick H, and Walker AM: Mortality among oral contraceptive users. Obstet Gynecol 70:29–32, 1987.

1604. Porter M and Jankovic J: Benign coital cephalgia. Differential diagnosis and treatment. Arch Neurol 38:710–712, 1981.

1605. Powers WJ, Grubb RL, and Raichle ME: Physiological responses to focal cerebral ischemia in humans. Ann Neurol 16:546–552, 1984.

1606. Pózniak-Patewicz E: "Cephalgic" spasm of head and neck muscles. Headache 15:261–266, 1976.

1607. Pradalier A, Clapin A, and Dry J: Non-steroidal anti-inflammatory drugs in the treatment and long-term prevention of migraine attacks. Headache 28:550–557, 1988.

1608. Pradalier A and Launay JM: 5-Hydroxytryptamine uptake by platelets from migrainous patients. Lancet i:862, 1982.

1609. Pradalier A, Rancurel G, Dordain G, Verdure L, Rascol A, and Dry J: Acute migraine attack therapy: Comparison of naproxen sodium and an ergotamine tartrate compound. Cephalalgia 5:107–113, 1985.

1610. Pradalier A, Weinman S, Launay JM, Baron JF, and Dry J: Total IgE, specific IgE and prick-tests against foods in common migraine—a prospective study. Cephalalgia 3:231–234, 1983.

1611. Pratt RTC: The Genetics of Neurological Disorders. London University Press, London, 1968.

1612. Prendes JL: Considerations on the use of propranolol in complicated migraine. Headache 20:93–95, 1980.

1613. Prensky AL: Migraine and migrainous variants in pediatric patients. Pediatr Clin North Am 23:461–471, 1976.

1614. Prensky AL: Migraine in children. In Blau JN (ed): Migraine. Clinical and Research Aspects. Johns Hopkins University Press, Baltimore, 1987, pp 31–53.

1615. Prensky AL and Sommer D: Diagnosis and treatment of migraine in children. Neurology 29:506–510, 1979.

1616. Prichard BNC: Pharmacologic aspects of intrinsic sympathomimetic activity in beta-blocking drugs. Am J Cardiol 59:13F–17F, 1987.

1617. Prusinski A and Kozubski W: Use of verapamil in the treatment of migraine. Wiad Lek 1:734–738, 1987.

1618. Pruyn SC, Phelan JP, and Buchanan GC: Long-term propranolol therapy in pregnancy: Maternal and fetal outcome. Am J Obstet Gynecol 135:485–489, 1979.

1619. Puca FM, de Tommaso M, Savarese MA, Genco S, and Prudenzano A: Topographic analysis of steady-state visual evoked potentials (SVEPs) in the medium frequency range in migraine with and without aura. Cephalalgia 12:244–249, 1992.

1620. Quinaux N, Scuvée-Moreau J, and Dresse A: Inhibition of in vitro and ex vivo uptake of noradrenaline and 5-hydroxytryptamine by five antidepressants: Correlation with reduction of spontaneous firing rate of central monoaminergic neurones. Naunyn-Schmiedebergs Arch Pharmacol 319:66–70, 1982.

1621. Rabe EF: Recurrent paroxysmal nonepileptic disorders. Curr Probl Pediatr 4:1–31, 1974.

1622. Rackham A and Ford-Hutchinson AW: Inflammation and pain sensitivity: Effects of leukotrienes D_4, B_4 and prostaglandin E_1 in the rat paw. Prostaglandins 25:193–203, 1983.

1623. Raichle ME, Eichling JO, Grubb RL, and Hartman BK: Central noradrenergic regulation of brain microcirculation. In Pappius HM and Feindel W (eds): Dynamics of Brain Edema. Springer-Verlag, New York, 1976, pp 11–17.

1624. Raichle ME, Hartman BK, Eichling JO, and Sharpe LG: Central noradrenergic regulation of cerebral blood flow and vascular permeability. Proc Natl Acad Sci USA 72:3726–3730, 1975.

1625. Raja SN, Meyer A, and Campbell JN: Peripheral mechanisms of somatic pain. Anesthesiology 68:571–590, 1988.

1626. Rall TW: Oxytocin, prostaglandins, ergot alkaloids and other drugs; tocolytic agents. In Gilman AG, Rall TW, Nies AS, and Taylor P (eds): The Pharmacological Basis of Therapeutics. Pergamon, New York, 1990, pp 933–953.

1627. Rando TA and Fishman RA: Spontaneous intracranial hypotension. Neurology 42:481–487, 1992.

1628. Ranson R, Igarashi H, MacGregor EA, and Wilkinson M: The similarities and differences of migraine with aura and migraine without aura: A preliminary study. Cephalalgia 11:189–192, 1991.

1629. Rao NS and Pearce J: Hypothalamic-pituitary-adrenal axis studies in migraine with special reference to insulin sensitivity. Brain 94:289–298, 1971.

1630. Rapoport AM: Analgesic rebound headache. Headache 28:662–665, 1988.

1631. Rapoport AM and Sheftell FD: Headaches. Runner's World 15:41–43, 1980.

1632. Rapoport AM, Weeks RE, Sheftell FD, Baskin SM, and Verdi J: Analgesic rebound headache: Theoretical and practical implications. Cephalalgia 5(Suppl 3):448–449, 1985.

1633. Rascol A, Cambier J, Guiraud B, Manelfe C, David J, and Clanet M: Accidents ischèmiques cèrèbraux au cours de crises migraineuses: a propos des migraines compliquèes. Rev Neurol (Paris) 135:867–884, 1979.

1634. Rascol A, Montastruc JL, and Rascol O: Flunarizine versus pizotifen: A double-blind study in the prophylaxis of migraine. Headache 26:83–85, 1986.

1635. Raskin NH: Repetitive intravenous dihydroergotamine as therapy for intractable migraine. Neurology 36:995–997, 1986.

1636. Raskin NH: Headache, 2nd ed. Churchill Livingstone, New York, 1988.

1637. Raskin NH: Treatment of status migrainosus: The American experience. Headache 30(Suppl 2):550–553, 1990.

1638. Raskin NH, Hosobuchi Y, and Lamb S: Headache may arise from perturbation of brain. Headache 27:416–420, 1987.

1639. Raskin NH and Knittle SC: Ice cream headache and orthostatic symptoms in patients with migraine. Headache 16:222–225, 1976.

1640. Raskin NH and Prusiner S: Carotidynia. Neurology 27:43–46, 1977.

1641. Raskin NH and Schwartz RK: Ice pick-like pain. Neurology 30:203–205, 1980.

1642. Raskin NH and Schwartz RK: Interval therapy of migraine: Long-term results. Headache 20:336–340, 1980.

1643. Rasmussen BK, Jensen R, and Olesen J: Questionnaire versus clinical interview in the diagnosis of headache. Headache 31:290–295, 1991.

1644. Rasmussen BK, Jensen R, Schroll M, and Olesen J: Epidemiology of headache in a general population—a prevalence study. J Clin Epidemiol 44:1147–1157, 1991.

1645. Rasmussen BK, Jensen R, Schroll M, and Olesen J: Interrelations between migraine and tension-type headache in the general population. Arch Neurol 49:914–918, 1992.

1646. Rasmussen BK and Olesen J: Migraine with aura and migraine without aura: An epidemiological study. Cephalalgia 12:221–228, 1992.

1647. Ray BS and Wolff HG: Experimental studies on headache: Pain sensitive structures of the head and their significance in headache. Arch Surg 41:813–856, 1940.

1648. Reddy RSV, Maderrut JL, and Yaksh TL: Spinal cord pharmacology of adrenergic agonist-mediated antinociception. J Pharmacol Exp Ther 213:525–533, 1980.

1649. Redfield MM, Nicholson WJ, Edwards WD, and Tajik AJ: Valve disease associated with ergot alkaloid use: Echocardiographic and pathologic correlations. Ann Intern Med 117:50–52, 1992.

1650. Redmond GP: Propranolol and fetal growth retardation. Semin Perinatol 6:142–147, 1982.

1651. Refsum S: Genetic aspects of migraine. In Baker AB (ed): Clinical Neurology, Vol 4, 2nd ed. Hoeber, New York, 1962, pp 2272–2316.

1652. Regan JF and Poletti BJ: Vascular adventitial fibrosis in a patient taking methysergide maleate. JAMA 203:1069–1071, 1968.

1653. Regoli D: Neurohumoral regulation of precapillary vessels: The kallikrein-kinin system. J Cardiovasc Pharmacol 6 (Suppl 2):S401–S412, 1984.

1654. Regoli D and Barabé J: Pharmacology of bradykinin and related kinins. Pharmacol Rev 32:1–46, 1980.

1655. Regoli D, Barabé J, and Park WK: Receptors for bradykinin in rabbit aortae. Can J Physiol Pharmacol 55:855–867, 1977.

1656. Reich B: Non-invasive treatment of vascular and muscle contraction headache: A comparative longitudinal clinical study. Headache 29:34–41, 1989.

1657. Reichling DB, Kwait GC, and Basbaum AI: Anatomy, physiology and pharmacology of the periaqueductal gray—contribution to antinocicep-

tive control. Prog Brain Res 77:31–46, 1988.

1658. Reid RL and Yen SS: Premenstrual syndrome. Am J Obstet Gynecol 139:85–104, 1981.

1659. Reif-Lehrer L: A questionnaire study of the prevalence of Chinese restaurant syndrome. Fed Proc 36:1617–1623, 1977.

1660. Reik L: Cluster headache after head injury. Headache 27:509–510, 1987.

1661. Reik L and Hale M: The temporomandibular joint pain–dysfunction syndrome: A frequent cause of headache. Headache 21:151–156, 1981.

1662. Reinhard JF, Liebmann JE, Schlosberg AJ, and Moskowitz MA: Serotonin neurons project to small blood vessels in the brain. Science 206:85–87, 1979.

1663. Reinhart JB, Evans SL, and McFadden DL: Cyclic vomiting in children: Seen through the psychiatrist's eye. Pediatrics 59:371–377, 1977.

1664. Reis DJ: Central nervous control of cerebral circulation and metabolism. In Mackenzie ET, Seylaz J, and Bes A (eds): Neurotransmitters and the Cerebral Circulation. Raven, New York, 1984, pp 91–119.

1665. Ricardo JA and Koh ET: Anatomical evidence of direct projections from the nucleus of the solitary tract to the hypothalamus, amygdala, and other forebrain structures in the rat. Brain Res 153:1–26, 1978.

1666. Rice SL, Eitenmiller BR, and Kohler PE: Biologically active amines in foods: A review. Journal of Milk and Food Technology 39:353, 1976.

1667. Richards W: The fortification illusions of migraines. Sci Am 224:88–96, 1971.

1668. Richardson DE: Analgesia produced by stimulation in various sites in the human beta-endorphin system. Appl Neurophysiol 45:116–122, 1982.

1669. Richelson E and Pfennig M: Blockade by antidepressants and related compounds of biogenic amine uptake into rat brain synaptosomes:

Most antidepressants selectively block norepinephrine uptake. Eur J Pharmacol 104:277–286, 1984.

1670. Richey ET, Kooi KA, and Waggoner RW: Visually evoked responses in migraine. Electroencephalogr Clin Neurophysiol 21:23–27, 1966.

1671. Richter AM and Banker VP: Carotid ergotism: A complication of migraine therapy. Radiology 106:339–340, 1973.

1672. Rickles WH, Onoda L, and Doyle CC: Task-force study section report: Biofeedback as an adjunct to psychotherapy. Biofeedback Self Regul 7:1–33, 1982.

1673. Riopelle R and McCans JL: A pilot study of the calcium antagonist diltiazem in migraine syndrome prophylaxis. Can J Neurol Sci 9:269, 1982.

1674. Robbins L: Migraine and anticardiolipin antibodies—case reports of 13 patients, and the prevalence of antiphospholipid antibodies in migraineurs. Headache 31:537–539, 1991.

1675. Robbins LD: Cryotherapy for headache. Headache 29:598–600, 1989.

1676. Robert M, Derbaudrenghien JP, Blampain JP, Lamy F, and Meyer P: Fibrotic processes associated with long-term ergotamine therapy. N Engl J Med 311:601–602, 1984.

1677. Roberts DJ: The pharmacological basis of the therapeutic activity of clebopride and related substituted benzamides. Curr Ther Res 31:S1–S44, 1982.

1678. Robertson WM, Welch KMA, Levine SR, and Schultz LR: The effects of aging on cerebral blood flow in migraine. Neurology 39:947–951, 1989.

1679. Robinson DS, Campbell IC, Walker M, Statham NJ, Lovenberg W, and Murphy DL: Effects of chronic monoamine oxidase inhibitor treatment on biogenic amine metabolism in rat brain. Neuropharmacology 18:771–776, 1979.

1680. Rolak LA: Headaches and multiple sclerosis. Headache Quarterly, Current Treatment and Research 3:39–44, 1992.

1681. Roldán-Montaud A, Jiménez-Jiménez FJ, Zancada F, Molina-Arjona JA, Fernández-Ballesteros A and Gutiérrez-Vivas A: Neurobrucellosis mimicking migraine. Eur Neurol 31:30–32, 1991.

1682. Rolf LH, Schlake HP, and Brune GG: Plasma factors and migraine. In Soyka D (ed): Migraine: Pathogenese-Pharmakologie-Therapie. Enke, Stuttgart, 1982, pp 79–97.

1683. Rompel H and Bauermeister P: Aetiology of migraine and prevention with carbamazepine (Tegretol). S African Med J 44:75–80, 1970.

1684. Román GC: Senile dementia of the Binswanger type. A vascular form of dementia in the elderly. JAMA 258:1782–1788, 1987.

1685. Roquebert J and Grenié B: α_2-Adrenergic agonist and α_1-adrenergic antagonist activity of ergotamine and dihydroergotamine in rats. Arch Int Pharmacodyn 284:30–37, 1986.

1686. Rosa R, Bellini V, Filippi MC, Taddei MT, Vitali T, and Conigliaro S: Hemodynamic studies by transcranial Doppler in primary headache. Cephalalgia 7 (Suppl 6):280–281, 1987.

1687. Roseman DM: Carotidynia. In Vinken PJ and Bruyn GW (eds): Handbook of Clinical Neurology, Vol 5. North-Holland, Amsterdam, 1968, pp 375–377.

1688. Rosen JA: Observations on the efficacy of propranolol for the prophylaxis of migraine. Ann Neurol 13:92–93, 1983.

1689. Rosen RC and Kostis JB: Biobehavioral sequelae associated with adrenergic-inhibiting antihypertensive agents: A critical review. Health Psychol 4:579–604, 1985.

1690. Rosen SM, O'Donnor K, and Shaldon S: Haemodialysis disequilibrium. Br Med J ii:672–675, 1964.

1691. Rosenbaum HE: Familial hemiplegic migraine. Neurology 10:164–170, 1960.

1692. Rosenberg CM: Drug maintenance in the outpatient treatment of chronic alcoholism. Arch Gen Psychiatry 30:373–377, 1974.

1693. Rosenblum WI: Constricting effect of leukotrienes on cerebral arterioles of mice. Stroke 16:262–263, 1985.

1694. Rosenblum WI: Endothelial dependent relaxation demonstrated *in vivo* in cerebral arterioles. Stroke 17:494–497, 1986.

1695. Rosenthaler J and Munzer H: 9-10-Dihydroergotamine production of antibodies and radioimmunoassay. Experientia 32:234–236, 1976.

1696. Rossi LN, Mumenthaler M, and Vassella F: Complicated migraine (migraine accompagnée) in children. Clinical characteristics and course in 40 personal cases. Neuropediatrics 11:27–35, 1980.

1697. Rossi LN, Vassella F, Bajc O, Tönz O, Lütschg J, and Mumenthaler M: Benign migraine-like syndrome with CSF pleocytosis in children. Develop Med Child Neurol 27:192–198, 1985.

1698. Ross-Lee L, Heazlewood V, Tyrer JH, and Eadie MS: Aspirin treatment of migraine attacks: Plasma drug level data. Cephalalgia 2:9–14, 1982.

1699. Rothrock JF, Walicke P, Swenson MR, Lyden PD, and Logan W: Migrainous stroke. Arch Neurol 45:63–67, 1988.

1700. Rotton WN, Sachtleben MR, and Friedman EA: Migraine and eclampsia. Obstet Gynecol 14:322–330, 1959.

1701. Round R and Keane JR: The minor symptoms of increased intracranial pressure: 101 patients with benign intracranial hypertension. Neurology 38:1461–1464, 1988.

1702. Rowbotham GR: Pain pathways in migraine. Br Med J ii:685–687, 1942.

1703. Rowbotham GR and Little E: New concepts on the aetiology and vascularization of meningiomata; the mechanism of migraine; the chemical processes of the cerebrospinal fluid; blood or fluid in the subdural space. Br J Surg 52:21–24, 1965.

1704. Rowland LP: Molecular genetics, pseudogenetics, and clinical neurology. Neurology 33:1179–1195, 1983.

1705. Rowsell AR, Neylan C, and Wilkinson M: Ergotamine induced headaches in migrainous patients. Headache 13:65–67, 1973.

1706. Rubin LS, Graham D, Pasker R, and Calhoun W: Autonomic nervous system dysfunction in common migraine. Headache 25:40–48, 1985.

1707. Rubin PC: Beta-blockers in pregnancy. N Engl J Med 305:1323–1326, 1981.

1708. Ruch TC: Visceral sensation and referred pain. In Fulton JF (ed): Howell's Textbook of Physiology, 15th ed. Saunders, Philadelphia, 1946, pp 385–401.

1709. Ruda MA, Coffield J, and Dubner R: Demonstration of postsynaptic opioid modulation of thalamic projection neurons by the combined techniques of retrograde horseradish peroxidase and enkephalin immunocytochemistry. J Neurosci 4: 2117–2132, 1984.

1710. Rudorfer MV and Young RC: Desipramine: Cardiovascular effects and plasma levels. Am J Psychiatry 137:984–986, 1980.

1711. Ruiz JS, du Boulay GH, Zilkha KJ, and Clifford Rose F: The abnormal CT scan in migraine patients. In Clifford Rose F and Amery WK (eds): Cerebral Hypoxia in the Pathogenesis of Migraine. Pitman, London, 1982 pp 105–109.

1712. Rushton JG and Rooke ED: Brain tumor headache. Headache 2:147–152, 1962.

1713. Ruskell GL: The tentorial nerve in monkeys is a branch of the cavernous plexus. J Anat 157:67–77, 1988.

1714. Ruskell GL and Simons T: Trigeminal nerve pathways to the cerebral arteries in monkeys. J Anat 155:23–37, 1987.

1715. Russell D: Cluster headache: Severity and temporal profile of attacks and patient activity prior to and during attacks. Cephalalgia 1:209–219, 1981.

1716. Russell D, Dahl A, Nyberg-Hansen R, and Rostwelt K: Reproducibility of simultaneous TCD and rCBF measurements. Cephalalgia 11(Suppl 11):46–47, 1991.

1717. Russell MB, Rasmussen BK, Breenum J, Iversen HK, Jensen RA, and Olesen J: Presentation of a new instrument: The diagnostic headache diary. Cephalalgia 12:369–374, 1992.

1718. Ryan RE: BC-105, a new preparation for the interval treatment of migraine—a double blind evaluation compared with a placebo. Headache 11:6–18, 1971.

1719. Ryan RE: A study of Midrin in the symptomatic relief of migraine headache. Headache 14:33–42, 1974.

1720. Ryan RE: A clinical study of tyramine as an etiology factor in migraine. Headache 14:43–48, 1974.

1721. Ryan RE: A controlled study of the effect of oral contraceptives on migraine. Headache 17:250–252, 1978.

1722. Ryan RE: Comparative study of nadolol and propranolol in prophylactic treatment of migraine. Am Heart J 108:1156–1159, 1984.

1723. Ryan RE, Diamond S, and Ryan RE: Double-blind study of clonidine and placebo for prophylactic treatment of migraine. Headache 15:202–210, 1975.

1724. Ryan RE, Ryan RE, and Sudilovsky A: Nadolol: Its use in the prophylactic treatment of migraine. Headache 23:26–31, 1983.

1725. Rydzewski W: Serotonin (5HT) in migraine: Levels in whole blood in and between attacks. Headache 16:16–19, 1976.

1726. Saadah HA: Abortive headache therapy in the office with intravenous dihydroergotamine plus prochlorperazine. Headache 32:143–146, 1992.

1727. Sabatini U, Rascol O, Rascol A, and Montastruc JL: Migraine attacks induced by subcutaneous apomorphine in two migrainous parkinsonian patients. Clin Neuropharmacol 13:264–267, 1990.

1728. Sachs H, Wolf A, Russell JAG, and Christman DR: Effect of reserpine on regional cerebral glucose metabolism in control and migraine subjects. Arch Neurol 43:1117–1123, 1986.

1729. Sacks O: Migraine. Understanding a Common Disorder. University of California Press, Berkeley, 1985.

1730. Sacquegna T, Andreoli A, Baldrati A, et al.: Ischemic stroke in young adults: The relevance of migrainous infarction. Cephalalgia 9:255–258, 1989.

1731. Safran AB, Kline LB, and Glaser JS: Positive visual phenomena in optic nerve and chiasm disease: Photopsias and photophobia. In Glaser JS (ed): Neuro-ophthalmology, Vol 10. Mosby, St. Louis, 1980, pp 225–231.

1732. Saito A, Shiba R, Yanagisawa M, et al.: Endothelins: Vasoconstrictor effects and localization in canine cerebral arteries. Br J Pharmacol 103:1129–1135, 1991.

1733. Saito K, Liu-Chen LY, and Moskowitz MA: Substance P-like immunoreactivity in rat forebrain leptomeninges and cerebral vessels originates from the trigeminal but not sympathetic ganglia. Brain Res 403:66–71, 1987.

1734. Saito K, Markowitz S, and Moskowitz MA: Ergot alkaloids block neurogenic extravasation in dura mater: Proposed action in vascular headaches. Ann Neurol 24:732–737, 1988.

1735. Saito K and Moskowitz MA: Contributions from the upper cervical dorsal roots and trigeminal ganglia to the feline circle of Willis. Stroke 20:524–526, 1989.

1736. Sakai F and Meyer JS: Regional cerebral hemodynamics during migraine and cluster headaches measured by the ^{133}Xe inhalation method. Headache 18:122–132, 1978.

1737. Sakai F and Meyer JS: Abnormal cerebrovascular reactivity in patients with migraine and cluster headache. Headache 19:257–266, 1979.

1738. Sakas DE, Moskowitz MA, Wei EP, Kontos HA, Kano M, and Oglivy CS: Trigeminovascular fibers increase blood flow in cortical gray matter by axon reflex-like mechanisms during acute severe hypertension or sei-zures. Proc Natl Acad Sci USA 86:1401–1405, 1989.

1739. Salmon MA: Diagnosis of abdominal migraine in children. In Wilson J (ed): Migraine in Childhood. Medi-cine Publishing Foundation, Oxford, 1983, pp 1–2.

1740. Salter M, Brooke RI, Merskey H, Fi-chter GF, and Kapusianyk DH: Is the temporo-mandibular pain and dys-function syndrome a disorder of the mind? Pain 17:151–166, 1983.

1741. Samuelsson B: Leukotrienes: Medi-ators of immediate hypersensitivity reactions and inflammation. Science 220:568–575, 1983.

1742. Samuelsson B, Dahlén SE, Lindgren JA, Rouzer CA, and Serhan CN: Leu-kotrienes and lipoxins: Structures, biosynthesis, and biological effects. Science 237:1171–1176, 1987.

1743. Samuelsson B, Goldyne M, Gran-ström E, Hamberg M, Hammarström S, and Malmsten C: Prostaglandins and thromboxanes. Annu Rev Bio-chem 47:997–1029, 1978.

1744. Sances G, Martignoni E, Fioroni L, Blandini F, Facchinetti F, and Nappi G: Naproxen sodium in menstrual migraine prophylaxis: A double-blind placebo controlled study. Headache 30:705–709, 1990.

1745. Sand T: EEG in migraine: A review of the literature. Funct Neurol 6:7–22, 1991.

1746. Sanders SW, Haering N, Mosberg H, and Jaeger H: Pharmacokinetics of ergotamine in healthy volunteers following oral and rectal dosing. Eur J Clin Pharmacol 30:331–334, 1986.

1747. Sandler M: Migraine: A pulmonary disease? Lancet *i*:618–619, 1972.

1748. Sandler M: Transitory platelet monoamine oxidase deficit in mi-graine: Some reflections. Headache 17:153–158, 1977.

1750. Sandler M, Youdim MBH, and Han-ington E: A phenylethylamine oxi-dising effect in migraine. Nature 250:335–337, 1974.

1751. Santoro G, Gernasconi F, Sessa F, and Venco A: Premonitory symp-

toms in migraine without aura: A clinical investigation. Funct Neurol 5:339–344, 1990.

1752. Santoro G, Curzio M, and Venco A: Abdominal migraine in adults: Case reports. Funct Neurol 5:61–64, 1990.

1753. Saper JR: The mixed headache syn-drome: A new perspective. Headache 22:284–286, 1982.

1754. Saper JR: Treating the headache pa-tient in the emergency room. In Saper JR: Headache Disorders. Cur-rent Concepts and Treatment Strat-egies. John Wright, Boston, 1983, pp 279–286.

1755. Saper JR: Treatment of migraine. In Saper JR: Headache Disorders. Cur-rent Concepts and Treatment Strat-egies. John Wright, Boston, 1983, pp 61–87.

1756. Saper JR: Ergotamine depen-dency—review. Headache 27:435–438, 1987.

1757. Saper JR: Daily chronic headache. Neurol Clin 8:891–901, 1990.

1758. Saper JR and Jones JM: Ergotamine tartrate dependency: Features and possible mechanism. Clin Neuro-pharmacol 9:244–256, 1986.

1759. Saper JR and Van Meter MJ: Ergot-amine headache—an analysis and profile. Headache 20:159, 1980.

1760. Sargent JD, Baumel B, Peters K, et al.: Aborting a migraine attack: Na-proxen sodium v. ergotamine plus caffeine. Headache 28:263–266, 1988.

1761. Sargent JD, Lawson RC, Solbach P, and Coyne L: Use of CT scans in an outpatient headache population: An evaluation. Headache 19:388–390, 1979.

1762. Sargent JD and Solbach P: Medical evaluation of migraineurs: Review of the value of laboratory and radi-ologic tests. Headache 23:62–65, 1983.

1763. Sargent JD, Solbach P, Damasio H, et al.: A comparison of naproxen so-dium to propranolol hydrochloride and a placebo control for the prophy-laxis of migraine headache. Head-ache 25:320–324, 1985.

1764. Satel SL and Gawin FH: Migrainelike headache and cocaine use. JAMA 261:2995–2996, 1989.

1765. Savoldi F, Tartara A, Manni R, and Maurelli M: Headache epilepsy: Two autonomous entities? Cephalalgia 4:39–44, 1984.

1766. Sawchenko PE and Swanson LW: Central noradrenergic pathways for the integration of hypothalamic neuroendocrine and autonomic responses. Science 214:685–687, 1981.

1767. Saxena PR: Selective vasoconstriction in carotid vascular bed by methysergide: Possible relevance to its antimigraine effect. Eur J Pharmacol 27:99–105, 1974.

1768. Scatton B, Duverger D, L'Heureux R, et al.: Neurochemical studies on the existence, origin and characteristics of the serotonergic innervation of small pial vessels. Brain Res 345:219–229, 1985.

1769. Scheinberg P and Jayne HW: Factors influencing cerebral blood flow and metabolism. Circulation 5:225–236, 1952.

1770. Scherf D and Schlachman M: Electrocardiographic and clinical studies on the action of ergotamine tartrate and dihydroergotamine 45. Am J Med Sci 216:673–679, 1948.

1771. Schiffman SS, Buckley CE, Sampson HA, et al.: Aspartame and susceptibility to headache. N Engl J Med 317:1181–1185, 1987.

1772. Schipper HM: Neurology of sex steroids and oral contraceptives. Neurol Clin 4:721–751, 1986.

1773. Schlake HP, Böttger IG, Grotemeyer KH, et al.: Single photon emission computed tomography with technetium-99m hexamethyl propylenamino oxime in the pain-free interval of migraine and cluster headache. Eur Neurol 30:153–156, 1990.

1774. Schlake HP, Böttger IG, Grotemeyer KH, Husstedt IW, and Schober O: Brain imaging with ^{99m}HMPAO and SPECT in migraine with aura: An interictal study. In Olesen J (ed): Migraine and Other Headaches. The

1775. Schlake HP, Grotemeyer KH, Böttger I, Husstedt IW, and Brune G: ^{123}I-amphetamine-SPECT in classical migraine and migraine accompagnée. Neurosurg Rev 10:191–196, 1987.

1776. Schlake HP, Grotemeyer KH, Husstedt IW, Schuierer G, and Brune GG: "Symptomatic migraine:" Intracranial lesions mimicking migrainous headache—a report of three cases. Headache 31:661–665, 1991.

1777. Schlesinger EB: Role of the cervical spine in headache. In Friedman AP and Merritt HH (eds): Headache: Diagnosis and Treatment. Davis, Philadelphia, 1959, pp 35–65.

1778. Schmidt AW and Peroutka SJ: 5-Hydroxytryptamine receptor "families." FASEB J 3:2242–2249, 1989.

1779. Schmidt R and Fanchamps A: Effect of caffeine on intestinal absorption of ergotamine in man. Eur J Clin Pharmacol 7:213–216, 1974.

1780. Schnarch DM and Hunter JE: Migraine incidence in clinical vs nonclinical populations. Psychosomatics 21:314–325, 1980.

1781. Schoeffter P and Hoyer D: How selective is GR 43175? Interactions with functional $5-HT_{1A}$, $5-HT_{1B}$, $5-HT_{1C}$ and $5-HT_{1D}$ receptors. Naunyn-Schmiedebergs Arch Pharmacol 340:135–138, 1989.

1782. Schoenen J, Jamart B, and Delwaide PJ: Electroencephalographic mapping in migraine during the critical and intercritical period. Rev Electroencephalogr Neurophysiol Clin 17:289–299, 1987.

1783. Schoenen J, Lenarduzzi P, and Sianard-Gainko J: Chronic headaches associated with analgesics and/or ergotamine abuse: A clinical survey of 434 consecutive out-patients. In Clifford Rose F (ed): New Advances in Headache Research. Smith-Gordon, London, 1989, pp 255–259.

1784. Schoenen J and Maertens de Noordhout A: The role of the sympathetic nervous system in migraine and cluster headache. In Olesen J and Edvinsson L (eds): Basic Mecha-

Vascular Mechanisms. Raven, New York, 1991, pp 61–64.

nisms of Headache. Elsevier, Amsterdam, 1988 pp 393–410.

1785. Schoenen J and Timsit-Berthier M: Contingent negative variation: Methods and potential interest in headache. Cephalalgia 13:28–32, 1993.

1786. Scholz E, Diener HC, and Geiselhart S: Does a critical dosage exist in drug-induced headache? In Diener HC and Wilkinson M (eds): Drug-Induced Headache. Springer-Verlag, Berlin, 1988, pp 29–43.

1787. Scholz E, Gerber WD, Bille A, Niederberger U, and Fahrner I: Plasma levels of metoprolol and propranolol in responders and non-responders to prophylactic treatment of migraine. Cephalalgia 7(Suppl 6):412–413, 1987.

1788. Schon F and Blau JN: Post-epileptic headache and migraine. J Neurol Neurosurg Psychiatry 50:1148–1152, 1987.

1789. Schon F and Harrison MJH: Can migraine cause multiple segmental cerebral artery constrictions? J Neurol Neurosurg Psychiatry 50:492–494, 1987.

1790. Schottstaedt WW and Wolff HG: Studies on headache: Variations in fluid and electrolyte excretion in association with vascular headache of the migraine type. Arch Neurol Psychiatry 73:158–164, 1955.

1791. Schraeder PL and Burns RA: Hemiplegic migraine associated with an aseptic meningeal reaction. Arch Neurol 37:377–379, 1980.

1792. Schuchman H and Thetford WN: A comparison of personality traits in ulcerative colitis and migraine patients. J Abnorm Psychol 76:443–452, 1970.

1793. Schuckit M, Robins E, and Feighner J: Tricyclic antidepressants and monoamine oxidase inhibitors. Arch Gen Psychiatry 24:509–514, 1971.

1794. Schulman EA and Rosenberg SB: Claudication: An unusual side effect of DHE administration. Headache 31:237–239, 1991.

1795. Schulman EA and Silberstein SD: Symptomatic and prophylactic treatment of migraine and tension-type headache. Neurology 42(Suppl 2):16–21, 1992.

1796. Schultz J and Luthe W: Autogenic Therapy: Medical Applications. Grune & Stratton, New York, 1969.

1797. Schumacher GA and Wolff HG: Experimental studies on headache. Arch Neurol Psychiatry 45:199–214, 1941.

1798. Schweitzer JW, Friedhoff AJ, and Schwartz R: Chocolate, β-phenylethylamine and migraine reexamined. Nature 257:256, 1975.

1799. Scopp AL: MSG and hydrolyzed vegetable protein induced headache: Review and case studies. Headache 31:107–110, 1991.

1800. Scott AK: Dihydroergotamine: A review of its use in the treatment of migraine and other headaches. Clin Neuropharmacol 15:289–296, 1992.

1801. Scott AK, Grimes S, Ng K, et al.: Sumatriptan and cerebral perfusion in healthy volunteers. Br J Clin Pharmacol 33:401–404, 1992.

1802. Scremin OU, Sonnenschein RR, and Rubinstein EH: Cholinergic cerebral vasodilatation: Lack of involvement of cranial parasympathetic nerves. J Cereb Blood Flow Metab 3:362–368, 1983.

1803. Scrutton MC and Thompson NT: Agonists and receptors: Serotonin. In Homson H (ed): Platelet Responses and Metabolism, Vol 2: Receptors and Metabolism. CRC, Boca Raton, 1987, pp 58–68.

1804. Sedman G: Trial of a sustained release form of amitriptyline (Lentizol) in the treatment of depressive illness. Br J Psychiatry 123:69–71, 1973.

1805. Selby G: Migraine and Its Variants. ADIS, Sydney, 1983.

1806. Selby G and Lance JW: Observations on 500 cases of migraine and allied vascular headache. J Neurol Neurosurg Psychiatry 23:23–32, 1960.

1807. Selman WR and Ratcheson RA: Arteriovenous malformations. In Bradley WG, Daroff RB, Fenichel GM, and Marsden CD (eds): Neurology in Clinical Practice, Vol II. Butterworth-Heinemann, Boston, 1989, pp 970–978.

1808. Sens NP: Analysis and significance of tyramine in foods. J Food Sci 34:22–26, 1969.

1809. Senter HJ, Lieberman AN, and Pinto R: Cerebral manifestations of ergotism. Report of a case and review of the literature. Stroke 7:88–92, 1976.

1810. Septien L and Giroud M: Centro-temporal epilepsy and migraine. A long-term controlled study. Headache Quarterly. Current Treatment and Research 2:297–299, 1991.

1811. Serafin WE and Austin KF: Mediators of immediate hypersensitivity reactions. New Engl J Med 317:30–34, 1987.

1812. Serdaru M, Chiras J, Cujas M, and Lhermitte F: Isolated benign cerebral vasculitis or migrainous vasospasm? J Neurol Neurosurg Psychiatry 47:73–76, 1984.

1813. Sethna ER: A study of refractory cases of depressive illnesses and their response to combined antidepressant treatment. Br J Psychiatry 124:265–272, 1974.

1814. Seylaz J, Pinard E, and Mraovitch S: Influence of specific intracerebral structures on the regulation of cerebral circulation. In Owman C and Hardebo JE (eds): Neural Regulation of Brain Circulation. Elsevier, Amsterdam, 1986, pp 147–167.

1815. Shapiro HM, Stromberg DD, Lee DR, and Wiederhielm CA: Dynamic pressures in the pial arterial microcirculation. Am J Physiol 221:279–283, 1971.

1816. Sharav Y, Tzukert A, and Refaeli B: Muscle pain index in relation to pain dysfunction and dizziness associated with myofascial pain–dysfunction syndrome. Oral Surgery 46:742–747, 1978.

1817. Sharbrough FW, Messick JM, and Sundt TM: Correlation of continuous electroencephalograms with cerebral blood flow measurements during carotid endarterectomy. Stroke 4:674–683, 1973.

1818. Shaw RW: Adverse long-term effects of oral contraceptives: A review. Br J Obstet Gynaecol 94:724–730, 1987.

1819. Sheard HM, Zolovick A, and Aghajanian GK: Raphe neurons: Effect of tricyclic antidepressant drugs. Brain Res 43:690–694, 1972.

1820. Sheftell FD: Chronic daily headache. Neurology 42(Suppl 2):32–36, 1992.

1821. Shigenaga Y, Chen IC, Suemune S, et al.: Oral and facial representation within the medullary and upper cervical dorsal horns in the cat. J Comp Neurol 243:388–408, 1986.

1822. Shimell CJ, Fritz VU, and Levien SL: A comparative trial of flunarizine and propranolol in the prevention of migraine. S African Med J 77:75–77, 1990.

1823. Short EM, Conn HO, Snodgrass PJ, Campbell AG, and Rosenberg LE: Evidence for X-linked dominant inheritance of ornithine transcarbamylase deficiency. N Engl J Med 299:7–12, 1973.

1824. Shuaib A: Stroke from other etiologies masquerading as migraine stroke. Stroke 22:1068–1074, 1991.

1825. Shuaib A, Barklay L, Lee MA, and Sucherowsky O: Migraine and antiphospholipid antibodies. Headache 29:42–45, 1989.

1826. Shuaib A and Hachinski VC: Migraine and the risks from angiography. Arch Neurol 45:911–912, 1988.

1827. Sicuteri F: Mast cells and their active substances: Their role in pathogenesis of migraine. Headache 3:86–92, 1963.

1828. Sicuteri F: Vasoneuroactive substances and their implication in vascular pain. Res Clin Stud Headache 1:19–33, 1973.

1829. Sicuteri F: Opioid receptor impairment—underlying mechanism in "pain disease"? Cephalalgia 1:77–82, 1981.

1830. Sicuteri F, Anselmi B, and Fanciullacci M: The serotonin theory of migraine. Adv Neurol 4:383–394, 1974.

1831. Sicuteri F, Buffoni F, Anselmi B, and del Bianco PL: An enzyme (MAO) defect on the platelets in migraine. Res Clin Stud Headache 3:245–251, 1972.

1832. Sicuteri F, Del Bene E, and Anselmi B: Fenfluramine headache. Headache 16:185–188, 1976.

1833. Sicuteri F, Franchi G, and Del Bianchi PL: An antaminic drug, BC 105, in the prophylaxis of migraine. Pharmacological, clinical, and therapeutic experiences. Int Arch Allerg 31:78–93, 1967.

1834. Sicuteri F, Franiciullacci M, and Del Bene E: Dopamine system and idiopathic headache. In Sicuteri F (ed): Headache New Vistas. Biomedical, Florence, 1977, pp 239–250.

1835. Sicuteri F, Franiciullacci M, Granchi G, and Del Bianco PL: Serotonin-bradykinin potentiation on the pain receptors in man. Life Sci 4:309–316, 1965.

1836. Sicuteri F, Testi A, and Anselmi B: Biochemical investigations in headache: Increases in hydroxyindoleacetic acid excretion during migraine attacks. Int Arch Allergy Appl Immun 19:55–58, 1961.

1837. Siegel AM, Smith JB, Silver MJ, Nicolaou KC, and Ahern D: Selective binding site for [^{3}H]prostacyclin on platelets. J Clin Invest 63:215–220, 1979.

1838. Silberstein SD: Twenty questions about headache in children and adolescents. Headache 30:716–724, 1990.

1839. Silberstein SD: Estrogens, progestins, and headache. Neurology 41:786–793, 1991.

1841. Silberstein SD, Schulman EA, and Hopkins MM: Repetitive intravenous DHE in the treatment of refractory headache. Headache 30:334–339, 1990.

1842. Silbert PL, Edis RH, Stewart-Wynne EG, and Gubbay SS: Benign vascular sexual headache and exertional headache: Interrelationships and long term prognosis. J Neurol Neurosurg Psychiatry 54:417–421, 1991.

1843. Sillanpää M: Prevalence of migraine and other headache in Finnish children starting school. Headache 15:288–290, 1976.

1844. Sillanpää M: Changes in the prevalence of migraine and other headaches during the first seven school years. Headache 23:15–19, 1983.

1845. Sillanpää M and Hillevi A: Epidemiology of headache in childhood and adolescence. In Gallai V and Guidotti V (eds): Juvenile Headache. Elsevier, Amsterdam, 1991, pp 99–104.

1846. Sillanpää M, Piekkala P, and Kero P: Prevalence of headache at preschool age in an unselected child population. Cephalalgia 11:239–242, 1991.

1847. Sills M, Congdon P, and Forsythe I: Clonidine and childhood migraine: A pilot and double-blind study. Develop Med Child Neurol 24:837–841, 1982.

1848. Silver BV, Blanchard EB, Williamson DA, Theobold DE, and Brown DA: Temperature biofeedback and relaxation training in the treatment of migraine headaches: One year follow-up. Biofeedback Self Regul 4:359–366, 1979.

1849. Simard D and Paulson OB: Cerebral vasomotor paralysis during migraine attack. Arch Neurol 29:207–209, 1973.

1850. Simon RH, Zimmerman AW, Sanderson P, and Tasman A: EEG markers of migraine in children and adults. Headache 23:201–205, 1983.

1851. Simon RH, Zimmerman AW, Tasman A, and Hale MS: Spectral analysis of photic stimulation in migraine. Electroencephalogr Clin Neurophysiol 53:270–276, 1982.

1852. Simonnet G, Taquet H, Floras P, et al.: Simultaneous determination of radio-immunoassayable methionine-enkephalin and radioreceptoractive opiate peptides in CSF of chronic pain suffering and nonsuffering patients. Neuropeptides 7:229–240, 1986.

1853. Simons A, Solbach P, Sargent J, and Malone L: A wellness program in the treatment of headache. Headache 26:343–352, 1986.

1854. Simons D: Muscular pain syndromes. Adv Pain Res Ther 17:1–41, 1990.

1855. Simons DJ and Wolff HG: Studies on headache: Mechanisms of chronic post-traumatic headache. Psychosom Med 8:227–242, 1946.

1856. Simons T and Ruskell GL: Distribution and termination of trigeminal nerves to the cerebral arteries in monkeys. J Anat 159:57–71, 1988.

1857. Sinclair DC, Weddell G, and Feindel WH: Referred pain and associated phenomena. Brain 71:184–211, 1948.

1858. Singh I, Singh I, and Singh D: Progesterone in the treatment of migraine. Lancet i:745–747, 1947.

1859. Sjaastad O: Chronic paroxysmal hemicrania (CPH). In Clifford Rose F (ed): Handbook of Clinical Neurology, Vol 4. Elsevier, Amsterdam, 1986, pp 257–266.

1860. Sjaastad O: Transitory, isolated global blindness and headache. The possible relationship to migraine. Funct Neurol 1:467–471, 1986.

1861. Sjaastad O: Chronic paroxysmal hemicrania: Recent developments. Cephalalgia 7:179–188, 1987.

1862. Sjaastad O: Cluster Headache Syndrome. Saunders, London, 1992.

1863. Sjaastad O, Fredriksen TA, and Stolt-Nielsen A: Cervicogenic headache. C2 rhizopathy and occipital neuralgia: A connection? Cephalalgia 6:189–195, 1986.

1864. Sjaastad O, Saunte C, Hovdahl H, Breivik H, and Grønbaek E: "Cervicogenic" headache. A hypothesis. Cephalalgia 3:249–256, 1983.

1865. Sjaastad O and Sjaastad OV: Urinary histamine excretion in migraine and cluster headache. J Neurol 216:91–104, 1977.

1866. Sjaastad O and Stensrud P: Appraisal of BC-105 in migraine prophylaxis. Acta Neurol Scand 45:594–600, 1969.

1867. Sjaastad O and Stensrud P: Clinical trial of a β-receptor blocking agent (LB 46) in migraine prophylaxis. Acta Neurol Scand 48:124–128, 1972.

1868. Sjaastad O, Torbjørn AF, Sand T, and Antonaci F: Unilaterality of headache in classic migraine. Cephalalgia 9:71–77, 1989.

1869. Skagerberg G and Björklund A: Topographic principles in the spinal projections of serotonergic and nonserotonergic brainstem neurons in the rat. Neuroscience 15:445–480, 1985.

1870. Skinhøj E: Hemodynamic studies within the brain during migraine. Arch Neurol 29:95–98, 1973.

1871. Skinhøj E and Paulson OB: Regional cerebral blood flow in internal carotid artery distribution during a migraine attack. Br Med J iii:569–570, 1969.

1872. Skinner DJ and Misbin RI: Uses of propranolol. N Engl J Med 293:1205, 1979.

1873. Skyhøj Olsen T: Migraine with and without aura: The same disease due to cerebral vasospasm of different intensity. A hypothesis based on CBF studies during migraine. Headache 30:269–272, 1990.

1874. Skyhøj Olsen T, Friberg L, and Lassen NA: Ischemia may be the primary cause of the neurologic deficits in classic migraine. Arch Neurol 44:156–161, 1987.

1875. Skyhøj Olsen T and Lassen NA: Blood flow and vascular reactivity during attacks of classic migraine— limitations of the Xe-133 intraarterial technique. Headache 29:15–20, 1989.

1876. Slater R: Benign recurrent vertigo. J Neurol Neurosurg Psychiatry 42:363–367, 1979.

1877. Slatter KH: Some clinical and EEG findings in patients with migraine. Brain 81:85–98, 1968.

1878. Slevin JT, Faught E, Hanna GR, and Lee SI: Temporal relationship of EEG abnormalities in migraine to headache and medication. Headache 21:251–254, 1981.

1879. Smith I, Kellow AH, and Hanington E: A clinical and biochemical correlation between tyramine and migraine headache. Headache 10:43–52, 1970.

1880. Smith R and Schwartz A: Diltiazem prophylaxis in refractory migraine. New Engl J Med 310:1327–1328, 1984.

1881. Smith WB: Biofeedback and relaxation training: The effect on headache and associated symptoms. Headache 27:511–514, 1987.

1882. Smith WL: The eicosanoids and their biochemical mechanisms of action. Biochem J 259:315–324, 1989.

1883. Smyth VOG and Winter AL: The EEG in migraine. Electroencephalogr Clin Neurophysiol 16:194–202, 1964.

1884. Snell NJ, Smith CR, and Coysh HC: Myocardial ischemia in migraine sufferers taking ergotamine. Postgrad Med J 54:37–39, 1978.

1885. Snyder BD and Ramirez-Lassepas M: Cerebral infarction in young adults. Long term prognosis. Stroke 11:149–153, 1980.

1886. Snyder CH: Paroxysmal torticollis in infancy: A possible form of labyrinthitis. Am J Dis Child 117:458–460, 1969.

1887. Soelberg Sørensen P, Hansen K, and Olesen J: A placebo-controlled, double-blind, cross-over trial of flunarizine in common migraine. Cephalalgia 6:7–14, 1986.

1888. Soelberg Sørensen P, Krogsaa B, and Gjerris F: Clinical course and prognosis of pseudotumor cerebri. A prospective study of 24 patients. Acta Neurol Scand 77:164–172, 1988.

1889. Soges LJ, Cacayorin ED, Petro GR, and Ramachandran TS: Migraine: evaluation by MR. AJNR 9:425–429, 1988.

1890. Solbach P and Sargent JD: A follow-up evaluation of the Menninger Pilot Migraine Study using thermal training. Headache 17:198–202, 1977.

1891. Solbach P, Sargent J, and Coyne L: Menstrual migraine headache: Results of a controlled, experimental outcome study of non-drug treatments. Headache 24:75–78, 1984.

1892. Soliman H, Pradalier A, Launay SM, Dry H, and Dreux C: Decreased phenol and tyramine sulphoconjugation by platelets in dietary migraine. In Clifford Rose F (ed): Advances in Headache Research, Vol 4. Libbey, London, 1987, pp 117–121.

1893. Solomon GD: Verapamil and propranolol in migraine prophylaxis: A double-blind, crossover study. Headache 26:325, 1986.

1894. Solomon GD: Circadian variation in the frequency of migraine. Cephalalgia 11(Suppl 11):179–180, 1991.

1895. Solomon GD: Concomitant medical disease and headache. Med Clin North Am 75:631–651, 1991.

1896. Solomon GD, Diamond S, and Freitag FG: Verapamil in migraine prophylaxis: Comparison of dosages. Clin Pharmacol Ther 41:202–207, 1987.

1897. Solomon GD, Kunkel RS, and Frame J: Demographics of headache in elderly patients. Headache 30:273–276, 1990.

1898. Solomon GD and Spaccavento LJ: Lateral medullary syndrome after basilar migraine. Headache 22:171–172, 1982.

1899. Solomon GD, Steel JG, and Spaccavento LJ: Verapamil prophylaxis of migraine: A double-blind, placebo-controlled study. JAMA 250:2500–2502, 1983.

1900. Solomon S and Cappa G: The headache of temporal arteritis. J Am Geriatr Soc 35:163–165, 1987.

1901. Somerville BW: The role of progesterone in menstrual migraine. Neurology 21:853–859, 1971.

1902. Somerville BW: The role of estradiol withdrawal in the etiology of menstrual migraine. Neurology 22:355–365, 1972.

1903. Somerville BW: A study of migraine in pregnancy. Neurology 22:824–828, 1972.

1904. Somerville BW: Estrogen withdrawal migraine. I. Duration of exposure required and attempted prophylaxis by premenstrual estrogen administration. Neurology 25:239–244, 1975.

1905. Somerville BW: Estrogen withdrawal migraine. II. Attempted prophylaxis by continuous estradiol administration. Neurology 25:245–250, 1975.

1906. Somerville BW: Platelet-bound and free serotonin levels in jugular and forearm venous blood during migraine. Neurology 26:41–45, 1976.

1907. Somjen GG: Extracellular potassium in the mammalian central nervous system. Annu Rev Physiol 41:159–177, 1979.

1908. Sorbi M and Tellegen B: Multimodal migraine treatment: Does thermal feedback add to the outcome? Headache 24:249–255, 1984.

1909. Sorensen KV: Valproate: A new drug in migraine prophylaxis. Acta Neurol Scand 78:46–48, 1988.

1910. Sorge F, DeSimone R, Marano R, Nolano M, Orefice G, and Carrieri P: Flunarazine in prophylaxis of childhood migraine. Cephalalgia 8:1–6, 1988.

1911. Sorge F and Marano E: Flunarizine v. placebo in childhood migraine: A double-blind study. Cephalalgia 5(Suppl 2):145–148, 1985.

1912. Sovak M, Kunzel M, Sternbach RA, and Dalessio DJ: Is volitional manipulation of hemodynamics a valid rationale for biofeedback therapy of migraine? Headache 18:197–202, 1978.

1913. Sovak M, Kunzel M, Sternbach RA, and Dalessio DJ: Mechanism of the biofeedback therapy of migraine: Volitional manipulation of the psychophysiological background. Headache 21:89–92, 1981.

1914. Soyka D, Taneri Z, Oestreich W, and Schmidt R: Flunarizine I.V. in the acute treatment of common or classical migraine attacks—a placebo controlled double blind trial. Headache 29:21–27, 1989.

1915. Spaccavento LJ and Solomon GD: Migraine as an etiology of stroke in young adults. Headache 24:19–22, 1984.

1916. Sparks JP: The incidence of migraine in school children: A survey by the medical officers of school associations. Practitioner 221:407–411, 1978.

1917. Speer F: The many facets of migraine. Ann Allergy 34:273–285, 1975.

1918. Spence JD, Amacher AL, and Willis NR: Cerebrospinal fluid (CSF) pressure monitoring in the management of benign intracranial hypertension without papilledema. Neurology 29:551, 1979.

1919. Sperber AD and Abarbanel JM: Migraine-induced epistaxis. Headache 26:517–518, 1986.

1920. Spierings ELH: The role of arteriovenous shunting in migraine. In Amery WK, Van Nueten JM, and Wauquier A (eds): The Pharmacological Basis of Migraine Therapy. Pitman, London, 1984, pp 36–49.

1921. Spierings ELH: Cardiac murmurs indicative of aortic valve disease with chronic and excessive intake of ergotamine. Headache 28:278–279, 1988.

1922. Spierings ELH: Episodic and chronic jabs and jolts syndrome. Headache Quarterly, Current Treatment and Research 1:299–302, 1990.

1923. Spierings ELH and Schellekens JAE: Headache in suburban high-school students. In Clifford Rose F (ed): New Advances in Headache Research: 2. Smith-Gordon, London, 1991, pp 15–22.

1924. Spinhoven P: Similarities and dissimilarities in hypnotic and nonhypnotic procedures for headache control: A review. Am J Clin Hypnosis 30:183–193, 1988.

1925. Spira PJ, Mylecharane EJ, and Lance JW: The effects of humoral agents and antimigraine drugs on the cranial circulation of the monkey. Res Clin Stud Headache 4:37–75, 1976.

1926. Spira PJ, Mylecharane EJ, Misbach J, Duckworth JW, and Lance JW: Internal and external carotid vascular responses to vasoactive agents in the monkey. Neurology 28:162–173, 1978.

1927. Sramka M, Brozek G, Bures J and Nádvorník P: Functional ablation by spreading depression: Possible use in human stereotactic neurosurgery. Appl Neurophysiol 40:48–61, 1977.

1928. Standaert DG, Watson SJ, Houghten RA, and Saper CB: Opioid peptide immunoreactivity in spinal and trigeminal dorsal horn neurons projecting to the parabrachial nucleus in the rat. J Neurosci 6:1220, 1986.

1929. Standnes B: The prophylactic effect of timolol versus propranolol and placebo in common migraine: Beta-blockers in migraine. Cephalalgia 2:165–170, 1982.

1930. Steardo L, Marano E, Barone P, Denman DW, Monteleone P, and Cardone G: Prophylaxis of migraine attacks with a calcium channel-blocker: Flunarazine versus methysergide. J Clin Pharmacol 26:524–528, 1986.

1931. Stecker JF, Rawls HP, Devine CJ, et al.: Retroperitoneal fibrosis and ergot derivatives. J Urol 112:30–32, 1974.

1932. Steer ML and Atlas D: Demonstration of human platelet beta-adrenergic receptors using ^{125}I-labeled cyanopindolol and ^{125}I-labeled hydroxybenzyl-pindolol. Biochem Biophys Acta 686:240–244, 1982.

1933. Steiger HJ and Meakin CJ: The meningeal representation in the trigeminal ganglion—an experimental study in the cat. Headache 24:305–309, 1984.

1934. Steiger HJ, Tew JM, and Keller JT: The sensory representation of the dura mater in the trigeminal ganglion of the cat. Neurosci Lett 31:231–236, 1982.

1935. Stein C, Millan MJ, Shippenberg TS, Peter K, and Herz A: Peripheral opioid receptors mediating antinociception in inflammation: Evidence for involvement of *mu, delta,* and *kappa* receptors. J Pharmacol Exp Ther 248:1269–1275, 1989.

1936. Stein GS: Headaches in the first postpartum week and their relationship to migraine. Headache 21:201–205, 1981.

1937. Stein GS, Morton J, Marsh A, et al.: Headaches after childbirth. Acta Neurol Scand 69:74–79, 1984.

1938. Stein M: Acute arterial spasm of the lower extremities after methysergide therapy. S African Med J 51:737, 1977.

1939. Steinbusch HWM: Distribution of serotonin-immunoreactivity in the central nervous system of the rat—cell bodies and terminals. Neuroscience 6:557–618, 1981.

1940. Steinbusch HWM and Nieuwenhuys R: The raphe nuclei of the rat brainstem: A cytoarchitectonic and immunohistochemical study. In Emson PC (ed): Chemical Neuroanatomy. Raven, New York, 1983, pp 131–207.

1941. Steiner TJ and Clifford Rose F: Problems encountered in the assessment of treatment of headache and migraine. In Hopkins A (ed): Headache. Problems in Diagnosis and Management. Saunders, London, 1988, pp 303–348.

1942. Steiner TJ, Clifford Rose F, and Joseph R: Migraine is not a platelet disorder. Headache 27:400–402, 1987.

1943. Steiner TJ, Cooke GE, Joseph R, and Clifford Rose F: Double-blind dose-ranging comparison of metoprolol with placebo in the prophylaxis of classical and common migraine. Cephalalgia 5(Suppl 3):558–559, 1985.

1944. Steiner TJ and Davies PTG: ^{99m}Tc-HMPAO studies in migraine without aura. In Olesen J (ed): Migraine and Other Headaches: The Vascular Mechanisms. Raven, New York, 1991, pp 221–226.

1945. Steiner TJ, Guha P, Capildeo R, and Clifford Rose F: Migraine in patients attending a migraine clinic: An analysis by computer of age, sex, and family history. Headache 20:190–195, 1980.

1946. Steiner TJ and Joseph R: Practical experience of beta-blockade in migraine: A personal view. Postgrad Med J 60(Suppl 2):56–60, 1984.

1947. Steiner TJ, Joseph R, Hedman JC, and Clifford Rose F: Metoprolol in the prophylaxis of migraine: Parallel-groups comparison with placebo and dose-ranging follow-up. Headache 28:15–23, 1988.

1948. Steingold KA, Lu JKH, Judd HI, and Meldrum DR: Danazole inhibits steroidogenesis by the human ovary in vivo. Fertil Steril 45:649–654, 1986.

1949. Stellar S, Ahrens SP, Meibohm AR, and Reines SA: Migraine prevention with timolol. A double-blind crossover study. JAMA 252:2576–2580, 1984.

1950. Stensrud P and Sjaastad O: Clinical trial of a new anti-bradykinin, anti-inflammatory drug, ketoprofen in migraine prophylaxis. Headache 14:96–100, 1974.

1951. Stensrud P and Sjaastad O: Short-term clinical trial of propranolol in racemic form (Inderal), d-propranolol, and placebo in migraine. Acta Neurol Scand 55:229–232, 1976.

1952. Stensrud P and Sjaastad O: Comparative trial of Tenormin (atenolol) and Inderal (propranolol) in migraine. Headache 20:204–207, 1980.

1953. Stephenson PE: Physiologic and psychotropic effects of caffeine on man. A review. J Am Diet Assoc 71:240–247, 1977.

1954. Steranka LR, Manning DC, DeHaas CJ, et al.: Bradykinin as a pain mediator: Receptors are localized to sensory neurons, and antagonists have analgesic actions. Proc Natl Acad Sci USA 85:3245–3249, 1988.

1955. Stevenson DD: Allergy and headache. Headache Quarterly, Current Treatment and Research 2:9–16, 1991.

1956. Stewart DJ, Gelston A, and Hakim A: Effect of prophylactic administration of nimodipine in patients with migraine. Headache 28:260–262, 1988.

1957. Stewart I, Newhall WF, and Edwards FJ: The isolation and identification of I-synephrine in the leaves and fruit of citrus. J Biol Chem 239:930–932, 1964.

1958. Stewart I and Wheaton TA: L-Octopamine in citrus: Isolation and identification. Science 145:60–61, 1964.

1959. Stewart RB and Cluff LE: A review of medication errors and compliance in ambulant patients. Clin Pharmacol Ther 13:463–467, 1972.

1960. Stewart TW: Idiopathic retroperitoneal fibrosis—past and present. NY State J Med 89:503–504, 1989.

1961. Stewart WF, Linet MS, and Celentano DD: Migraine headaches and panic attacks. Psychosom Med 51:559–569, 1989.

1962. Stewart WF, Linet MS, Celentano DD, Natta MV, and Ziegler D: Age- and sex-specific incidence rates of migraine with and without visual aura. Am J Epidemiol 134:1111–1120, 1991.

1963. Stewart WF, Lipton RB, Celentano DD, and Read ML: Prevalence of migraine headache in the United States. Relation to age, income, race, and other sociodemographic factors. JAMA 267:64–69, 1992.

1964. Strassman A, Mason P, Moskowitz M, and Maciewicz R: Response of brainstem trigeminal neurons to electrical stimulation of the dura. Brain Res 379:242–250, 1986.

1965. Straus SE: The chronic mononucleosis syndrome. J Infect Dis 157:405–412, 1988.

1966. Stromberg DD and Fox JR: Pressures in the pial arterial microcirculation of the cat during changes in systemic arterial blood pressure. Circ Res 31:229–239, 1972.

1967. Strum JM and Junod AF: Radioautographic demonstration of 5-hydroxytryptamine-^{3}H uptake by pulmonary endothelial cells. J Cell Biol 54:456–467, 1972.

1968. Stuart MJ, Gross SJ, Elrad H, and Graeber JE: Effects of acetylsalicylic-acid ingestion on maternal and neonatal hemostasis. N Engl J Med 307:909–912, 1982.

1969. Sturzenegger MH and Meienberg O: Basilar artery migraine: A follow-up study of 82 cases. Headache 25:408–415, 1985.

1970. Su C: Neurogenic release of purine compounds in blood vessels. J Pharmacol Exp Ther 195:159–166, 1975.

1971. Sudilovsky A, Elkind AH, Ryan RE, Saper JR, Stern MA, and Meyer JH: Comparative efficacy of nadolol and propranolol in the management of migraine. Headache 27:421–426, 1987.

1972. Sumner MJ and Humphrey PPA: Sumatriptan (GR 43175) inhibits cyclic-AMP accumulation in dog isolated saphenous vein. Br J Pharmacol 99:219–220, 1990.

1973. Sutherland JM and Eadie MJ: The drug therapy of migraine. Med J Aust ii:740–742, 1961.

1974. Sutherland JM and Eadie MJ: Cluster headache. Res Clin Stud Headache 3:92–125, 1972.

1975. Sutherland JM, Hopper WD, Eadie MJ, Tyrer JH: Buccal absorption of ergotamine. J Neurol Neurosurg Psychiatry 37:1116–1120, 1974.

1976. Suzuki N, Hardebo JE, and Owman C: Origins and pathways of cerebrovascular vasoactive intestinal polypeptide-positive nerves in rat. J Cereb Blood Flow Metab 8:697–712, 1988.

1977. Swanson JW and Vick NA: Basilar artery migraine. Neurology 29:782–786, 1978.

1978. Swanson LW, Connelly MA, and Hartman BK: Ultrastructural evidence for central monoaminergic innervation of blood vessels in the paraventricular nucleus of the hypothalamus. Brain Res 136:166–173, 1977.

1979. Swerdlow B and Dieter JN: The validity of the vascular "cold patch" in the diagnosis of chronic headache. Headache 26:22–26, 1986.

1980. Swerdlow B and Dieter JN: The vascular cold patch is not a prognostic index for headache. Headache 29:562–568, 1989.

1981. Swerdlow B and Dieter JN: The value of medical thermography for the diagnosis of chronic headache. Headache Quarterly, Current Treatment and Research 2:96–104, 1991.

1982. Sylvälahti E, Kangasniemi P, and Ross SB: Migraine headache and blood serotonin levels after administration of zimelidine, a selective inhibitor of serotonin uptake. Curr Ther Res 25:299–310, 1979.

1983. Symon DNK: Is there a place for "abdominal migraine" as a separate entity in the IHS classification? Yes! Cephalalgia 12:345–346, 1992.

1984. Symon DNK and Russell G: Abdominal migraine: A childhood syndrome defined. Cephalalgia 6:223–228, 1986.

1985. Symonds C: Migrainous variants. Trans Med Soc Lond 67:237–250, 1951.

1986. Symonds C: Concussion and contusion of the brain and their sequelae. In Feiring EH (ed): Brock's Injuries of the Brain and Their Coverings, 5th ed. Springer-Verlag, New York, 1974, pp 100–161.

1987. Szczeklik A, Gryglewski RJ, Nizankowski R, Skawinski S, Gluszko P, and Korbut R: Prostacyclin therapy in peripheral arterial disease. Thromb Res 19:191–199, 1980.

1988. Szczudlik A and Lypka A: The short metyrapone test in chronic headache patients. Funct Neurol 3:245–252, 1986.

1989. Szekely B, Botwin D, Eidelman BH, Becker M, Elman N, and Schemm R: Nonpharmacological treatment of menstrual headache: Relaxation-biofeedback behavior therapy and person-centered insight therapy. Headache 26:86–92, 1986.

1990. Taal BG, Spierings ELH, and Hilvering C: Pleuropulmonary fibrosis associated with chronic and excessive intake of ergotamine. Thorax 38:396–398, 1983.

1991. Tal Y, Dunn HG, and Chrichton JU: Childhood migraine—a dangerous diagnosis? Acta Paediatr Scand 73:55–59, 1984.

1992. Tatemichi TK and Mohr JP: Migraine and stroke. In Barnett HJM, Stein BM, Mohr JP, and Yatsu FM (eds): Stroke: Pathophysiology, Diagnosis, and Management. Churchill Livingstone, New York, 1986, pp 845–868.

1993. Tek DS, McClellan DS, Olshaker JS, Allen CL, and Arthur DC: A prospective, double-blind study of metoclopramide hydrochloride for the control of migraine in the emergency department. Ann Emer Med 19:1083–1087, 1990.

1994. Teng P and Papatheodorou C: Primary cerebrospinal fluid hypotension. Bull Los Angeles Neurol Soc 33:121–128, 1968.

1995. Ten Holter J and Tijssen C: Cheiro-oral syndrome: Does it have a specific localizing value? Eur Neurol 28:326–330, 1988.

1996. Terasaki T, Yamatogi Y, and Ohtahara S: Electroclinical delineation of occipital lobe epilepsy in childhood. In Andermann F and Lugaresi E (eds): Migraine and Epilepsy. Butterworth, Boston, 1987, pp 125–138.

1997. Terenghi G, Polak JM, Ghatei MA, et al.: Distribution and origin of calcitonin gene-related peptide (CGRP) immunoreactivity in the sensory innervation of the mammalian eye. J Comp Neurol 233:506–516, 1985.

1998. Terzano MG, Manzoni GC, and Parrino L: Benign epilepsy with occipital paroxysms and migraine: The question of intercalated attacks. In Andermann F and Lugaresi E (eds): Migraine and Epilepsy. Butterworth, Boston, 1987, pp 83–96.

1999. Tfelt-Hansen P: Clinical pharmacology of ergotamine. An overview. In Diener HC and Wilkinson M (eds): Drug-Induced Headache. Springer-Verlag, Berlin, 1988, pp 105–116.

2000. Tfelt-Hansen P, Brand J, Dano P, et al.: Early clinical experience with subcutaneous GR43175 in acute migraine: An overview. Cephalalgia 9(Suppl 9):73–77, 1989.

2001. Tfelt-Hansen P and Krabbe AE: Ergotamine abuse. Do patients benefit from withdrawal? Cephalalgia 1:29–32, 1981.

2002. Tfelt-Hansen P, Lous I, and Olesen J: Prevalence and significance of muscle tenderness during common migraine attacks. Headache 21:49–54, 1981.

2003. Tfelt-Hansen P and Olesen J: Effervescent metoclopramide and aspirin (Migravess) versus effervescent aspirin or placebo for migraine attacks: A double-blind study. Cephalalgia 4:107–111, 1984.

2004. Tfelt-Hansen P and Paalzow L: Intramuscular ergotamine: Plasma levels and dynamic activity. Clin Pharmacol Ther 37:29–35, 1985.

2005. Tfelt-Hansen P, Paalzow L, and Ibraheem JJ: Bioavailability of sublingual ergotamine. Br J Clin Pharmacol 13:239–240, 1982.

2006. Tfelt-Hansen P, Sperling B, and Andersen AR: The effect of ergotamine on human cerebral blood flow and cerebral arteries. In Olesen J (ed): Migraine and Other Headaches: The Vascular Mechanisms. Raven, New York, 1991, pp 339–343.

2007. Tfelt-Hansen P, Standnes B, Kangasniemi P, Hakkarainen H, and Olesen J: Timolol vs propranolol vs placebo in common migraine prophylaxis: A double-blind multicenter trial. Acta Neurol Scand 69:1–8, 1984.

2008. The Multinational Oral Sumatriptan and Cafergot Study Group: A randomized, double-blind comparison of sumatriptan and cafergot in the acute treatment of migraine. Eur Neurol 31:314–322, 1991.

2009. The Oral Sumatriptan Dose-defining Study Group: Sumatriptan—an oral dose-defining study. Eur Neurol 31:300–305, 1991.

2010. The Subcutaneous Sumatriptan International Study Group: Treatment of migraine attacks with Sumatriptan. N Engl J Med 325:316–321, 1991.

2011. Theoharides TC: Mast cells: The immune gate to the brain. Life Sci 46:607–617, 1990.

2012. Theoharides TC, Bondy PK, Tsakalos ND, and Askenase PW: Differential release of serotonin and histamine from mast cells. Nature 297:229–231, 1982.

2013. Thie A, Fuhlendorf A, Spitzer K, and Kunze K: Transcranial Doppler evaluation of common and classic migraine. Part I. Ultrasonic features during the headache-free period. Headache 30:201–208, 1990.

2014. Thomas DP and Vane JR: 5-Hydroxytryptamine in the circulation of the dog. Nature 216:335–338, 1967.

2015. Thomas JE, Rooke ED, and Kvale WF: The neurologist's experience with pheochromocytoma. JAMA 197:754–758, 1966.

2016. Thompson JH: Serotonin and the alimentary tract. Res Commun Chem Pathol Pharmacol 2:687–781, 1971.

2017. Thonnard-Neurmann E: Heparin. In Diamond S, Dalessio DJ, Graham JR, and Medina JL (eds): Vasoactive Substances Relevant to Migraine. Thomas, Springfield, 1975, pp 67–72.

2018. Thorneycroft IH, Mishell DR, Stone SC, Kharma KM, and Nakamura RM: The relationship of serum 17-hydroxyprogesterone and estradiol-17β levels during the human menstrual cycle. Am J Obstet Gynecol 111:947–951, 1971.

2019. Tillgren N: Treatment of headache with dihydroergotamine tartrate. Acta Med Scand 196(Suppl):222–228, 1947.

2020. Toda N: Relaxant responses to transmural stimulation and nicotine of dog and monkey cerebral arteries. Am J Physiol 243:H145–H153, 1982.

2021. Toda N: Alpha-adrenergic receptor subtypes in human, monkey and dog cerebral arteries. J Pharmacol Exp Ther 226:861–868, 1983.

2022. Toda N, Okamura T, and Miyazaki M: Heterogeneity in the response to vasoconstrictors of isolated dog proximal and distal middle cerebral arteries. Eur J Pharmacol 106:291–299, 1984.

2023. Tokola RA and Hokkanen E: Propranolol for acute migraine. Br Med J ii:1089, 1978.

2024. Tokola RA and Neuvonen PJ: Effects of migraine attack and metoclopramide on the absorption of tolfenamic acid. Br J Clin Pharmacol 17:67–75, 1984.

2025. Toller PA: Ultrastructure of the condylar articular surface in severe mandibular pain dysfunction syndrome. Int J Oral Surg 6:297, 1977.

2026. Tomsak RL: Ophthalmologic aspects of headache. Med Clin North Am 75:693–706, 1991.

2027. Tran Dinh YR, Thurel C, Cunin G, Serrie G, and Seylaz J: Cerebral vasodilatation after the thermocoagulation of the trigeminal ganglion in humans. Neurosurgery 31:658–663, 1992.

2028. Traub YM and Korczyn AD: Headache in patients with hypertension. Headache 17:245–247, 1978.

2029. Traum E: Beiträge zur Innervation der Dura mater cerebri. Z Ges Anat 77:488–492, 1925.

2030. Travell J: Temporomandibular joint pain referred from muscles of the head and neck. J Prosthet Dent 10:745–763, 1960.

2031. Travell J and Rinzler SH: The myofascial genesis of pain. Postgrad Med J 11:425–434, 1952.

2032. Travell JG and Simons DG: Myofascial Pain and Dysfunction. The Trigger Point Manual. Williams & Wilkins, Baltimore, 1983.

2033. Treiser SL, Cascia CS, O'Donohue TL, Thoa NB, Jacobowitz DM, and Kellar KJ: Lithium increases serotonin release and decreases serotonin receptors in the hippocampus. Science 213:1529–1531, 1981.

2034. Treves TA, Korizyn AD, and Streifler M: Naproxen in the treatment of acute migraine attacks. Neurology 36:101, 1986.

2035. Treves TA, Streiffer M, and Korczyn AD: Naproxen sodium versus ergotamine tartrate in the treatment of acute migraine attacks. Headache 32:280–282, 1992.

2036. Trojaborg W and Boysen G: Relation between EEG, regional cerebral blood flow and internal carotid artery pressure during carotid endarterectomy. Electroencephalogr Clin Neurophysiol 34:61–69, 1973.

2037. Troost BT: Migraine and other headaches. In Glaser JS (ed): Neuro-ophthalmology. Vol 10. Aeolus Press, Amsterdam, 1990, pp 487–517.

2038. Troost BT, Mark LE, and Maroon JC: Resolution of classic migraine after removal of an occipital lobe AVM. Ann Neurol 5:199–201, 1979.

2039. Troost BT and Newton TH: Occipital lobe arteriovenous malformations. Clinical and radiologic features in 26 cases with comments on differentiation from migraine. Arch Ophthalmol 93:250–256, 1975.

2040. Tropper PJ and Petrie RH: Antiepileptics. In Eskes TKAB and Finster M (eds): Drug Therapy in Pregnancy. Butterworth, London, 1985, pp 100–109.

2041. Tsai SH, Tew JM, Mclean JG, and Shipley M: Cerebral arterial innervation by nerve fibers containing calcitonin gene-related peptide (CGRP): I. Distribution and origin of CGRP perivascular innervation in the rat. J Comp Neurol 271:435–444, 1988.

2042. Tucker RM: Sublingual nifedipine relieves migraine prodromes. Headache 24:285, 1984.

2043. Tunis M, Clark RG, Lee R, and Wolff HG: Studies on headache: Further observations on cranial and conjunctival vessels during and between vascular headache attacks. Trans Am Neurol Assoc 76:67–69, 1951.

2044. Tunis MM and Wolff HG: Analysis of cranial artery pulse waves in patients with vascular headache of the migraine type. Am J Med Sci 224:565–568, 1952.

2045. Tunis MM and Wolff HG: Studies of headache. Arch Neurol Psychiatry 70:551–557, 1953.

2046. Turk DC and Meichenbaum DH: A cognitive-behavioural approach to pain management. In Wall PD and Melzack R (eds): Textbook of Pain, 2nd ed. Churchill Livingstone, Edinburgh, 1989, pp 1001–1009.

2047. Turk DC, Meichenbaum DH, and Berman WH: Application of biofeedback for the regulation of pain: A critical review. Psychol Bull 86:1322–1328, 1979.

2048. Turner JA and Chapman CR: Psychological interventions for chronic pain: A critical review. I. Relaxation training and biofeedback. Pain 12:1–21, 1982.

2049. Uddman R, Edvinsson L, Ekman R, Kingman T, and McCulloch J: Innervation of the feline cerebral vasculature by nerve fibers containing calcitonin gene-related peptide: Trigeminal origin and co-existence with substance P. Neuroscience Lett 62:131–136, 1985.

2050. Udenfriend S, Lovenberg W, and Sjoerdsma A: Physiologically active amines in common fruits and vegetables. Arch Biochem Biophys 85:487–490, 1959.

2051. Ulett GA, Gleser G, Winokur G, and Lawler A: The EEG and reaction to photic stimulation as an index of anxiety proneness. Electroencephalogr Clin Neurophysiol 5:23–32, 1953.

2052. Uski TK: Cerebrovascular smooth muscle effects of prostanoids. In Owman C and Hardebo JE (eds): Neural Regulation of Brain Circulation. Elsevier, Amsterdam, 1986, pp 245–260.

2053. Usui H, Fujiwara M, Tsukahara T, Taniguchi T, and Kurahashi K: Differences in contractile responses to electrical stimulation and α-adrenergic binding sites in isolated cerebral arteries of humans, cows, dogs, and monkeys. J Cardiovascular Pharmacol 7:S47–S52, 1985.

2054. Vahlquist B: Migraine in children. Int Arch Allergy 7:348–355, 1955.

2055. Vahlquist B and Hackzell G: Migraine of early onset: A study of thirty-one cases in which the disease first appeared between one and four years of age. Acta Paediatr Scand 38:622–636, 1949.

2056. Vanast WJ, Diaz-Mitoma F, and Tyrell DLJ: Hypothesis—Epstein-Barr virus-related syndromes: Implications for headache research. Headache 27:321–324, 1987.

2057. Van den Berg E, Walterbusch G, Gotzen L, Rumpf KD, Otten B, and Fröhlich H: Ergotism leading to threatened limb amputation or to death in two patients given heparin-dihydroergotamine prophylaxis. Lancet i:955–956, 1982.

2058. Van den Bergh V, Amery WK, and Waelkens J: Trigger factors in migraine: A study conducted by the Belgian Migraine Society. Headache 27:191–196, 1987.

2059. VanderWende C and Spoerlein MT: Role of dopaminergic receptors in morphine analgesia and tolerance. Res Commun Chem Pathol Pharmacol 5:35–43, 1973.

2060. Van Dijk JG, Dorresteijn M, Haan J, and Ferrari MD: No confirmation of visual evoked potential diagnostic test for migraine. Lancet 337:517–518, 1991.

2061. Van Dijk JG, Haan J, and Ferrari MD: Photic stimulation and the diagnosis of migraine. Headache Quarterly. Current Treatment and Research 3:387–397, 1992.

2062. Vane JR: The evolution of non-steroidal antiinflammatory drugs and their mechanisms of action. Drugs 33(Suppl 1):18–27, 1987.

2063. Van Harreveld A: Compounds in brain extracts causing spreading depression of cerebral cortical activity and contraction of crustacean muscle. J Neurochem 3:300–315, 1959.

2064. Van Houdenhove B: Interpersonal and psychodynamic links between pain and depression. Eur J Psychiat 5:177–185, 1991.

2065. Vanhoutte PM: 5-Hydroxytryptamine and vascular disease. Fed Proc 42:233–237, 1983.

2066. Vécsei L, Widerlöv E, Ekman R, et al.: Suboccipital cerebrospinal fluid and plasma concentrations of somatostatin, neuropeptide Y and beta-endorphin in patients with common migraine. Neuropeptides 22:111–116, 1992.

2067. Ver Brugghen A: Pathogenesis of ophthalmoplegic migraine. Neurology 5:311–318, 1955.

2068. Verret S and Steele JC: Alternating hemiplegia in childhood: A report of eight patients with complicated migraine beginning in infancy. Pediatrics 47:675–680, 1971.

2069. Vestal RE, Wood AJJ, Branch RA, Shand DG, and Wilkinson GR: Effects of age and cigarette smoking on propranolol disposition. Clin Pharmacol Ther 26:8–15, 1979.

2070. Vestal RE, Wood AJJ, and Shand DG: Reduced β-adrenoceptor sensitivity in the elderly. Clin Pharmacol Ther 26:181–186, 1979.

2071. Vestergaard P, Amdison A, and Schou M: Clinically significant side effects of lithium treatment: A survey of 237 patients in long-term treatment. Acta Psychiatr Scand 62:193–200, 1980.

2072. Vetulani J, Antkiewicz-Michaluk L, and Rokosz-Pelc A: Chronic administration of antidepressant drugs increases the density of cortical [^{3}H] prazosin binding sites in the rat. Brain Res 310:360–362, 1984.

2073. Vijayan N: Ophthalmoplegic migraine: Ischemic or compressive neuropathy. Headache 20:300–304, 1980.

2074. Vijayan N, Gould S, and Watson C: Exposure to sun and precipitation of migraine. Headache 20:42–43, 1980.

2075. Volans GN: Migraine and drug absorption. Clin Pharmacokinet 3:313–318, 1978.

2076. Volans GN and Castleden CM: The relationship between smoking and migraine. Postgrad Med J 52:80–82, 1976.

2077. Volta GD and Anzola GP: Are there objective criteria to follow up migrainous patients? A prospective study with thermography and evoked potentials. Headache 28:423–425, 1988.

2078. Volta GD, Anzola GP, and Di Monda V: The disappearance of the "cold patch" in recovered migraine patients: Thermographic findings. Headache 31:305–309, 1991.

2079. Volta GD, Di Monda V, Bariselli M, and Anzola GP: Headache and dialysis: What kind of relationship? Headache Quarterly, Current Treatment and Research 2:292–296, 1991.

2080. von Euler C, Hayward JN, Martilla I, and Wayman RJ: Respiratory neurons of the ventrolateral nucleus of the solitary tract of the cat: Vagal input, spinal connections and morphological identification. Brain Res 61:1–11, 1983.

2081. von Storch TJC and Merritt HH: The cerebrospinal fluid during and between attacks of migraine headaches. Am J Med Sci 190:226–231, 1935.

2082. Waeber C, Hoyer D, and Palacios JM: GR 43175: A preferential 5-HT$_{1D}$ agent in monkey and human brains as shown by autoradiography. Synapse 4:168–170, 1989.

2083. Waelkens J: Warning symptoms in migraine: Characteristics and therapeutic implications. Cephalalgia 5:223–228, 1985.

2084. Waga S, Otsuka K, and Handa H: Warning signs of intracranial aneurysms. Surg Neurol 3:15–20, 1975.

2085. Wahl M: The effect of opiate-like substances and bradykinin on cerebrovascular resistance in cats. In Heistad DD and Marcus ML (eds): Cerebral Blood Flow: Effects of Nerves and Neurotransmitters. Elsevier, New York, 1982, pp 235–241.

2086. Wahl M and Kuschinsky W: The dilating effect of histamine on pial arteries of cats and its mediation by H$_2$ receptors. Circ Res 44:161–165, 1979.

2087. Wahl M, Unterberg A, Whalley ET, et al.: Cerebrovascular effects of bradykinin. In Owman C and Hardebo JE (eds): Neural Regulation of Brain Circulation. Elsevier, Amsterdam, 1986, pp 419–430.

2088. Wainscott G, Kaspi T, and Volans GN: The influence of thiethylperazine on the absorption of effervescent aspirin in migraine. Br J Clin Pharmacol 3:1015–1021, 1976.

2089. Wainscott G, Sullivan FM, Volans GN, and Wilkinson M: The outcome of pregnancy in women suffering from migraine. Postgrad Med J 54:98–102, 1978.

2090. Waiquier A, Ashton D, and Marannes R: The effects of flunarazine in experimental models related to the pathogenesis of migraine. Cephalalgia 5(Suppl 2):119–123, 1985.

2091. Waldenlind E, Ross SB, Sääf J, Ekbom K, and Wetterberg L: Concentration and uptake of 5-hydroxytryptamine in platelets from cluster headache and migraine patients. Cephalalgia 5:45–54, 1985.

2092. Walker CH: Migraine and its relationship to hypertension. Br Med J ii:1430–1433, 1959.

2093. Walser H and Isler H: Frontal intermittent rhythmic delta activity. Impairment of consciousness and migraine. Headache 22:74–80, 1982.

2094. Walsh JP and O'Doherty DS: A possible explanation of the mechanism of ophthalmoplegic migraine. Neurology 10:1079–1084, 1960.

2095. Walsh TT: Antidepressants in chronic pain. Clin Neuropharmacol 6:271–295, 1983.

2096. Walters BB, Gillespie SA, and Moskowitz MA: Cerebrovascular projections from the sphenopalatine and otic ganglia to the middle cerebral artery of the cat. Stroke 17:488–494, 1986.

2097. Waltimo O, Hokkanen E, and Pirskanen R: Intracranial arteriovenous malformations and headache. Headache 15:133–135, 1975.

2098. Wanaka A, Matsuyama T, Yoneda S, et al.: Origins and distribution of calcitonin gene-related peptide-containing nerves in the wall of the cerebral arteries of the guinea pig with special reference to the coexistence with substance P. Brain Res 369:185–192, 1986.

2099. Wang SC and Borison HL: The vomiting center: A critical experimental analysis. Arch Neurol Psychiat 63:928–941, 1950.

2100. Ward N, Whitney C, Avery D, and Dunner D: The analgesic effects of caffeine in headache. Pain 44:151–155, 1991.

2101. Washton AM and Gold MS: Chronic

cocaine abuse: Evidence for adverse effects on health and functioning. Psychiatric Ann 14:733–743, 1984.

2102. Waters WE: Community studies of the prevalence of migraine. Headache 9:178–186, 1970.

2103. Waters WE: Controlled clinical trial of ergotamine tartrate. Br Med J ii:325, 1970.

2104. Waters WE: Headache and blood pressure in the community. Br Med J i:142–143, 1971.

2105. Waters WE: Migraine: Intelligence, social class and familial prevalence. Br Med J ii:277–281, 1971.

2106. Waters WE: The epidemiological enigma of migraine. Int J Epidemiol 2:189–194, 1973.

2107. Waters WE: The Pontypridd headache survey. Headache 14:81–90, 1974.

2108. Waters WE: Headache. Series in Clinical Epidemiology. PSG Publishing Company, Littleton, 1986.

2109. Waters WE and O'Connor PJ: Prevalence of migraine. J Neurol Neurosurg Psychiatry 38:613–616, 1975.

2110. Watson P and Steele JC: Paroxysmal dysequilibrium in the migraine syndrome of childhood. Arch Otolaryngol 99:177–179, 1974.

2111. Watt DM: Temporomandibular joint sounds. J Dent 8:119–127, 1980.

2112. Watts PG, Peet KM, and Juniper RP: Migraine and the temporomandibular joint: The final answer? Br Dent J 6:170–173, 1986.

2113. Wayne VS: A possible relationship between migraine and coronary artery spasm. Aust NZ J Med 16:708–710, 1986.

2114. Weber RB and Reinmuth OM: The treatment of migraine with propranolol. Neurology 22:366–369, 1972.

2115. Weerasuriya K, Patel L, and Turner P: β-Adrenoceptor blockade and migraine. Cephalalgia 2:33–45, 1982.

2116. Wei EP, Raper AJ, Kontos HA, and Patterson JL: Determinants of response of pial arteries to norepinephrine and sympathetic nerve stimulation. Stroke 6:654–658, 1975.

2117. Wei ET, Tseng LF, Loh HH, and Li CH: Comparison of the behavioral effects of beta-endorphin and enkephalin analogs. Life Sci 21:321–327, 1977.

2118. Weil AA: The EEG findings in a certain type of psychosomatic headache: Dysrhythmic migraine. Electroencephagr Clin Neurophysiol 4:181–186, 1952.

2119. Weil AA: Observations on "dysrhythmic" migraine. J Nerv Ment Dis 134:277–281, 1962.

2120. Weingarten S, Kleinman M, Elperin L, and Larson EB: The effectiveness of cerebral imaging in the diagnosis of chronic headache. Arch Intern Med 152:2457–2462, 1992.

2121. Weisberg LA: Benign intracranial hypertension. Medicine 54:197–207, 1975.

2122. Weiss HD, Stern BJ, and Goldberg J: Post-traumatic migraine: Chronic migraine precipitated by minor head or neck trauma. Headache 31:451–456, 1991.

2123. Weiss NS: Relation of high blood pressure to headache, epistaxis and selected other symptoms. The United States health examination survey of adults. N Engl J Med 287:631–633, 1972.

2124. Welch KMA: Naproxen sodium in the treatment of migraine. Cephalalgia 6(Suppl 4):85–92, 1986.

2125. Welch KMA: Migraine. A biobehavioral disorder. Arch Neurol 44:323–327, 1987.

2126. Welch KMA, Chabi E, Bartosh K, Achar VS, and Meyer JS: Cerebrospinal fluid γ-aminobutyric acid levels in migraine. Br Med J iii:516–517, 1975.

2127. Welch KMA, Chabi E, Nell JH, et al.: Biochemical comparison of migraine and stroke. Headache 16:160–167, 1976.

2128. Welch KMA, Ellis DJ, and Keenan PA: Successful migraine prophylaxis with naproxen sodium. Neurology 35:1304–1310, 1985.

2129. Welch KMA, Levine SR, and D'Andrea G: The pathogenesis of migraine. Curr Opinion Neurol Neurosurg 1:183–188, 1988.

2130. Welch KMA, Levine SR, D'Andrea G, Schultz LR, and Helpern JA: Preliminary observations on brain energy metabolism in migraine studied by in vivo phosphorus[31] NMR spectroscopy. Neurology 39:532–541, 1989.

2131. Welch KMA, Spira PJ, Knowles L, and Lance JW: Effects of prostaglandins on the internal and external carotid blood flow in the monkey. Neurology 24:705–710, 1974.

2132. Welling PG: Drug kinetics. In Hathway DE (ed): Foreign Compound Metabolism in Mammals, Vol 3. The Chemical Society, London, 1975, pp 107–200.

2133. Werbach MR and Sandweiss JH: Peripheral temperatures of migraineurs undergoing relaxation training. Headache 18:211–214, 1978.

2134. Werder DS and Sargent JD: A study of childhood headache using biofeedback as a treatment alternative. Headache 24:122–126, 1984.

2135. Wessely P, Suess E, Koch G, and Podreka I: [99m]-d,l-HMPAO SPECT in migraine without aura. In Olesen J (ed): Migraine and Other Headaches. The Vascular Mechanisms. Raven, New York, 1991, pp 203–207.

2136. West TET, Davies RJ, and Kelly RE: Horner's syndrome and headache due to carotid artery disease. Br Med J i:818–820, 1976.

2137. Westlund KN, Bowker RM, Ziegler MG, and Coulter JD: Origins and terminations of descending noradrenergic projections to the spinal cord of the monkey. Brain Res 292:1–16, 1984.

2138. Whalley ET, Amure YO, and Lye RH: Analysis of the mechanism of action of bradykinin on human basilar artery in vitro. Naunyn-Schmiedebergs Arch Pharmacol 335:433–437, 1987.

2139. Whalley ET and Wahl M: Analysis of bradykinin receptor mediating relaxation of cat cerebral arteries in vivo and in vitro. Naunyn-Schmiedebergs Arch Pharmacol 323:66–71, 1983.

2140. White JC and Sweet WH: Pain and the Neurosurgeon: A Forty-year Experience. Thomas, Springfield, 1969.

2141. White K and Simpson G: Combined MAO-tricyclic antidepressant treatment: A reevaluation. J Clin Psychopharmacol 1:264–282, 1981.

2142. White RP and Hagen AA: Cerebrovascular actions of prostaglandins. Pharmac Ther 18:313–331, 1982.

2143. Whitty CWM: Familial hemiplegic migraine. J Neurol Neurosurg Psychiatry 16:172–177, 1953.

2144. Whitty CWM: Migraine without headache. Lancet ii:283–285, 1967.

2145. Whitty CWM: Familial hemiplegic migraine. In Clifford Rose F (ed): Handbook of Clinical Neurology, Vol 4. Elsevier, Amsterdam, 1986, pp 141–153.

2146. Whitty CWM and Hockaday JM: Migraine: A follow-up study of 92 patients. Br Med J i:735–736, 1968.

2147. Whitty CWM, Hockaday JM, and Whitty MM: The effects of oral contraceptives on migraine. Lancet i:856–859, 1966.

2148. Wiberg M, Westman J, and Blomqvist A: The projection to the mesencephalon from the sensory trigeminal nuclei. An anatomical study in the cat. Brain Res 399:51–68, 1986.

2149. Widerøe TE and Vigander T: Propranolol in the treatment of migraine. Br Med J ii:699–701, 1974.

2150. Wijdicks EFM, Kerkhoff H, and Van Gijn J: Long term follow-up of 71 patients with thunderclap headache mimicking subarachnoid hemorrhage. Lancet ii:68–70, 1988.

2151. Wilkinson M: The treatment of acute migraine attacks. Headache 15:291–292, 1976.

2152. Wilkinson M: Treatment of the acute migraine attack—current status. Cephalalgia 3:61–67, 1983.

2153. Wilkinson M and Blau JN: Are classical and common migraine different entities? Headache 25:211–213, 1985.

2154. Wilkinson M, Williams K, and Leyton M: Observations on the treatment of an acute attack of migraine. Res Clin Stud Headache 6:141–146, 1978.

2155. Wilkinson M and Woodrow J: Migraine and weather. Headache 19:375–378, 1979.

2156. Willet F, Curzon N, Adams J, and Armitage M: Coronary vasospasm induced by subcutaneous sumatriptan. Br Med J 304:1415, 1992.

2157. Williams L and Lowenthal DT: Drug therapy in the elderly. Southern Med J 85:127–131, 1992.

2158. Williamson DA: Behavioral treatment of migraine and muscle-contraction headaches: Outcome and theoretical explanations. In Hersen M, Eisler RM, and Miller PM (eds): Progress in Behavior Modification, Vol 11. Academic, New York, 1981, pp 163–201.

2159. Willis WD: Control of nociceptive transmission in the spinal cord. Prog Sensory Physiol 3:1–159, 1982.

2160. Winston KR: Whiplash and its relationship to migraine. Headache 27:452–457, 1987.

2161. Winther K and Hedman C: Platelet function and migraine. In Olesen J and Edvinsson L (eds): Basic Mechanisms of Headache. Elsevier, Amsterdam, 1988, pp 301–312.

2162. Winther K, Klysner R, Geisler A, and Andersen PH: Characterization of human platelet beta-adrenoceptors. Thromb Res 40:757–767, 1985.

2163. Wirth FP and Van Buren JM: Referral of pain from dural stimulation in man. J Neurosurg 34:630–642, 1971.

2164. Wober C, Wober-Bingol, Koch G, and Wessely P: Long-term results of migraine prophylaxis with flunarazine and beta-blockers. Cephalalgia 11:251–256, 1991.

2165. Wolf S and Wolff HG: Intermittent fever of unknown origin. Arch Intern Med 70:293–302, 1942.

2166. Wolff HG: Personality features and reactions of subjects with migraine. Arch Neurol Psychiatry 37:895–921, 1937.

2167. Wolff HG: Headache and Other Head Pain, 2nd ed. Oxford University Press, New York, 1963.

2168. Wolff HG and Tunis MM: Analysis of cranial artery pressure pulse waves in patients with vascular headache of the migraine type. Trans Assoc Am Phys 65:240–244, 1952.

2169. Wolff HG, Tunis MM, and Goodell H: Evidence of tissue damage and changes in pain sensitivity in subjects with vascular headaches of the migraine type. Arch Intern Med 92:478–485, 1953.

2170. Wolter JR and Burchfield WJ: Ocular migraine in a young man resulting in unilateral transient blindness and retinal edema. J Pediatr Ophthalmol 8:173–176, 1971.

2171. Wong RL and Korn JH: Temporal arteritis without an elevated erythrocyte sedimentation rate. Am J Med 80:959–964, 1986.

2172. Woodforde JM and Mersky H: Personality traits of patients with chronic pain. J Psychosom Res 16:167–172, 1972.

2173. Woods NF, Most A, and Dery GK: Prevalence of perimenstrual symptoms. Am J Public Health 72:1257–1264, 1982.

2174. World Federation of Neurology: Definition of Migraine. In Cochrane AL (ed): Background to Migraine: Third Migraine Symposium. Heinemann, London, 1970, pp 181–182.

2175. Wright AD, Barber SG, Kendall MJ, and Poole PH: Beta-adrenoceptor blocking drugs and blood sugar control in diabetes mellitus. Br Med J i:159–161, 1979.

2176. Wright GDS and Patel MK: Focal migraine and pregnancy. Br Med J 293:1557–1558, 1986.

2177. Yaksh TL: Direct evidence that spinal serotonin and noradrenaline terminals mediate the spinal antinociceptive effects of morphine in the periaqueductal gray. Brain Res 160:180–185, 1979.

2178. Yaksh TL: Opioid receptor systems and the endorphins: A review of their spinal organization. J Neurosurg 67:157–176, 1987.

2179. Yaksh TL, Plant RL, and Rudy TA: Studies on the antagonism by raphe lesions of the antinociceptive action of systemic morphine. Eur J Pharmacol 41:399–408, 1977.

2180. Yaksh TL and Rudy TA: Studies on the direct spinal action of narcotics in the production of analgesia in the rat. J Pharmacol Exp Ther 202:411–428, 1977.

2181. Yaksh TL and Tyce GM: Microinjection of morphine into the periaqueductal gray evokes the release of serotonin from spinal cord. Brain Res 171:176–181, 1979.

2182. Yaksh TL and Wilson PR: Spinal serotinin terminal system mediates antinociception. J Pharmacol Exp Ther 208:446–453, 1979.

2183. Yaksh TL, Yeung JC, and Rudy TA: Systematic examination in the rat of brain sites sensitive to the direct application of morphine: Observation of differential effects within the periaqueductal gray. Brain Res 114:83–103, 1976.

2184. Yamamoto K, Matsuyama T, Shiosaka S, et al.: Overall distribution of substance P-containing nerves in the wall of cerebral arteries of the guinea pig and its origins. J Comp Neurol 215:421–426, 1983.

2185. Yamamoto M and Meyer JS: Hemicranial disorder of vasomotor adrenoceptors in migraine and cluster headache. Headache 20:231–235, 1980.

2186. Yanagisawa M, Inoue A, Ishikawa T, et al.: Primary structure, synthesis, and biological activity of rat endothelin, an endothelium-derived vasoconstrictor peptide. Proc Natl Acad Sci USA 85:6964–6967, 1988.

2187. Yanigasawa M, Otsuka M, and Garcia-Arraras JE: E-type prostaglandins depolarize primary afferent neurons of the neonatal rat. Neuroscience Lett 68:351–355, 1986.

2188. el-Yassir N, Fleetwood-Walker SM, and Mitchell R: Heterogeneous effects of serotonin in the dorsal horn of the rat: The involvement of $5HT_1$ receptor subtypes. Brain Res 456:147–158, 1988.

2189. Yasue H, Omote S, Takizawa A, and Nagoe M: Acute myocardial infarction induced by ergotamine tartrate: Possible role of coronary arterial spasm. Angiology 32:414–418, 1981.

2190. Young WB and Silberstein SD: Transcranial doppler: Techniques and application to headache. Headache 32:136–142, 1992.

2191. Yuill GM, Swinburn WR, and Liversedge LA: A double-blind crossover trial of isometheptene mucate compound and ergotamine in migraine. Br J Clin Pract 26:76–79, 1972.

2192. Zagami AS, Goadsby PJ, and Edvinsson L: Stimulation of the superior sagittal sinus in the cat causes release of vasoactive peptides. Neuropeptides 16:69–75, 1990.

2193. Zagami AS and Lambert GA: Stimulation of cranial vessels excites nociceptive neurones in several thalamic nuclei of the cat. Exp Brain Res 81:552–566, 1990.

2194. Zeitlin C and Oddy M: Cognitive impairment in patients with severe migraine. Br J Clin Psychol 23:27–35, 1984.

2195. Zetterstrom T, Vernet L, Ungerstadt U, Tossman U, Jonzon BF, and Fredholm BB: Purine levels in the intact rat brain. Studies with an implanted hollow fiber. Neurosci Lett 29:111–115, 1982.

2196. Ziegler DK: Headache syndromes: Problems of definition. Psychosomatics 20:443–447, 1979.

2197. Ziegler DK: Epidemiology of migraine. In Clifford Rose F (ed): Handbook of Clinical Neurology, Vol 48. Elsevier, Amsterdam, 1986, pp 13–22.

2198. Ziegler DK, Batnitzky S, Barter R, and McMillan JH: Magnetic resonance image abnormality in migraine with aura. Cephalalgia 11:147–150, 1991.

2199. Ziegler DK and Ellis DJ: Naproxen in prophylaxis of migraine. Arch Neur 42:582–584, 1985.

2200. Ziegler DK, Hassanien RS, and Couch JR: Characteristics of life headache histories in a nonclinic population. Neurology 27:265–269, 1977.

2201. Zeigler DK, Hassanein RS, and Couch JR: Headache syndromes suggested by statistical analysis of headache symptoms. Cephalalgia 2:125–134, 1982.

2202. Ziegler DK, Hassanein RS, Harris D, and Stewart R: Headache in a non-clinic twin population. Headache 14:213–218, 1975.

2203. Ziegler DK, Hassanein R, and Hassanein K: Headache syndromes suggested by factor analysis of symptom variables in a headache prone population. J Chron Dis 25:353–363, 1972.

2204. Ziegler DK, Hurwitz A, Hassanein RS, Kodanaz HA, Preskorn SH, and Mason J: Migraine prophylaxis. A comparison of propranolol and amitryptiline. Arch Neurol 44:486–489, 1987.

2205. Ziegler DK and Stewart R: Failure of tyramine to induce migraine. Neurology 27:725–726, 1977.

2206. Ziegler DK and Wong G: Migraine in children: Clinical and electroencephalographic study of families. The possible relation to epilepsy. Epilepsia 8:171–187, 1967.

2207. Ziegler VE, Clayton PJ, and Biggs JT: A comparison study of amitriptyline and nortriptyline with plasma levels. Arch Gen Psychiatry 34:607–612, 1977.

2208. Zieglgansberger W and Tulloch IF: The effects of methionine- and leucine-enkephalin on spinal neurones of the cat. Brain Res 167:53–64, 1979.

2209. Zieleniewski AM, Murphy RM, and Semlan FP: Behavioral effects of 5-HT$_1$ agonist administration on spinal reflexes. Soc Neurosci Abstr 15:546, 1989.

2210. Zwestloot CP, Caekebeke JFV, Jansen JC, Odink J, and Ferrari MD: Blood flow velocities in the vertebrobasilar system during migraine attacks—a transcranial Doppler study. Cephalalgia 12:29–32, 1992.

INDEX

A "t" following a page number indicates a table; an "f" indicates a figure.